The Elbow and Wrist

AANA Advanced Arthroscopic Surgical Techniques

AANA Advanced Arthroscopic Surgical Techniques
SERIES

SERIES EDITORS, RICHARD K. N. RYU, MD
AND JEFFREY S. ABRAMS, MD

The Elbow and Wrist

AANA Advanced Arthroscopic Surgical Techniques

EDITED BY

FELIX H. SAVOIE III, MD
Professor and Chief of Sports Medicine
Vice Chairman, Department of Orthopaedics
Tulane University School of Medicine
New Orleans, Louisiana

LARRY D. FIELD, MD
Mississippi Sports Medicine and Orthopedic Center
Jackson, Mississippi

SCOTT P. STEINMANN, MD
Professor of Orthopedics
Mayo Clinic
Rochester, Minnesota

CRC Press
Taylor & Francis Group
Boca Raton London New York

CRC Press is an imprint of the
Taylor & Francis Group, an **informa** business

First published 2016 by SLACK Incorporated

Published 2024 by CRC Press
2385 NW Executive Center Drive, Suite 320, Boca Raton FL 33431

and by CRC Press
4 Park Square, Milton Park, Abingdon, Oxon, OX14 4RN

CRC Press is an imprint of Taylor & Francis Group, LLC

Library of Congress Cataloging-in-Publication Data

AANA advanced arthroscopic surgical techniques. The elbow and wrist / edited by Felix H. Savoie III, Larry D. Field, Scott P. Steinmann.
p. ; cm.
Advanced arthroscopic surgical techniques
Elbow and wrist
Preceded by: AANA advanced arthroscopy. The elbow and wrist / [edited by] Felix H. Savoie III., Larry D. Field. Philadelphia : Saunders/Elsevier, c2010.
Includes bibliographical references and index.
ISBN 9781630910013 (alk. paper)
I. Savoie, Felix H., III, editor. II. Field, Larry D., editor. III. Steinmann, S. (Scott), editor. IV. Arthroscopy Association of North America, issuing body. V. AANA advanced arthroscopy. The elbow and wrist. Preceded by (work): VI. Title: Advanced arthroscopic surgical techniques. VII. Title: Elbow and wrist.
[DNLM: 1. Elbow Joint--surgery. 2. Wrist Joint--surgery. 3. Arthroscopy--methods. WE 820]
RD686
617.4'720597--dc23
2015024359

ISBN: 9781630910013 (hbk)
ISBN: 9781003523963 (ebk)

DOI: 10.1201/9781003523963

Dedication

To my wonderful wife, Amy, for her patience and understanding in allowing me to pursue this—and many other—projects. We really are a great team; thank you.
Felix H. Savoie III, MD

To my wife, Cindy, and our three children, Eric, Evelyn, and Adam. Your love and support make everything possible.
Larry D. Field, MD

To my wife, Julie, and my daughter, Sarah; they are the light of my life.
Scott P. Steinmann, MD

Contents

Acknowledgments

To Ms. Rita Richardson of Tulane Department of Orthopedic Surgery for her invaluable assistance with manuscript editing and creating hundreds of figures and numerous videos. This would not be a book without her.

About the Editors

Felix H. "Buddy" Savoie III, MD is an internationally recognized expert in the areas of Shoulder and Elbow Surgery and Sports Medicine. He is American Board of Orthopaedic Surgery certified in Orthopedic Surgery and Sports Medicine. A graduate of the Louisiana State University School of Medicine in New Orleans, he completed his internship and residency at the University of Mississippi Medical Center in Jackson. After completing AO, Hand and Microvascular Surgery, and Arthroscopy fellowships, he returned to Jackson to enter private practice and as an Assistant Professor of Orthopedic Surgery at the University of Mississippi. Dr. Savoie came to the Tulane University School of Medicine in New Orleans in 2007 after Hurricane Katrina to take on the mantle of Professor of Clinical Orthopedics, Chief of the Division of Sports Medicine, and Director of the Tulane Institute of Sports Medicine. In July 2015, he was named Chairman of the Department of Orthopedics.

Larry D. Field, MD is an orthopedic sports medicine surgeon specializing in shoulder and elbow surgery and serves as program director for the ACGME-accredited Sports Medicine and Arthroscopy Fellowship Program at the Mississippi Sports Medicine Center in Jackson, Mississippi. He completed his orthopedic surgical training at the University of Mississippi with additional fellowship training with Dr. Bruno Noesberger in Interlaken, Switzerland and with Professor Ulrich Holz in Stuttgart, Germany. Dr. Field also completed a sports medicine fellowship training program at the Hospital for Special Surgery in New York. He is active in clinical research related to shoulder and elbow disorders and has written and edited several books on these conditions. In addition, Dr. Field has published over 150 peer-reviewed scientific papers, review articles, and book chapters on shoulder- and elbow-related topics and lectures nationally and internationally regarding shoulder and elbow problems. Dr. Field is actively involved in a number of professional orthopedic organizations and societies including the International Society of Arthroscopy, Knee Surgery and Orthopaedic Sports Medicine, the American Orthopaedic Society for Sports Medicine, the American Shoulder and Elbow Surgeons, the American Orthopaedic Association, the American Academy of Orthopaedic Surgeons, and the Arthroscopy Association of North America, where he currently serves on the Board of Directors. Dr. Field also participates as an editorial board member for the *Journal of Shoulder and Elbow Surgery* and *Techniques in Shoulder and Elbow Surgery*.

Scott P. Steinmann, MD received his undergraduate degree from Columbia University in New York, New York and his MD degree from Cornell University in Ithaca, New York. He completed an orthopedic residency at New York Orthopedic Hospital, followed by a shoulder fellowship at Columbia and a hand fellowship at Mayo Clinic. He is a member of the American Shoulder and Elbow Surgeons, the American Society for Surgery of the Hand, the Arthroscopy Association of North America, the American Academy of Orthopedic Surgeons, the American Association for Hand Surgery, the International Society of Arthroscopy, Knee Surgery and Orthopaedic Sports Medicine, and the Minnesota Orthopedic Society. Dr. Steinmann has participated in numerous meetings as course chair, faculty, and moderator. He also continues to be very active as a scientific reviewer and editor of various journals. Dr. Steinmann holds the position of Professor of Orthopedics at the Mayo Clinic in Rochester, Minnesota and is a member of various committees at Mayo Clinic regarding research, focusing on elbow, shoulder, and hand surgery.

Contributing Authors

Julie E. Adams, MD (Chapters 31, 37)
Department of Orthopedic Surgery
Mayo Clinic
Rochester and Austin, Minnesota

David W. Altchek, MD (Chapter 15)
Sports Medicine and Shoulder Service
The Hospital for Special Surgery
New York, New York

James R. Andrews, MD (Chapter 16)
Medical Director, The Andrews Institute
President & Chairman of the Board, Andrews Research & Education Foundation (AREF)
Gulf Breeze, Florida
Chairman of the Board and Medical Director, American Sports Medicine Institute (ASMI)
Birmingham, Alabama

Alejandro Badia, MD, FACS (Chapter 38)
Hand and Upper Limb Surgeon
Badia Hand to Shoulder Center
OrthoNOW
International Society for Sport Traumatology of the Hand (ISSPORTH)
Doral, Miami, Florida

Gregory Bain, MBBS, FRACS, FA (Ortho)A, PhD (Chapters 17, 23, 40)
Department of Orthopaedic Surgery
Flinders University and Flinders Medical Centre
Adelaide, Australia

Champ L. Baker III, MD (Chapter 3)
The Hughston Clinic
Columbus, Georgia

Champ L. Baker Jr, MD (Chapter 3)
Director of Sports Medicine Fellowship
President of the Hughston Foundation
Columbus, Georgia

Jonathan D. Brown, MD (Chapter 19)
Resident
Tulane University
Tulane Institute of Sports Medicine
New Orleans, Louisiana

James C. Y. Chow, MD (Chapter 41)
Cocoa Beach, Florida

Tyler R. Clark, MD (Chapter 6)
Department of Orthopaedics
Tulane University School of Medicine
New Orleans, Louisiana

Mark S. Cohen, MD (Chapter 9)
Hand, Elbow and Microsurgery Service
Department of Orthopaedic Surgery
Rush University Medical Center
Chicago, Illinois

Randall W. Culp, MD (Chapters 34, 36)
The Philadelphia Hand Center
Thomas Jefferson University
King of Prussia, Pennsylvania

D. Nicole Deal, MD (Chapter 42)
University of Virginia School of Medicine
University of Virginia Hand Center
Charlottesville, Virginia

William Desloges, MD, FRCSC (Chapter 12)
Hull Hospital
Gatineau, Québec

Joshua S. Dines, MD (Chapter 15)
Sports Medicine and Shoulder Service
The Hospital for Special Surgery
New York, New York

Brandon P. Donnelly, MD (Chapters 26, 27)
Pontchartrain Orthopedics and Sports Medicine
Metairie, Louisiana

Michael P. Gaspar, MD (Chapters 34, 36)
The Philadelphia Hand Center, P.C.
Thomas Jefferson University
Philadelphia, Pennsylvania

William B. Geissler, MD (Chapters 33, 39)
Alan E. Freeland Chair of Hand Surgery
Division of Hand and Upper Extremity Surgery
Section of Arthroscopic Surgery and Sports Medicine
Hand and Upper Extremity Fellowship
Department of Orthopaedic Surgery and Rehabilitation
University of Mississippi Medical Center
Jackson, Mississippi

Benjamin Graves, MD (Chapter 42)
Hand and Upper Extremity Surgery
Department of Orthopaedic Surgery
Wake Forest Baptist Health
Winston-Salem, North Carolina

Bikramjit S. Grewal, MD (Chapter 3)
Cape Fear Orthopedics
Fayetteville, North Carolina

Timothy Griffith, MD (Chapter 15)
Sports Medicine Service
Peachtree Orthopaedic Clinic
Atlanta, Georgia

Jennifer A. Hertz, MD (Chapter 36)
Hand and Upper Extremity Surgeon
L.A. Wilshire Orthopaedic and Medical Associates
Los Angeles, California

E. Rhett Hobgood, MD (Chapter 24)
Mississippi Sports Medicine and Orthopaedic Center
Jackson, Mississippi

Bhavin Jadav, MBBS, MS (Ortho) (Chapter 40)
Department of Orthopaedics
Flinders Medical Centre
Adelaide, Australia

Graham J. W. King, MD, MSc, FRCSC (Chapters 11, 12)
Roth|McFarlane Hand and Upper Limb Centre
Professor
Western University
London, Ontario, Canada

Brian Klika, MD (Chapter 10)
Mayo Clinic
Rochester, Minnesota

Rudy Kovachevich, MD (Chapter 22)
Hand Surgery Associates
Englewood, Colorado

Leonard C. Macrina, MSPT, SCS, CSCS (Chapter 21)
Champion Physical Therapy and Performance
Waltham, Massachusetts

Michael L. Mangonon, DO (Chapter 35)
Plancher Orthopaedics and Sports Medicine
New York, New York

Murphy P. Martin III, MD (Chapter 18)
Resident
Department of Orthopaedic Surgery
Tulane University School of Medicine
New Orleans, Louisiana

Brent V. McCarty, MD (Chapter 20)
Chief Resident
Department of Orthopaedics
Tulane University
New Orleans, Louisiana

Robert Nelson Mead, MD, MBA (Chapter 8)
Orthopaedic Surgery Resident
Department of Orthopaedic Surgery
Tulane School of Medicine
New Orleans, Louisiana

Bernard F. Morrey, MD (Chapters 4, 5)
Professor of Orthopaedic Surgery
Mayo Clinic
Rochester, Minnesota
Professor of Orthopaedic Surgery
University of Texas Health Science Center
San Antonio, Texas

Mike Moskal, MD (Chapter 30)
Sellersburg, Indiana

Daniel J. Nagle, MD, FACS, FAAOS (Chapter 28)
Professor of Clinical Orthopedics
Northwestern Feinberg School of Medicine
Chicago, Illinois

Brian D. Norton, MD (Chapter 34)
Hand and Upper Extremity Surgeon
Arkansas Specialty Orthopaedics
Little Rock, Arkansas

Michael J. O'Brien, MD (Chapters 2, 6, 8, 14, 18, 19, 20, 25)
Assistant Professor
Tulane University School of Medicine
Department of Orthopedic Surgery
New Orleans, Louisiana

Patrick M. O'Brien, MD (Chapter 24)
Carolina Orthopaedic Specialists
Hickory, North Carolina

Daryl C. Osbahr, MD (Chapter 16)
Chief of Sports Medicine
Orlando Health Orthopedic Institute
Medical Director, Orlando City Soccer Club
Orlando, Florida
Assistant Team Physician, Washington Nationals
Washington, DC

A. Lee Osterman, MD (Chapters 29, 34)
Professor of Hand and Orthopedics
Thomas Jefferson University
President of the Philadelphia Hand Center
Philadelphia, Pennsylvania

Stephanie C. Petterson, MPT, PhD (Chapters 13, 35)
Director of Research
Orthopaedic Foundation
Stamford, Connecticut

Joideep Phadnis, MBChB, MRCS, Dip Sports Med, FRCS (Tr&Orth) (Chapters 17, 23)
Department of Orthopaedic Surgery
Flinders Medical Centre
Adelaide, Australia

Kevin D. Plancher, MD, MS (Chapters 13, 35)
Clinical Professor
Albert Einstein College of Medicine
Plancher Orthopaedics and Sports Medicine
New York, New York

Gary Poehling, MD (Chapter 42)
Wake Forest University School of Medicine
Winston-Salem, North Carolina

Marc Prud'homme-Foster, MD, FRCSC (Chapter 11)
University of Ottawa
Ottawa, Ontario, Canada

Matthew L. Ramsey, MD (Chapter 7)
Professor and Vice Chairman
Department of Orthopaedic Surgery
Sidney Kimmel College of Medicine
Chief, Shoulder and Elbow Service
Rothman Institute
Philadelphia, Pennsylvania

Ashkon Razavi, MD (Chapter 29)
Hand, Wrist, Upper Extremity Surgery
Orthopedic Center of Illinois
Springfield, Illinois

Juan Manuel Ríos Ruh, MD (Chapter 38)
Orthopedic Surgery
Consorci Sanitari Integral
Barcelona, Spain

Akash Sabharwal, MBBS, MS, M.Ch Orthopedics (Chapter 23)
Department of Orthopaedic Surgery
Flinders Medical Centre
Adelaide, Australia

David J. Slutsky, MD (Chapter 32)
The Hand and Wrist Institute
Associate Clinical Professor
Department of Orthopedics
Harbor UCLA Medical Center
Torrance, California

Alex Soneru, MD (Chapter 28)
Northwestern Feinberg School Medicine
Department of Orthopedic Surgery
Chicago, Illinois

Sarah Stelma, MD (Chapter 13)
Orthopaedic Foundation
Stamford, Connecticut
Albert Einstein College of Medicine
New York, New York

William B. Stetson, MD (Chapter 1)
Stetson Powell Orthopedics and Sports Medicine
Burbank, California
University of Southern California Keck School of Medicine
Los Angeles, California

Philipp N. Streubel, MD (Chapter 9)
Department of Orthopaedic Surgery and Rehabilitation
University of Nebraska Medical Center
Omaha, Nebraska

Cuney Tamam, MD (Chapter 42)
Wake Forest University School of Medicine
Winston-Salem, North Carolina

Lucas H. B. Walschot, MD, PhD (Chapter 17)
Flinders Medical Centre
Adelaide, Australia

Chris S. Warrell, MD (Chapter 16)
Orlando Health Orthopedic Institute
Orlando, Florida

Aaron M. Weber, DO (Chapters 33, 39)
Hand and Upper Extremity Fellow
Department of Orthopaedic Surgery and Rehabilitation
University of Mississippi Medical Center
Jackson, Mississippi

Matthew Wert, MD (Chapter 25)
Director of Sports Medicine/Orthopaedic Surgeon
New York Methodist Hospital
Brooklyn, New York

Kevin E. Wilk, PT, DPT, FAPTA (Chapter 21)
Champion Sports Medicine
A Physiotherapy Associates Clinic
American Sports Medicine Institute
Birmingham, Alabama

Jeffrey B. Witty, MD (Chapters 26, 27)
Mississippi Sports Medicine and Orthopaedic Center
Jackson, Mississippi

Eric S. Wroten, MD (Chapter 36)
Orthopaedic Hand Surgery
Fort Worth Hand Center
Fort Worth, Texas

Foreword

It is always a challenge to develop a textbook regarding surgical technique when the subject matter is constantly in flux. To provide a useful contribution to the body of knowledge, the identity of a relevant topic is critical, and the editors have certainly accomplished this with an update on elbow and wrist arthroscopy. However, the successful completion of this undertaking resides both in content but also of equal importance in the composition and experience of the pool of contributors. Once again, in this regard, the editors have assembled an excellent contributing faculty with a great breadth and depth of experience. Ultimately, it is the reputation of the editors and their ability to recognize and accomplish the above goals that makes this volume a success.

Based on these three considerations, I must commend the editors, Drs. Savoie, Field, and Steinmann, for this outstanding contribution to the orthopedic arthroscopic literature. The editors are all internationally recognized not just for their expertise; they also are known to be effective communicators and educators. These attributes are well represented in this book. I have been fortunate to have worked with and to have been associated with each of these individuals over the years and can think of no better combination of editors capable of producing the product such as they have successfully done. The fact that over 40 chapters are dedicated to exploring the challenging clinical dimensions of elbow and wrist arthroscopy is a testament to the comprehensiveness of the vision as well as the effectiveness of its execution. As a contributor to this volume, I can personally attest to the care and detail with which the editors have guided and assembled the material enclosed here in. I am convinced this is the most current and useful guide to assist the orthopedic surgeon in the execution of these procedures.

The basic format of the text is particularly relevant as it is simple and straightforward and includes technical tips as well as pitfalls and pearls. This focused approach to teaching surgical techniques is precisely what is desired by the surgeon and delivered by this text. The subject matter is thoughtfully organized and logically structured. The contributors to the chapters as mentioned are well known clinicians and well recognized educators. Of interest, and as a further reflection of the high quality of this effort, it should be noted that the editors themselves have participated in almost 40% of the content, and Dr. Savoie himself serves as a coauthor of almost 25% of the chapters.

In summary, this is a significant contribution to the orthopedic library focusing on advanced as well as basic techniques applied to joints for which there is generally less familiarity in the orthopedic community. As such, it is an invaluable guide and directory for the management of the full constellation of afflictions amenable to arthroscopic diagnosis and treatment. I personally feel privileged to have been asked to participate in this outstanding contribution.

Bernard F. Morrey, MD
Professor of Orthopaedic Surgery
Mayo Clinic
Rochester, Minnesota
Professor of Orthopaedic Surgery
University of Texas Health Science Center
San Antonio, Texas

INTRODUCTION

The *AANA Advanced Arthroscopic Surgical Techniques Series* represents the very best that AANA has to offer the practicing orthopedic surgeon. With premier arthroscopic surgeons taking the lead, each book in the series presents the latest diagnostic, therapeutic, and reconstructive techniques available in arthroscopic surgery today.

Each technique-based chapter is consistently organized with a user-friendly interface allowing for a quick reference or for prolonged study. Bulleted lists of easily accessed, high-yield information, including preoperative planning, patient selection, equipment checklists, step-by-step descriptions of procedures, and essential technical pearls, in addition to indications, contraindications, postoperative protocols, and potential complications, make this an invaluable resource for surgeons who want to improve not only their skill level, but also their mastery of the fundamentals that define arthroscopic surgery. Well-edited videos, accompanied by narration, further serve to support the materials systematically outlined in each chapter for each volume.

Education and innovation continue to be the top priority for AANA and its leadership. As such, all proceeds from this Series will be donated to the AANA Education Foundation, which, among other endeavors, helps support resident education at the Orthopedic Learning Center, The Traveling Fellowship, the Society of Military Orthopedic Surgeons (SOMOS)–AANA collaboration, resident scholarships to the Annual Meeting, as well as numerous research grants and awards. With the purchase of this textbook series, AANA will also provide free electronic access to the text and videos from the same book in their initial series, *AANA Advanced Arthroscopy* (2010).

We believe that this 5-volume series is a "must have" resource for those who rely on their arthroscopic skills and knowledge to improve patient outcomes. Concise, current, and cogent help describe the impact that these textbooks will have on your practice and in your clinical successes. AANA is delighted to have again taken on this critical leadership position in surgeon education, and is proud of the quality and immediacy of these 5 outstanding volumes.

Richard K. N. Ryu, MD
Jeffrey S. Abrams, MD
Series Co-Editors

Section I

THE ELBOW
Basics

1

Elbow Arthroscopy
Positioning, Setup, Anatomy, and Portals

William B. Stetson, MD

Introduction

Elbow arthroscopy is a technically demanding procedure, and extensive hands-on training and supervised experience are needed to acquire proficiency. When performed with appropriate judgment and technique, elbow arthroscopy is an excellent tool for the correction of many lesions of the elbow joint with minimal risk However, it poses greater technical challenges and neurological risks than knee or shoulder arthroscopy because of the small size of the elbow joint and the proximity of portals to neurovascular structures, and it has the potential for causing injury to important nearby nerves and vessels (Figure 1-1). Intimate knowledge and familiarity with the normal elbow anatomy and portals will decrease the risk of damage to important structures. Elbow arthroscopy provides an opportunity for diagnostic and therapeutic intervention with little morbidity and has advantages over open surgery, including decreased scarring, decreased risk of infection, less postoperative pain, and a more thorough visualization of the elbow joint than is possible with arthrotomy.[1]

In 1985, Andrews and Carson[2] described the patient-supine technique and the use of various portals for elbow arthroscopy. In 1989, Poehling et al[3] described the patient-prone position for elbow arthroscopy. Since then, the techniques and indications for elbow arthroscopy have expanded, and many more reports have described variations in operative technique.

This chapter gives an overview of the positioning, setup, anatomy, and portals used for elbow arthroscopy.

Indications

In 1992, O'Driscoll and Morrey[4] described the early indications for elbow arthroscopy, which were pain or symptoms that were substantial enough to interfere with work, daily activities, sports, or sleep and did not resolve after conservative treatment. In this early study, they analyzed their results of 71 elbow arthroscopies as the indications for such a procedure were evolving. The best

Savoie FH III, Field LD, Steinmann SP, eds. *The Elbow and Wrist: AANA Advanced Arthroscopic Surgical Techniques* (pp 3-20).

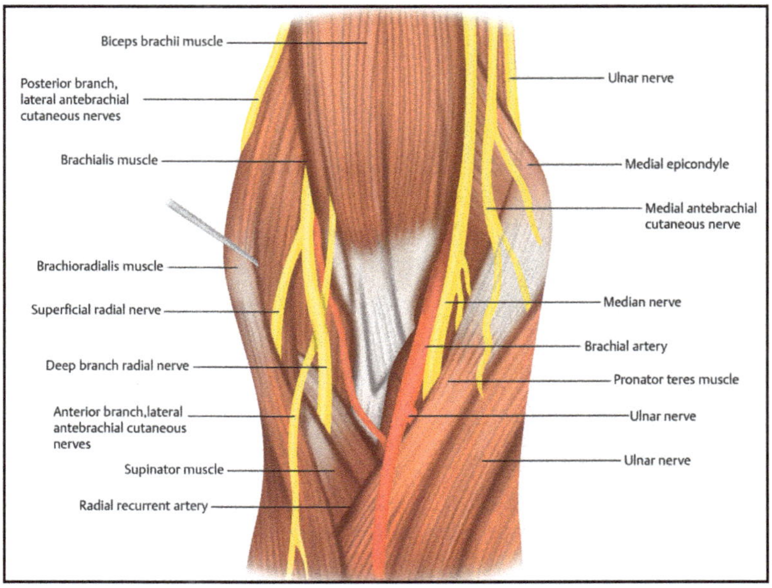

Figure 1-1. The antecubital fossa with important neurovascular structures.

early results were seen with arthroscopic removal of loose bodies, assessment of undiagnosed snapping, idiopathic flexion contractures, local debridement of damaged articular surfaces, and synovectomy. They found that the patients least likely to benefit were the ones in whom there was a disparity between objective and subjective findings.[4]

Since then, the indications for elbow arthroscopy have evolved. In 1994, Poehling and Ekman[5] further refined the indications, which included use for the diagnosis of intra-articular lesions of the elbow, the removal of loose and foreign bodies, irrigation of the joint, debridement of an infected joint, excision of osteophytes, synovectomy, capsular release, excision of the radial head, and treatment of acute fractures of the elbow. The indications for elbow arthroscopy are outlined in Table 1-1.

Controversial Indications

The controversial indications for elbow arthroscopy include the treatment of lateral and medial epicondylitis, endoscopic distal biceps tendon repair, and arthroscopic ulnar nerve release.

Contraindications

The primary contraindication to elbow arthroscopy is any significant distortion of normal bony or soft tissue anatomy that precludes safe entry of the arthroscope into the joint.[4,6] For example, a previous ulnar nerve transposition that is submuscular or subcutaneous would interfere with safe proximal, anteromedial portal placement and is a relative contraindication for safe introduction of the arthroscope through the medial side of the elbow.[7,8] In these cases, identification of the ulnar nerve is necessary before establishing a medial portal.[8]

Another relative contraindication is a severely ankylosed joint may distort normal anatomy and place important neurovascular structures at risk. This may not allow for adequate joint distension and may not allow proper displacement of neurovascular structures away from portal sites and within the joint from instrumentation.[7] As with any other procedure, a localized infection in the area of portal placement is also a contraindication to the elbow arthroscopy.

Appropriate conservative measures should always be tried before making the decision to proceed with elbow arthroscopy. However, the diagnosis is often not often clear until the time

Table 1-1. Indications

Indications	Symptoms	Chapter
Pain, swelling of unknown etiology	Pain and swelling	2
Infection	Pain, swelling, fevers, chills	2
Osteophyte removal	Loss of motion, primarily in extension	2
Recurrent posterolateral instability	Pain, instability	13
Acute repair of ligamentous avulsion	History of trauma, pain, swelling	13
Synovitis and synovial biopsy	Pain, swelling of unknown etiology	11
Osteochondritis dissecans of the capitellum	Pain, swelling, limited ROM	8
Degenerative osteoarthritis	Pain, swelling, mechanical symptoms of locking and catching, loss of ROM	10
Arthrofibrosis	Loss of ROM	9
Controversial Indications	*Symptoms*	*Chapter*
Lateral epicondylitis	Lateral elbow pain	3
Medial epicondylitis	Medial elbow pain	4
Radial head excision	Posttraumatic arthritis of radiocapitellar joint secondary to a radial head fracture	12
Elbow fracture, including radial head, capitellum, coronoid process	History of trauma with pain, swelling, and radiographic evidence of fracture	19
Olecranon bursitis	Pain, swelling of olecranon bursa	6
Repair of torn distal biceps tendon	History of trauma with pain, swelling, and clinical evidence of distal biceps rupture	16
Repair of torn distal triceps tendon	History of trauma with pain, swelling, and clinical evidence of a distal triceps rupture	18
Cubital tunnel release	Numbness, tingling in ulnar nerve distribution of hand with clinical evidence of ulnar neuropathy	21

of diagnostic arthroscopy as loose bodies, articular cartilage damage, or other pathology cannot always be detected by physical examination, x-ray, or magnetic resonance imaging (MRI). When conservative measures have failed, elbow arthroscopy is a useful tool in the treatment of simple and complex elbow disorders. However, it does not replace a careful history, physical examination, diagnostic testing, or adequate course of nonoperative treatment. When the decision is made to proceed with elbow arthroscopy, it is important to discuss with the patient the risks and benefits of the procedure, including the remote risk of blood vessel and nerve damage, and what realistic results can be expected after the surgery. The documentation of this discussion and in the medical record and proper informed consent is critical before proceeding with this or any other surgical procedure.

Pertinent Physical Findings

A careful physical examination of all 3 compartments of the elbow is critical to determine the correct diagnosis. Each compartment should be examined individually to fully evaluate the elbow. The physical examination starts with careful inspection of the skin and soft tissues to make sure there are no surgical scars, swelling, ecchymosis, soft tissue masses, or bony abnormalities. The alignment of the elbow should also be inspected, noting any significant varus or valgus deformities. Range of motion (ROM) of the elbow in flexion, extension, supination, and pronation should be noted and compared to the contralateral side. A careful neurovascular examination should be done on every patient, paying close attention to the ulnar nerve medially. The ulnar nerve should also be palpated as the elbow is also flexed and extended to determine whether the nerve subluxes. A subluxing ulnar nerve or a previous ulnar nerve transposition places the ulnar nerve at risk with proximal anteromedial portal placement. Specific physical examination findings are detailed in the following chapters for each specific diagnosis.

Pertinent Imaging

Routine diagnostic x-rays include an anteroposterior view with the elbow in full extension and a lateral view with the joint in 90 degrees of flexion. An axial view can also be obtained to outline the olecranon and its medial and lateral articulations. This is the best view for identifying and assessing a posteromedial osteophyte. When there is a history of trauma, an oblique view should also be done, and careful attention should be paid to the radial head and the coronoid process for subtle fracture lines. Also, x-rays should be reviewed for more obvious anterior or posterior elbow dislocations along with more subtle degenerative changes, osteophytes, and loose bodies. However, plain x-rays are not always able to demonstrate all loose bodies.

A gravity stress test x-ray can be used to detect valgus laxity of the elbow. The patient is placed in a supine position and the shoulder is abducted and brought to maximum external rotation so that the elbow is parallel to the floor. If there is an injury to the ligament or bony attachment, increased joint space can be seen on x-rays.[7]

MRI and computed tomography (CT) arthrogram have been found to be accurate in diagnosing a complete tear of the ulnar collateral ligament (UCL) as described by Timmerman et al in 1994.[9] However, in early studies of Timmerman and Andrews,[10] CT arthrogram was more sensitive in detecting a partial undersurface tear of the UCL. This was described as a "T sign" lesion by Timmerman and Andrews[10] that represents "dye leaking around the detachment of the deep portion of the UCL from its bony insertion, but remaining within the intact superficial layer, UCL, and capsule."[10(33-36)]

MRI is useful for evaluating osteochondral lesions in the radiocapitellar joint and for demonstrating early vascular changes not yet apparent on plain x-rays, and it can be used to assess the extent of the lesion and displacement of fragments.[7] MRI is also helpful for evaluating the soft tissue structures of the elbow, including the tendinous insertions of the flexor and extensor musculature to help in diagnosing medial and lateral epicondylitis, the triceps insertion, and associated musculature to evaluate for triceps tendonitis, and for evaluating the medial and lateral collateral ligaments for possible tears. However, MRI may not demonstrate subtle undersurface tears of the UCL. Magnetic resonance arthrography with saline contrast or gadolinium, however, can increase the sensitivity for detecting undersurface tears of the UCL and has become the test of choice to detect these tears.

Equipment

The following standard equipment is needed for elbow arthroscopy:

- 4.0-mm, 30-degree arthroscope
- Metal cannulas with blunt trocars and no side vents
- Plastic disposable cannulas
- Arthroscopic shaver and burr
- Handheld instruments: grasper, forceps, probe, punches
- Smooth switching stick
- Mechanical pump
- Sterile tourniquet

A standard 4.0-mm, 30-degree arthroscope permits excellent visualization of the elbow joint. A smaller 2.7-mm arthroscope is usually not necessary but can be useful for viewing small spaces, such as the lateral compartment from the direct lateral portal, and for arthroscopy in adolescent patients.[7,8] The use of cannulas allows one to switch viewing and working portals without repeated joint capsule injuries. This also minimizes the risk of injury to neurovascular structures and decreases the chance of fluid extravasation into the soft tissues, swelling, and possible compartment syndrome.[7] A metal cannula is usually used for the arthroscope. In the working portal, a disposable plastic cannula is typically used with a diaphragm, which allows instruments to be introduced without loss of joint distension.

Side-vented inflow cannulas should be avoided in elbow arthroscopy because the distance between the skin and the joint capsule is often slight. With side-vented cannulas, the cannula can be intra-articular while the side vents remain extra-articular, resulting in fluid extravasation into the surrounding soft tissues. Inflow cannulas should be devoid of side vents, with fluid flow occurring directly at the end of the cannula.

All trocars should be conical and blunt tipped to decrease the possibility of neurovascular and articular cartilage injury. A variety of handheld instruments, such as probes, grasping forceps, and punches, along with motorized instruments, such as synovial resectors and burrs, are also used during elbow arthroscopy.[7,8]

If a mechanical pump is used, an inflow pressure of 35 mm Hg is usually used to maintain joint distension.[7] Some surgeons prefer the use of gravity inflow and feel that it gives adequate joint distension without the risk of fluid extravasation. If a tourniquet is used, it can be set at 250 mm Hg and inflated if needed.

Step-by-Step Description of the Procedure

A clear understanding of the anatomy of the elbow is important before proceeding with arthroscopy. Without having a thorough understanding of the anatomy of the elbow, improper portal placement can cause significant complications to neurovascular structures. It is important to know and review superficial elbow anatomy before beginning elbow arthroscopy. The bony landmarks provide the key to avoiding damage to important neurovascular structures. Important bony anatomic landmarks should be palpated, including the lateral and medial epicondyle, olecranon process, and the radial head (Figure 1-2). On the lateral side, the lateral epicondyle, olecranon process, and the radial head form a triangle. Located in the center of this triangle is a soft spot called the *anconeus triangle*. This is often used to inflate the joint with fluid before introducing any instruments or cannulas and can also be the landmarks for a direct lateral portal (Figure 1-3). Posteriorly, important structures include the triceps muscle, tendon, and the tip of the olecranon.

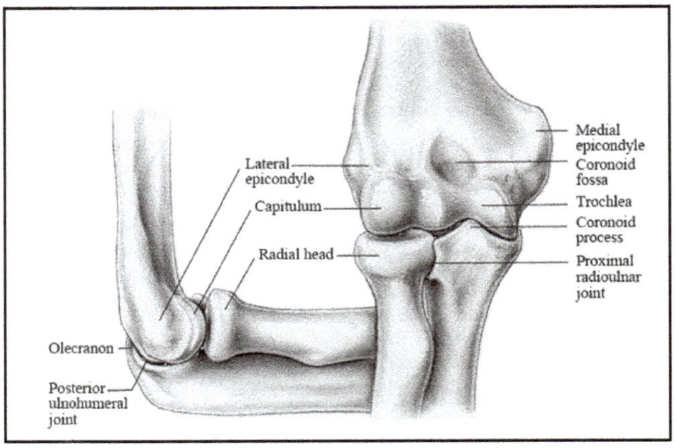

Figure 1-2. Bony landmarks of the elbow joint.

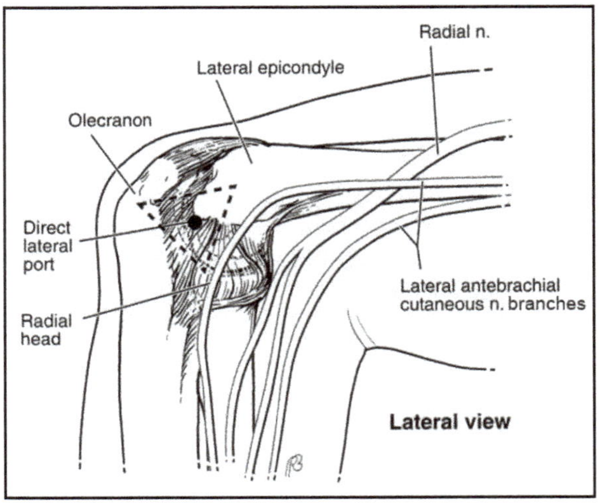

Figure 1-3. Lateral view in the prone position.

Anteriorly, the antecubital fossa is formed by the following 3 muscular borders: laterally by the "mobile wad of 3" (the brachioradialis, the extensor carpi radialis brevis, and the extensor carpi radialis longus muscles), medially by the pronator teres muscle, and superiorly by the biceps muscle. The anconeus muscle, which is located on the posterolateral aspect of the joint, originates on the lateral epicondyle and posterior elbow capsule and inserts on the proximal ulna.

Sensory nerves around the elbow include the medial brachial cutaneous, the medial antebrachial cutaneous, the lateral antebrachial cutaneous, and the posterior antebrachial cutaneous nerves.[6] The medial brachial cutaneous nerve penetrates the deep fascia midway down the arm on the medial side and supplies skin sensation to the posteromedial aspect of the arm to the level of the olecranon. The medial antebrachial cutaneous nerve supplies sensation to the medial side of the elbow and forearm. The lateral antebrachial cutaneous nerve is a branch of the musculocutaneous nerve, which exits between the biceps and brachialis muscles laterally to supply sensation to the elbow and lateral aspect of the forearm. Finally, the posterior antebrachial cutaneous nerve branches from the radial nerve and courses down the lateral aspect of the arm to supply sensation to the posterolateral elbow and posterior forearm.[7]

The main neurovascular structures about the elbow are the median nerve, radial nerve, ulnar nerve, and brachial artery.[6] The radial nerve spirals around the posterior humeral shaft, penetrates the lateral intermuscular septum, and descends anteriorly to the lateral epicondyle between the brachioradialis and brachialis muscles. The radial nerve then branches to form the superficial radial nerve, which supplies sensation to the dorsoradial wrist and posterior surface of the radial

3.5 digits, and the posterior interosseous nerve, which provides motor branches to the wrists, thumb, and finger extensors. The ulnar nerve penetrates the medial intermuscular septum in the distal one-third of the arm, courses posteriorly to the median epicondyle, and then descends distally between the flexor carpi ulnaris and flexor digitorum superficialis muscles. Finally, the brachial artery courses just medial to the biceps tendon in the antecubital fossa and then descends to the level of the radial head, where it bifurcates into the radial and ulnar arteries (see Figure 1-1).[7]

Most surgeons prefer to use general endotracheal anesthesia for patients undergoing elbow arthroscopy because it provides total muscle relaxation and is more comfortable for the patient.[7,8] The use of regional anesthesia is advocated by some, including the use of an axillary nerve block or an interscalene nerve block. These can be administered safely and successfully by a trained anesthesiologist, but there is an inherent risk in these blocks not seen with general anesthesia.

There is apprehension among some surgeons about using local and intravenous blocks because the patient's postoperative neurologic status cannot be assessed and may be compromised by an extended axillary or interscalene nerve block.[7] If a neurological deficit is found after the procedure, it may be difficult to determine how it occurred and there may be finger pointing between the anesthesiologist and the surgeon.

The use of local anesthetics for postoperative pain control is also not commonly used because of the difficulty in assessing the patient's postoperative neurological status. However, there is no strict rule against the use of local anesthetics for postoperative pain control; it should be left to the discretion of the operating surgeon.

Traditionally, elbow arthroscopy was performed with the patient resting supine on the operating table[2] until use of the prone position was introduced in 1989 by Poehling.[3] The prone position improves the mobility of the arthroscope within the joint, facilitates manipulation of the joint, provides for a more complete intra-articular inspection (especially in the posterior aspect of the joint), and eliminates the need for an overhead suspension device to support the elbow. The main disadvantage to this position is that it is more difficult to access the patient's airway.[5] The supine position should be avoided as it is difficult to access the posterior compartment.

After an appropriate level of anesthesia (general endotracheal or axillary block) has been achieved, the patient is placed prone with large chest rolls under the torso. It is important that these chest rolls are large enough to raise the patient's torso up from the operating room table. If these rolls are not large enough, it makes it difficult to position the arm and elbow to access the proximal anteromedial portal. An arm board is placed on the operative side of the table and parallel to it. To increase the mobility of the upper extremity intraoperatively, a sandbag, block, or firm bump of towels is placed under the shoulder to further elevate the arm away from the table. The forearm is then allowed to hang in a dependent position over the arm board at 90 degrees (Figure 1-4). A sterile tourniquet may be placed around the proximal aspect of the arm to help control bleeding during the procedure, but it is not always necessary to inflate when using a mechanical irrigation system.[5] After the extremity is prepped and draped, a large sterile bump is placed under the arm proximal to the elbow to keep the shoulder abducted to 90 degrees and to keep the elbow at approximately 90 degrees of flexion (Figure 1-5).

Other authors prefer the lateral decubitus position because they feel it provides improved stability of the extremity, is more convenient for the anesthesiologist, and allows posterior elbow joint access without compromising airway access.[4,8] O'Driscoll and Morrey[4] prefer the lateral decubitus position because it has the advantages of the prone positioning without compromising the anesthesiologist's access to the airway. The patient is placed in the lateral decubitus position with the involved extremity facing upward. The arm is then supported on a well-padded bolster with the forearm hanging free and the elbow flexed to 90 degrees. In this position, the elbow is supported in front of the surgeon, who then has access to the various portal sites.

Whether using the prone or lateral decubitus position, the forearm is prepped from the proximal arm to the tip of the fingers, and the extremity is wrapped with an elastic bandage from the fingers to just below the elbow to minimize fluid extravasation into the forearm.[8]

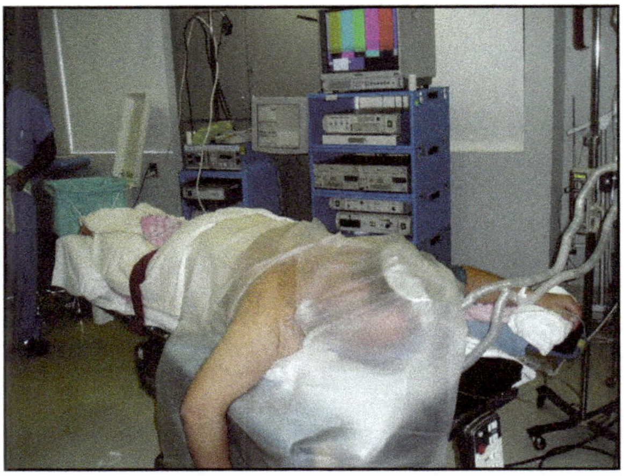

Figure 1-4. The prone position with the right elbow resting over an arm board, which is parallel to the operating room table. A nonsterile U-drape is placed proximally. A sterile bump is placed under the arm for support after the extremity is prepped.

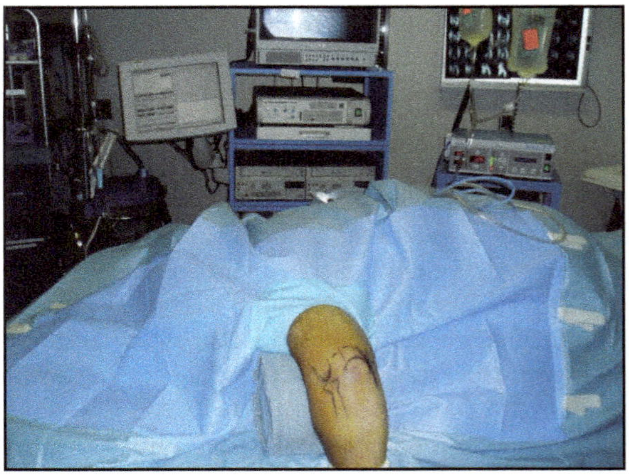

Figure 1-5. A left elbow is shown in the prone position. Anesthesia is at the head (left) of the patient, and all equipment is on the opposite side of the table. Note the sterile bump under the arm, which helps stabilize the elbow during the procedure. This rests on the arm board, which has been placed parallel to the table.

When using the prone position, the anesthesiologist is positioned at the head of the table, the surgeon stands directly lateral to the flexed elbow, and the assistant stands toward the head of the patient. The ancillary scrub personnel stand toward the foot of the patient or behind the surgeon and the assistant. One Mayo stand is placed behind the surgeon and the other Mayo stand is on the opposite side of the table. All tubing and electrical cords run from this Mayo stand to run to the video monitor, recorder, light source, camera, fluid bags, and mechanical irrigation system, which are placed on the opposite side of the patient (see Figure 1-5).

Elbow arthroscopy has a significant potential for complications, particularly neurovascular injury.[7] The key to avoiding complications is to have a clear understanding of the relationship of the neurovascular structures to the soft tissue and bony anatomy. With the patient positioned in the lateral decubitus or prone position, it is important to identify and mark landmarks. This includes the tip of the olecranon, the medial and lateral epicondyle, the radial head, the soft spot of the elbow, the medial intermuscular septum, and the ulnar nerve (Figure 1-6). Some authors recommend distending the joint with 20 to 40 cc of fluid through the lateral soft spot before establishing the initial portal.[11] Cadaveric studies have demonstrated that joint insufflation significantly increases the distance between the joint surfaces and neurovascular structures, thus helping to protect them from injury during joint entry.

In a different cadaveric study looking at the role of joint insufflation before portal placement, Miller et al[12] demonstrated that there is a small distance (as narrow as 6 mm) between the joint capsule and neurovascular structures and that joint insufflation does not increase the capsule-to-nerve distance. The authors of this chapter have found joint insufflation not necessary before

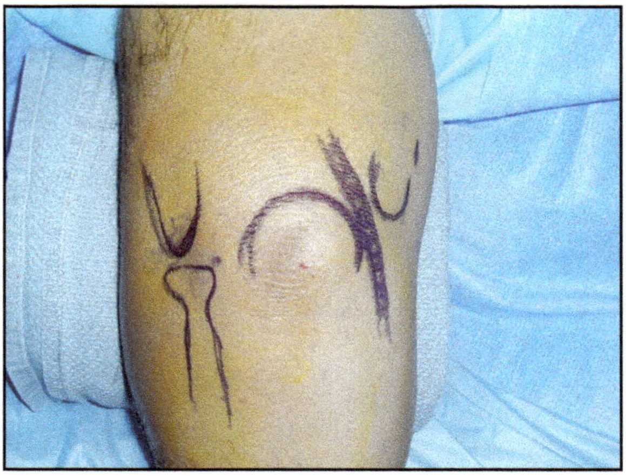

Figure 1-6. Anatomic landmarks are identified on the left elbow in the prone position, including the medial epicondyle (right), the lateral epicondyle (left), the radial head, the olecranon, and the ulnar nerve (dark blue line on right). The intermuscular septum is also identified on the medial aspect of the elbow just anterior to the medial epicondyle.

making the proximal anteromedial portal, the first portal that they typically establish. If one pays close attention to anatomic landmarks, the elbow joint can be safely entered into without having to inflate the joint with fluid.

When creating portals, the surgeon should avoid penetrating the subcutaneous tissue, thereby helping to prevent injury to the superficial cutaneous nerves. A hemostat or mosquito clamp should be used to spread tissues down to the capsule.[7] When the arthroscope is introduced, the elbow should be flexed to 90 degrees to relax and protect the anterior neurovascular structures, and only blunt trocars should be used.

Whether the anteromedial or anterolateral portal should be created first has been an issue of some debate. Many surgeons create a lateral portal initially and then establish a medial portal with a spinal needle by direct visualization from within the joint. Alternatively, an inside-out technique may be used in which a switching stick is used to establish the medial portal from inside the joint. Other surgeons, using the same techniques, establish the medial portal first. Cadaveric studies have found that it is safer to establish the proximal anteromedial portal first rather than the lateral portal.[13]

The senior author believes, and many others agree, that the proximal anteromedial portal should be created first as it is the safest as long as the surgeon has identified and outlined the important soft tissue and bony landmarks, including the intermuscular septum.[7,8,13] The most important landmark is the medial intermuscular septum as it protects the ulnar nerve, and, by staying anterior to it, the nerve is safe. There is less fluid extravasation when starting medially because a superomedial portal traverses predominately tendinous tissue and a tough portion of the forearm flexor muscles. The thicker tissues minimize fluid extravasation more effectively than the softer, thinner radial capsule.[6,14] Finally, most elbow disorders are located in the lateral compartment, which is best visualized from the proximal anteromedial portal.[7]

For the anterior compartment, the proximal anteromedial portal is established first and was first described by Poehling.[3] It is located approximately 2 cm proximal to the medial epicondyle and just anterior to the intermuscular septum (Figure 1-7). Prior to establishing this portal, the location and the stability of the ulnar nerve should be assessed. The prevalence rate of ulnar nerve subluxation anterior to the cubital tunnel is approximately 17%. Blunt dissection is carried out until the anterior aspect of the humerus is palpated, again staying anterior to the intermuscular septum. The arthroscopic sheath is then inserted anterior to the intermuscular septum while maintaining contact with the anterior aspect of the humerus and directing the trocar toward the radial head. Use of the anterior surface of the humerus as a constant guide helps prevent injury to the median nerve and the brachial artery, which are anterior to the capsule. The ulnar nerve is located approximately 3 to 4 mm from this portal, posterior to the intermuscular septum (Figure 1-8). Palpating the septum and making sure that the portal is established anterior to the

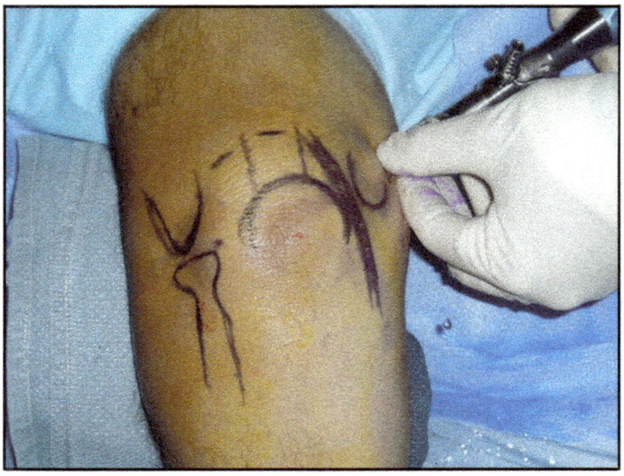

Figure 1-7. The proximal anteromedial portal is the first to be established. It is located just anterior to the intermuscular septum and 2 cm proximal to the medial epicondyle.

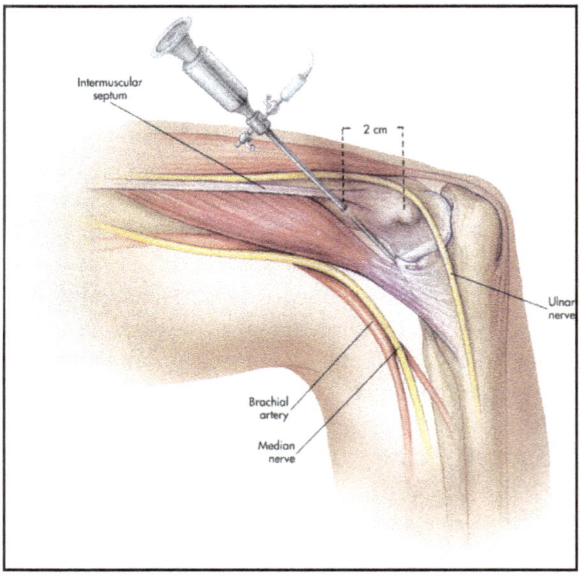

Figure 1-8. The arthroscope is inserted 2 cm proximal to the medial epicondyle and just anterior to the intermuscular septum on the medial aspect of the arm. In the prone position, the brachial artery and median nerve fall away from the joint capsule, allowing for safe portal placement.

septum minimizes the risk of injury to the nerve while providing excellent visualization. If the trocar is placed posterior to the intermuscular septum, injury to the ulnar nerve can occur. This portal provides excellent visualization of the anterior compartment of the elbow, particularly the radiocapitellar joint, humeroulnar joints, coronoid fossa, and superior joint capsule.[5,7]

Careful attention should be paid to the medial aspect of the elbow and the ulnar nerve should be carefully examined to make sure it does not sublux. If there is any question, the ulnar nerve should be dissected out and identified and then the trocar placed carefully around it. Another option is for 2 lateral portals to be used or a transfossa portal with a 70-degree scope to view into the anterior compartment.

The anteromedial portal, as described by Lynch et al,[15] is located 2 cm distal and 2 cm anterior to the medial epicondyle and is at or near the distal extent of the elbow capsule. Because of the location of this portal, the cannula can enter the joint only by being advanced straight laterally toward the median nerve.[13] The proximal anteromedial portal is recommended as it is safer because the more proximal position allows the arthroscope to be directed distally, resulting in the arthroscope being almost parallel to the median nerve in the anteroposterior plane.[7,13]

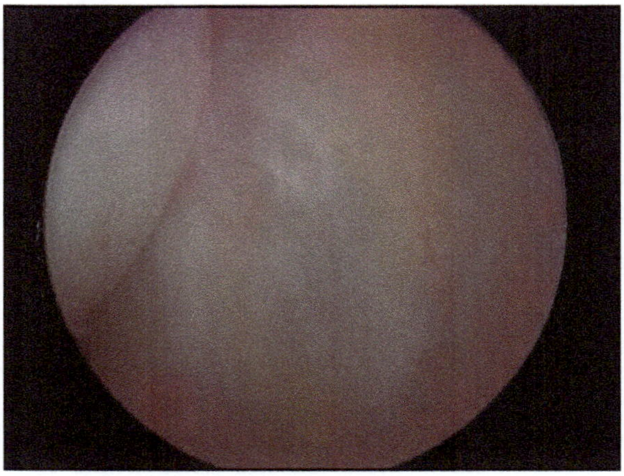

Figure 1-9. The lateral capsule is seen from the proximal anteromedial portal. This is the location where a spinal needle is introduced for the proximal anterolateral portal.

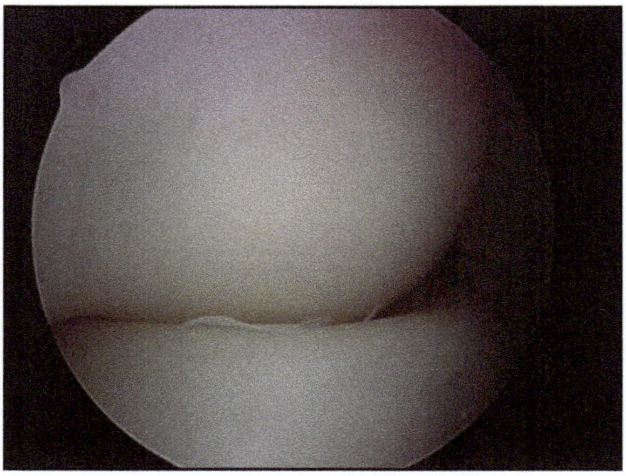

Figure 1-10. Viewing from the proximal anteromedial portal, the radial head and the capitellum are easily visualized.

The anterolateral portal was originally described as being located 3 cm distal and 2 cm anterior to the lateral epicondyle.[2] However, this portal location places the radial nerve at significant risk for iatrogenic injury. Lindenfeld[13] demonstrated that the radial nerve could be as close as 3 mm to this portal. To decrease risk of injury to the radial nerve, several investigators have stressed the importance of avoiding the distal placement of this portal in favor of a more proximal placement of the anterolateral portal.[11] Field et al[11] compared the following 3 lateral portals: a proximal anterolateral portal (located 2 cm proximal and 1 cm anterior to the lateral epicondyle); a distal anterolateral portal,[2] and a middle anterolateral portal (located 1 cm directly anterior to the lateral epicondyle). The authors found that the proximal anterolateral portal was the safest and the radiohumeral joint visualization was most complete and technically easiest using this most proximal portal.

After creating the proximal anteromedial portal and using it as viewing portal, creating the proximal anterolateral portal is best done using an outside-in technique localizing the position with a spinal needle. This portal is created 2 cm proximal and 1 cm anterior to the lateral epicondyle as described by Field et al.[11] The exact entry can vary depending on the pathology to be addressed. Visualizing from the proximal anteromedial portal, the lateral capsule is visualized and palpation of the skin will help localize the exact location of the spinal needle to aid in portal placement (Figure 1-9). It is important to direct the cannula toward the humerus while penetrating the capsule so that the portal placement is not too far anterior and medial. Viewing from the proximal anteromedial portal, the radiocapitellar joint is easily visualized (Figure 1-10). The trochlea and the coronoid process can also be seen from the proximal anteromedial portal (Figure 1-11).

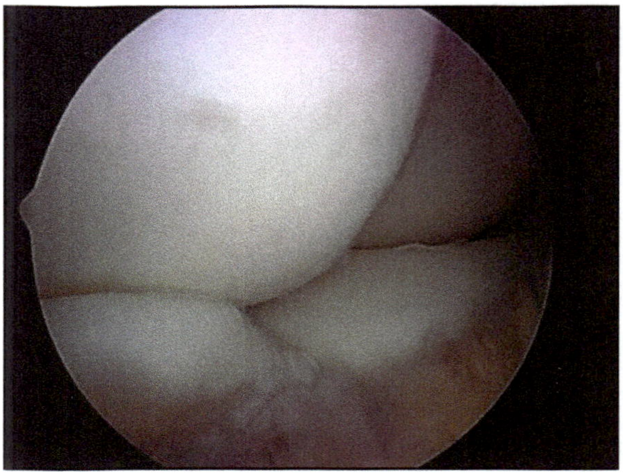

Figure 1-11. The trochlea (top left) and the coronoid process (lower left) can also be seen from the proximal anteromedial portal.

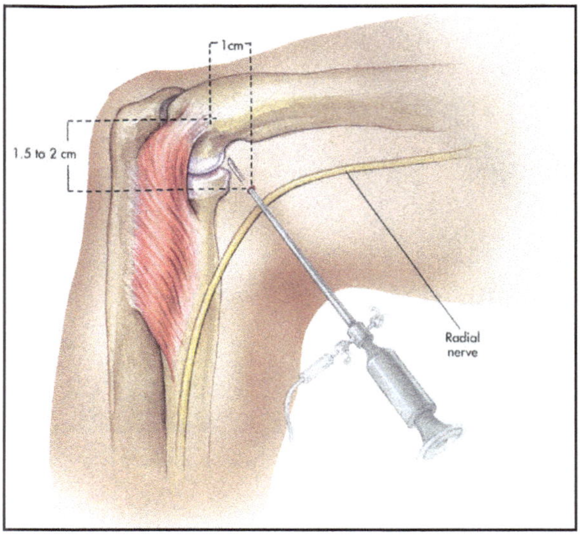

Figure 1-12. The proximal anterolateral portal is created 1 to 2 cm proximal to the lateral epicondyle and 1 to 2 cm anterior to the lateral epicondyle. Placing the arthroscope in the proximal anterolateral portal allows visualization of anterior compartment looking medially.

The proximal anterolateral portal is often a working portal and is ideal for arthroscopic lateral epicondyle release and for debridement of the radiocapitellar joint. Viewing from this portal permits visualization of the anterior compartment (Figure 1-12) and is particularly good in evaluating medial structures, such as the trochlea, coronoid tip, and medial capsule (Figure 1-13).

For the posterior compartment, the straight posterior portal is located 3 cm proximal to the tip of the olecranon and can be used as a viewing portal or as a working portal. When it is the first portal created, a cannula with a blunt trocar is inserted. The cannula pierces the triceps muscle just above the musculotendinous junction and is bluntly maneuvered in a circular motion, manipulating the soft tissues from the olecranon fossa for better visualization. When used as a working portal, it is helpful for removal of impinging olecranon osteophytes and loose bodies from the posterior elbow joint.[16] It is also needed when a complete synovectomy of the elbow is done.[7] The straight posterior portal passes within 25 mm of the ulnar nerve and within 23 mm of the posterior antebrachial cutaneous nerve.[6]

The posterolateral portal is located 2 to 3 cm proximal to the tip of olecranon at the lateral border of the triceps tendon. This is created while visualizing from the straight posterior portal using a spinal needle directed toward the olecranon fossa (Figure 1-14). Initial visualization is often difficult due to scarring, fat pad hypertrophy, and synovitis. A trocar is then directed toward the olecranon fossa, passing through the triceps muscle to reach the capsule. A shaver is then

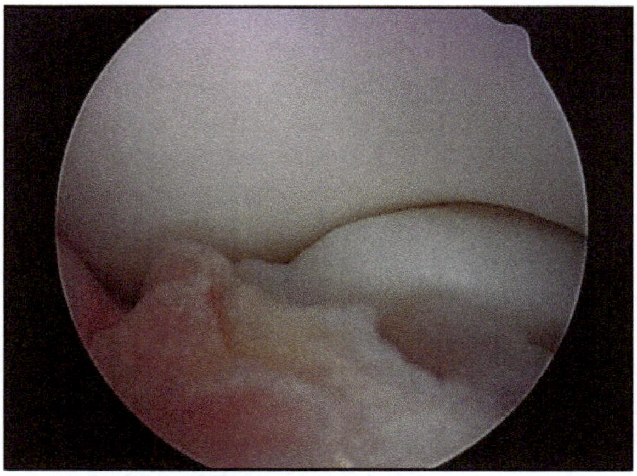

Figure 1-13. Viewing from the proximal anterolateral portal, the trochlea and the coronoid process can also be seen.

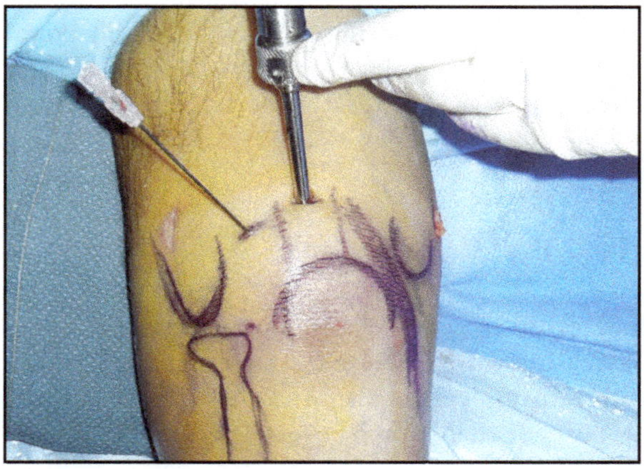

Figure 1-14. The arthroscope is introduced into the posterior compartment using a straight posterior portal, 3 cm proximal from the tip of the olecranon. A spinal needle is introduced lateral to the triceps tendon toward the olecranon fossa for the posterolateral portal.

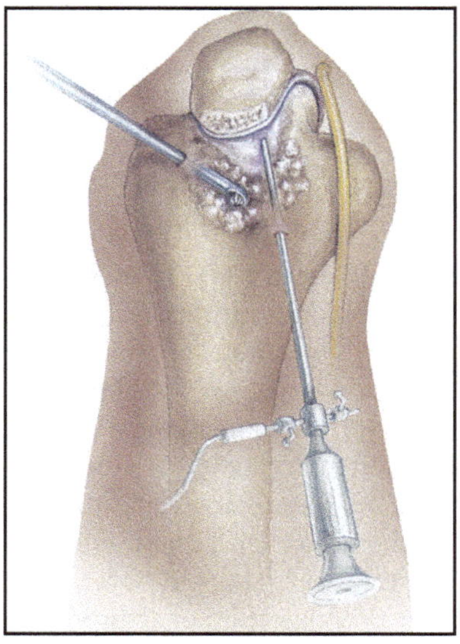

Figure 1-15. The posterior lateral portal is used as a working portal to remove osteophytes and loose bodies from the posterior compartment.

introduced to improve visualization of the posterior compartment. This portal permits visualization of the olecranon tip, olecranon fossa, and posterior trochlea and can be used as a working portal to remove osteophytes and loose bodies from the posterior compartment (Figure 1-15). However, the posterior capitellum is not well seen from this portal.[7] The medial and posterior antebrachial cutaneous nerves are the 2 neurovascular structures at most risk; they are an average of 25 mm from this portal. The ulnar nerve is also approximately 25 mm from this portal, but as long as the cannula is kept lateral to the posterior midline, the nerve is not at risk.[6] Initial visualization of the posterior compartment can be difficult because of synovitis, scar tissue, and fat pad hypertrophy. It is important to patiently triangulate with the arthroscope and shaver within the olecranon fossa to debride tissues in order to gain adequate visualization. The tip of the olecranon is one of the first landmarks to be identified. Blindly debriding in the posterior compartment and straying outside of the olecranon fossa can cause severe iatrogenic nerve injury.

The posterolateral anatomy of the elbow allows for portal placement anywhere from the proximal posterolateral portal to the lateral soft spot. Altering the portal position along the line between the posterolateral portal and lateral soft spot changes the orientation of the portal relative to the joint.[8] These portals are particularly useful for gaining access to the posterolateral recess.

The direct lateral portal is located at the soft spot, which is the triangle formed by the radial head, lateral epicondyle, and olecranon. It is developed under direct visualization using a spinal needle. It is useful as a viewing portal for working in the posterior compartment, viewing the radiocapitellar joint, and for a working portal for radial head resection.[17] This is the only portal that provides easy access to the posterior capitellum and radioulnar joint and can be useful for lesions of the radiocapitellar joint.[7] A full description of the arthroscopic portals are outlined in Table 1-2.

Postoperative Protocol

The postoperative treatment following elbow arthroscopy depends on the particular procedure that has been performed. In general, early active-assisted ROM exercises are instituted within the first 24 to 48 hours after surgery along with early gripping of the hand and wrist to facilitate circulation and reduce swelling. However, one must be careful not to be too exuberant in the early postoperative period until the portal sites are well healed to prevent persistent portal drainage primarily from the lateral portal. Once the portal sites are healed, passive, active-assisted, and active ROM exercises are instituted to prevent stiffness. The particulars of this, including when to institute strengthening exercises, depend on the exact procedure that was performed.

Potential Complications

Complications due to elbow arthroscopy can be minimized if the surgeon has a sound knowledge of the anatomy of the elbow and uses proper equipment and meticulous operative technique.[3] One of the most common complications is neurological injury,[1,5,18-20] including transient nerve palsies involving the radial nerve, posterior interosseous nerve, and ulnar nerve.[1,19,20] The most significant risk factors for the development of a temporary nerve palsy are an underlying diagnosis of rheumatoid arthritis and a contracture.[1] Injury can be caused by direct laceration of a nerve by a knife penetrating deep to the skin, from the arthroscopic shaver, or from the cannula trocar.[21] Compression from a cannula, from fluid extravasation, or from the use of local anesthetics has also been reported to cause neurological injuries[1,4] but is usually transient. Delayed-onset ulnar neuritis after elbow arthroscopy has also been reported and can be a complication of arthroscopic elbow contracture release. Its incidence and severity can be reduced by limited open ulnar nerve compression or transposition. Transection of the posterior interosseous nerve, median nerve, ulnar nerve, and radial nerve has also been reported in the literature. Neurological complications are more common than reported in the literature and can be devastating not only for the patient, but also for the surgeon.[1,5,18-20] It is vitally important that the surgeon discuss the risks and benefits of elbow arthroscopic procedure with the patient and this is well documented in the medical record.

Table 1-2. Elbow Arthroscopic Portals

PORTAL	ANATOMY	NEUROVASCULAR RISK
Proximal anteromedial	2 cm proximal to medial epicondyle, anterior to intermuscular septum, deep to brachialis	Median nerve: 12.4 mm (7 to 20 mm) Brachial artery: 18 mm Ulnar nerve: 12 mm (7 to 18 mm)
Proximal anterolateral	~2 cm proximal to lateral epicondyle, 1 cm anterior to humerus, through brachioradialis	Posterior branch of antebrachial cutaneous nerve: 6.1 mm (0 to 14 mm) Radial nerve: 2x further away vs anterolateral 9.9 mm away
Anteromedial	2 cm distal, 2 cm anterior to medial epicondyle, passes through common flexor origin, then passes through brachialis and capsule	Anterior branch of medial antebrachial cutaneous nerve: average 1 mm away (0 to 5 mm) Median nerve: protected by the brachialis muscle, average 7 mm (5 to 13 mm) Brachial artery: protected by brachialis muscle, average 15 mm (8 to 20 mm)
Anterolateral	3 cm distal, 1 cm anterior to lateral epicondyle, penetrates extensor carpi radialis muscles, portal is inappropriately placed below joint line in most patients if only measured guidelines are followed	Anterior branch of posterior antebrachial cutaneous nerve: average 7.6 mm away (0 to 20 mm) Radial nerve: at extreme risk, average 4.9 mm away in flexion (2 to 10 mm) Posterior interosseous nerve: relatively fixed as it passes under the arcade of Frohse, just distal to the joint line, poorly protected even with elbow flexion. Ensure placement of portal is proximal to radial head
Anterosuperolateral	Directly anterior to lateral epicondyle	Risk to radial nerve between anterolateral and proximal anterolateral portal
Posterior soft spot	Traverses anconeus, posterolateral capsule	No neurovascular risk in this safe portal
Posterocentral	3 cm directly proximal to olecranon tip in midline, penetrates triceps near muscle/tendon junction	Safe, distance to ulnar nerve averages 19.1 mm (15 to 25 mm)
Posterolateral	3 cm proximal to olecranon tip along lateral tendinous edge, passes through triceps muscle, then capsule	Radial nerve proximity averages 4.8 mm (3 to 8 mm)

In a 2001 report of 473 elbow arthroscopies performed by experienced arthroscopists,[1] 4 types of minor complications, including infection, nerve injury, prolonged drainage, and contracture, were identified in 50 cases. The most common complication was persistent portal drainage, especially from the lateral portal. There is little subcutaneous tissue separating the skin from the capsule. Portal drainage can be reduced by using a side box stay suture, which closes the portal securely and minimizes drainage.[1] Subcutaneous emphysema of the upper extremity has also been reported after elbow arthroscopy, as have heterotopic ossification and minor flexion contractures.[1]

Superficial and deep wound infections can also occur. Superficial wound infections are easily treated, but deep infections can be serious if not recognized early. The rate of deep infections ranges from 0.8% to 2.2%.[1,20] Two studies have found that the use of intraoperative steroid injections significantly increases the risk of deep infection vs those that did not receive steroid injections, so their use during surgery should be avoided or minimized.[1,20] However, it is up to the discretion of the surgeon as intraoperative steroid injections have been shown to reduce the risk of heterotopic bone ossification in the postoperative period.[20]

Many of the complications associated with elbow arthroscopy are the result of inexperience, poor technique, and lack of knowledge in regard to the anatomy about the elbow. However, even in the most experienced hands, complications such as nerve injuries, transient or permanent, can occur. It is crucial that the surgeon who wishes to perform elbow arthroscopy safely and effectively adhere to strict surgical technique and portal placement to avoid possible complications.[21] If a nerve injury is suspected in the early postoperative period, careful monitoring is required; if it does not resolve, early wound exploration is recommended within the first 4 to 6 weeks after surgery as early primary repair of nerve injuries gives the best results. Electromyography and nerve conduction studies typically do not show changes until approximately 6 weeks after an injury, but if a nerve injury is suspected, the author recommends early exploration even before electromyography can be done.

Arthroscopic surgery of the elbow is a technically demanding procedure. Attention to detail, including careful portal placement, is necessary to avoid injury to neurovascular structures around the elbow joint. In every clinical case, the bony anatomy should be drawn on the elbow of the patient, and an 18-gauge spinal needle should be used to confirm the correct portal location before introducing larger arthroscopic instruments.[21] With new innovations in techniques and technology, it is possible to treat a variety of lesions of the elbow. As with any operative procedure, careful preoperative planning, including a detailed history and physical examination along with proper imaging studies is necessary, along with sound clinical judgment to ensure a successful procedure.

Top Technical Pearls for the Procedure

1. Elbow arthroscopy poses greater technical challenges and neurological risks than knee or shoulder arthroscopy because of the small size of the elbow joint and the proximity of the portals to neurovascular structures, and it has the potential for causing injury to important nearby nerves and vessels. Intimate knowledge and familiarity with the normal elbow anatomy and portals will decrease the risk of damage to important structures.
2. Elbow arthroscopy is useful for the diagnosis of intra-articular lesions of the elbow, the removal of loose and foreign bodies, irrigation of the joint, debridement of an infected joint, excision of osteophytes, synovectomy, capsular release, excision of the radial head, and treatment of acute fractures of the elbow. The indications for elbow arthroscopy have been extended to include the treatment of lateral and medial epicondylitis, endoscopic distal biceps tendon repair, and arthroscopic ulnar nerve release.

(continued)

3. Without having a thorough understanding of the anatomy of the elbow, improper portal placement can cause significant complications to neurovascular structures. It is vitally important to know and review superficial anatomy of the elbow before beginning elbow arthroscopy. The bony landmarks provide the key to avoiding damage to important neurovascular structures.
4. The proximal anteromedial portal should be created first as it is the safest as long as the surgeon has identified and outlined the important soft tissue and bony landmarks, including the intermuscular septum. The most important landmark is the medial intermuscular septum as it protects the ulnar nerve; by staying anterior to it, the nerve is safe. Palpating the septum and making sure that the portal is established anterior to the septum minimizes the risk of injury to the nerve while providing excellent visualization. Preoperatively, it is important to check for a subluxing ulnar nerve.
5. Initial visualization of the posterior compartment can be difficult because of synovitis, scar tissue, and fat pad hypertrophy. It is important to patiently triangulate with the arthroscope and shaver within the olecranon fossa to debride tissues to gain adequate visualization. The tip of the olecranon is one of the first landmarks to be identified. Blindly debriding in the posterior compartment and straying outside of the olecranon fossa can cause severe nerve injury.

References

1. Kelly EW, Morrey BF, O'Driscoll SW. Complications of elbow arthroscopy. *J Bone Joint Surg Am.* 2001;83(1):25-34.
2. Andrews JR, Carson WG. Arthroscopy of the elbow. *Arthroscopy.* 1985;1(2):97-107.
3. Poehling GG, Whipple TL, Sisco L, Goldman B. Elbow arthroscopy: a new technique. *Arthroscopy.* 1989;5:220-224.
4. O'Driscoll SW, Morrey BF. Arthroscopy of the elbow. Diagnostic and therapeutic benefits and hazards. *J Bone Joint Surg Am.* 1992;74(1):84-94.
5. Poehling GG, Ekman EF. Arthroscopy of the elbow. *J Bone Joint Surg Am.* 1994;76(8):1265-1271.
6. Baker CL, Brooks AA. Arthroscopy of the elbow. *Clin Sports Med.* 1996;15(2):261-281.
7. Baker CL Jr, Jones GL. Arthroscopy of the elbow. *Am J Sports Med.* 1999;27(2):251-264.
8. Abboud JA, Ricchette ET, Tjoumakaris F, Ramsey ML. Elbow arthroscopy: basic setup and portal placement. *J Am Acad Orthop Surg.* 2006;14(5):312-318.
9. Timmerman LA, Schwartz ML, Andrews JR. Preoperative evaluation of the ulnar ligament by magnetic resonance imaging and computed tomography arthrography. Evaluation in 25 baseball players with surgical confirmation. *Am J Sports Med.* 1994;22:26-32.
10. Timmerman LA, Andrews JR. Undersurface tear of the ulnar collateral ligament in baseball players. A newly recognized lesion. *Am J Sports Med.* 1994;22:33-36.
11. Field LD, Altchek DW, Warren RF, O'Brien SJ, Skyhar MJ, Wickiewicz TL. Arthroscopic anatomy of the lateral elbow: a comparison of 3 portals. *Arthroscopy.* 1994;10(6):602-607.
12. Miller CD, Jobe CM, Wright MH. Neuroanatomy in elbow arthroscopy. *J Shoulder Elbow Surg.* 1995;4:168-174.
13. Lindenfeld TN. Medial approach in elbow arthroscopy. *Am J Sports Med.* 1990;18(4):413-417.
14. McLaughlin RE II, Savoie FH III, Field LF, Ramsey JR. Arthroscopic treatment of the arthritic elbow due to primary radiocapitellar arthritis. *Arthroscopy.* 2006;22(1):63-69.
15. Lynch GJ, Meyers JF, Whipple TL, Caspari RB. Neurovascular anatomy and elbow arthroscopy: inherent risks. *Arthroscopy.* 1986;2:190-197.
16. Andrews JR, St. Pierre RK, Carson WG Jr. Arthroscopy of the elbow. *Clin Sports Med.* 1986;5(4):653-662.

17. Savoie FH III, Nunley PD, Field LD. Arthroscopic management of the arthritic elbow: indications, technique, and results. *J Shoulder Elbow Surg.* 1999;8(3):214-219.
18. Byram IR, Kim HM, Levine WN, Ahmad CS. Elbow arthroscopic surgery update for sports medicine conditions. *Am J Sports Med.* 2013;41(9):2191-2202.
19. Elfeddali R, Schreuder MH, Eygendall D. Arthroscopic elbow surgery, is it safe? *J Shoulder Elbow Surg.* 2013;22(5):647-652.
20. Nelson GN, Wu T, Galatz LM, Yamaguchi K, Keener JD. Elbow arthroscopy: early complications and associated risk factors. *J Shoulder Elbow Surg.* 2014;23(2):273-278.
21. Dodson CC, Nho SJ, Williams RJ III, Altchek DW. Elbow arthroscopy. *J Am Acad Orthop Surg.* 2008;16(10):574-585.

Please see videos on the accompanying website at

www.routledge.com/9781630910013

2

Diagnostic Arthroscopy and Loose Body Removal

Michael J. O'Brien, MD and Felix H. Savoie III, MD

Introduction

The indications for elbow arthroscopy have advanced drastically in the last 20 years. Originally used as a tool for diagnostic purposes, removal of loose bodies,[1] synovectomy,[2] and lysis of adhesions,[3,4] the indications have evolved to treat myriad elbow conditions. Elbow arthroscopy is now routinely used for the treatment of lateral epicondylitis,[5,6] osteochondritis dissecans (OCD),[7,8] osteoarthritis and osteophyte resection,[9,10] radial head resection,[11] plica excision,[12,13] septic arthritis,[14] and contracture release.[4,15,16] Pioneers in the field continually develop innovative ideas and new surgical techniques to treat a growing list of conditions, including arthroscopic reduction and fixation of fractures,[17-19] ligament repair,[20,21] ulnar nerve decompression,[22] and elbow arthroplasty.

Diagnostic arthroscopy and loose body removal will always remain basic tenants to elbow arthroscopy. Removal of loose bodies is one of the most common and rewarding arthroscopic procedures in the elbow. Loose bodies in the elbow typically manifest with mechanical symptoms that block range of motion (ROM) and predispose to arthritic changes. Therefore, conservative treatment plays a limited role. These procedures allow novice arthroscopists to gain familiarity and confidence in the elbow, and they can be used as stepping stones to more advanced procedures. As one becomes more comfortable and facile using the arthroscope in the elbow joint, it allows the treating surgeon to use the scope as a diagnostic tool to confirm instability patterns, assess articular cartilage congruence during fracture reduction, and confirm stability after fracture fixation or ligament reconstruction.

As with all elbow arthroscopic procedures, a 3-dimensional understanding of the neurovascular anatomy is paramount for safety and success. A concrete preoperative plan is essential. The surgery should be performed with speed and precision, with adjustments made to account for intraoperative findings, as swelling will increase throughout the case.

This chapter highlights indications for diagnostic elbow arthroscopy, patient positioning, and the key steps to perform during the procedure. Several methods for loose body removal are discussed. Hopefully this information will allow young orthopedic surgeons and novice

Savoie FH III, Field LD, Steinmann SP, eds. *The Elbow and Wrist: AANA Advanced Arthroscopic Surgical Techniques* (pp 21-30).

arthroscopists to perform the procedure with safety, speed, and confidence and build upon this knowledge to perform more complex arthroscopic procedures in the elbow.

Anatomy

The elbow is a complex joint that allows flexion and extension through the ulnohumeral articulation and pronation and supination at the radiocapitellar joint. Stability is provided by the medial collateral ligament complex, the lateral collateral ligament complex, and the ulnohumeral articulation. Numerous portals have been described and are discussed in greater detail elsewhere in this text. Standard arthroscopy portals include proximal anteromedial and proximal anterolateral portals to access the anterior compartment and posterior central (or posterior transtendon) and posterolateral portals to enter the posterior compartment.

A thorough understanding of 3-dimensional neurovascular anatomy is crucial to safely perform elbow arthroscopy. All described portals allow access to the joint through safe zones. In general, proximal portals are safer than distal portals as they are further away from the neurovascular structures. The radial nerve and posterior interosseous nerve are at risk on the lateral side of the elbow, the median nerve is at risk on the anteromedial side, and the ulnar nerve is at risk on the posteromedial side. It is important never to stray medial to midline when establishing portals on the posterior aspect of the elbow to avoid injury to the ulnar nerve. Blunt trocars and cannulas can help to protect neurovascular structures and limit iatrogenic injury.

Indications

- Loose body secondary to arthritis or trauma
- Synovial chondromatosis
- OCD with a displaced cartilage cap
- To debride OCD or an osteochondral lesion prior to an open grafting procedure
- To confirm instability patterns prior to ligament repair or reconstruction
- To remove hematoma or cartilage fragments from irreducible elbow dislocation
- Arthroscopic irrigation and debridement for septic arthritis
- Arthroscopic assistance with fracture reduction
- To confirm articular cartilage congruence during open reduction and internal fixation

Controversial Indications

- To diagnose or rule out intra-articular pathology in the painful elbow. With the availability of magnetic resonance imaging (MRI) and computed tomography, elbow arthroscopy is rarely indicated as a purely diagnostic procedure. The diagnosis should be made prior to surgery based on patient history, physical examination, x-rays, and advanced imaging studies.

Pertinent Physical Findings

Patients with loose bodies in the elbow will often complain of intermittent pain and feelings of clicking, catching, or locking in the joint. They may report stiffness and a gradual loss of motion, most commonly loss of terminal flexion or extension. A traumatic injury may precede the symptoms, although there is often no history of trauma. It is important to inquire about any previous surgery for ulnar nerve decompression or transposition.

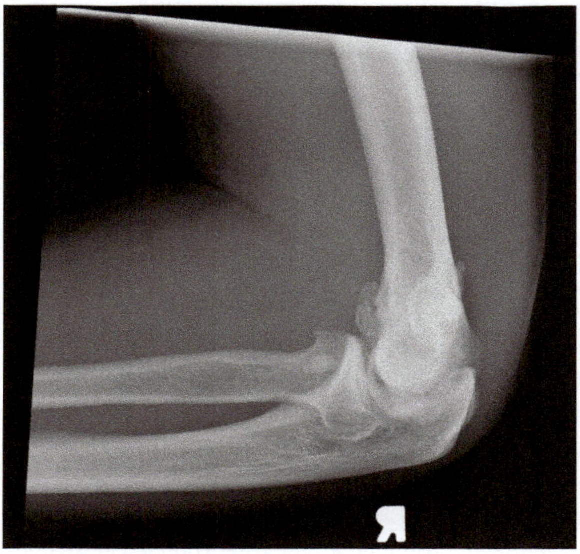

Figure 2-1. Lateral x-ray of a right elbow demonstrating spurring of the radial head, osteophytes on the tip of the coronoid and olecranon, and loose bodies in the anterior and posterior compartments. Loose bodies will typically be found in the coronoid fossa anteriorly and olecranon fossa posteriorly.

- Inspect the elbow for any scars or obvious deformity. Surgical scars on the medial side may alert the orthopedic surgeon to previous ulnar nerve surgery.
- Elbows with isolated loose bodies may have an effusion with subtle swelling in the posterolateral gutter.
- ROM in flexion, extension, and pronosupination should be measured and compared to the contralateral side.
- Elbows with arthritis and osteophytes may show loss of motion, most notably terminal flexion and extension. These elbows will have a firm end point at terminal flexion and extension due to osteophyte impingement.
- Palpate the radiocapitellar joint and lateral gutter for palpable loose bodies.
- On the medial side, the ulnar nerve and medial epicondyle should be palpated during flexion and extension to evaluate for a subluxating ulnar nerve. A subluxated or dislocated ulnar nerve can be found in 16% of the normal population.[23]
- It is crucial to know the location and status of the ulnar nerve prior to any arthroscopic procedure to avoid iatrogenic injury to the nerve. Previous ulnar nerve transposition is a relative contraindication to elbow arthroscopy. Prior to accessing the joint from the medial side, an open ulnar nerve exploration should be performed to identify and protect the nerve.
- Assess stability on the medial and lateral sides of the elbow with varus and valgus stress testing.
- Recommended best test: Palpation of the radiocapitellar joint during simultaneous valgus load and pronation/supination of the forearm can assess for crepitus and arthritis or palpable loose bodies in the lateral gutter.
- Finally, a thorough neurovascular examination should be performed and documented.

Pertinent Imaging

- Routine elbow x-rays, including anteroposterior, lateral, and oblique projections are routinely obtained. The lateral projection is most helpful to identify osteophytes or loose bodies in the anterior or posterior compartments (Figure 2-1).

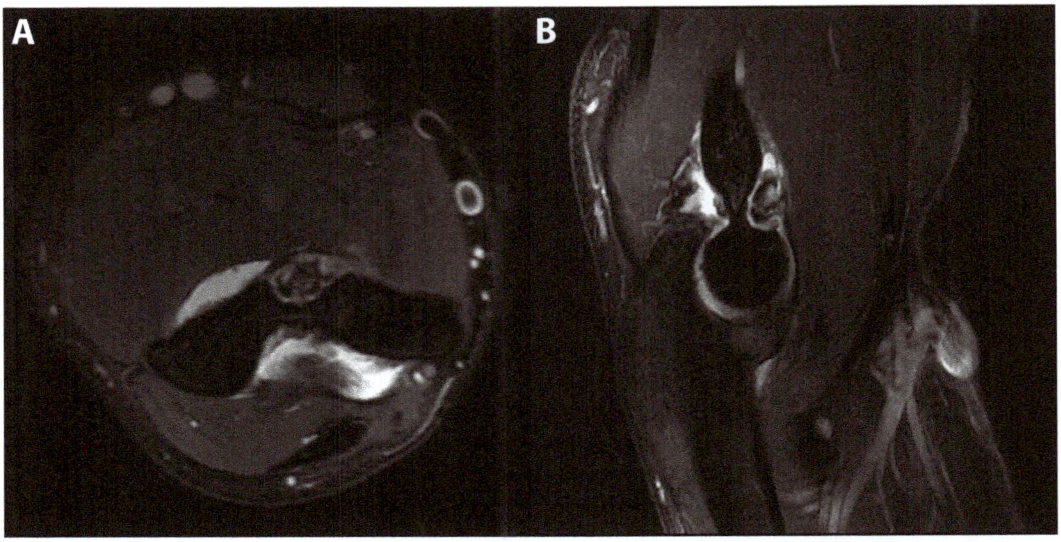

Figure 2-2. (A) Axial and (B) sagittal T2-weighted MRIs demonstrating a large osteochondral loose body in the coronoid fossa in the anterior compartment of the elbow.

- Standard imaging fails to identify loose bodies in almost 30% of cases.[1,23] In these instances, when history and physical examination is consistent with intra-articular loose body, advanced imaging such as computed tomography or MRI may be warranted.
- Even when loose bodies are identified on x-rays, advanced imaging can be very helpful to identify the number and size of loose bodies as well as the specific location of osteophytes that may be resected at the time of surgery.
- Loose bodies are often identified in the coronoid fossa, olecranon fossa, and posterolateral gutter (Figure 2-2).

Equipment

- Standard arthroscopy equipment
- Standard 4-mm arthroscope
- Arthroscopic cannulas to limit extravasation of fluid into the soft tissues
- Spinal needle
- Arthroscopic graspers of different sizes, arthroscopic biter
- Motorized shaver, motorized burr

Positioning and Portals

- Arthroscopic surgery can be performed in the supine, prone, or lateral decubitus position.
- The authors prefer the prone position with the arm on a bolster, which stabilizes the humerus and provides excellent access to the posterior compartment of the elbow.
- On the operative side, an arm board is placed parallel to the operating room table at shoulder level. A nonsterile arm tourniquet is applied, and the arm is placed in 90 degrees of shoulder abduction and neutral rotation. The arm is supported at the midhumerus level by a padded

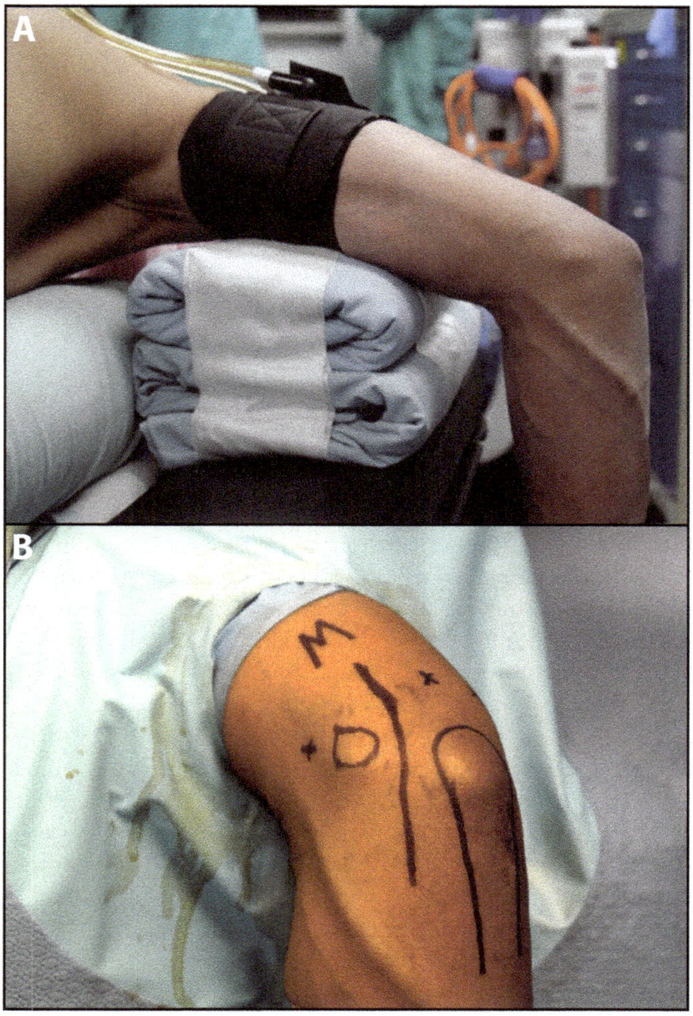

Figure 2-3. (A) In the prone position, the arm is supported by a bump positioned on top of the arm board, which suspends the elbow in 90 degrees of flexion and allows excellent access to the posterior compartment. (B) All bony landmarks can be marked with a pen.

bolster attached to the operating table or a bump positioned on top of the arm board, which suspends the elbow in 90 degrees of flexion (Figure 2-3).

- Advantages of the prone position include excellent access to the posterior compartment, easy manipulation of the elbow from flexion to extension and forearm rotation, and direct access to medial and lateral structures if an open approach is necessary. In addition, flexion of the elbow allows the neurovascular structures to safely sag anteriorly, farther away from arthroscopic portals.
- Disadvantages include airway access for the anesthesia provider and difficulty in accessing the anterior compartment if an open anterior approach is undertaken.
- Standard arthroscopic portals are used.
- The anterior compartment is accessed through proximal anteromedial and proximal anterolateral portals.
- The proximal anteromedial portal is located 2 cm proximal and 1 cm anterior to the medial epicondyle.
- The proximal anterolateral portal is located 2 cm proximal and 2 cm anterior to the lateral epicondyle.

- The posterior compartment is accessed via a posterior central viewing portal and a posterolateral working portal.
- The posterior central portal is located 2 to 3 cm proximal to the tip of the olecranon and traverses the triceps tendon, whereas the posterolateral portal is located just lateral to the triceps tendon.
- It is paramount not to stray medial to midline when making the posterior central portal for risk of injury to the ulnar nerve.
- A posterolateral soft spot portal may be used to remove loose bodies from the posterolateral gutter and access the posterior radiocapitellar joint.

Step-by-Step Description of the Procedure

Step 1

After the adequate induction of general endotracheal anesthesia and secure control of the airway, the patient is placed in the prone position on the operating table. The patient is placed on 2 gel rolls to support the chest, and all bony prominences are well padded. A nonsterile tourniquet is applied to the upper arm and the arm is placed in 90 degrees of shoulder abduction. The arm is supported by a bump on an arm board parallel to the operating table to allow the elbow to freely hang at 90 degrees of flexion.

All bony landmarks are palpated and marked with a marking pen, including the tip of the olecranon and medial and lateral epicondyles. Special attention is given to the course of the ulnar nerve, which is also marked with a marking pen. Confirm that the ulnar nerve does not subluxate over the medial epicondyle with elbow flexion. The hand and forearm are wrapped with a sterile impervious stocking and wrapped with self-adherent Coban wrap. The arm is exsanguinated with an Esmarch bandage and the tourniquet is inflated. The elbow joint is insufflated with 20 to 30 mL of sterile saline through a direct posterior portal or soft spot portal. Insufflation expands the joint capsule and safely moves the neurovascular structures in a more anterior position.

Step 2

A proximal anteromedial portal is established for the arthroscope, 2 cm proximal and 1 cm anterior to the medial epicondyle and immediately anterior to the medial intermuscular septum. A small incision is made just through skin with a #11 blade. A small hemostat may be used to spread the subcutaneous tissue until the medial intermuscular septum is palpable. A blunt trocar is advanced anterior to the medial intermuscular septum to avoid injury to the ulnar nerve. The blunt trocar is advanced in direct contact with the anterior cortex of the humerus in the direction of the radiocapitellar joint, which ensures protection of the anterior neurovascular structures by the overlying brachialis muscle. The anterior capsule is pierced to gain access to the elbow joint. An egress of fluid with removal of the trocar confirms intra-articular placement. The 30-degree, 4-mm arthroscope is introduced, and diagnostic arthroscopy of the anterior compartment ensues.

Step 3

The proximal anteromedial portal permits a systematic evaluation of the lateral gutter, capitellum, radial head, anterior capsule, trochlea, coronoid process, and medial gutter. The radiocapitellar joint is assessed for instability and cartilage defects, with pronation and supination of the forearm aiding in the evaluation. Laxity of the annular ligament on the radial head and subluxation of the radial head with forearm supination is indicative of posterolateral rotatory instability

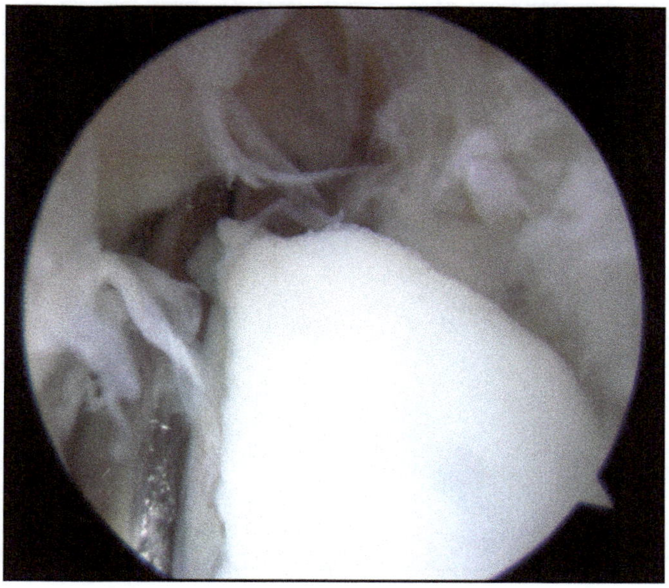

Figure 2-4. A loose body in the anterior compartment of the elbow. The loose body can be skewered with a spinal needle and removed with a grasper, a biter, or a motorized shaver.

of the elbow. The lateral capsule and extensor carpi radialis brevis origin are inspected. Tearing in this region is indicative of lateral epicondylitis. By slightly withdrawing the arthroscope and rotating the lens of the arthroscope, the anterior capsule and tip of the coronoid is evaluated next. By moving the arthroscope more medially, the medial ulnohumeral articulation can be visualized. An arthroscopic valgus stress test[24] is performed. Gapping of the medial ulnohumeral articulation may indicate incompetence of the medial ulnar collateral ligament.

Step 4

A proximal anterolateral portal is established next, using an outside-in technique with a spinal needle or a direct inside-out technique. This portal is located 2 cm proximal and 2 cm anterior to the lateral epicondyle. The skin is incised with a #11 blade. A blunt trocar or switching stick is advanced on the anterior cortex of the humerus gaining access to the elbow joint. A cannula is then advanced over the trocar or switching stick, minimizing the risk to the radial nerve on traversing the soft tissues.

Loose bodies in the anterior compartment are frequently found in the coronoid fossa (Figure 2-4). An arthroscopic grasper is placed through the proximal anterolateral portal and used to remove any loose bodies. Small loose bodies may be evacuated with a motorized shaver. Take great care to use limited suction with the motorized shaver. Full suction can inadvertently pull the anterior capsule into the shaver teeth and risk iatrogenic injury to the neurovascular structures. For large loose fragments that will not fit through the cannula, the fragment can be removed in piecemeal by using an arthroscopic biter or the motorized shaver. Alternatively, the grasper and cannula can be removed together with the loose fragment. This can be accomplished by rotating the grasper through the soft tissues while maintaining a firm grasp on the fragment. In addition, a spinal needle may be used to skewer the loose fragment until it can be secured and removed with the grasper. Once removed, loose bodies can be measured and photographed on the back table to document their size (Figure 2-5).

Step 5

After thorough evaluation and removal of all loose bodies from the anterior compartment, attention is directed to the posterior compartment. A posterior central portal is established for

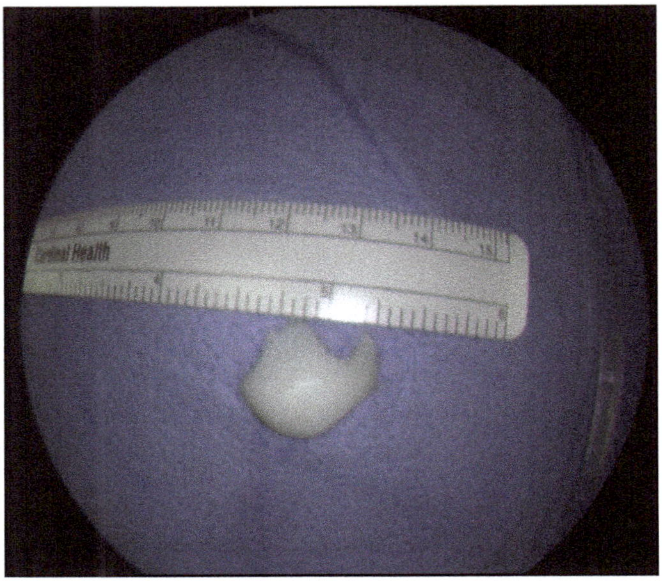

Figure 2-5. Once the loose body has been removed, an arthroscopic photo can be taken to document the size of the fragment.

the arthroscope, 3 cm proximal to the tip of the olecranon. When establishing this portal, it is important not to stray medial to the midline to avoid injury to the ulnar nerve. A #11 blade is used to incise the skin and is advanced straight down through the triceps tendon and into the olecranon fossa. The blunt trocar is then advanced down the same path into the olecranon fossa. A posterolateral portal is established as a working portal. This portal is made 3 cm proximal to the tip of the olecranon, just lateral to the triceps tendon. Initial visualization may be difficult in the posterior compartment due to the posterior fat pad in the olecranon fossa. In order to safely excise this bursa, triangulate with the arthroscope and the shaver. Use the shaver as a probe to confirm that it is centered in the olecranon fossa and feel the tip of the scope with the shaver. Running the shaver with intermittent suction will clear the posterior fat pad and create a working space. The entire posterior bursa is excised until the tip of the olecranon is visualized.

The elbow can be extended to bring the tip of the olecranon into better view. Osteophytes on the tip of the olecranon can be visualized and resected with the shaver or high-speed burr. Loose bodies can be skewered with a spinal needle until they are secured with a grasper. Next the medial and lateral gutters are inspected. Small loose bodies can often be identified in the gutters. The elbow is extended and held in approximately 45 degrees of flexion. This relaxes the triceps and posterior capsule and allows the arthroscope to maneuver medial to the tip of the olecranon and into the medial gutter. The posterior capsule is inspected and loose bodies identified. Loose bodies can be removed with a grasper or motorized shaver. It is critical not to use suction while the shaver is running in the posteromedial gutter. The use of suction in the medial gutter can inadvertently pull the posteromedial capsule into the shaver and injure the ulnar nerve.

Step 6

Next, the arthroscope is advanced lateral to the tip of the olecranon and down the lateral gutter. The lateral gutter is a favorite hiding place for loose bodies. The scope can be advanced down the lateral gutter to the level of the posterior radiocapitellar joint. The forearm can be pronated and supinated to bring the posterior radial head into view. If loose bodies or chondral flaps are identified in the posterior radiocapitellar joint, a posterior soft spot portal can be established with a spinal needle and outside-in technique. In some cases, a lateral plica may obscure the view of the radial head and may be excised with the shaver. Switching to a 70-degree arthroscope may allow better visualization, especially for OCD lesions in the posterior capitellum in adolescent patients.

Following a standard protocol for diagnostic elbow arthroscopy permits full visualization and evaluation of the entire joint. All important anatomic structures can be critically assessed and the operative plan can be adjusted for arthroscopic findings. The tourniquet is deflated. Portals are closed with interrupted nylon sutures. A sterile dressing is applied that allows full ROM in flexion/extension and pronation/supination.

Postoperative Protocol

The patient is typically seen back in the office 5 to 7 days postoperatively. The wound is assessed and the sutures are removed. The first goal in the postoperative period is to obtain full ROM. Loss of terminal extension is a known complication of elbow arthroscopic procedures,[25] and obtaining full terminal extension should be stressed with patients. Patients are discouraged from wearing splints or braces and are encouraged to use the operative extremity immediately after surgery, with pain as their guide to activity limitations. Physical therapy is initiated at the first postoperative visit, with goals of aggressive ROM and edema control. Strengthening is initiated as ROM improves, usually at 4 weeks postoperatively.

Potential Complications

Nerve injury is a potential complication of any elbow arthroscopic procedure. When establishing portals, only incise the skin with the scalpel, and always use a blunt trocar to gain access to the joint. The use of cannulas can help prevent swelling and protect neurovascular structures. Use great caution when working in the posteromedial compartment and medial gutter to avoid injury to the ulnar nerve. Use limited suction on the shaver in the anterior compartment and medial gutter to avoid damage to the capsule and overlying nerves.

Top Technical Pearls for the Procedure

1. Define and mark all surface landmarks, especially the course of the ulnar nerve. This helps to identify safe zones for portal placement as the elbow swells and bony landmarks become more difficult to palpate.
2. Always palpate the ulnar nerve during elbow flexion and extension to ensure that the nerve does not subluxate or dislocate with the elbow flexed.
3. Use a spinal needle to hold the loose body while grasping it for removal.
4. Carefully evaluate the posterolateral gutter and the ulnohumeral articulation adjacent to the radial head as this is a common area for mobile loose bodies to be found.
5. Use limited suction when running the shaver in the anterior compartment and medial gutter to limit injury to the capsule and overlying neurovascular structures.

References

1. O'Driscoll SW. Elbow arthroscopy for loose bodies. *Orthopedics*. 1992;15(7):855-859.
2. Andrews JR, Baumgarten TE. Arthroscopic anatomy of the elbow. *Orthop Clin North Am*. 1995;26(4):671-677.
3. Byrd JW. Elbow arthroscopy for arthrofibrosis after type I radial head fractures. *Arthroscopy*. 1994;10(2):162-165.
4. Jones GS, Savoie FH III. Arthroscopic capsular release of flexion contractures (arthrofibrosis) of the elbow. *Arthroscopy*. 1993;9(3):277-283.
5. Baker CL Jr, Murphy KP, Gottlob CA, Curd DT. Arthroscopic classification and treatment of lateral epicondylitis: two-year clinical results. *J Shoulder Elbow Surg*. 2000;9(6):475-482.
6. Baker CL Jr, Baker CL III. Long-term follow-up of arthroscopic treatment of lateral epicondylitis. *Am J Sports Med*. 2008;36(2):254-260.
7. Baumgarten TE, Andrews JR, Satterwhite YE. The arthroscopic classification and treatment of osteochondritis dissecans of the capitellum. *Am J Sports Med*. 1998;26(4):520-523.
8. Ruch DS, Cory JW, Poehling GG. The arthroscopic management of osteochondritis dissecans of the adolescent elbow. *Arthroscopy*. 1998;14(8):797-803.
9. O'Driscoll SW. Arthroscopic treatment for osteoarthritis of the elbow. *Orthop Clin North Am*. 1995;26(4):691-706.
10. Ogilvie-Harris DJ, Gordon R, MacKay M. Arthroscopic treatment for posterior impingement in degenerative arthritis of the elbow. *Arthroscopy*. 1995;11(4):437-443.
11. Menth-Chiari WA, Poehling GG, Ruch DS. Arthroscopic resection of the radial head. *Arthroscopy*. 1999;15(2):226-230.
12. Clarke RP. Symptomatic, lateral synovial fringe (plica) of the elbow joint. *Arthroscopy*. 1988;4(2):112-116.
13. Ruch DS, Papadonikolakis A, Campolattaro RM. The posterolateral plica: a cause of refractory lateral elbow pain. *J Shoulder Elbow Surg*. 2006;15(3):367-370.
14. Thomas MA, Fast A, Shapiro D. Radial nerve damage as a complication of elbow arthroscopy. *Clin Orthop Relat Res*. 1987;(215):130-131.
15. Kim SJ, Kim HK, Lee JW. Arthroscopy for limitation of motion of the elbow. *Arthroscopy*. 1995;11(6):680-683.
16. Phillips BB, Strasburger S. Arthroscopic treatment of arthrofibrosis of the elbow joint. *Arthroscopy*. 1998;14(1):38-44.
17. Hardy P, Menguy F, Guillot S. Arthroscopic treatment of capitellum fracture of the humerus. *Arthroscopy*. 2002;18(4):422-426.
18. Holt MS, Savoie FH III, Field LD, Ramsey JR. Arthroscopic management of elbow trauma. *Hand Clin*. 2004;20(4):485-495.
19. Rolla PR, Surace MF, Bini A, Pilato G. Arthroscopic treatment of fractures of the radial head. *Arthroscopy*. 2006;22(2):233.e1-233.e6.
20. Savoie FH III, Field LD, Gurley DJ. Arthroscopic and open radial ulnohumeral ligament reconstruction for posterolateral rotatory instability of the elbow. *Hand Clin*. 2009;25(3):323-329.
21. O'Brien MJ, Lee Murphy R, Savoie FH III. A preliminary report of acute and subacute arthroscopic repair of the radial ulnohumeral ligament after elbow dislocation in the high-demand patient. *Arthroscopy*. 2014;30(6):679-687.
22. Kovachevich R, Steinmann SP. Arthroscopic ulnar nerve decompression in the setting of elbow osteoarthritis. *J Hand Surg Am*. 2012;37(4):663-668.
23. Savoie FH III, Nunley PD, Field LD. Arthroscopic management of the arthritic elbow: indications, technique, and results. *J Shoulder Elbow Surg*. 1999;8(3):214-219.
24. O'Driscoll SW, Lawton RL, Smith AM. The "moving valgus stress test" for medial collateral ligament tears of the elbow. *Am J Sports Med*. 2005;33(2):231-239.
25. Anakwe RE, Middleton SD, Jenkins PJ, McQueen MM, Court-Brown CM. Patient-reported outcomes after simple dislocation of the elbow. *J Bone Joint Surg Am*. 2011;93(13):1220-1226.

3

Lateral Epicondylitis
Debridement, Repair, and Evaluation of Associated Pathology

Champ L. Baker III, MD; Bikramjit S. Grewal, MD; and Champ L. Baker Jr, MD

Introduction

Clinical outcomes of arthroscopic treatment of lateral epicondylitis have been reported,[1-11] and the authors of this chapter found high rates of clinical success in their patients with lateral epicondylitis treated arthroscopically using the technique described here.[3,4]

Anatomy and Pathoanatomy

Nirschl and Pettrone[12,13] detailed the most commonly accepted theory of the pathogenesis of lateral epicondylitis. Building on the previous findings of Cyriax,[14] Goldie,[15] and Coonrad and Hooper,[16] Nirschl[13] noted the basic underlying lesion is in the origin of the extensor carpi radialis brevis (ECRB) tendon. Repetitive overuse leads to microtears in the ECRB origin. Subsequent tendinous nonrepair and replacement with immature reparative tissue follows. Histopathology reveals an absence of inflammatory cells and the presence of a degenerative process with tissue characterized as angiofibroblastic hyperplasia, later modified to angiofibroblastic tendinosis.[12,13,17,18]

In a cadaveric study, Cohen et al[19] characterized the ECRB origin as diamond shaped and beginning just anterior to the most distal aspect of the lateral supracondylar ridge. The anatomical ECRB footprint is located between the most proximal aspect of the capitellum and the midline of the radiocapitellar joint. The lateral collateral ligamentous complex, consisting of the radial collateral ligament, annular ligament, accessory collateral ligament, and lateral ulnar collateral ligament, lies posterior to the ECRB origin. This lateral collateral ligamentous complex is not disrupted during arthroscopy as long as resection of the ECRB and elbow capsule is kept anterior to a line bisecting the radial head.[20]

Savoie FH III, Field LD, Steinmann SP, eds. *The Elbow and Wrist: AANA Advanced Arthroscopic Surgical Techniques* (pp 31-38).

Indications

Indications for surgical intervention for lateral epicondylitis include persistent, disabling symptoms despite an appropriate course of nonoperative management.

Contraindications

Relative contraindications to the arthroscopic technique include the following:

- Previous medial elbow surgery with an ulnar nerve transposition
- The presence of a subluxating ulnar nerve. (In these instances, the ulnar nerve should be exposed and protected before the creation of the proximal medial portal to prevent iatrogenic injury.)

An absolute contraindication is the presence of an active infection.

Pertinent Physical Findings

- Tenderness to palpation, anterior and distal to lateral epicondyle
- Lateral elbow pain with grip or handshake
- Pain resisted wrist extension
- Must evaluate cervical spine for cervical radiculopathy

Pertinent Imaging

- Plain anteroposterior, lateral, and axial x rays
- X-rays may show soft tissue calcification adjacent to lateral epicondyle in 25% of cases
- MRI can provide additional information regarding intra-articular pathology, integrity of lateral ligamentous complex, and the presence and extent of extensor tendon tearing.[21]

Equipment

- Arm holder, compressive dressing, marking pen
- 30-degree arthroscope (70-degree arthroscope is optional equipment)
- Soft tissue resector
- Gravity only for joint distention (no pressurized infusion)
- Spinal needle
- Knife
- Hemostat
- Radiofrequency probe
- Trocar and cannula
- Nonabsorbable sutures (to close the portals)

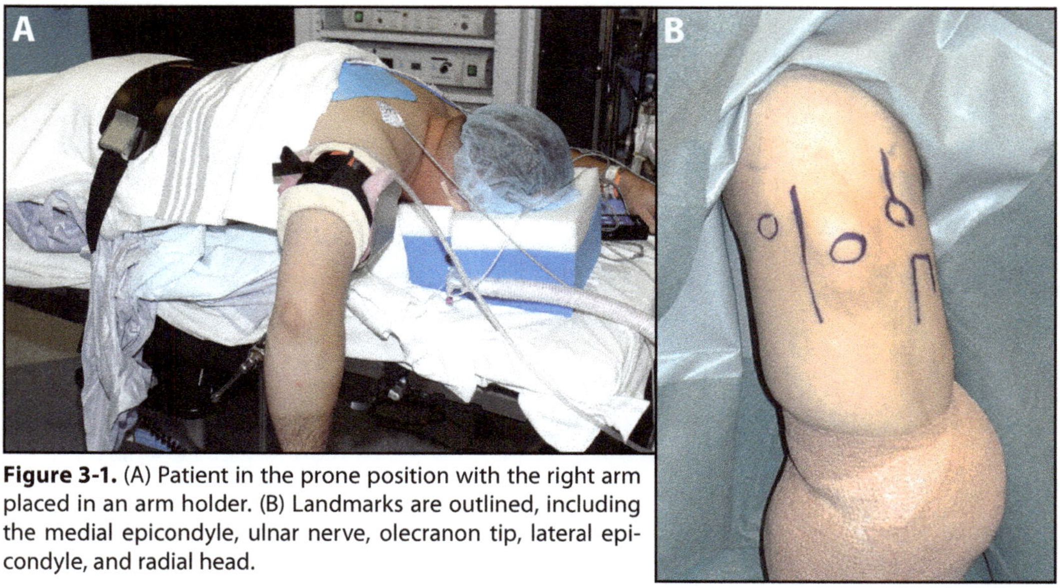

Figure 3-1. (A) Patient in the prone position with the right arm placed in an arm holder. (B) Landmarks are outlined, including the medial epicondyle, ulnar nerve, olecranon tip, lateral epicondyle, and radial head.

Positioning and Portals

The patient can be placed in the supine, lateral decubitus, or prone position. The authors prefer the prone position with the use of a general anesthetic to allow for an accurate postoperative neurovascular assessment. A well-padded tourniquet is applied to the upper arm, which is then placed into a commercially available arm holder. The extremity is then prepared and draped in standard fashion. A compressive dressing is wrapped around the forearm to help prevent leakage of fluid into the distal soft tissues. The following bony anatomic landmarks and important structures are outlined with a marking pen to assist in proper portal creation: medial and lateral epicondyles, radial head, olecranon tip, and ulnar nerve (Figure 3-1).

Step-by-Step Description of the Procedure

The limb is exsanguinated and the tourniquet is inflated to 250 mm Hg. An 18-gauge spinal needle is introduced into the lateral soft spot, which can be found in the center of a triangle formed by the palpable radial head, lateral epicondyle, and olecranon. Approximately 20 to 30 mL of saline are injected into the joint. Joint distention pushes the neurovascular structures more anterior, thereby protecting them from iatrogenic injury. Next, the proximal medial portal is created approximately 2 cm proximal to the medial epicondyle and 1 cm anterior to the medial intermuscular septum (Figure 3-2). To protect against injury to the sensory nerves, the authors use a nick-and-spread technique in which only the skin is incised and a hemostat is used to spread the subcutaneous tissues. Stothers et al[22] found the proximal medial portal to be, on average, 2.3 mm away from the medial antebrachial cutaneous nerve, 7.6 mm away from the median nerve, and 18 mm away from the brachial artery with the elbow in flexion. The ulnar nerve is typically located 12 mm from this portal and lies anterior to and is protected by the medial intermuscular septum. A blunt trocar is inserted through the portal. The surgeon should aim toward the center of the joint and maintain contact with the anterior surface of the humerus. Backflow of fluid through the cannula confirms entry into the joint.

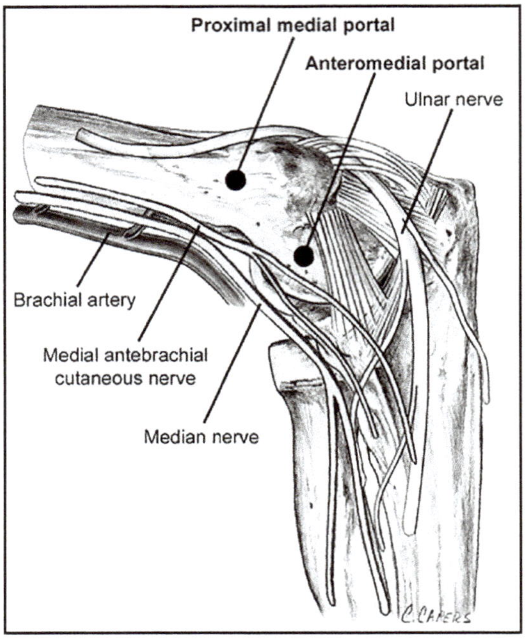

Figure 3-2. Relationship of the proximal medial portal to the surrounding neurovascular structures.

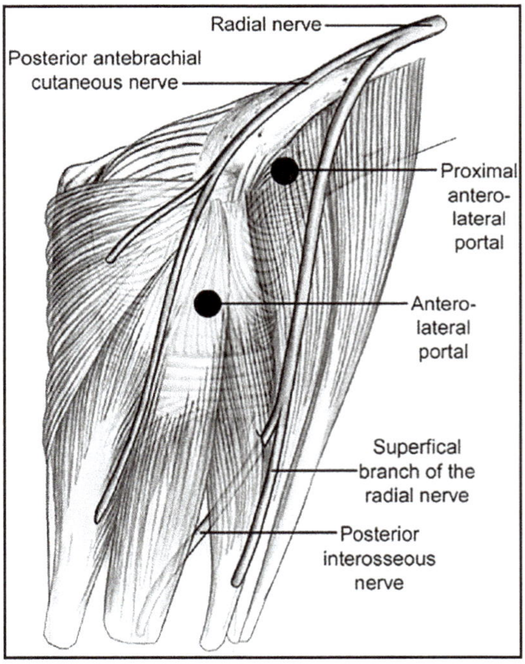

Figure 3-3. Relationship of the proximal lateral portal to the surrounding neurovascular structures.

Next, the 4-mm, 30-degree arthroscope is inserted into the joint. The lateral capsule and radiocapitellar articulation are easily inspected. Irregular extension of the annular ligament overlying the radial head, or synovial fringe, can be appreciated, if present. The authors believe that this structure can be a source of lateral elbow symptoms often mimicking lateral epicondylitis and should be removed concomitant with the ECRB resection.[8] The proximal lateral portal is typically located 1 to 2 cm proximal to the lateral epicondyle along the anterior humeral surface (Figure 3-3). This portal is then established after needle localization using an outside-in technique (Figure 3-4). Stothers et al[22] found the radial nerve to be 9.9 mm away from this portal and the

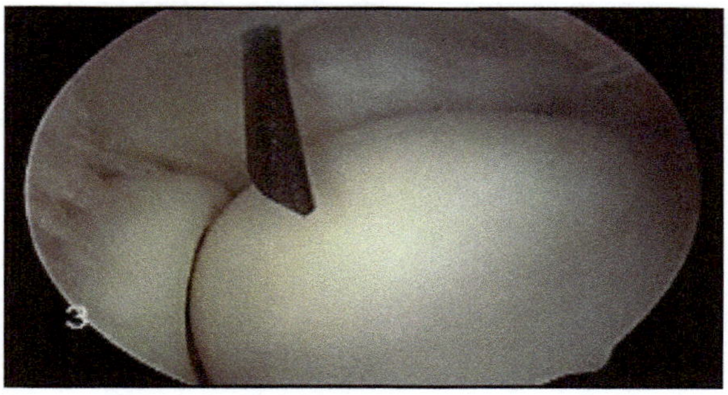

Figure 3-4. The proximal lateral portal is created with an outside-in technique for correct portal localization.

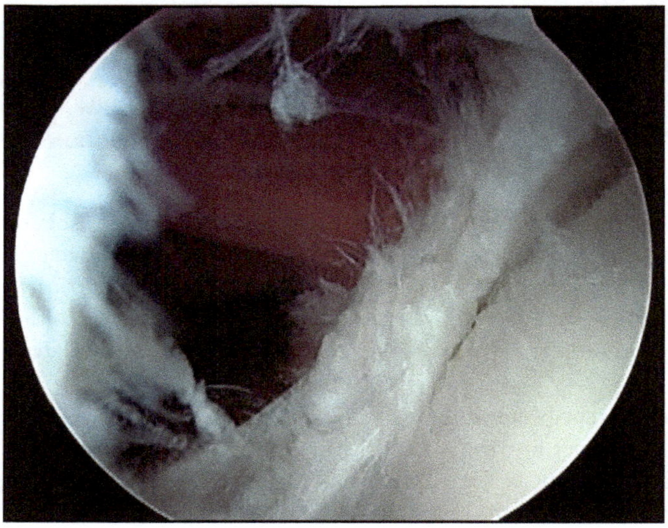

Figure 3-5. A portion of the lateral capsule is removed to reveal the underlying ECRB tendon.

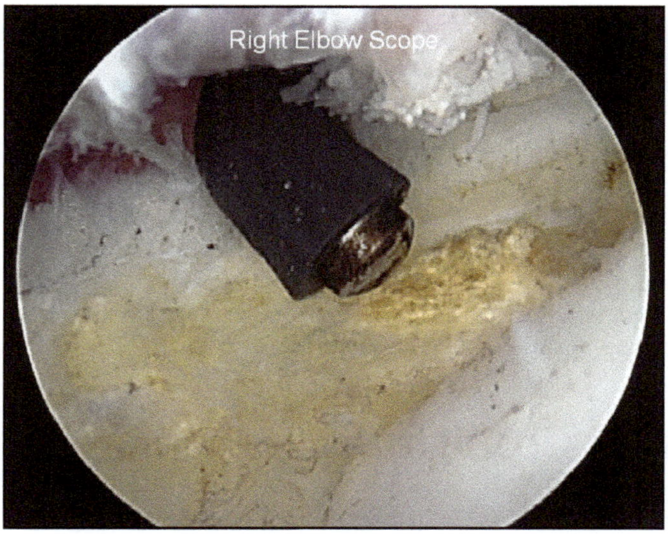

Figure 3-6. A radiofrequency device is used to resect the ECRB origin from its insertion.

posterior branch of the antebrachial cutaneous nerve to be an average of 6.6 mm away from the portal with the elbow flexed. A blunt trocar is used to enter the joint, followed by a small motorized shaver. A portion of the lateral capsule is resected to reveal the underlying common extensor origin (Figure 3-5). The ECRB tendon lies between the common extensor origin and the removed capsule. The shaver is exchanged for a monopolar radiofrequency device (Figure 3-6).

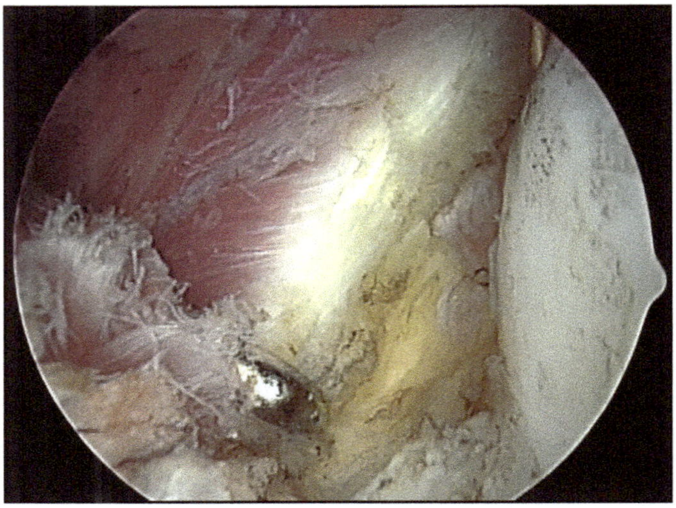

Figure 3-7. Completed resection.

The ECRB origin is then completely released from its insertion and the tendinosis tissue is ablated (Figure 3-7). To protect the lateral ligamentous structures, care is taken not to extend the release posterior to a line bisecting the radial head. Early in the authors' experience, they decorticated the lateral epicondyle; however, several patients developed a postoperative bony tenderness that was not present preoperatively. The authors therefore no longer routinely decorticate the lateral epicondyle.

If the patient has preoperative concurrent posterior or posterolateral pain on terminal elbow extension, the authors then inspect the posterior compartment through the posterior and direct lateral portals. If no such symptoms are present at the preoperative evaluation, they do not routinely examine the posterior compartment. The portal sites are closed with simple nylon sutures, and a sterile dressing is applied.

Postoperative Protocol

All procedures are performed on an outpatient basis. Initially, the arm is placed into a sling for comfort only. The patient is encouraged to begin immediate active and passive range of motion exercises of the elbow. The first postoperative visit is within 7 days of surgery. Sutures are removed at that time. If potential motion loss is a concern or if the patient has difficulty regaining full extension, then formal physical therapy is prescribed. Home exercises, including simple stretching and strengthening, are initiated as patient symptoms allow. Patients typically return to light activities 2 weeks after surgery and to sports approximately 6 weeks postoperatively.

Potential Complications

It is important to identify the presence of a previous ulnar nerve transfer or subluxating ulnar nerve preoperatively to avoid iatrogenic injury to the nerve. The ulnar nerve, median nerve, medial antebrachial nerve, and brachial artery are at risk while establishing the anteromedial portal. The radial nerve is at risk while establishing the anterolateral portal. These can be avoided by using the nick-and-spread method. Intraoperative extravasation of the fluid into the soft tissues can be prevented by using cannulas without sideports. To prevent iatrogenic posterolateral rotatory instability, resection should not extend posterior to a line bisecting the radial head with the elbow in 90 degrees of flexion.

Top Technical Pearls for the Procedure

1. The tourniquet and arm holder should be placed as far proximally as possible to allow easy joint access with instrumentation.
2. The nick-and-spread technique decreases potential injury to the medial sensory nerves during the creation of the proximal medial portal.
3. Annular ligament extension with synovial tissue can become entrapped between the radial head and capitellum and can be a source of lateral elbow pain. It should be excised concurrently with the tendinosis resection.
4. If visualization becomes difficult, a second more proximal lateral portal can be created to insert a retractor.
5. If a concurrent open procedure is planned, a side board can be affixed to the table.

References

1. Szabo SJ, Savoie FH III, Field LD, Ramsey JR, Hosemann CD. Tendinosis of the extensor carpi radialis brevis: an evaluation of three methods of operative treatment. *J Shoulder Elbow Surg.* 2006;15(6):721-727.
2. Peart RE, Strickler SS, Schweitzer KM Jr. Lateral epicondylitis: a comparative study of open and arthroscopic lateral release. *Am J Orthop (Belle Mead NJ).* 2004;33(11):565-567.
3. Baker CL Jr, Murphy KP, Gottlob CA, Curd DT. Arthroscopic classification and treatment of lateral epicondylitis: two-year clinical results. *J Shoulder Elbow Surg.* 2000;9(6):475-482.
4. Baker CL Jr, Baker CL III. Long-term follow-up of arthroscopic treatment of lateral epicondylitis. *Am J Sports Med.* 2008;36(2):254-260.
5. Brooks-Hill AL, Regan RD. Extra-articular arthroscopic lateral elbow release. *Arthroscopy.* 2008;24(4):483-485.
6. Cummins CA. Lateral epicondylitis: in vivo assessment of arthroscopic debridement and correlation with patient outcomes. *Am J Sports Med.* 2006;34(9):1486-1491.
7. Jerosch J, Schunck J. Arthroscopic treatment of lateral epicondylitis: indications, technique and early results. *Knee Surg Sports Traumatol Arthrosc.* 2006;14(4):379-382.
8. Mullett H, Sprague M, Brown G, Hausman M. Arthroscopic treatment of lateral epicondylitis: clinical and cadaveric studies. *Clin Orthop Relat Res.* 2005;(439):123-128.
9. Owens BD, Murphy KP, Kuklo TR. Arthroscopic release for lateral epicondylitis. *Arthroscopy.* 2001;17(6):582-587.
10. Romeo AA, Fox JA. Arthroscopic treatment of lateral epicondylitis: the 4-step technique. *Orthop Tech Review.* 2002;4:206.
11. Sennoune B, Costa V, Dumontier C. Arthroscopic treatment of tennis elbow: preliminary experience with 14 patients [in French]. *Rev Chir Orthop Reparatric Appar Mot.* 2005;91(2):158-164.
12. Nirschl RP, Pettrone FA. Tennis elbow: the surgical treatment of lateral epicondylitis. *J Bone Joint Surg Am.* 1979;61(6):832-839.
13. Nirschl RP. Elbow tendinosis/tennis elbow. *Clin Sports Med.* 1992;11(4):851-870.
14. Cyriax JH. The pathology and treatment of tennis elbow. *J Bone Joint Surg Am.* 1936;18:921-940.
15. Goldie I. Epicondylitis lateralis humeri (epicondylalgia or tennis elbow). A pathogenetical study. *Acta Chir Scand Suppl.* 1964;57(suppl 339):1+.
16. Coonrad RW, Hooper WR. Tennis elbow: its course, natural history, conservative and surgical management. *J Bone Joint Surg Am.* 1973;55(6):1177-1182.

17. Kraushaar BS, Nirschl RP. Tendinosis of the elbow (tennis elbow). Clinical features and findings of histological, immunohistochemical, and electron microscopy studies. *J Bone Joint Surg Am.* 1999;81(2):259-278.
18. Regan W, Wold LE, Coonrad R, Morrey BF. Microscopic histopathology of chronic refractory lateral epicondylitis. *Am J Sports Med.* 1992;20(6):746-749.
19. Cohen MS, Romeo AA, Hennigan SP, Gordon M. Lateral epicondylitis: anatomic relationships of the extensor tendon origins and implications for arthroscopic treatment. *J Shoulder Elbow Surg.* 2008;17(6):954-960.
20. Smith AM, Castle JA, Ruch DS. Arthroscopic resection of the common extensor origin: anatomic considerations. *J Shoulder Elbow Surg.* 2003;12(4):375-379.
21. Calfee RP, Patel A, DaSilva MF, Akelman E. Management of lateral epicondylitis: current concepts. *J Am Acad Orthop Surg.* 2008;16(1):19-29.
22. Stothers K, Day B, Regan WR. Arthroscopy of the elbow: anatomy, portal sites, and a description of the proximal lateral portal. *Arthroscopy.* 1995;11(4):449-457.

Please see videos on the accompanying website at

www.routledge.com/9781630910013

4

Management of Medial Epicondylitis

Bernard F. Morrey, MD

Introduction

Over the last several years, a number of common features have emerged as trends in the treatment of chronic tendinopathy from a patient and from a physician perspective (Table 4-1). A common feature to these trends is the goal to first more accurately define and isolate the lesion by ultrasound or magnetic resonance imaging (MRI)[1,2] and then to definitively treat the patient earlier in the disease process in a less invasive fashion that is well tolerated with minimal morbidity, few complications, and a high chance of success. The author considers satisfying these goals to be treatment nirvana.

Diagnosis

This is a clinical diagnosis in the author's opinion. Accurate diagnosis is dependent upon a thorough understanding of the anatomic and pathophysiologic factors that can lead to medial epicondylitis and differentiate it from other medial elbow conditions. The diagnosis of medial epicondylitis requires a thorough patient history and detailed physical examination, along with radiographic studies to accurately identify medial epicondylitis and distinguish it from ulnar neuritis and medial collateral ligament injury, all of which can occur concurrently.

Medial epicondylitis is characterized by pain that is usually of insidious onset along the medial elbow that is made worse by resistance to forearm pronation and wrist flexion. Tenderness to palpation usually occurs over the pronator teres and the flexor carpi radialis. The maximum tenderness is usually identified by palpation approximately 5 to 10 mm distal and anterior to the midpoint of the medial epicondyle.

When examining for medial epicondylitis, it is also essential to carefully assess for ulnar neuritis and ulnar collateral ligament (UCL) instability, especially in overhead athletes. These may coexist as a result of the repetitive valgus forces imparted to the medial elbow with throwing. Ulnar neuritis is identified by a positive Tinel's sign, as indicated by local pain and numbness or tingling radiating distally with the direct compression of the ulnar nerve at the elbow. Another test valuable in helping to recognize ulnar neuritis is the elbow flexion test for ulnar neuritis,

Savoie FH III, Field LD, Steinmann SP, eds. *The Elbow and Wrist: AANA Advanced Arthroscopic Surgical Techniques* (pp 39-49).

Table 4-1. Patient and Physician Expectations for Definitive Intervention for Tendinopathy

1	Intervene earlier rather than later
2	Minimal discomfort, well tolerated
3	Rapid recovery, return to normalcy
4	Office based
5	Objective effectiveness data
6	Cost effective
7	Safe

performed by placing the elbow in maximum flexion, the forearm in pronation, and the wrist in extension for approximately 60 seconds. If the patient develops numbness or tingling in the ring and little fingers, the test is considered positive for ulnar neuritis. UCL instability is best identified by performing the valgus stress test with the elbow at 30 degrees of flexion or by using the moving valgus stress test. Both of these cause medial elbow pain at the UCL and often reproduce the symptoms experienced by overhead athletes in the late acceleration phase of throwing.

If soft tissue imaging is felt to be necessary before intervention is offered, the authors favor ultrasound to MRI because it is as reliable and is much more convenient and inexpensive. In recent years, there has been considerable growth and interest in the use of ultrasound image guidance to more accurately direct injections.[3,4] Ultrasound-guided percutaneous tenotomy was described as early as 1999 for the treatment of patellar tendinopathy,[5,6] and the utility of ultrasound-guided percutaneous tenotomy with a needle or knife blade has been subsequently documented.[7,8]

Arthroscopic Treatment

Because of the presence of the ulnar nerve, the most experienced elbow arthroscopists feel that arthroscopic treatment of medial epicondylitis is probably not indicated (Baker, O'Driscoll, oral communication, 2014). Hence, the definitive treatment of chronic refractory medial epicondylitis remains open debridement or, more recently, percutaneous ultrasonic tenotomy.

Open Treatment

In contrast to lateral involvement, there is relatively little information regarding surgical debridement and excision for medial epicondyle tendinopathy. What is known is the poorer prognosis associated with concurrent ulnar nerve symptoms and poorer results than is the case with lateral epicondyle involvement.[9]

Percutaneous Ultrasonic Tenotomy: Rationale

Cataract Management

The successful introduction of ultrasound as a treatment for cataracts—phacoemulsification—has revolutionized the management of this condition.[10] Referable to tendinopathy, this concept has been extrapolated to result in a novel technology that delivers focused ultrasound energy specifically designed to cut, debride, and remove diseased tendon tissue. In this sense, it has features that characterize open or arthroscopic surgical procedures. It is felt that the pain evoked by the necrotic tendon is mediated by cytokines, which are removed by the process. Hence, some improvement in pain is recognized immediately by cutting and removing the necrotic tissue. In addition, it is hypothesized that with subsequent support in animal experiments, the anatomic void created by the ultrasonic treatment allows a more normal and rapid healing response.[11]

Indications

- The indications for definitive treatment of this disease are that of chronic involvement that has been refractory to nonoperative management and is having a major impact on the individual's ability to work or conduct daily activities.
- When the process is more of a nuisance or one that the patient can tolerate, the intervention is deferred.

Pertinent Physical Findings

- Tenderness to palpation adjacent and immediately distal to the medial epicondyle is consistently demonstrated.
- Medial elbow discomfort is often worsened by resistance to forearm pronation and wrist flexion.
- Local swelling and warmth may be present in very symptomatic cases.
- Careful assessment is required to identify and distinguish symptoms related to UCL damage and ulnar neuritis from those symptoms attributable to medial epicondylitis.

Pertinent Imaging

- Standard anteroposterior and lateral x-rays should be obtained in patients with symptoms compatible with medial epicondylitis, although these x-rays are not diagnostic. Calcifications adjacent to the medial epicondyle, suggestive of medial epicondylitis, may occasionally be visualized.
- MRI can more accurately identify the location and extent of the pathologic tissue but is not routinely obtained in patients with suspected medial epicondylitis in whom no other significant pathologic conditions are anticipated.
- Ultrasound can reliably identify the location and extent of medial epicondylar tissue disease and is much more convenient and inexpensive compared to MRI.

Equipment for the Open Medial Epicondylitis Release Technique

- A straightforward open surgical approach is carried out for open medial epicondylitis release and requires only standard surgical equipment.
- A rongeur may be valuable to debride the affected tissue, and a drill with small drill bits may be helpful in stimulating the medial epicondyle bone prior to reapproximation of the soft tissues.

Step-by-Step Description of the Open Medial Epicondylitis Release Technique

Nonsurgical management is the standard of care for medial epicondylitis after the diagnosis is confirmed. The goal of such conservative care is to eliminate symptoms, allowing patients to return to their preinjury levels of function. Although this treatment has been described as successful, there remains little information concerning the long-term outcome of nonsurgical treatment. The available literature suggests that between 5% and 15% of patients suffer recurrent symptoms.[12] In a prospective review of the nonoperative treatment, Binder and Hazleman[13] reported that 26% of patients experience a recurrence of symptoms, and over 40% had prolonged minor discomfort. Thus, the previously reported success rates for nonoperative management may be less successful than commonly quoted. Nonetheless, nonsurgical treatment remains the mainstay of treatment for medial epicondylitis.

For patients failing to respond to an organized and compliant nonoperative treatment program for 3 to 6 months and in whom all other causes for their symptoms has been eliminated, surgical treatment is recommended. Currently, the standard and most commonly performed surgical intervention consists of excision of the pathologic portion of the tendon, enhancement of local vascularity to stimulate a healing response, reapproximation of any elevated tendon back to the epicondylar origin, and repair of the resultant defect.

With the patient in the supine position, the arm is placed on an arm board and a tourniquet is applied. After exsanguination of the arm and elevation of the tourniquet, a 5-cm oblique incision is then made just anterior to the medial epicondyle. The surgeon must take care to identify the medial antebrachial cutaneous nerve within the subcutaneous tissues during the surgical approach. The common flexor-pronator origin is identified, along with the ulnar nerve, which is palpated within the ulnar groove. A longitudinal split in the fascia and excision of any identified abnormal flexor-pronator tendinous tissue is performed. Preparation of the medial epicondyle origin for reattachment of the common flexor-pronator tissue often includes rongeuring any fibrous tissue followed by drilling multiple small holes in the surface to create a sufficient vascular bed. The released flexor-pronator tendon is then reattached to healthy, attached adjacent flexor-pronator tissue using absorbable interrupted sutures, thus reapproximating this tissue to the bleeding surface. Alternatively, drill holes placed through the medial epicondyle (or a suture anchor) can be used to reattach flexor-pronator tissue. Finally, routine subcutaneous and skin closures are performed and a soft compressive dressing or a posterior plaster splint is then applied to the elbow and wrist.

Postoperative Protocol Following Open Medial Epicondylitis Release

At approximately 1 week postoperatively, the splint and skin sutures are removed. At this point, gentle passive and active hand, wrist, and elbow exercises are begun. Gentle isometrics are undertaken at 3 weeks postoperatively, with more rigorous, resistive exercise, including wrist flexion and forearm pronation, beginning at 6 weeks. A progressive strengthening program follows, with patients allowed to return to normal activities by 3 to 6 months postoperatively.

Surgical Results

Vangsness and Jobe[14] evaluated 35 patients with medial epicondylitis unresponsive to nonoperative treatment who underwent surgical treatment with a standard technique using the aforementioned surgical principles. After 6 years of follow-up, they reported 88% good-to-excellent results. Fourteen percent of their patients also had ulnar nerve submuscular transposition. Nineteen of 20 athletes returned to their previous level of sport. Gabel and Morrey[9] reviewed their results in 26 patients (30 elbows) using several different surgical techniques to manage medial epicondylitis, including partial and complete elevation of the flexor-pronator mass with or without complete reattachment. After an average follow-up of 7 years, they reported 87% good-to-excellent results. Despite the limited literature on the surgical treatment of medial epicondylitis, techniques such as these are generally reported to yield reliable pain relief and relatively high patient satisfaction.

Potential Complications Following Open Medial Epicondylitis Release

- The UCL can be inadvertently damaged (causing medial elbow instability) during flexor-pronator debridement. A detailed knowledge of the ligamentous anatomy is important in preventing iatrogenic injury to this ligament.
- The ulnar nerve courses adjacent to and around the medial epicondyle and is at significant risk of injury during open medial epicondylitis release. Palpation of the nerve and confirmation that it resides in the cubital tunnel and cannot be manually subluxated into the operative field is important prior to beginning the surgical approach.

Top Technical Pearls for the Procedure

1. An adequately sized incision ensures that the entire flexor-pronator tendon can be clearly visualized making appropriate resection of diseased tissue more reliably performed.
2. Thorough debridement of all identified affected tendinous tissue increases the chances of a successful outcome following surgical intervention. However, careful attention should be paid to the anatomy of the origin and course of the UCL in order to protect the ligament during the procedure.
3. Following resection of the flexor-pronator tissue, stimulation of the bony origin of the tendon at the medial epicondyle should be accomplished using a curette or drill bits to encourage healing.
4. Securely reapproximating the tendon using sutures, drill holes, or anchors likely improves the chances that uneventful healing will occur postoperatively.
5. Confirmation of the location and stability of the ulnar nerve at the beginning of the surgical approach protects the nerve from inadvertent injury.

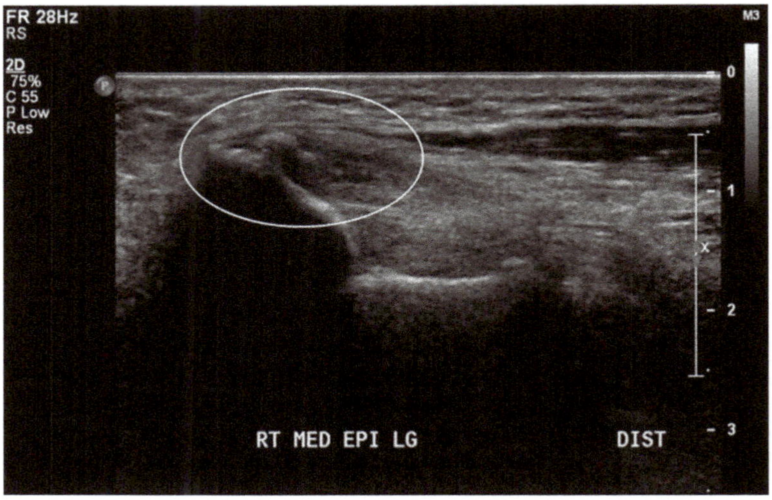

Figure 4-1. Typical ultrasonic image of medial epicondylitis revealing the hypoechoic area at the site of tendinous attachment with calcification. This degree of pathology is not always observed.

Equipment for the Ultrasonic-Guided Percutaneous Tenotomy Technique

Facility

Ultrasonic-guided percutaneous tenotomy with the TX1 device (Tenex Health) may be performed in a clinical or ambulatory surgical center.

Ultrasound Confirmation of the Lesion

The pathology of a diseased tendon has been well characterized as loss of contour and the presence of edema, often with a hypoechoic area that is felt to represent the degenerative portion of the process. Blinded studies using ultrasound have revealed a sensitivity of 90%, specificity of 89%, and diagnostic accuracy of 94%.[15] Extensive experience with ultrasound as a diagnostic tool is not required. The ability to visualize the medial epicondyle is straightforward. The normal tendon appears more homogenous and more uniform in appearance by ultrasound image. Tendinopathy exhibits a hypoechoic image, which appears as a black defect in the tendon; in some instances, calcific deposits confirm the site of pathology (Figure 4-1).

Positioning and Portals for the Ultrasonic-Guided Percutaneous Tenotomy Technique

The elbow is examined to determine the stability of the ulnar nerve in its groove. The patient lies on the involved side with the medial elbow resting on the table. If the ulnar nerve does not sublux, the elbow is treated in 90 degrees of flexion. If there is a tendency toward subluxation of the nerve, the treatment is carried out with the arm in extension (Figure 4-2).

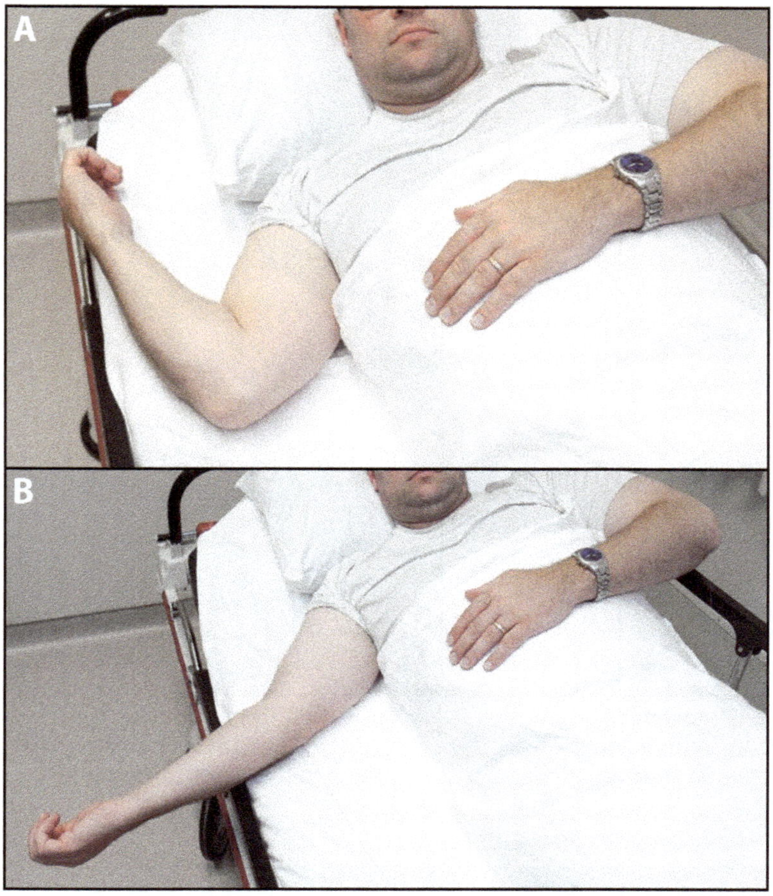

Figure 4-2. (A) Ideally, the patient rests on the involved side with the elbow flexed. (B) If the ulnar nerve has a tendency to sublux during flexion, the elbow is treated in extension.

Reassessment and Examination

The site of maximum tenderness is identified by the patient and confirmed by the physician. An ultrasonic examination of the medial or lateral elbow is performed and the point of maximum tenderness is marked and assessed referable to the ultrasonic image (Figure 4-3). In patients who do not have the hypoechoic area, calcification and irregularity of the cortical surface of the epicondyle is usually present.[16] If there is any question regarding the status of the ulnar nerve, it may readily be visualized to assure it is safely out of the field of treatment.

Prep and Drape

The area is prepped as if an injection is to be performed. The epicondyle is squared off with sterile towels. The sensor is then placed in a sterile sleeve (Figure 4-4). It is important to place a thin layer of gel over the sensor prior to placing it in the sterile sleeve. The area of maximum tenderness is again confirmed. A fast-acting local anesthetic is used to create a skin wheal approximately 1.5 cm from the point of maximum tenderness. The needle is then advanced through the skin wheal to the precise area of maximum tenderness, which corresponds to the hypoechoic region. The ultrasonic sensor may or may not be used to guide the injection. Approximately 2 to 4 cc of a fast-acting local anesthetic are injected into the region. The needle is used to tap the epicondyle to assure that this area is also insensate during the procedure. The local anesthetic does not typically interfere with the ultrasonic image.

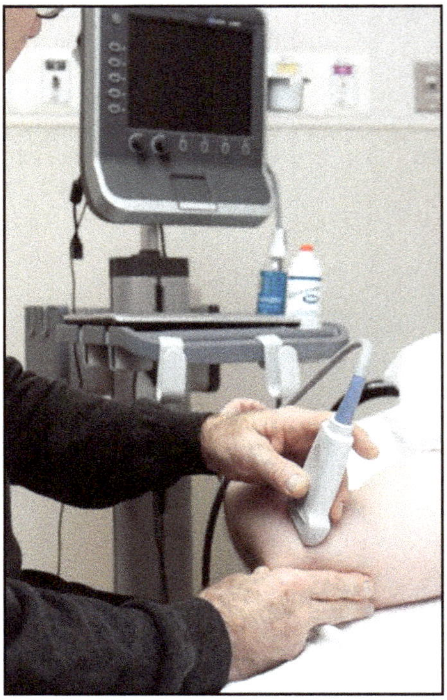

Figure 4-3. The pathology is identified by palpation and confirmed by ultrasonic assessment prior to the procedure.

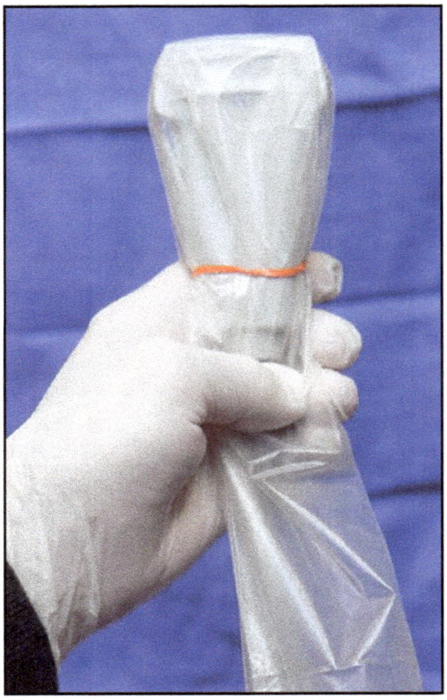

Figure 4-4. After the elbow has been prepped and draped as if for a steroid injection, the ultrasonic sensor is placed in a sterile sleeve.

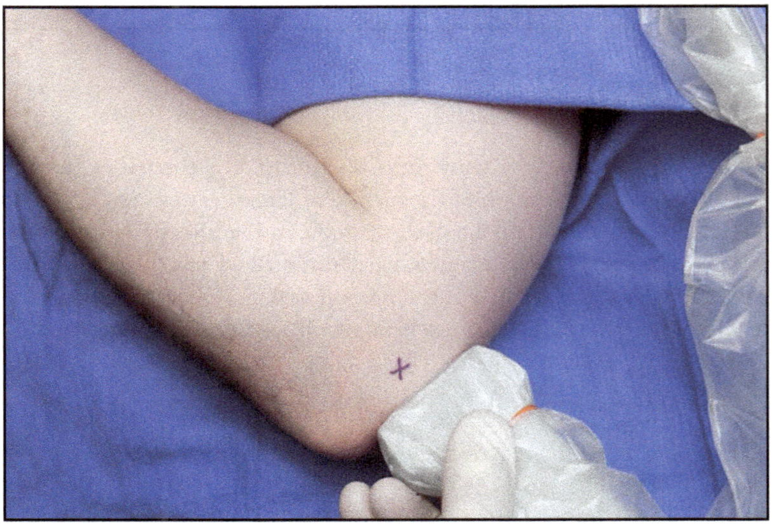

Figure 4-5. The site of maximum tenderness is marked and the pathology is again confirmed.

Insertion of the Ultrasonic Instrument

A #11 blade knife is used to create a puncture site through the skin wheal about 1.5 cm distal to the site of maximum tenderness (Figure 4-5). The blade continues through the subcutaneous tissue and incises the fascia. This facilitates the entry of the probe to the site of disease. The ultrasonic probe, which is the size of a 16-gauge needle, is then introduced through the puncture site and, under ultrasonic guidance, the probe is introduced into the hypoechoic region (Figure 4-6).

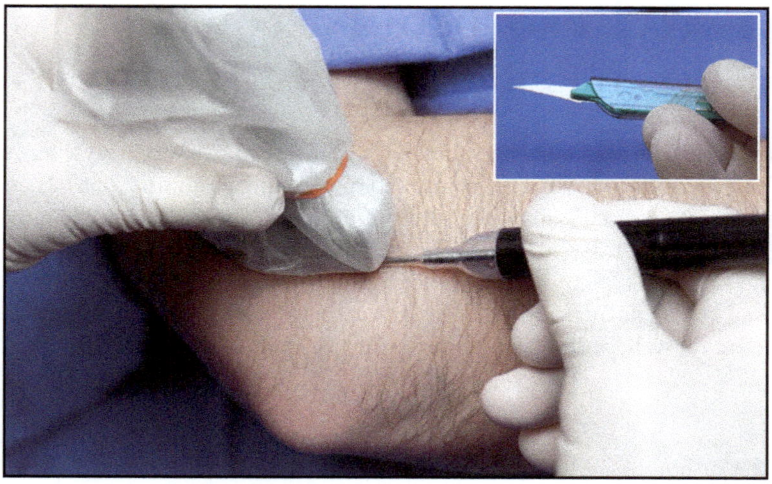

Figure 4-6. After the area has been anesthetized, a #11 blade knife punctures the skin and the fascia, and the ultrasonic probe is introduced into the site of pathology under ultrasound visualization.

Step-by-Step Description of the Ultrasonic-Guided Percutaneous Tenotomy Technique

Technical tips following the ultrasonic-guided percutaneous tenotomy technique are as follows:

1. Assure that the ulnar nerve does not sublux anteriorly during elbow flexion. If this occurs, the procedure should be performed with the elbow in extension.
2. The clinician confirms and marks the site of maximum tenderness.
3. Confirm the pathology with a diagnostic ultrasound.
4. When anesthetizing the area, include the attachment of the diseased tendon to the epicondyle when anesthetizing the area.
5. Be sure not to initiate the puncture site too distal to the site of pathology (the current probe is 1.3 inches in length).
6. Typically, 60 to 90 seconds of activation is adequate to treat most pathologic conditions.

Treatment of the Pathology

Once the pathologic area is identified, the ultrasonic energy to the TX1 handpiece is activated with a foot pedal. An auditory signal is emitted, which indicates that the ultrasonic energy is being expended. Irrigation flows during the ultrasonic activation concurrent with aspiration of the tenotomized diseased tendon tissue.

If the irrigation ceases or the aspiration becomes clogged, the energy is automatically discontinued until the irrigation resumes. This usually takes 1 to 2 seconds.

The probe is moved in a linear fashion in and out of the lesion. In doing so, the hypoechoic region is visually altered, indicating that the lesion has been treated. The probe typically is tapped against the osseous attachment at the site of the necrotic process. In most instances, 60 to 100 seconds of ultrasonic energy is adequate to appropriately treat the lesion.

Dressing

The wound is closed with a Steri-Strip (3M) and covered with an occlusive dressing. The authors prefer a compressive stockinette for added comfort. The dressing is removed in 2 days and the Steri-Strip is removed in 5 to 7 days.

Postoperative Protocol Following Ultrasonic-Guided Percutaneous Tenotomy

The patient is advised to use the elbow in a very minimal fashion for the next 1 to 2 days. Ice is recommended the night of surgery and pain is usually controlled by Tylenol (acetaminophen). If on the third day the patient is having minimal symptoms, resumption of routine, normal, sedentary daily activities is allowed. If after 14 to 21 days the symptoms remain resolved or very minimal, the patient may gradually resume a normal type of activity. After 5 to 6 weeks, if the patient continues to be markedly improved, then a more normal type of daily activity may be introduced. If after this period the patients continues to do well, resumption of normal activities is allowed as tolerated.

Surgical Results

A formal assessment of the author's results has not yet been performed. No patient has requested additional treatment. In a recent report, Barnes et al[17] reported a similar success rate of greater than 80%, which is similar to the author's experience.

Potential Complications Following Ultrasonic-Guided Percutaneous Tenotomy

There have been no complications in the author's experience after approximately 35 procedures. No complications have been reported to the company after more than 1000 procedures.

Top Technical Pearls for the Procedure

1. Mark the point of maximum tenderness at flexion angle of treatment.
2. Avoid the puncture site being too distal.
3. Incise skin and fascia.
4. Probe back and forth in about 5 mm of motion.
5. Calcification need not be removed.

References

1. Miller TT, Shapiro MA, Schultz E, Kalish PE. Comparison of sonography and MRI for diagnosing epicondylitis. *J Clin Ultrasound*. 2002;30(4):193-202.
2. Poltawski L, Ali S, Jayaram V, Watson T. Reliability of sonographic assessment of tendinopathy in tennis elbow. *Skeletal Radiol*. 2012;41(1):83-89.
3. Blankstein A. Ultrasound in the diagnosis of clinical orthopedics: the orthopedic stethoscope. *World J Orthop*. 2011;18(2):13-24.
4. Patil P, Dasgupta B. Role of diagnostic ultrasound in the assessment of musculoskeletal diseases. *Ther Adv Musculoskeletal Dis*. 2012;4(5):341-355.

5. Royall NA, Farrin E, Bahner DP, Stawicki SP. Ultrasound-assisted musculoskeletal procedures: a practical overview of current literature. *World J Orthop.* 2011;2(7):57-66.
6. Testa V, Capasso G, Maffulli N, Bifulco G. Ultrasound-guided percutaneous longitudinal tenotomy for the management of patellar tendinopathy. *Med Sci Sports Exerc.* 1999;31(11):1509-1515.
7. Dunkow PD, Jatti M, Muddu BN. A comparison of open and percutaneous techniques in the surgical treatment of tennis elbow. *J Bone Joint Surg Br.* 2004;86(5):701-704.
8. McShane JM, Nazarian LN, Harwood MI. Sonographically guided percutaneous needle tenotomy for treatment of common extensor tendinosis in the elbow. *J Ultrasound Med.* 2006;25(10):1281-1289.
9. Gabel GT, Morrey BF. Operative treatment of medial epicondylitis. Influence of concomitant ulnar neuropathy at the elbow. *J Bone Joint Surg Am.* 1995;77(7):1065-1069.
10. Kelman CD. The history and development of phacoemulsification. *Int Ophthalmol Clin.* 1994;34(2):1-12.
11. Kamineni S, Butterfield T, Sinai A, Butterfield T. *Percutaneous Ultrasounic Debridement for Chronic Achilles Tendinopathy: A Pilot Rabbit Mode.* (Submitted to CORR) 2014.
12. Jobe FW, Ciccotti MG. Lateral and medial epicondylitis of the elbow. *J Am Acad Orthop Surg.* 1994;2(1):1-8.
13. Binder AI, Hazleman BL. Lateral humeral epicondylitis--a study of natural history and the effect of conservative therapy. *Br J Rheumatol.* 1983;22(2):73-76.
14. Vangsness CT Jr, Jobe FW. Surgical technique of medial epicondylitis. Results in 35 elbows. *J Bone Joint Surg Br.* 1991;73(3):409-411.
15. Crass J, Karl R. Bedside drainage of abscesses with sonographic guidance in the desperately ill. *AJR Am J Roentgenol.* 1982;139(1):183-185.
16. Jaén-Díaz JI, Cerezo-López E, López-de Castro F, et al. Sonographic findings for the common extensor tendon of the elbow in the general population. *J Ultrasound Med.* 2010;29(12):1717-1724.
17. Barnes DE, Beckley JM, Smith J. Percutaneous ultrasonic tenotomy for chronic elbow tendinosis: a prospective study. *J Shoulder Elbow Surg.* 2015;24(1):67-73.

Please see videos on the accompanying website at

www.routledge.com/9781630910013

5

Plica Synovialis of the Elbow

Bernard F. Morrey, MD

Introduction

An awareness and documentation of a synovial plica as an anatomic structure dates back at least to 1912 when Testut described the humeral radialis labrum.[1,2] Descriptions of this as a pathologic condition date back to the 1950s.[3-5] Since then, the pathologic condition has been variably described as the lateral synovial fringe,[6] snapping plica,[7] and synovial fold of the humeral radial joint.[1] That the plica could represent a pathologic condition can be traced to individual case reports within the last 30 years with description of symptomatology, clinical presentation, and treatment. The true significance has been dramatically enhanced with the advent of arthroscopy.

Pathoanatomy

Most of the anatomic descriptions of this structure come from the Japanese or French literature.[8-12] A capsular fold has been documented to be present in the embryo and in the adult elbow, thus giving rise to the recognition of this as a normal anatomic structure (Figure 5-1).[13] The pathologic condition occurs with the development of a hard fibrous type of tissue that has a circumferential distribution around the radial head (Figure 5-2). Duparc et al[1] correlated this type of structure with degenerative changes of the radial head. A German investigation recently documented the magnetic resonance image (MRI) to detect the presence of a plica in all 88 specimens examined and classified 31% as small, 57% as medium, and 12% as large. Of interest and consistent with the observations of Duparc et al,[1] they also correlated degenerative changes with the larger plicae.

Clinical Presentation

In the early descriptions, the pain was confused with that of tennis elbow. Some patients have no snapping but have a vague pain that is felt primarily in the region of the lateral epicondyle. It may well have been confusion with this presentation of the lesion that prompted the so-called *Bosworth approach* to tennis elbow.[14] In this procedure, arthrotomy and inspection of the joint

Savoie FH III, Field LD, Steinmann SP, eds. *The Elbow and Wrist: AANA Advanced Arthroscopic Surgical Techniques* (pp 51-57).

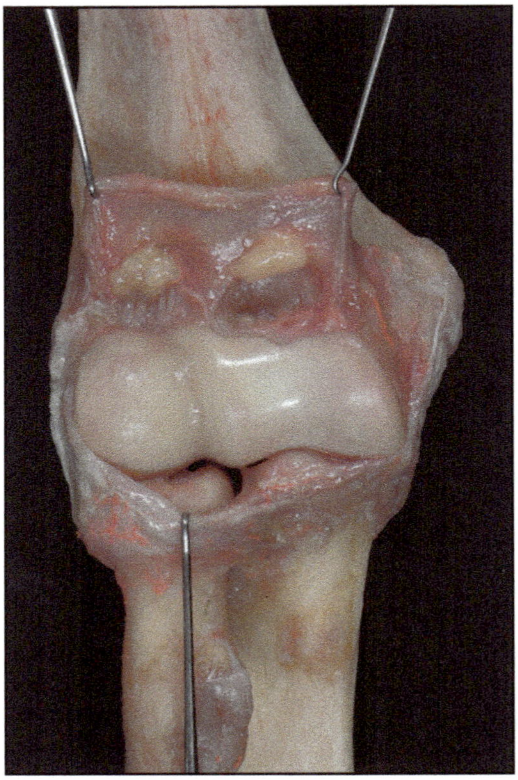

Figure 5-1. The capsule consists of several folds, including one from anterolateral that drapes over the radial head when it becomes thickened as in the pathologic state. Typically, this normal structure does not cause symptoms. (Reprinted with permission from Llusá Pérez M. *Atlas de Disección Anatomoquirúrgica del Codo*. Barcelona, Spain: Elsevier Masson; 2009.)

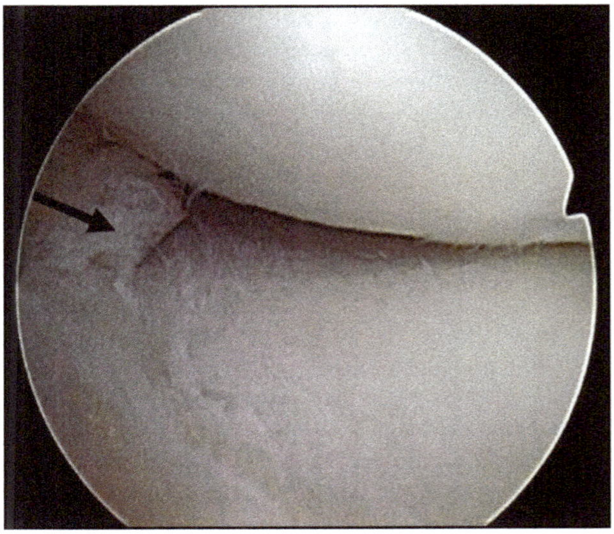

Figure 5-2. A thickened plica is seen draping over the anterolateral margin of the radial head (arrow). The normal plica is thin and filamentous and often translucent in distinction to the pathologic process.

and resection of the annular ligament was recommended as it was felt the annular ligament was associated with lateral elbow pain. Numerous authors have subsequently pointed out the difficulty of differentiating a nonsnapping pathologic plica from lateral epicondylitis.[1,6,15] The diagnosis becomes simpler when the clinical presentation is not so much lateral or posterolateral joint pain, but rather catching, snapping, and locking. Thus, the differential diagnosis may be tennis elbow or loose body depending on the presence or absence of the mechanical features.[6,7,15]

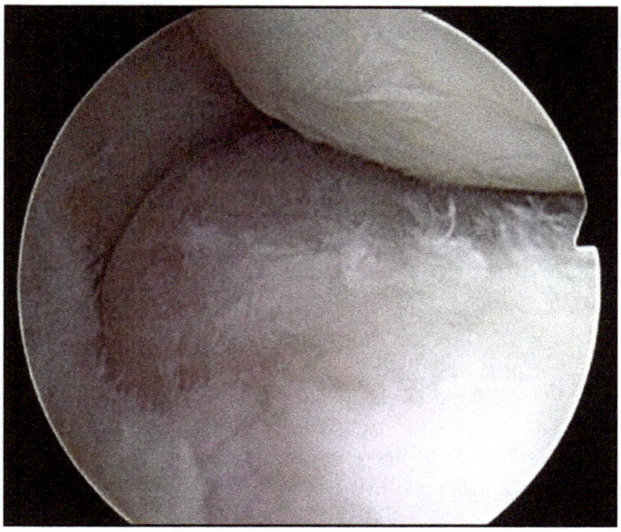

Figure 5-3. After the plica has been resected, the effect of the snapping over the radial head is often visualized and identified as chondromalacia of the involved portion of the head.

Early recognition of the potential pathologic features of this tissue has appeared in the form of case reports.[3,6,8,9,12] The intra-articular fold slips over the radial head in flexion around 90 to 100 degrees and then slides over the radial neck with extension past 90 degrees.[6,7] This translation results in a well-recognized chondromalacia of the margin of the radial head (Figure 5-3). Others have speculated that there is also an association with this lesion and subtle posterolateral rotatory instability.[10,15] As of yet, this relationship has not been confirmed.

Outcome

Several studies have demonstrated experience with relatively large sample sizes of 10 to 14 patients.[7,11,15] These authors universally demonstrate a high likelihood of success with arthroscopic resection, with more than 90% being free of all symptoms with a short postoperative surveillance period. There is minimal postoperative morbidity. However, it should be noted that Antuna and O'Driscoll[7] observed that 2 of 14 patients (15%) had some residual discomfort and 1 patient developed recurrence of the snapping several months after resolution of symptoms following the original procedure. The articular changes that frequently occur at the radial head may develop arthritic symptoms in the future

Indications

- Persistent snapping or catching at the anterior or posterior aspect of the lateral elbow usually occurs. These symptoms are most often reproducible around 90 degrees of flexion and are particularly noted when the forearm is placed into full pronation.
- Symptoms consistent with a symptomatic plica (but in the absence of reproducible catching or snapping) when an MRI demonstrates the characteristic thickened synovial fold after other causes, such as lateral epicondylitis, have been ruled out. However, lateral epicondylitis and a symptomatic plica can occur concurrently.

Pertinent Physical Findings

- The patient will typically present with some form of trauma, either chronic from repetitive use or acute from a single traumatic event.
- The most common complaint is that of a snapping or catching sensation, which occurs around 90 degrees and is often exacerbated by pronation.[7,11,15]
- A painful sensation over the lateral epicondyle as an isolated complaint is also sometimes seen. This has increased confusion with lateral epicondylitis.

Pertinent Imaging

- Anteroposterior and lateral elbow x-rays should be routinely obtained but are rarely helpful in making the diagnosis. Plain x-rays, however, can serve to identify other pathologic conditions that can occur concomitantly.
- MRI will identify a fold in most individuals but is not necessarily specific as a diagnostic test.[16] The diagnosis is usually made clinically and confirmed arthroscopically

Equipment

Standard arthroscopic equipment typically used for elbow arthroscopy and including an arthroscopic shaver is all that is required to complete the procedure. Handheld arthroscopic biters and other sharp arthroscopic instruments may also be helpful in incising and removing this sometimes very thickened plica tissue. Also, because of the proximity of the radial nerve and its branches when removing some anterior lateral plicae, these handheld instruments may offer added protection compared to the arthroscopic power shaver with its attached suction.

Positioning and Portals

The patient is positioned according to surgeon preference. The author prefers lateral decubitus positioning on the table (Figure 5-4).

Step-by-Step Description of the Procedure

1. The patient is placed in the lateral decubitus position.
2. An anteromedial insertion of the scope is used for the initial, and often the only, diagnostic portal. The plica is usually readily demonstrated to be present as investing the radial head when the elbow is flexed around 90 degrees. Observing the altered position of the plica with flexion and extension provides absolute confirmation of the diagnosis.
3. The working portal for the resection occurs through an anterior lateral portal, but resection may be somewhat difficult because the hardened fibrous tissue may require a sharp incision into the plica in order to provide an edge against which the shaver can be more effective (Figure 5-5).

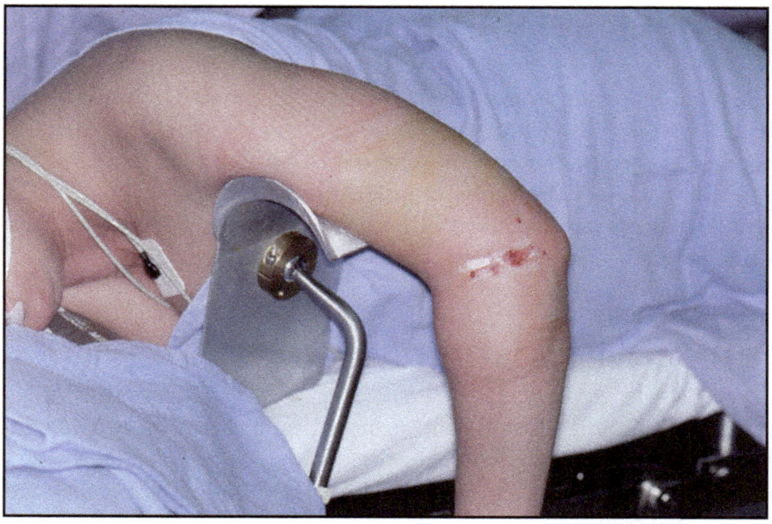

Figure 5-4. The arthroscopic position of choice for the author is lateral decubitus position. The arm is well padded with the support shown in this figure. This positioning allows excellent working distance for the anterior joint.

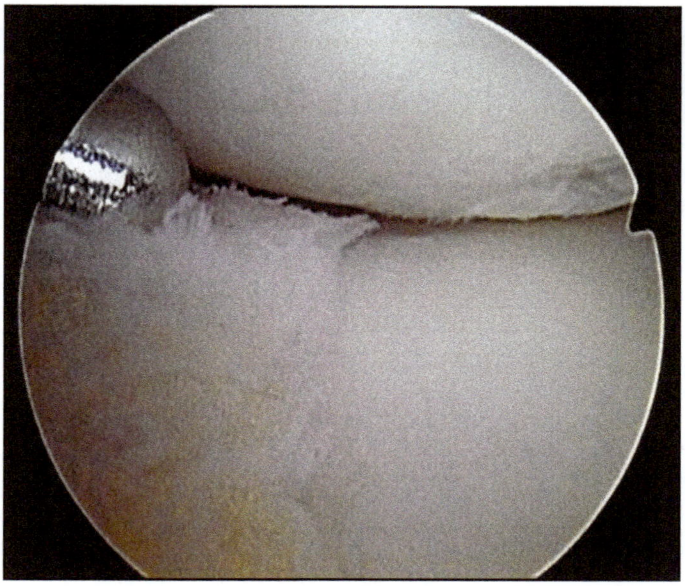

Figure 5-5. The initiation of the resection is facilitated by incising the margin of the plica. Once this is accomplished, the remainder of the excision is carried out with a shaver.

4. In some instances, a second midlateral and posterior lateral or distal lateral portal may be needed for completion of the resection of the posterior lateral portions of the plica. Davis et al[17] described the use and value of dual direct lateral portals and noted that it affords excellent investigation for osteochondritis dissecans and lateral elbow plica.
5. Removing the plica is all that is required to relieve the symptoms, but this should be thorough and demonstrate no tendency for residual snapping of capsular tissue during flexion and extension. The resection must remove, not just release, the plica. However, care should be taken not to continue the resection too posterior to the margin of the radial head as it is possible to violate the lateral collateral ligament complex if the resection proceeds posterior to the meridian of the radial head.

Postoperative Protocol

A soft tissue dressing is applied following isolated resection of a symptomatic plica, and the patient is seen at approximately 1 week postoperatively. Gentle active range of motion exercises are encouraged. Organized physical therapy is sometimes prescribed based on evaluation of the patient at the initial postoperative visit. Avoiding excessive or repetitive activities for 2 to 4 weeks is also recommended. Generally, patients have achieved full range of motion by 4 weeks and are released to full activities at that time.

Potential Complications

The most likely potential complication is development of instability from an aggressive capsular release, which violates the lateral ulnar collateral ligament causing posterior lateral rotatory instability. Injury to the posterior interosseous nerve is also a concern, so proper placement and visualization of the shaver is essential to avoid this problem.

Top Technical Pearls for the Procedure

1. Obtain visualization from the medial portal; the working portal should be such that the shaver can effectively reach the anterior aspect and the lateral margin of the radial head.
2. Incise the fibrotic margin to allow effective resection with the shaver.
3. The excision should be complete and elimination of snapping should be confirmed arthroscopically.
4. Avoid resection past the meridian of the radial head to avoid injury to the collateral ligament.
5. If the process extends posteriorly, a midlateral visualization and working portal are necessary to effect complete resection.

References

1. Duparc F, Putz R, Michot C, Muller JM, Fréger P. The synovial fold of the humeroradial joint: anatomical and histological features, and clinical relevance in lateral epicondylalgia of the elbow. *Surg Radiol Anat.* 2002;24(5):302-307.
2. Testut L, Latarjet A. *Traite' d'Anatomie Humaine.* Paris, France: Doin; 1928.
3. Miyazaki K, Murakami H. Report of a case of snapping elbow. *J Jpn Orthop Assoc.* 1958;32:250-254.
4. Paturet G. *Traite d'Anatomie Humaine. Vol II. Membres Superieur et Inferieur.* Paris, France: Masson et Cie; 1951.
5. Wightman JAK. Clicking elbow from a torn annular ligament: report of a case. *J Bone Joint Surg Br.* 1963;45:380-381.
6. Clarke RP. Symptomatic, lateral synovial fringe (plica) of the elbow joint. *Arthroscopy.* 1988;4(2):112-116.
7. Antuna SA, O'Driscoll SW. Snapping plicae associated with radiocapitellar chondromalacia. *Arthroscopy.* 2001;17(5):491-495.
8. Akagi M, Nakamura T. Snapping elbow caused by the synovial fold in the radiohumeral joint. *J Shoulder Elbow Surg.* 1998;7(4):427-429.

9. Commandre FA, Taillan B, Benezis C, Follacci FM, Hammou JC. Plica synovialis (synovial fold) of the elbow. Report on one case. *J Sports Med Phys Fitness*. 1988;28(2):209-210.
10. Isogai S, Murakami G, Wada T, Ishii S. Which morphologies of synovial folds result from degeneration and/or aging of the radiohumeral joint: an anatomic study with cadavers and embryos. *J Shoulder Elbow Surg*. 2001;10(2):169-181.
11. Kim DH, Gambardella RA, Elattrache NS, Yocum LA, Jobe FW. Arthroscopic treatment of posterolateral elbow impingement from lateral synovial plicae in throwing athletes and golfers. *Am J Sports Med*. 2006;34(3):438-444.
12. Kurosawa H, Koide S, Yaoita T, Nakajima H. Snapping elbow caused by the plica synovialis patellaris [in Japanese]. *Rinsyo Seikei Geka (Clin Orthop Surg)*. 1976;11:231-237.
13. Llusá Pérez M. *Atlas de Disección Anatomoquirúrgica del Codo*. Barcelona, Spain: Elsevier Masson; 2009.
14. Bosworth DM. The role of the orbicular ligament in tennis elbow. *J Bone Joint Surg Am*. 1955;37(3):527-533.
15. Ruch DS, Papadonikolakis A, Campolattaro RM. The posterolateral plica: a cause of refractory lateral elbow pain. *J Shoulder Elbow Surg*. 2006;15(3):367-370.
16. Vahlensieck M, Wiche U, Schmidt HM. Humeroradial plica: frequency and visualization on MRI [in German]. *Rofo*. 2004;176(7):959-964.
17. Davis JT, Idjadi JA, Siskosky MJ, ElAttrache NS. Dual direct lateral portals for treatment of osteochondritis dissecans of the capitellum: an anatomic study. *Arthroscopy*. 2007;23(7):723-728.

Please see videos on the accompanying website at

www.routledge.com/9781630910013

6

Olecranon Bursa Excision via Arthroscopy

Tyler R. Clark, MD; Michael J. O'Brien, MD; and Felix H. Savoie III, MD

Introduction

Olecranon bursitis is a common condition that most often is incited by repetitive trauma but also includes infection, autoimmune disorders, or idiopathic etiology.[1-10] It is the most common superficial bursitis, with noninfectious causes accounting for 80% of cases.[11] A fluid-secreting membrane lines the subcutaneous space making up the olecranon bursa that allows low-friction mobility between the olecranon surface and skin.[1,2,6,7,12,13] The bursa develops after the age of 7 years and is usually larger on the dominant arm. Olecranon bursitis usually occurs in males of the 30- to 60-year age group.[4,14] It can cause pain and distress and interfere with daily life. Most patients respond to conservative management, including anti-inflammatory drugs, antibiotics, rest, splinting, compressive dressings, aspiration, or corticosteroid injection.[1,2,4-9,11,13,15,16] Surgeons are reluctant to operate on this condition secondary to the high risks of complications, particularly wound healing issues with open incisions and high success rates of nonoperative management.[10] However, there is a subset of patients that benefits from this surgery.[9,13] Open vs arthroscopic techniques have been used, with arthroscopic techniques displaying better cosmetic results, lower morbidity, fewer wound complications, and a faster recovery.[2,10,17,18]

Indications

- It may be used for septic and aseptic bursitis if there is a failure of nonoperative management with continued pain and disruption of daily activity.
- Once patients have failed multiple conservative modalities (anti-inflammatory drugs, compressive dressings, splinting, physiotherapy, and aspiration), they can be considered for surgical excision.[19]
- Patients for whom bursitis is incited by autoimmune disorders and who have had prior surgical intervention have reported less than satisfactory results.[18]

Savoie FH III, Field LD, Steinmann SP, eds. *The Elbow and Wrist: AANA Advanced Arthroscopic Surgical Techniques* (pp 59-64).

Controversial Indications

- Most patients who develop septic bursitis can be cured with solely antibiotic therapy, most of which respond to several weeks of oral antibiotics.[20]
- However, in patients who have persisting bursitis symptomatology after at least 10 days of antibiotics and several repeat percutaneous aspirations, bursectomy should be considered in the treatment algorithim.[2]

To differentiate between aseptic and septic bursitis, aspiration should be performed with fluid sent for analysis, including Gram stain, culture, white blood cell count, glucose, and crystals, and lactate dehydrogenase.[4,9,11] Aseptic bursitis tends to present with either a clear, milky, or hemorrhagic aspirate.[2] A white blood cell count greater than 10,000/mm^3 is consistent with septic bursitis, whereas counts less than 1000/mm^3 are associated with aseptic bursitis.[11] The most common pathogen isolated from septic bursitis is *Staphylococcus aureus*.[20,21]

Pertinent Physical Findings

- Patients presenting with olecranon bursitis tend to show a uniform distention of the bursal sac of the olecranon, with symptoms including tenderness, bursal warmth, and redness.[2,4,6,7,11,19] The distended bursal sac can be up to 2.5 cm wide and 7 cm long.[11]

Pertinent Imaging

Multiple imaging modalities have been used in the initial medical workup for olecranon bursitis:

- Elbow x-rays tend to show no abnormalities, except for the possible bony spur.[19]
- Ultrasound has been used in the diagnosis for bursitis as it can reveal collections of fluid in the bursal sac.[3]
- Magnetic resonance imaging (MRI) of an olecranon bursitis will show a hypointensity on T1-weighted images, variable signals intensity in T2-weighed images, and contrast enhancement of bursal margins.[4] MRI can be indicated for evaluation of possible abscesses or osteomyelitis; however, ultrasound and MRI have been unable to provide diagnostic value for distinguishing septic from aseptic bursitis.[2,4,12]

Equipment

Equipment that is recommended for successful completion for this surgery includes a 30-degree, 4.0-mm diameter arthroscope; basket forceps; 4.5-mm, full-radius motorized shaver; arthroscopic grasper; and gravity fed in-flow cannula or pressure pump.[18,22]

Positioning and Portals

For olecranon bursal excision, the prone or lateral decubitus position is preferred. Place the elbow in 90 degrees of flexion to obtain maximal visualization of the bursa.[10,17,18] A sterile or nonsterile tourniquet may be used.[17]

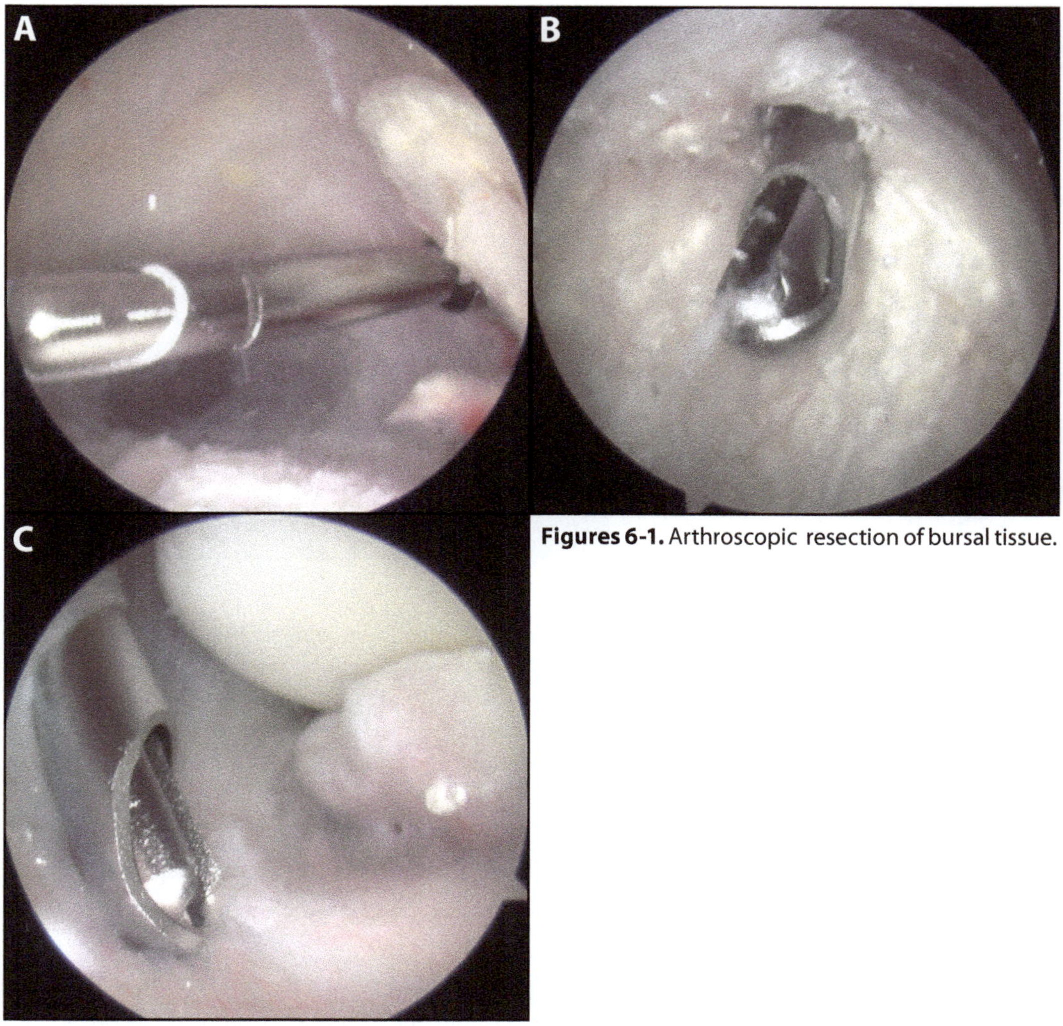

Figures 6-1. Arthroscopic resection of bursal tissue.

Step-by-Step Description of the Procedure

The bursa is usually large. The ulnar nerve is carefully marked, and then a portal superior and inferior to the bursa is established. The authors prefer to view from inferiorly and resect from superior to inferior. The arthroscope is introduced into the inferior portal and the bursa is visualized. A spinal needle is inserted to mark the superior portal and the shaver is introduced. It is sometimes helpful to place a spinal needle posterior to the ulnar nerve and into the bursa to prevent straying too far medially. The shaver is used to begin the excision from superior to inferior under direct visualization (Figure 6-1). Loose bodies may be found on initial exploration of the bursa and removed with forceps or suction. Complete and full resection of the bursa requires viewing from both portals. The authors usually excise the majority of the bursa while viewing from inferiorly, then place the arthroscope into the superior portal and the shaver into the inferior portal to complete the resection. Complete resection is obtained when the fibers of the triceps are observed (Figure 6-2). Avoid resecting subcutaneous fat on superficial resection. If there are osteophytes, a bony shaver may be introduced to resect the bony protuberance while protecting the triceps tendon.

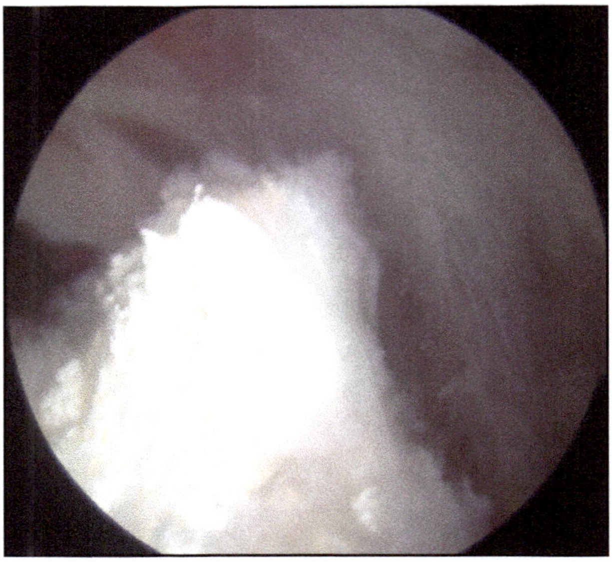

Figure 6-2. Triceps tendon fibers.

Upon completion of the procedure, deflate the tourniquet and suction out the remaining arthroscopic insufflation fluid. An incisional wound vacuum device (Prevena Incision Management System, KCI) is placed to maintain the decompression of the bursa. A compressive bandage is then placed over the wound vacuum device.

The following is the procedure listed in bullet point format for surgical planning and preparation:

- Prep, drape, and insufflate the tourniquet on the planned surgical extremity.
- Identify and mark the ulnar nerve, and mark and establish the inferior and superior portals.
- Place the arthroscope in the inferior portal and the spinal needle in the superior portal to establish the correct position.
- Place the shaver in the superior portal and begin excising superiorly to inferiorly.
- Switch the arthroscope into the superior portal and the shaver into the inferior portal and complete excision.
- One may remove loose bodies and perform bony resection of osteophytes.
- Remove the instrumentation, drain the elbow, deflate the tourniquet, and place incisional wound vacuum dressing and compressive dressing.

Postoperative Protocol

The wound vacuum and a removable splint are maintained for the first 2 to 3 days. Once the portals are healed, the wound vacuum and splint are discontinued and a compressive sleeve is placed on the elbow. Physical therapy for cryocompression and range of motion is used shortly following surgery to prevent stiffness. At 14 days, patients should begin to increase elbow activity.

Potential Complications

Complications following surgery have been well documented and include prolonged exudation from surgical sites, infection, intermittent recurrent swelling, recurrence of bursitis (documented as high as 1 in 5 patients), skin necrosis at the surgical site secondary to poor blood supply (more common in open vs arthroscopic procedures), and, rarely, complex regional pain syndrome.[1,2,4,9] Necrosis of the skin can lead to the patient requiring a skin flap.[1]

Top Technical Pearls for the Procedure

1. Use the prone position with elbow flexed to 90 degrees to distend the bursa.
2. Use portals away from the center of the bursa.
3. Have a systematic excision plan in order to perform a timely and complete excision.
4. Carefully mark and protect the ulnar nerve to prevent damage during the procedure and, if necessary, protect it with a spinal needle inserted in the area between the nerve and the bursa.
5. Use an incisional wound vacuum to minimize the risk of wound complications and recurrence.

References

1. Degreef I, Smet L. Complications following resection of the olecranon bursa. *Acta Orthop Belg.* 2006;72(4):400-403.
2. Baumbach SF, Lobo CM, Badyine I, Mutschler W, Kanz KG. *Arch Orthop Trauma Surg.* 2014;134(3):359-370.
3. Blankstein A, Ganel A, Givon U, Mirovski Y, Chechick A. Ultrasonographic findings in patients olecranon bursitis. *Ultraschall Med.* 2006;27(6):568-571.
4. Del Buono A, Franceschi F, Palumbo A, Denaro V, Maffulli N. Diagnosis and management of olecranon bursitis. *Surgeon.* 2012;10(5):297-300.
5. Ip TC, Jones NF. Treatment of chronic infected olecranon bursitis by radical excision and radial forearm flap coverage. *Tech Hand Up Extrem Surg.* 2001;5(2):112-116.
6. McAfee JH, Smith DL. Olecranon and prepatellar bursitis. Diagnosis and treatment. *West J Med.* 1988;149(5):607-610.
7. Salzman KL, Lillegard WA, Butcher JD. Upper extremity bursitis. *Am Fam Physician.* 1997;56(7):1797-1806.
8. Smith DL, McAfee JH, Lucas LM, Kumar KL, Romney DM. Treatment of nonseptic olecranon bursitis. A controlled, blinded prospective trial. *Arch Intern Med.* 1989;149(11):2527-2530.
9. Stewart NJ, Manzanares JB, Morrey BF. Surgical treatment of olecranon bursitis. *J Shoulder Elbow Surg.* 1997;6(1):49-54.
10. Tu CG, McGuire DT, Morse LP, Bain GI. Olecranon extrabursal endoscopic bursectomy. *Tech Hand Up Extrem Surg.* 2013;17(3):173-175.
11. Aaron DL, Patel A, Kayiaros S, Calfee R. Four common types of bursitis: diagnosis and management. *J Am Acad Orthop Surg.* 2011;19(6):359-367.
12. Floemer F, Morrison WB, Bongartz G, Ledermann HP. MRI characteristics of olecranon bursitis. *AJR Am J Roentgenol.* 2004;183(1):29-34.
13. McFarland EG, Mamanee P, Queale WS, Cosgarea AJ. Olecranon and prepatellar bursitis: treating acute, chronic, and inflamed. *Phys Sportsmed.* 2000;28(3):40-52.
14. Chen J, Alk D, Eventov I, Wientroub S. Development of the olecranon bursa. An anatomic cadaver study. *Acta Orthop Scand.* 1987;58(4):408-409.
15. Herrera FA, Meals RA. Chronic olecranon bursitis. *J Hand Surg Am.* 2011;36(4):708-709.
16. Weinstein PS, Canoso JJ, Wohlgethan JR. Long-term follow-up of corticosteroid injection for traumatic olecranon bursitis. *Ann Rheum Dis.* 1984;43(1):44-46.
17. Kerr DR. Prepatellar and olecranon arthroscopic bursectomy. *Clin Sports Med.* 1993;12(1):137-142.

18. Ogilvie-Harris DJ, Gilbart M. Endoscopic bursal resection: the olecranon bursa and prepatellar bursa. *Arthroscopy.* 2000;16(3):249-253.
19. Sferopoulos NK. A new approach to the surgical treatment of olecranon bursitis. *Br J Med Medical Res.* 2013;4(1):272-278.
20. Pien Fd, Ching D, Kim E. Septic bursitis: experience in a community practice. *Orthopedics.* 1991;14(9): 981-984.
21. Garcia-Porrua C, Gonzalez-Gay MA, Ibanez D, Garcia-Pais MJ. The clinic spectrum of severe septic bursitis in northwestern Spain: a 10 year study. *J Rheumatol.* 1999;26(3):663-667.
22. Kerr DR, Carpenter CW. Arthroscopic resection of olecranon and prepatellar bursae. *Arthroscopy.* 1990;6(2):86-88.

Please see videos on the accompanying website at

www.routledge.com/9781630910013

SECTION II

THE ELBOW
Advanced Procedures

7

Arthroscopic Osteocapsular Arthroplasty

Matthew L. Ramsey, MD

Introduction

The indications for elbow arthroscopy have expanded rapidly to include more complex pathologies.[1-7] This chapter discusses arthroscopic osteocapsular arthroplasty (AOCA), which remains one of the more difficult arthroscopic procedures of the elbow. The goal is to present appropriate patient selection, the technical aspects of the procedure, and postsurgical considerations while focusing on safety.

Indications

The indications for AOCA depend on the underlying pathology and vary with the skill level of the surgeon. The ideal pathologic indication includes the following:

- Pain and functional limitations as a result of osteoarthritis
- Posttraumatic and rheumatoid involvement of the elbow

Pertinent Physical Findings

A complete general physical examination of the elbow should include the following:

- Visual inspection
- Palpation of bony and soft tissues about the elbow
- Evaluation of passive and active range of motion
- Careful neurovascular examination
- Crepitus against resisted flexion/extension and pronation/supination give a sense of the degree of articular involvement.
- End range pain in forced flexion and extension is the result of osteophyte impingement.

Savoie FH III, Field LD, Steinmann SP, eds. *The Elbow and Wrist: AANA Advanced Arthroscopic Surgical Techniques* (pp 67-74).

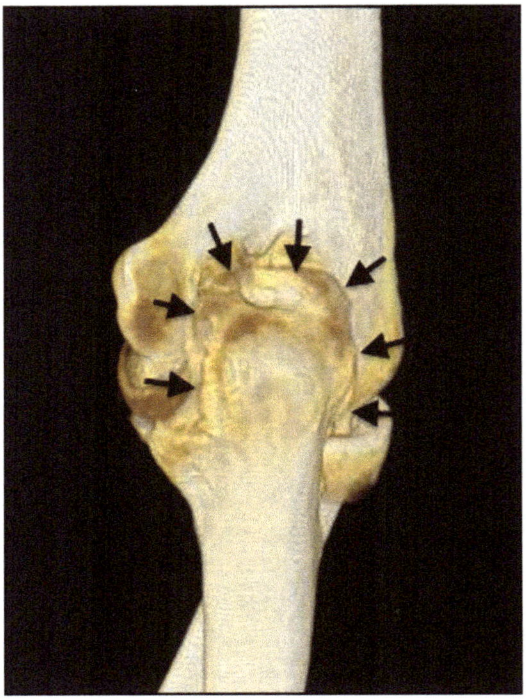

Figure 7-1. CT scan demonstrating 3-dimensional formation of osteophytes. CT scans provide the best detail on the location and extent of osteophyte formation.

Pertinent Imaging

- Standard anteroposterior, lateral, and oblique x-rays provide gross assessment of the arthritic changes.
- Computed tomography (CT) scans with 2-dimensional coronal and sagittal reconstructions and 3-dimensional reconstructions provide assessment of the surface anatomy and are an important tool in mapping osteophyte excision (Figure 7-1).

Equipment

A standard 4.0-mm, 30-degree arthroscope is used with nonvented inflow cannulas to avoid fluid extravasation into the surrounding soft tissues. An inflow pump is used with pump pressures set at 30 mm Hg or less. All trocars are conical and blunt tipped to prevent neurovascular and articular injury.

Handheld instruments (probes, grasping forceps, and blunt-tipped punches) and motorized instruments (shaver and burr) are used. Retractors are used to maintain the joint space.

General Considerations

Technical refinements in how AOCA is performed have been introduced with safety as the driving force for change. Fluid distension displaces the capsule and neurovascular structures away from the bone, tamponades bleeding, and aids in washing away the bone debris. The use of intra-articular retractors allows the capsule and neurovascular structures to be displaced away from bone. The combination of low-pressure inflow and retractors maintains visualization and reduces the risk of neurovascular injury.

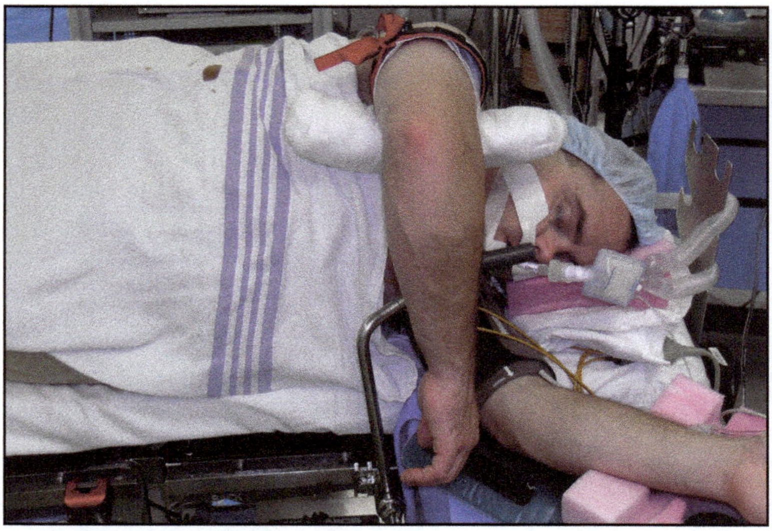

Figure 7-2. Lateral decubitus positioning. The patient is maintained on a bean bag with an axillary roll. The arm is draped free and maintained on a post or arm positioner.

Anesthesia

The choice of anesthesia is driven by the desire to perform a neurovascular examination following the surgery. If the surgeon prefers to evaluate the neurologic status of the patient following surgery, general anesthesia is used. Once the neurologic status of the operative extremity is confirmed postoperatively, regional blockade can be administered for postoperative pain control.

Positioning and Portals

The patient can be positioned supine, prone, or lateral decubitus. The operation can be performed with the patient in any position. The author prefers the lateral decubitus position. The arm is maintained in an elbow arthroscopy positioner with the shoulder perpendicular to the body and the elbow positioned above the level of the shoulder (Figure 7-2). The patient is maintained on a bean bag with an axillary roll. A nonsterile tourniquet is applied high on the arm and inflated to 250 mm Hg. The extremity is prepped and draped free to allow intraoperative manipulation.

Surface landmarks help localize deep bone and neurovascular structures. Prior to instrumenting the elbow, the topographical anatomy of the elbow is carefully outlined (Figure 7-3).

The elbow is divided into the following 3 regions: the anterior joint, posterior joint, and lateral gutter. The locations of the various portals used to instrument each of these regions were previously described in Chapter 1.

Three portals are typically used in the anterior joint, including the proximal anterolateral portal, the anterolateral portal, and the proximal anteromedial portal. These portals are used interchangeably for visualization and instrumentation as needed. An accessory anteromedial portal is occasionally used but is not routine.

Two portals are typically used in the posterior joint compartment (including the medial gutter): the posterolateral portal and the posterocentral portal. Accessory portals for retractor placement include the proximal posterolateral portal and the accessory medial portal to protect the ulnar nerve if one is working in the medial gutter.

The lateral gutter is considered by some to be an extension of the posterior joint compartment. Work in the lateral gutter uses the posterolateral portal and the direct lateral (soft spot) portal.

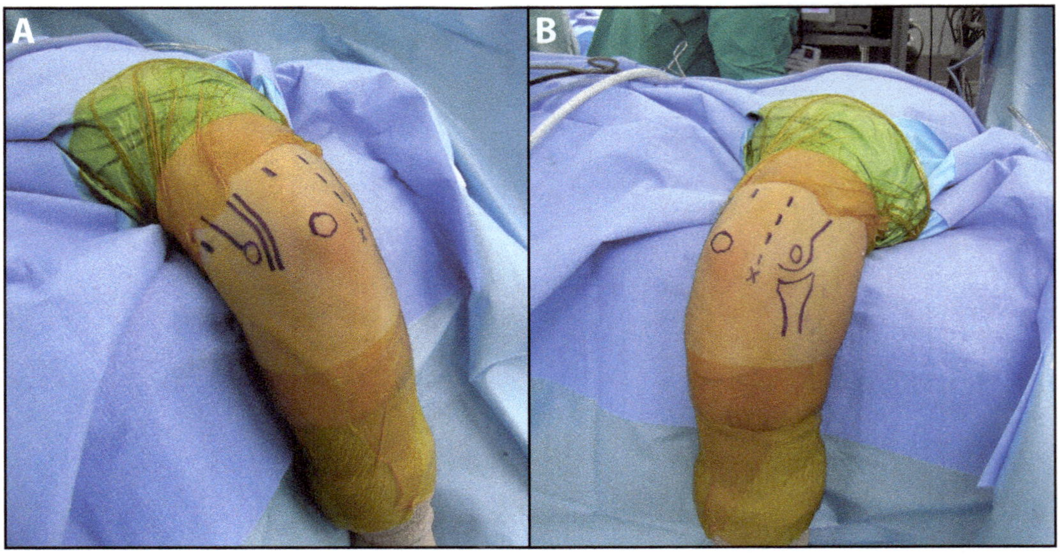

Figure 7-3. Surface landmarks drawn on the skin prior to surgery. (A) Medial and (B) lateral aspect of the elbow.

Step-by-Step Description of the Procedure

General Considerations

Safely performing AOCA requires a sequential surgical routine for each compartment of the elbow. This safety-driven strategy stresses establishing a view in the compartment, creating a space to work within, bone removal, and capsular excision.[8] If you cannot adequately complete one step, you must not proceed to the next step. It is best at that point to abandon the arthroscopy and convert to an open release.

Anterior Joint Compartment

The arthroscope is inserted through a proximal anteromedial portal and a shaver is inserted through an anterolateral portal. With the scope and shaver confirmed within the anterior joint space, any scar tissue and synovium are debrided, creating the working space (Figure 7-4). It is important to start proximally with the resection to decrease risk to the neurovascular structures. Once the capsule is released off the humerus, it can safely be resected while maintaining visualization of the brachialis muscle. The brachialis protects the anterior neurovascular structures and should not be violated. The arthroscope is switched to the anterolateral portal and the shaver is transferred to the proximal anteromedial portal to finish creating the working space anteriorly. A retractor can be placed in the proximal anterolateral portal to hold the capsule and brachialis away from the humerus, thereby maintaining the working space.

The arthroscope is replaced in the proximal anteromedial portal and the shaver is placed in the anterolateral portal. The retractor is placed against the anterior soft tissues in the region of the resection to maintain visualization. Osteophyte excision begins at the lateral-most extent of the supracondylar column. The end point to osteophyte excision is the cortical bone that represents the native humerus. The arthroscope is moved to the anterolateral portal and the shaver and/or burr are placed in the proximal anteromedial portal to complete osteophytes excision in the coronoid fossa. The elbow is flexed and impinging osteophytes on the tip and medial wall of the coronoid process are removed.

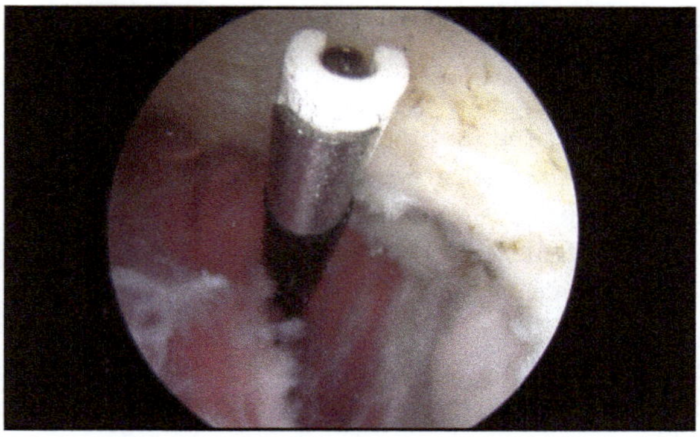

Figure 7-4. Removing intra-articular scar tissue from the humerus with electrocautery. Dissection is carried out proximally in the joint to increase the margin for safety.

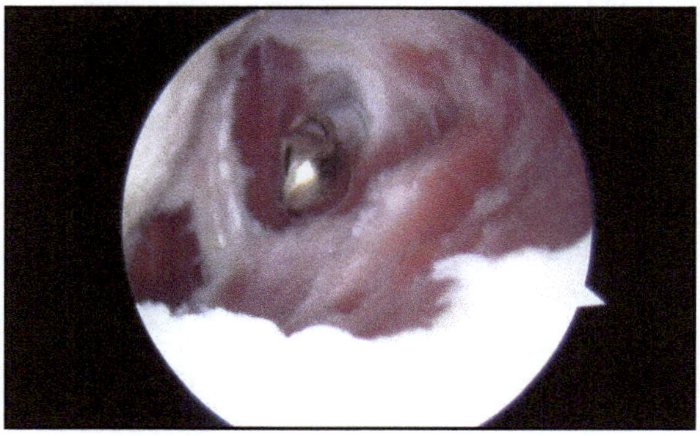

Figure 7-5. With the arthroscope in the proximal anterolateral portal, the shaver is placed in the proximal anteromedial portal to complete the capsular excision.

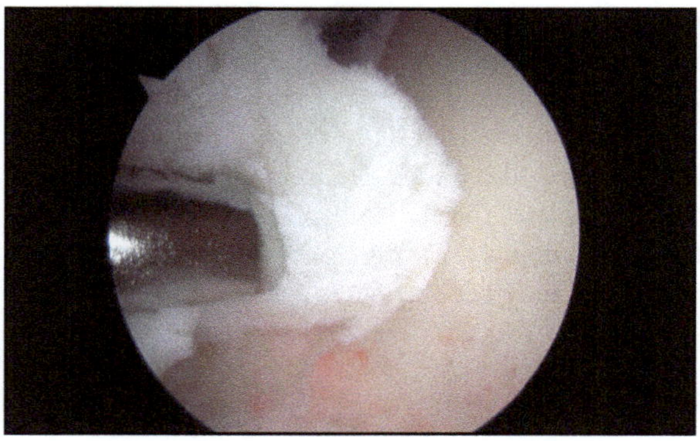

Figure 7-6. Scar tissue is removed from the olecranon fossa to improve visualization.

With the arthroscope moved back to the anterolateral portal, a capsulotomy is made in the mid-distal portion from medial to lateral. Tension is maintained on the tissues with the retractor while a blunt-tipped capsular release punch is advanced from medial to lateral. The portion of the capsule proximal to the capsulotomy is resected with a motorized shaver with no suction applied (Figure 7-5). The arthroscope is moved to the proximal anterolateral portal and the capsular release punch completes the mid-distal capsulectomy from the lateral column. The remaining capsular tissue superiorly is teased away from the underlying brachialis and resected.

Posterior Joint Compartment

The posterior compartment of the elbow is initially visualized with the arthroscope in the posterolateral portal and the shaver in the posterocentral portal. The arthroscope and shaver are directed centrally into the olecranon fossa. Once the arthroscope and shaver are confirmed in the posterior compartment, the fat pad, scar tissue, and loose bodies are removed (Figure 7-6).

A retractor is placed in a proximal posterolateral portal and directed toward the medial gutter to retract the tissues and protect the posteromedial capsule. The final step in creating working space is to strip the capsule off of the humerus proximally.

Osteophyte excision posteriorly begins proximally at the roof of the olecranon fossa and progresses distally until the normal margins and depth of the fossa are re-established. The retractor is placed at the entrance to the medial gutter and the capsule is retracted away from the posteromedial aspect of the ulnohumeral joint. The osteophytes that expand the width of the medial walls of the ulna and trochlea are removed. Only once the native anatomy is restored can the shaver and/or burr be introduced into the medial gutter. The retractor can be passed into the medial gutter to retract the capsule and nerve. The posteromedial capsule is not violated in the arthroscopic portion of this procedure. The arthroscope is then moved to the posterocentral portal and the shaver and/or burr is moved to the posterolateral portal. The retractor in the proximal posterolateral portal is used to retract the posterolateral capsule away from the bone to allow removal of the osteophytes on the posterolateral tip of the olecranon and posterior aspect of the lateral supracondylar column. This completes the bone excision in the posterior compartment of the elbow. The posterior capsule in now resected. The author does not resect any capsule medial to the medial most extent of the olecranon in order to protect the ulnar nerve. This portion of the capsule is removed during the open ulnar nerve decompression.

Lateral Gutter

The entrance to the lateral gutter begins at the posterolateral corner of the olecranon. The arthroscope is placed in the posterolateral portal and driven into the lateral gutter. The location of the direct lateral (soft spot) portal is identified using a spinal needle, and a shaver is introduced. With the arthroscope and shaver at the posterolateral corner of the ulna, visualization in the gutter is achieved by removing any synovium, scar tissue, redundant capsular tissue, and loose bodies. Once the view is established, osteophytes are removed from the lateral wall of the olecranon and trochlea. Osteophyte excision proceeds from the posterolateral corner of the olecranon into the lateral gutter. The final and critical aspect of osteophyte excision is performed on the posterior aspect of the capitellum from the sulcus between the trochlea and capitellum out to the far lateral aspect of the capitellum. Lateral capsular excision completes the arthroscopic portion of the operation. Excision of the capsule at the posterolateral olecranon is critically important in regaining full flexion. The more distal aspects of the lateral capsule only need to be resected with high-degree loss of elbow flexion.

Ulnar Nerve Management

Ulnar nerve management evolved with the realization that there was a relatively high incidence of delayed onset ulnar neuritis, noted with gains in flexion and extension. An open decompression of the ulnar nerve is performed instead of performing this arthroscopically. This is typically performed before the arthroscopic portion of the procedure but can be done at the conclusion of the operation. If performed before the AOCA, the author leaves the posterior bundle of the ulnar collateral ligament intact to protect the nerve and resect it at the completion of the arthroscopic procedure.

Postoperative Protocol

The postoperative management of patients begins preoperatively. A prescription for therapy is provided and the patient is directed to a therapist with experience in managing elbow patients. Patients are given a prescription for indomethacin to be taken for the first 3 weeks following surgery to reduce the risk of heterotopic bone formation. Postoperative radiation is not routinely used but is considered if heterotopic ossification is excised as part of the surgery.

All of these surgeries are performed in an outpatient setting. Patients are placed in a bulky dressing with a loosely applied elastic wrap for swelling. Patients are instructed to remove the dressing on the second postoperative day and to apply a compression sleeve. Continuous passive motion can be used to maintain motion achieved through surgery. If used, it needs to be arranged preoperatively and be available for use immediately postoperatively. Outpatient therapy begins on the second postoperative day. Active and active assisted range of motion with end range overpressure concentrates on maintaining the motion that was achieved in the operating room. Edema control and management of pain and inflammation are critical to the successful progression in therapy.

The patient is seen within the first week of surgery to determine the response to the first few days of therapy and for an initial wound check. Careful neurovascular examination is performed, with particular attention to the ulnar nerve. If ulnar nerve function is compromised at rest, therapy is discontinued temporarily. The patient is seen again in follow-up 2 weeks after surgery for suture removal and reevaluation. Follow-up is scheduled for 4 and 8 weeks postoperatively to assess the progress.

Potential Complications

Following a reproducible routine through a safety-driven approach minimizes but never eliminates complications. The most common immediate complication following elbow arthroscopy is nerve injury.[9-11] This complication is rare and most often transient.[12-14] Nerve injuries can be the result of direct injury, overaggressive joint distention/fluid extravasation, compression caused by arthroscopic sheaths, or the use of local anesthesia.[12,13]

Persistent wound drainage is reported as the most common delayed complication following arthroscopic elbow surgery, noted predominantly from the anterolateral and direct lateral portals.[15,16] Deep infection is a rare but devastating complication. The use of intra-articular corticosteroid injection following surgery has been associated with infectious complications, and its use should be avoided.[15,16]

Heterotopic bone following surgery has been rarely reported.[17-19] Intra-articular steroid injections have been demonstrated to reduce the risk of heterotopic bone.[16] However, because its use been associated with postoperative infectious complications, the routine use of intra-articular corticosteroid injections is not encouraged.

Top Technical Pearls for the Procedure

1. Never perform an arthroscopic procedure above your level of expertise.
2. Draw the topographical landmarks on the skin before beginning surgery.
3. Fluid distention or the use of retractors increases the distance between the bone and the joint capsule but not the bone-to-nerve distance.
4. Use retractors liberally. Retractors maintain visualization with low-pressure fluid inflow while protecting nerves.
5. Know where the nerves live and, if necessary, specifically identify their locations.

References

1. Moskal MJ, Savoie FH III, Field LD. Elbow arthroscopy in trauma and reconstruction. *Orthop Clin North Am.* 1999;30(1):163-177.
2. Byrd JW, Elrod BF, Jones KS. Elbow arthroscopy for neglected osteochondritis dissecans of the capitellum. *J South Orthop Assoc.* 2001;10(1):12-16.
3. Geib TM, Savoie FH III. Elbow arthroscopy for posttraumatic arthrosis. *Instr Course Lect.* 2009;58:473-480.
4. Hsu JW, Gould JL, Fonseca-Sabune H, Hausman MH. The emerging role of elbow arthroscopy in chronic use injuries and fracture care. *Hand Clin.* 2009;25(3):305-321.
5. DeGreef I, Samorjai N, De Smet L. The Outerbridge-Kashiwaghi procedure in elbow arthroscopy. *Acta Orthop Belg.* 2010;76(4):468-471.
6. Ahmad CS, Vitale MA, ElAttrache NS. Elbow arthroscopy: capitellar osteochondritis dissecans and radiocapitellar plica. *Instr Course Lect.* 2011;60:181-190.
7. Pederzini LA, Nicoletta F, Tosi M, Prandini M, Tripoli E, Cossio A. Elbow arthroscopy in stiff elbow. *Knee Surg Sports Traumatol Arthrosc.* 2014;22(2):467-473.
8. Blonna D, Wolf JM, Fitzsimmons JS, O'Driscoll SW. Prevention of nerve injury during arthroscopic capsulectomy of the elbow utilizing a safety-driven strategy. *J Bone Joint Surg Am.* 2013;95(15):1373-1381.
9. Thomas MA, Fast A, Shapiro D. Radial nerve damage as a complication of elbow arthroscopy. *Clin Orthop Relat Res.* 1987;(215):130-131.
10. Ruch DS, Poehling GG. Anterior interosseus nerve injury following elbow arthroscopy. *Arthroscopy.* 1997;13(6):756-758.
11. Hahn M, Grossman JA. Ulnar nerve laceration as a result of elbow arthroscopy. *J Hand Surg Br.* 1998;23(1):109.
12. Andrews JR, Carson WG. Arthroscopy of the elbow. *Arthroscopy.* 1985;1(2):97-107.
13. Lynch GJ, Meyers JF, Whipple TL, Caspari RB. Neurovascular anatomy and elbow arthroscopy: inherent risks. *Arthroscopy.* 1986;2(3):190-197.
14. Poehling GG, Ekman EF. Arthroscopy of the elbow. *Instr Course Lect.* 1995;44:217-223.
15. Kelly EW, Morrey BF, O'Driscoll SW. Complications of elbow arthroscopy. *J Bone Joint Surg Am.* 2001;83(1):25-34.
16. Nelson GN, Wu T, Galatz LM, Yamaguchi K, Keener JD. Elbow arthroscopy: early complications and associated risk factors. *J Shoulder Elbow Surg.* 2014;23(2):273-278.
17. Gofton WT, King GJ. Heterotopic ossification following elbow arthroscopy. *Arthroscopy.* 2001;17(1):E2.
18. Sodha S, Nagda SH, Sennett BJ. Heterotopic ossification in a throwing athlete after elbow arthroscopy. *Arthroscopy.* 2006;22(7):802.e1-802.e3.
19. Hughes SC, Hildebrand KA. Heterotopic ossification--a complication of elbow arthroscopy: a case report. *J Shoulder Elbow Surg.* 2010;19(1):e1-e5.

Please see videos on the accompanying website at

www.routledge.com/9781630910013

8

Osteochondritis Dissecans of the Elbow, Including Grafts via Arthroscopic and Mini-Open Techniques

Robert Nelson Mead, MD, MBA; Michael J. O'Brien, MD; and Felix H. Savoie III, MD

Introduction

Osteochondritis dissecans (OCD) is a focal defect in articular cartilage and subchondral bone.[1,2] Repetitive microtrauma injures the blood supply to the cartilage and subchondral bone leading to necrosis and fragmentation.[3] OCD lesions often occur in the elbows of young athletes whose activities result in repetitive microtrauma to the elbow, such as overhead throwing or gymnastics.[1,3,4] OCD lesions of the elbow are most commonly located at the capitellum but can occur in the trochlea, radial head, olecranon, and olecranon fossa.[2,5,6] OCD lesions are not to be confused with Panner's disease, which affects children 9 to 10 years old and spontaneously resolves. OCD lesions of the elbow typically occur in patients aged 11 to 21 years, with symptomatic lesions requiring treatment.[3]

Young athletes afflicted with an OCD lesion in the capitellum initially present with mild pain after the inciting activity.[7] The pain slowly progresses. They usually present with lateral-sided elbow pain that increases with activity and a loss of terminal extension.[3]

Nonoperative treatment consists of physical therapy, rest, and a brace that offloads the radiocapitellar joint.[1-3,8] The most common operative treatments are diagnostic arthroscopy with debridement, fragment excision, and microfracture; fragment fixation; and osteochondral graft transfer from the olecranon or the lateral femoral condyle.[9] These surgeries can be done arthroscopically or openly.[1-3,7,8] The characteristics of the lesion determine the type of procedure the surgeon performs. The surgeon's comfort level with the procedure dictates whether the surgery is done arthroscopically or openly.

Indications

- The presence of an intact cartilage cap determines nonoperative vs operative treatment.[1-3,8,10]
- Pain and functional impairment that has failed appropriate nonoperative management

Savoie FH III, Field LD, Steinmann SP, eds. *The Elbow and Wrist: AANA Advanced Arthroscopic Surgical Techniques* (pp 75-81).

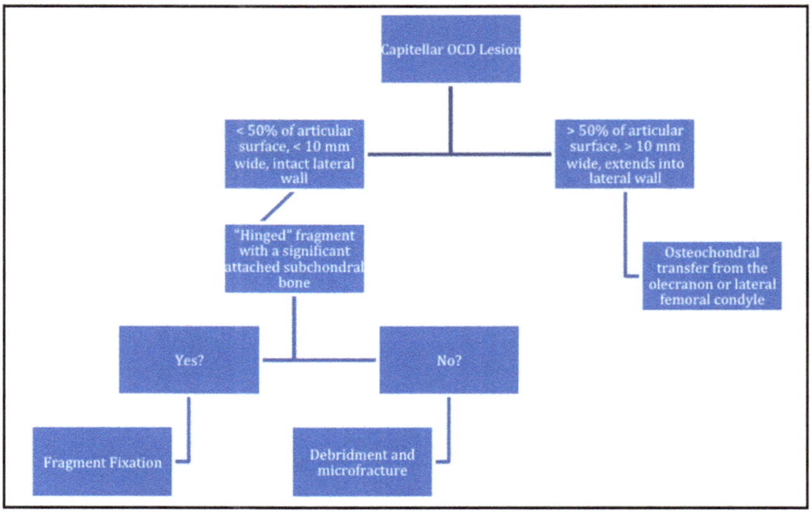

Figure 8-1. Treatment algorithm.

- A loose or unstable cartilage cap is treated with arthroscopic or mini-open fragment fixation vs debridement and microfracture.
- A dislodged cartilage cap resulting in an intra-articular loose body is treated with arthroscopic loose body removal and microfracture of the OCD bed.
- Osteochondral autograft transfer (OATS) from the femur or olecranon is reserved for large OCD lesions that are greater than 50% of the capitellar width[8,10] or more than 10 mm wide and involve the lateral aspect of the capitellum (Figure 8-1).[8,11]

Pertinent Physical Findings

- Inspection of the elbow may demonstrate an effusion or swelling in the lateral gutter.[1,3]
- Loss of terminal extension[1,3]
- Tenderness to palpation at the radiocapitellar joint
- A palpable thickening of the posterolateral plica, which may be tender
- Crepitus felt with flexion, pronation, and supination may indicate the presence of loose bodies.[2]
- Lateral pain and loss of motion with the moving valgus stress test and the active radiocapitellar compression test
- Recommended "BEST" test: The active radiocapitellar compression test, which was first described by Baumgarten,[12] consists of passive forearm pronation and supination during midrange elbow flexion and extension with an axial load applied to the radiocapitellar joint.[2] A positive test occurs when this maneuver recreates the patient's symptoms.

Pertinent Imaging

- Routine x-rays, including anteroposterior, lateral, and 2 oblique projections of the elbow, to evaluate for OCD lesions or loose bodies
- An anteroposterior x-ray of the elbow at 45 degrees of flexion may better visualize the joint.[1-3,10,13]

- An OCD lesion appears as an area of radiolucency and rarefaction with an irregular articular surface.[1,2,7]
- Magnetic resonance imaging should be obtained once an OCD lesion is suspected on x-ray.
- Magnetic resonance imaging provides the extent of bone involvement, integrity of the cartilage cap, and presence of loose bodies that are often not seen on plain x-rays.[1-3,10]
  - Early lesions, which often have an intact cartilage cap, will have low signal intensity on T1-weighted imaging in the superficial aspect of the capitellum. Late lesions will light up on both T1- and T2-weighted images.
  - The intervening fluid around late lesions will give a high-intensity signal on T2-weighted images, which indicates an unstable OCD.[1,3,10]

Equipment

- Standard 4-mm arthroscope
- Arm holder or bolster
- Spinal needle
- Motorized shaver
- Arthroscopic graspers, punches, and biters
- Steadman microfracture awls
- K-wires and wire driver, power drill
- Metal or bioabsorbable screws or anchors if fragment fixation is attempted

Positioning and Portals

Prone (Authors' Preferred Position)

The prone position enables easier access to the posterior compartment than supine or lateral decubitus. The anesthesiologist intubates the patient and then rolls the patient into the prone position. Appropriate padding is placed to support the head and face, and chest rolls are inserted to aid with ventilation. The shoulder of the nonoperative arm is placed in 90 degrees of abduction and neutral rotation with the elbow at 90 degrees of flexion. The surgeon then supports the elbow and wrist with a padded arm board. The surgeon places a padded arm board parallel to the table and centered at the shoulder of the operative side. A tourniquet is applied and the shoulder is placed in 90 degrees of abduction and neutral rotation. A rolled towel bump or padded bolster attached to the table supports the arm at the mid-humerus level. This suspends the elbow in 90 degrees of flexion.[14]

The advantages of the prone position are that the surgeon can easily manipulate the elbow into full flexion and extension and that the surgeon has access to the posterior compartment of the elbow. The disadvantage is that the prone position limits access to the airway.

Lateral Decubitus

The surgeon secures the patient in the lateral decubitus position with a bean bag. He or she then inserts an axillary roll. The operative arm is placed over an arm holder or a padded bolster with the shoulder internally rotated and flexed to 90 degrees. The elbow is also flexed at 90 degrees.[15]

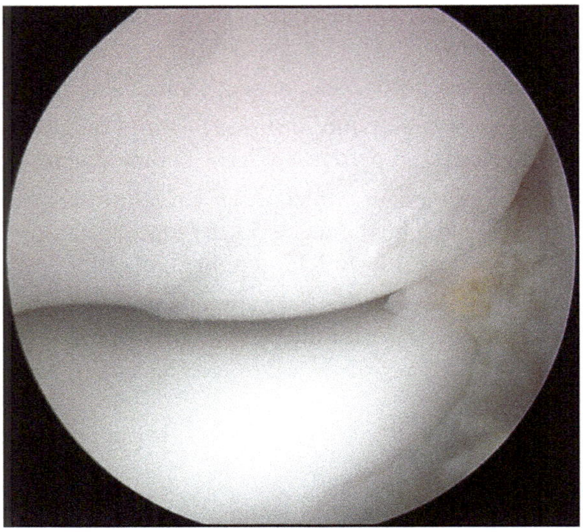

Figure 8-2. Panoramic view of the radiocapitellar joint.

The advantage of the lateral decubitus position is that the surgeon has access to the anterior and posterior compartments of the elbow without the anesthetic difficulties associated with positioning the patient prone.

Step-by-Step Description of the Procedure

Arthroscopic Exploration, Debridement, and Microfracture

The diagnostic arthroscopy begins with creating the proximal anteromedial portal and evaluating the anterior compartment of the elbow for lesions and loose bodies.[3] If loose bodies are present, an anterolateral portal is established to remove them.[3]

Once the anterior compartment has been evaluated, the arthroscope is moved to the posterior central portal and the posterior compartment is evaluated. In most cases, the olecranon fossa and medial gutter will be normal but should be checked for loose bodies. The posterolateral gutter is then evaluated to allow visualization of the OCD lesion and associated posterolateral plica.

A soft spot portal is used to remove the plica. A 70-degree arthroscope may be substituted for the 30-degree one to get a panoramic view of the radiocapitellar joint (Figure 8-2). The lesion is then probed for stability and a distal soft spot portal is used to microfracture the base if excision is necessary.[3]

Arthroscopic in Situ Fragment Fixation

If the surgeon encounters a viable cap for fixation, the inferior soft spot portal can be used to secure the fragment. The fragment is hinged open and the base of the lesion is debrided (Figure 8-3). The fragment is secured using a headless compression screw or a suture anchor.[3] If an absorbable anchor is used, the regular suture is replaced with a monofilament synthetic absorbable suture. A pilot hole is drilled and the anchor is placed into the base of the defect. The sutures are then retrieved through the fragment in a crossing pattern such that the fragment is compressed into the defect. This technique can even be used for fragments with minimal to no bone in the fragment.

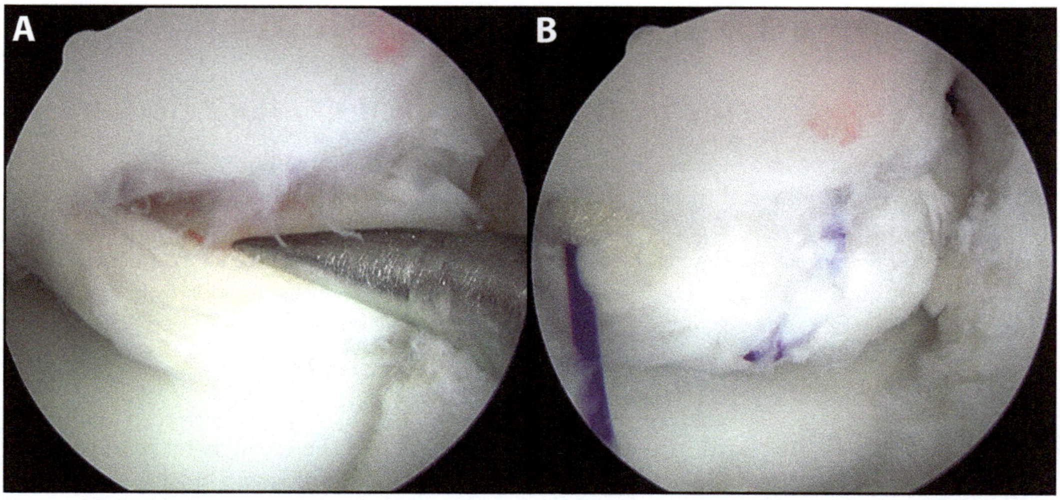

Figure 8-3. (A) Arthroscopic view of a hinged fragment amenable to fixation. (B) Arthroscopic view of the secured fragment demonstrating the suture knots within the fixation.

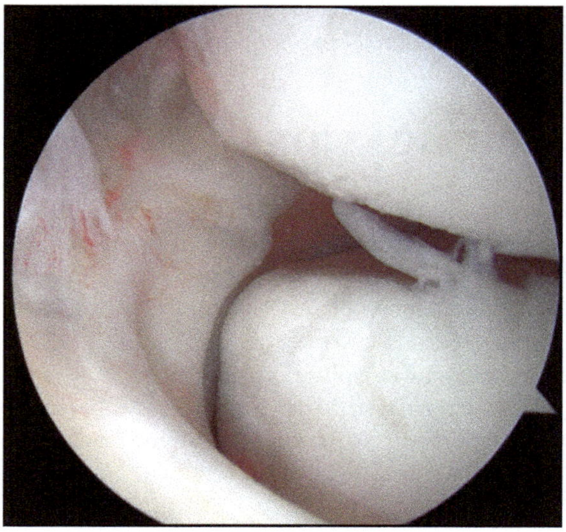

Figure 8-4. Advanced OCD lesion with extension into the lateral wall. These lesions require extensive reconstruction with a peg transfer or OATS procedure.

Arthroscopic Osteochondral Transfer from the Olecranon

The surgeon begins with the standard diagnostic arthroscopy of the elbow with management of associated injuries. The OCD lesion is evaluated and debrided with the arthroscope in the posterior central portal and the instrumentation in the soft spot and distal soft spot portals. The bed of the lesion is debrided until a healthy bed is created with stable borders. The sizing guide is used to confirm the size of the defect and the appropriate size and depth recipient hole is drilled into the center of the defect. Occasionally with lateral defects, the straight lateral portal can be used to place the recipient hole horizontally into the central part of the residual capitellum.[16] The graft is then harvested from the posterolateral corner of the olecranon tip by visualizing from the posterior central portal and harvesting via the posterolateral portal with the elbow slightly extended. The scope is brought back down the lateral gutter, the elbow is hyperflexed, and the osteochondral graft is inserted via the same distal soft spot portal that was used to drill the recipient hole. It is important not to overinsert the graft but to keep it flush with the normal contour of the capitellum (Figure 8-4).[3]

Postoperative Protocol

Arthroscopic Debridement and Excision of Loose Bodies

The patient is placed in a hinged elbow brace that offloads the capitellum, and early motion is initiated immediately. Physical therapy is initiated within 1 week for stretching exercises, edema reduction, and hand and wrist exercises.[7] The patient is started on general conditioning within the next 3 weeks. The patient is allowed to resume normal activity in the brace as tolerated, and the brace is discontinued by 6 weeks postoperatively. The patient can return to sports once he or she achieves full, pain-free range of motion (ROM) and acceptable strength.[7]

Fragment Fixation and Osteochondral Grafting

The patient is initially placed in a splint for 7 to 10 days until he or she is ready to have the sutures removed. The patient is placed in a contoured brace with hinges and begins a supervised physical therapy program focused on reducing pain and swelling and gently regaining ROM. The patient starts resistance exercises at 6 to 10 weeks and is gradually progressed to full activity while graft or fragment incorporation is closely monitored on x-rays, usually by 4 months.[10,17] If the patient has no pain, his or her ROM has returned to preoperative levels, and x-ray demonstrates a healed lesion, the patient can return to full activity at that time (4 to 5 months).[10,18]

Potential Complications

Three of the most common complications are lesion progression, elbow stiffness, and heterotopic ossification. Arthrofibrosis typically responds to nonoperative treatment but sometimes requires release or resection of the capsule.[3,7] Heterotopic ossification is more common in open procedures than arthroscopic ones and is amenable to arthroscopic excision and radiation in its early stages. Later stages require arthroscopic or open excision and radiation.[7]

Incongruent graft placement and donor site morbidity are complications specific to osteochondral grafting. An incongruent graft can result in an irregular articular surface that experiences uneven forces during motion.[15] Patients sometimes report pain at the knee when surgeons use the lateral femoral condyle or intercondylar notch as the donor site.[1]

Top Technical Pearls for the Procedure

1. Use a 70-degree arthroscope via a posterior central or posterolateral portal, placed down the lateral gutter to get a bird's eye view of the lesion.
2. Debride, microfracture, or graft via a distal soft spot portal from posterior with the elbow flexed more than 90 degrees to protect the radial head.
3. Lateral uncontained lesions with bone loss of the lateral shoulder require bone grafting with restoration of the cartilage cap.
4. If doing an OATS procedure, try to match the contour of the graft to the surrounding cartilaginous surface to avoid an uneven capitellar surface.
5. During OATS procedure, keep the tube harvester at 90 degrees perpendicular to articular surface during donor and recipient harvesting.

References

1. Ruchelsman DE, Hall MP, Youm T. Osteochondritis dissecans of the capitellum: current concepts. *J Am Acad Orthop Surg.* 2010;18(9):557-567.
2. Stubbs MJ, Field LD, Savoie FH III. Osteochondritis dissecans of the elbow. *Clin Sports Med.* 2001;20(1):1-9.
3. Savoie FH III. Osteochondritis dissecans of the elbow. *Oper Tech Sports Med.* 2008;16:187-193.
4. Peterson RK, Savoie FH III, Field LD. Osteochondritis dissecans of the elbow. *Instr Course Lect.* 1999;48:393-398.
5. Baker CL III, Baker CL Jr, Romeo AA. Osteochondritis dissecans of the capitellum. *J Shoulder Elbow Surg.* 2010;19(2 suppl):76-82.
6. Jones KJ, Wiesel BB, Sankar WN, Ganley TJ. Arthroscopic management of osteochondritis dissecans of the capitellum: mid-term results in adolescent athletes. *J Pediatr Orthop.* 2010;30(1):8-13.
7. Rubin CJ. Prone or lateral decubitus position. In: Savoie FH III, Field L, eds. *Arthroscopy of the Elbow.* New York, NY: Churchill Livingstone; 1996:41-47.
8. Maruyama M, Takahara M, Harada M, Satake H, Takagi M. Outcomes of an open autologous osteochondral plug graft for capitellar osteochondritis dissecans: time to return to sports. *Am J Sports Med.* 2014;42(9):2122-2127.
9. de Graaff F, Krijnen MR, Poolman RW, Willems WJ. Arthroscopic surgery in athletes with osteochondritis dissecans of the elbow. *Arthroscopy.* 2011;27(7):986-993.
10. Takahara M, Mura N, Sasaki J, Harada M, Ogino T. Classification, treatment, and outcome of osteochondritis dissecans of the humeral capitellum. Surgical technique. *J Bone Joint Surg Am.* 2008;90(suppl 2 pt 1):47-62.
11. Iwasaki N, Kato H, Ishikawa J, Masuko T, Funakoshi T, Minami A. Autologous osteochondral mosaicplasty for osteochondritis dissecans of the elbow in teenage athletes. *J Bone Joint Surg Am.* 2009;91(10):2359-2366.
12. Baumgarten TE. Osteochondritis dissecans of the capitellum. *Sports Med Arthrosc Rev.* 1995;3:219-223.
13. Kosaka M, Nakase J, Takahashi R, et al. Outcomes and failure factors in surgical treatment for osteochondritis dissecans of the capitellum. *J Pediatr Orthop.* 2013;33(7):719-724.
14. Poehling GG, Ekman EF. Arthroscopy of the elbow. *Instr Course Lect.* 1995;44:217-223.
15. O'Driscoll SW, Morrey BF. Arthroscopy of the elbow. Morrey B, ed. *The Elbow and Its Disorders.* 2nd ed. Philadelphia, PA: WB Saunders; 1993:120.
16. Ahmad CS, ElAttrache NS. Arthroscopy in the throwing athlete. In: Morrey B, Sanchez-Sotelo J, eds. *The Elbow and Its Disorders.* 4th ed. Philadelphia, PA: Saunders Elsevier; 2009:587-595.
17. McClung GA, Field L, Savoie FH III. Diagnostic arthroscopy and loose body removal. In: ElAttrache NS, Harner CD, Mirzayan R, Sekiya JK, eds. *Surgical Techniques in Sports Medicine.* Philadelphia, PA: Lippincott Williams & Wilkins; 2007:211-220.
18. Takeda H, Watarai K, Matsushita T, Saito T, Terashima Y. A surgical treatment for unstable osteochondritis dissecans lesions of the humeral capitellum in adolescent baseball players. *Am J Sports Med.* 2002;30(5):713-717.

Please see videos on the accompanying website at

www.routledge.com/9781630910013

9

Arthrofibrosis of the Elbow
Management via Arthroscopic and Arthroscopically Assisted Techniques

Philipp N. Streubel, MD and Mark S. Cohen, MD

Introduction

Arthroscopic surgery has gained increasing attention over the last decade as a viable alternative to open elbow release, with similar improvements in range of motion (ROM) and low complication rates.[1] Arthroscopic elbow release has the benefit of decreased soft tissue disruption. However, arthroscopic elbow release requires advanced skills and a thorough understanding of the normal and pathologic anatomy of the elbow. Given the complexity of arthroscopic elbow anatomy, it is recommended that a learning curve be established, with less complex procedures being mastered before one attempts arthroscopic release of the stiff elbow. In addition, for this operation, prior experience with open elbow releases will provide a valuable understanding of the spatial location of impinging and tethering structures. Unlike open surgery, in which the surgical field is visualized 3-dimensionally, during arthroscopy, elbow anatomy is assessed on a 2-dimensional level via the monitor. Prior experience with open surgery will also allow for the potential conversion to an open procedure if deemed necessary.

Indications

- Arthroscopic elbow release is indicated in patients with posttraumatic elbow stiffness that has not improved after a course of therapy and splinting (static progressive or dynamic).[2]
- Hypertrophic osteoarthritis with a congruous central ulnohumeral joint
- Loss of more than 30 degrees of extension and/or flexion of less than 110 to 120 degrees of elbow flexion is commonly accepted as the threshold to proceed with elbow surgery.[3-5]

Controversial Indications

- Patients with a prior history of surgery should be considered cautiously for arthroscopic release.

Savoie FH III, Field LD, Steinmann SP, eds. *The Elbow and Wrist: AANA Advanced Arthroscopic Surgical Techniques* (pp 83-92).

- A reliable understanding of the location of the ulnar nerve should exist. A subluxating ulnar nerve, although not a contraindication to arthroscopy, should be identified and considered when establishing the anteromedial portal.
- Arthroscopic elbow surgery should be done with great caution in patients with a prior ulnar nerve transposition.[6,7] In this setting, the nerve should be explored and protected prior to proceeding with instrument placement.
- Especially in the setting of a submuscular transposition, the ulnar nerve is at increased risk of injury during anteromedial portal placement and anterior capsulectomy.

Contraindications

- It is not advisable to perform elbow arthroscopy on an incongruous joint or in the presence of congenital abnormalities because neurovascular structures will be in an unpredictable position, precluding safe portal placement.[6]

Pertinent Physical Findings

- Patients with elbow stiffness most frequently complain of loss of terminal flexion. Occasionally, terminal extension may be functionally limiting, especially in gymnasts and other high-level athletes.[8]
- Pain may be present at the extremes of motion secondary to anterior and posterior bony impingement.
- Pain during the mid arc of motion suggests arthritic changes of the central ulnohumeral joint surfaces and may lead to less predictable pain relief after surgery.

Ulnar Nerve

Location and stability of the ulnar nerve should be carefully inspected. Prior scars may point toward a history of surgery and transposition of the nerve. Ulnar nerve subluxation should be identified as it may influence the decision making between open and arthroscopic surgery as well as between ulnar nerve release and transposition in the presence of ulnar nerve symptoms. Occasionally, upon palpation, the nerve is found to be scarred onto the underlying posteromedial capsule. Under this circumstance, an open cubital tunnel release and placement of a protective nerve loop is recommended prior to proceeding with arthroscopic capsular release. Ulnar nerve dysfunction should be suspected in patients complaining of tingling and numbness affecting the ring and small finger. Two-point discrimination should be assessed to quantify sensory disturbance. Furthermore, in more advanced stages, hand weakness and clumsiness can be present secondary to motor dysfunction of the intrinsic hand muscles. On physical examination, patients may exhibit a positive Tinel's sign over the course of the nerve at the elbow. Ulnar neuropathy can be further confirmed with a positive elbow flexion test. Atrophy of the first web space may be seen in advanced stages of ulnar neuropathy. Evaluating strength of the first dorsal interosseous muscle through index finger abduction further tests motor function and is confirmed with a positive Froment's sign. Of note, ulnar nerve compression may not always manifest as tingling and numbness. Especially in the setting of limited elbow flexion, patients occasionally only report medial elbow pain that can be precipitated by elbow flexion. Commonly in these patients, the nerve is sensitive and a positive Tinel's sign can often be elicited with nerve percussion.

Pertinent Imaging

- Routine anteroposterior, oblique, and lateral elbow x-rays are obtained to confirm joint congruency and to identify bony lesions that may be limiting motion.
- Computed tomography with reformatting in the sagittal and coronal plane as well as 3-dimensional surface renderings can be of great benefit to achieve a detailed understanding of the pathologic anatomy present.[9]
- In the setting of ulnar nerve–related symptoms, electromyography and nerve conduction studies can be useful to confirm the diagnosis.

Equipment

- Nonvented straight cannulas
- Radiofrequency probe with a 90-degree head
- Arthroscope: 4.5-mm, 30-degree viewing angle
- Soft tissue retractors or elevators
- Full-radius, 5.5-mm shaver (4.8- and 3.5-mm shavers available as needed for tighter spaces)
- Round 4.0-mm burr
- Auger burr
- Fluid pump (or pressure-assisted flow)
- Scissors

Positioning and Portals

After typically undergoing regional or general anesthesia, the patient is positioned prone with careful padding of the face, chest, pelvis, knees, and feet. Alternatively, the patient may be placed in the lateral decubitus position on a bean bag with the nonoperative elbow and shoulder flexed to avoid interfering with full flexion of the operative extremity during the procedure. The prone position optimizes working space around the elbow and can be safely used with the use of regional anesthesia. An arm holder is placed so that the arm is tilted 10 degrees from proximal inferior to distal superior. This will aid in gaining maximum elbow flexion during the procedure. The extremity is prepared and draped and a sterile tourniquet is applied. Bony landmarks are drawn, including the epicondyles, radiocapitellar joint, and olecranon. The ulnar nerve is checked for possible subluxation and its path is drawn. Proximally, this is posterior to the medial intermuscular septum, which can be palpated as it runs proximally from the medial epicondyle.

In order to regain elbow ROM, a step-wise approach has to be followed to resect impinging and tethering structures. Flexion is improved by releasing the posterior capsule and by resecting anterior impinging structures between the tip of the coronoid and the radial head and their respective fossae along the anterior humerus. Extension, however, requires release of the anterior capsule and resection of posterior impinging structures between the olecranon and its fossa.

Anterior Portals

- Anteromedial portal: 2 cm proximal to the medial epicondyle and 1 cm anterior to the intermuscular septum

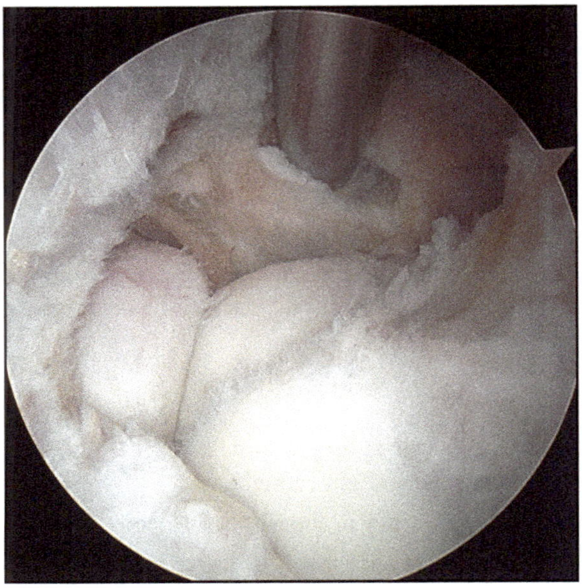

Figure 9-1. Anterior segment seen from the anteromedial portal. A shaver has been introduced through the anterolateral portal located anterior to the radiocapitellar joint. The radial head is seen to the left, articulating with the capitellum to the right. Note bony overgrowth of the coronoid in the lower left corner. Tissue overgrowth overlying the radial and coronoid fossae can also be noted.

- Anterolateral portal: This portal is established under direct visualization using an outside-in technique with localizing spinal needle. It is positioned anterior to the radiocapitellar joint (Figure 9-1).
- Proximal anteromedial portal: This portal is used for placement of a soft tissue retractor. It is located just anterior to the medial septum and 4 to 6 cm proximal to the medial epicondyle.

Posterior Portals

- Straight posterior portal: 3 to 4 cm proximal to tip of olecranon in midline of the arm
- Posterolateral portal: 1 cm proximal to midpoint from tip of olecranon to lateral epicondyle
- Proximal posterolateral portal: 4 to 6 cm proximal to the tip of the olecranon along the lateral triceps tendon. This portal is used for placement of a soft tissue retractor.
- Direct midlateral portal (soft spot): Located in the center of a triangle formed by the tip of the olecranon, lateral epicondyle, and the radial head. An outside-in technique is recommended with the use of a localizing spinal needle.

Step-by-Step Description of the Procedure

- If ulnar nerve symptoms (or sensitivity) are present or preoperative elbow flexion is limited, the ulnar nerve is released or transposed. The nerve is carefully retracted and the floor of the cubital tunnel, comprised by the posteromedial capsule of the ulnohumeral joint, is incised longitudinally. This may aid in improving elbow flexion and will expose any underlying osteophytes that can be excised under direct visualization. The ulnar nerve may be tagged with a moist Penrose drain for protection during arthroscopy.
- Joint insufflation is performed with saline using a 30-cc syringe through an 18-gauge needle inserted in the soft spot portal. If adequately placed, backflow through the needle should be obtained when removing the syringe from the inserted needle. Furthermore, from the 90-degree position, maximum joint insufflation will be confirmed by passive extension of the elbow by approximately 10 to 20 degrees, which will allow slightly more fluid to be injected.

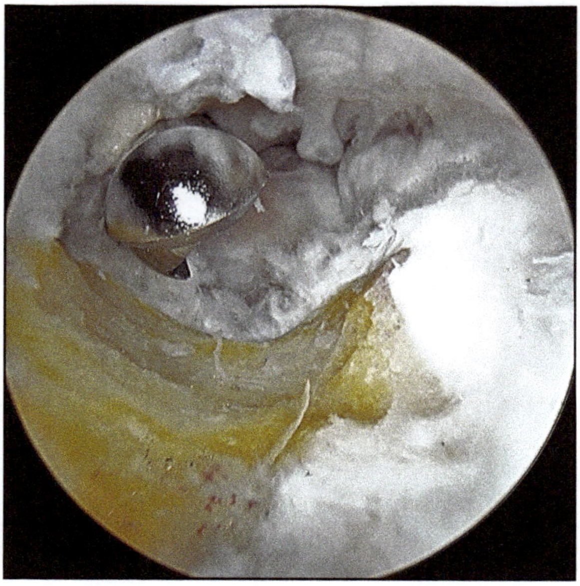

Figure 9-2. Anterior segment seen from the anterolateral portal. A shaver has been introduced through the anteromedial portal. Soft tissue has been removed followed by initial bone resection from the coronoid and radial fossae. The humerus is seen to the left and the articular surface facing anteriorly to the right.

Joint insufflation will increase the distance from the bony skeleton to the neurovascular structures running superficial to the joint capsule. In the setting of advanced scarring or post-traumatic contracture, minimal joint distension will often be achieved.

Anterior Segment

- The anteromedial portal is established. Portal placement requires incision of the skin only to avoid any possible injury to branches of the medial antebrachial cutaneous nerve. A blunt trochar or Wissinger rod (switching stick) is then introduced, aiming toward the radiocapitellar joint. The joint capsule should be pierced anterior to the medial aspect of the trochlea. Entering too lateral will make visualization difficult. In the presence of marked fibrosis, the trocar will skive anteriorly, making penetration of the capsule difficult. In this setting, bony contact with the anterior humerus should be felt to ensure penetration of the capsule. The arthroscope is introduced. As a convention, the camera is oriented so that the humerus is visualized vertically on the monitor (see Figure 9-1).
- Under direct visualization, the anterolateral portal is established by using a spinal needle piercing the joint anterior to the radiocapitellar joint. Care should be made to try to direct the needle perpendicular to the skin to allow for the shortest path possible through the soft tissues. After the skin incision, the knife can be advanced into the joint (with the cutting edge turned proximally) with care not to injure the articular cartilage. This allows one to open a nice sized defect in the joint capsule. A shaver is introduced (see Figure 9-1). If marked scarring is present, a small retractor may be used to strip the anterior capsule off of the humerus to establish a space in which to work.
- Once reliable orientation has been gained and under direct visualization of instruments, synovitis and adhesions are removed using a combination of a shaver and a thermal device. Before proceeding with removal of bony overgrowth, the coronoid and radial fossae are debrided, removing overlying scar tissue and soft tissue attachments (Figure 9-2). When using a thermal device, fluid flow is increased to avoid the risk of thermal chondral injury. Also, it is best to use only short bursts of energy to decrease heat generation within the joint.
- Bony overgrowth is removed with the use of burrs. A preoperative computed tomography scan can provide guidance on the location and amount of bone to be removed. Care is taken to

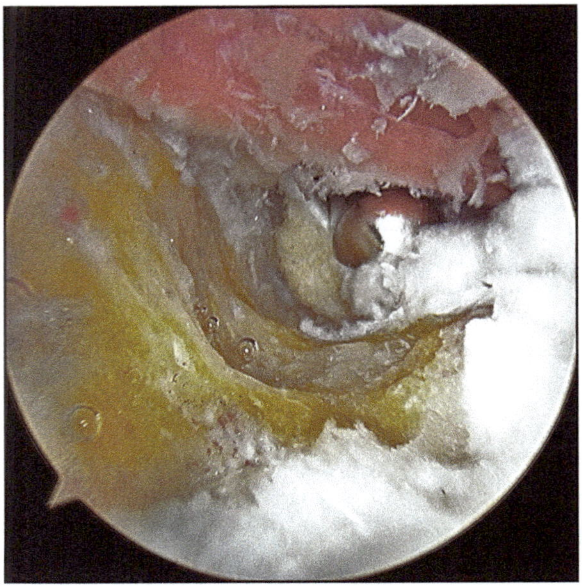

Figure 9-3. Anterior segment seen from the anterolateral portal. A shaver has been introduced through the anteromedial portal. Following bony work, anterior capsulectomy has been completed. Note visible fibers of the brachialis muscle on the upper part of the image. The humerus is seen to the left and the articular surface facing anteriorly to the right.

recreate a concavity above the entire humeral articular surface, including the coronoid fossa and the radial fossa, which is located above the capitellum (see Figures 9-2 and 9-3).

- Once all intra-articular work has been done, the anterior capsule is resected with the use of a shaver along its medial half. The lateral half is best cut by using scissors entering from the lateral portal. The radial nerve is located on the anterior joint capsule at the level of the radio-capitellar joint. Using scissors at this level allows for a controlled manner to cut into capsule only. Shavers and thermal devices should be avoided at this level.[10] It is safest to remove the capsule proximal to the joint line, where the radial nerve is farthest from potential injury.
- Switching the instruments and camera from the medial to lateral portal is routinely required and best achieved with the use of a switching stick. It is important not to lose the medial portal as it is difficult to regain control of it once all instruments are removed (see Figures 9-2 and 9-3).

Posterior Segment

- Posterior work is started with the camera in the straight posterior portal. The posterior portal can be established using a #15 blade from the skin straight down onto bone. The camera is introduced with the goal to visualize the ulnohumeral joint horizontally on the monitor (Figure 9-4). The camera now has to be oriented with the viewing window looking distally. Often, it is helpful to blindly strip the olecranon fossa clean of soft tissue with an elevator. This is done with the elbow extended to protect the articular surface.
- The posterolateral portal is then established in a similar manner and a shaver is introduced. The posterior capsule can be further stripped off of the humerus.
- Once reliable visualization of the shaver is achieved, the olecranon fossa is debrided. Again, soft tissue is first removed to allow for proper visualization of the bony contours.
- In the presence of advanced scarring, an accessory proximal posterolateral portal can be used for the introduction of a retractor.
- The posteromedial and posterolateral gutters are examined for the presence of loose bodies. Viewing in the posterolateral gutter often requires removal of the fat pad that is typically

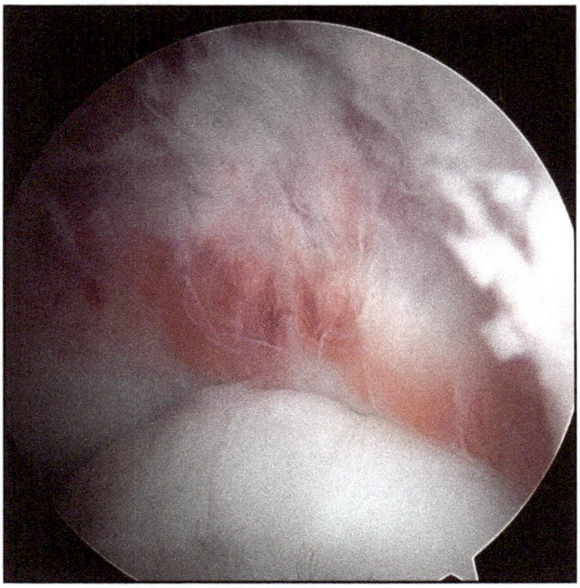

Figure 9-4. Posterior segment seen from the posterior portal. The tip of the olecranon is seen on the inferior aspect of the image, articulating with the posterior aspect of the trochlea. Note osteophytic overgrowth at the tip of the olecranon and soft tissue obliterating the olecranon fossa.

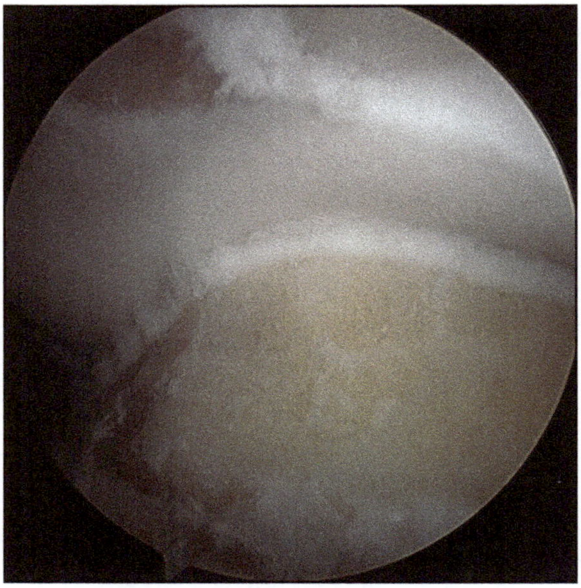

Figure 9-5. Posterior segment seen from the posterior portal. Bony overgrowth at the tip of the olecranon (bottom of image) and at the transition from the articular surface of the trochlea to the distal aspect of the olecranon fossa (top of image) have been resected.

located in this region. In addition, use of the direct midlateral (soft spot) portal can help provide a more direct view of this aspect of the joint.

- With the use of a burr, bony overgrowth at the tip of the olecranon and olecranon fossa is removed, including the medial and lateral corners (Figure 9-5). Care is taken not to use a burr when working on the posteromedial corner of the olecranon. A shaver is safest due to the proximity of the ulnar nerve.
- Once debridement has concluded, ROM is carefully assessed. Gentle progressive flexion and extension is performed with a sustained force over several minutes. This allows for stretching of the underlying myostatic contracture of the elbow flexors and extensors, respectively.

Postoperative Protocol

Postoperatively, patients are started on continuous passive motion (CPM) while the regional block is still present. This aids in early management of edema and theoretically helps maintain the motion gained at surgery. Formal therapy is begun on postoperative day 1. Active and gentle passive elbow motion is combined with intermittent CPM. To maintain extension, passive stretches with a 2-lb wrist weight are performed with the elbow placed over a bolster. These are performed for 10 to 15 minutes several times daily as tolerated.

After discharge, patients continue with daily home therapy, including active and passive exercises and weighted stretches. CPM is typically discontinued at 3 to 4 weeks. A static progressive brace is started early in the postoperative period and continued for several months. The brace is applied 2 to 3 times per day for 30-minute periods, alternating between flexion and extension. Prophylaxis against heterotopic ossification is commonly used. Indomethacin is taken orally for 3 weeks after surgery.[11] Single fraction radiation therapy in a dose of 700 cGy can be used in selected cases after resection of extensive heterotopic ossification.[12]

Potential Complications

Delayed-onset ulnar neuritis after arthroscopic elbow release occurs in approximately 10% of patients undergoing arthroscopic elbow release.[13,14] This incidence can be reduced to 3% by prophylactically releasing or transposing the ulnar nerve during surgery.[14] Patients with preoperative flexion loss are at an increased risk for delayed-onset ulnar neuritis.[13] In most instances, ulnar nerve release is the preferred strategy as it is associated with a lower risk of wound complications compared to transposition.[14] A low threshold for nerve release is recommended.

Arthroscopic elbow release is rarely associated with permanent nerve damage. In one of the largest reported series of 502 elbow releases,[15] no permanent nerve injuries were reported. Five percent of patients had nerve dysfunction that resolved within 1 day to 24 months after surgery. However, isolated reports of complete nerve injuries have been reported in the literature, including ulnar, median, radial, anterior interosseous, and posterior interosseous nerves.[6,16-19]

Top Technical Pearls for the Procedure

1. Fluid management: Fluid management plays the following 3 key roles in arthroscopy: joint space distension, cooling of the joint space during the use of thermal devices, and flushing of debris. During elbow arthroscopy, joint distension should not rely on fluid pressure. Rather, in order to allow prolonged surgery on the elbow during arthroscopy, low pressure should be maintained at all times to avoid extravasation into the surrounding soft tissues. A low-pressure pump should control fluid flow. Two types of fluid pumps are commonly used. One consists of a manual control that is adjusted according to acoustic feedback of a hydraulically assisted pump (a pulse lavage system hooked up to an intravenous tubing with a roller valve). This requires flow adjustment by a surgical assistant. The most frequently used pump consists of a rotary piston that regulates inflow according to pressure. Pressure settings should be kept to a minimum and flow increased only during the use of thermal devices and bony debridement. An outflow portal, through a separate cannula or through the shaver, should be used to avoid over-distension and ensure fluid outflow.

(continued)

2. Tissue retractors: The use of retractors introduced through accessory portals plays a key role in allowing distension of the working space during elbow arthroscopy while maintaining low fluid pressures.
3. Switching of portals: The use of a switching stick (Wissinger rod), allows for changing the position of the camera and instruments from one side to the other without losing the portal. This is of special importance for the anteromedial portal and in the setting of posttraumatic stiffness. Capsular thickening and progressive edema of the soft tissues may render this portal to become irrecoverable if lost.
4. Understanding of nerve location: The 2 nerves mostly at risk during arthroscopic elbow surgery are the motor branch of the radial nerve and the ulnar nerve. The radial nerve crosses the elbow anterior to approximately the midline of the radiocapitellar joint. At the joint line and distally at the level of the radial head and neck, the radial nerve most frequently lies directly on the capsule.[20] Thus, capsular resection performed more proximally is safest. The ulnar nerve is separated from the joint by the posteromedial capsule. Inadvertent dissection through the capsule at this level, especially while using a burr with suction, can lead to devastating nerve injury. Furthermore, the medial antebrachial cutaneous nerve may be injured when creating the anteromedial portal. This can be prevented by incising only the skin and completing the portal with a blunt trochar or switching stick.
5. Limited use of suction: The most devastating complication of elbow arthroscopy is nerve injury. Due to the tight space in which elbow arthroscopy is performed, soft tissues harboring vital structures may be inadvertently pulled into the surgical instruments if suction is used. Intermittent use of low-pressure suction is recommended if at all necessary. In general, sufficient outflow can be generated through the shaver by disconnecting the suction tubing from the instrument and leaving the outflow in the open position. Pressure generated by the fluid pump will generate sufficient flow to flush out the debris.

References

1. Kodde IF, van Rijn J, van den Bekerom MP, Eygendaal D. Surgical treatment of post-traumatic elbow stiffness: a systematic review. *J Shoulder Elbow Surg.* 2013;22(4):574-580.
2. Lindenhovius AL, Doornberg JN, Brouwer KM, Jupiter JB, Mudgal CS, Ring D. A prospective randomized controlled trial of dynamic versus static progressive elbow splinting for posttraumatic elbow stiffness. *J Bone Joint Surg Am.* 2012;94(8):694-700.
3. Singh H, Nam KY, Moon YL. Arthroscopic management of stiff elbow. *Orthopedics.* 2011;34(6):167.
4. Degreef I, De Smet L. Elbow arthrolysis for traumatic arthrofibrosis: a shift towards minimally invasive surgery. *Acta Orthop Belg.* 2011;77(6):758-764.
5. Morrey BF, Askew LJ, Chao EY. A biomechanical study of normal functional elbow motion. *J Bone Joint Surg Am.* 1981;63(6):872-877.
6. Gay DM, Raphael BS, Weiland AJ. Revision arthroscopic contracture release in the elbow resulting in an ulnar nerve transection: a case report. *J Bone Joint Surg Am.* 2010;92(5):1246-1249.
7. Dodson CC, Nho SJ, Williams RJ III, Altchek DW. Elbow arthroscopy. *J Am Acad Orthop Surg.* 2008;16(10):574-585.
8. Blonna D, Lee GC, O'Driscoll SW. Arthroscopic restoration of terminal elbow extension in high-level athletes. *Am J Sports Med.* 2010;38(12):2509-2515.
9. Miyake J, Shimada K, Oka K, et al. Arthroscopic debridement in the treatment of patients with osteoarthritis of the elbow, based on computer simulation. *Bone Joint J.* 2014;96(2):237-241.

10. Park JY, Cho CH, Choi JH, Lee ST, Kang CH. Radial nerve palsy after arthroscopic anterior capsular release for degenerative elbow contracture. *Arthroscopy.* 2007;23(12):1360.e1-1360.e3.
11. Cohen MS. Heterotopic ossification of the elbow. In: Jupiter J, ed. *The Stiff Elbow.* Rosemont, IL: American Academy of Orthopaedic Surgeons; 2006:31-40.
12. Heyd R, Strassmann G, Schopohl B, Zamboglou N. Radiation therapy for the prevention of heterotopic ossification at the elbow. *J Bone Joint Surg Br.* 2001;83(3):332-334.
13. Williams BG, Sotereanos DG, Baratz ME, Jarrett CD, Venouziou AI, Miller MC. The contracted elbow: is ulnar nerve release necessary? *J Shoulder Elbow Surg.* 2012;21(12):1632-1636.
14. Blonna D, O'Driscoll SW. Delayed-onset ulnar neuritis after release of elbow contracture: preventive strategies derived from a study of 563 cases. *Arthroscopy.* 2014;30(8):947-956.
15. Blonna D, Wolf JM, Fitzsimmons JS, O'Driscoll SW. Prevention of nerve injury during arthroscopic capsulectomy of the elbow utilizing a safety-driven strategy. *J Bone Joint Surg Am.* 2013;95(15):1373-1381.
16. Haapaniemi T, Berggren M, Adolfsson L. Complete transection of the median and radial nerves during arthroscopic release of post-traumatic elbow contracture. *Arthroscopy.* 1999;15(7):784-787.
17. Ruch DS, Poehling GG. Anterior interosseus nerve injury following elbow arthroscopy. *Arthroscopy.* 1997;13(6):756-758.
18. Jones GS, Savoie FH III. Arthroscopic capsular release of flexion contractures (arthrofibrosis) of the elbow. *Arthroscopy.* 1993;9(3):277-283.
19. Hahn M, Grossman JA. Ulnar nerve laceration as a result of elbow arthroscopy. *J Hand Surg Br.* 1998;23(1):109.
20. Omid R, Hamid N, Keener JD, Galatz LM, Yamaguchi K. Relation of the radial nerve to the anterior capsule of the elbow: anatomy with correlation to arthroscopy. *Arthroscopy.* 2012;28(12):1800-1804.

10

Degenerative Joint Disease of the Elbow

Arthroscopic Management

Scott P. Steinmann, MD and Brian Klika, MD

Introduction

Elbow arthroscopy has steadily gained popularity in the past 3 decades as clinical applications have expanded. Significant improvements in instrumentation and surgical technique have allowed it to become a safe and reproducible procedure. Previous indications have been limited to diagnostic arthroscopy and loose body removal, yet elbow arthroscopy has recently proved to be an essential tool in managing elbow arthritis, stiffness, trauma, and soft tissue pathology. An accurate history and physical examination are paramount in determining case selection, whereas many of the intraoperative positioning and surgical techniques outlined in this section remain essential in helping to provide safe and successful patient outcomes.

Indications

The indications for elbow arthroscopy are numerous. In the setting of arthritis, indications include extraction of loose bodies, debridement of osteoarthritis, synovectomy of rheumatoid arthritis, and contracture release.

Contraindications

Relative contraindications include submuscular or intramuscular transposition of the ulnar nerve. If these procedures have been performed previously, magnetic resonance imaging or ultrasound imaging of the ulnar nerve should be performed prior to arthroscopy to determine the exact location of the nerve. Instead of a standard portal on the medial side, a small incision is used to ensure that any exposure of the nerve is identified. Although not necessarily a contraindication, prior subcutaneous nerve transposition necessitates nerve path inspection via palpation, ultrasound, or exposure prior to incision.[1] Previous surgery, especially in the setting of an anterolateral

Savoie FH III, Field LD, Steinmann SP, eds. *The Elbow and Wrist: AANA Advanced Arthroscopic Surgical Techniques* (pp 93-98).

incision, may result in anatomical distortion and radial nerve scarring and tethering. In this situation, care should be taken in establishing all anterolateral portals.

Pertinent Physical Findings

On physical examination, inspection should include palpation of the ulnar nerve behind the medial epicondyle and posteromedial olecranon. The surgeon should examine for any subluxation of the ulnar nerve as the elbow is moved from extension to flexion. Elbow active range of motion (ROM) and passive ROM for flexion, extension, supination, and pronation should be performed and compared to the contralateral elbow. Lack of full elbow ROM may be secondary to a tight capsule or osteophytes. Painful clicking of the elbow may represent a plica that can be treated by arthroscopic resection. Stability testing with both varus and valgus forces in flexion and extension can identify any inherent medial or lateral elbow instability.[2]

Pertinent Imaging

Anteroposterior, lateral, and oblique x-rays are useful in determining whether joint degeneration, osteophytes, loose bodies, or previous fractures are present. Advanced degenerative and posttraumatic arthritis can best be characterized by computed tomography. Three-dimensional computerized reconstructions can further identify subchondral erosions or osteophytes and ultimately provide a roadmap for arthroscopic debridement.

Equipment

Arthroscopic equipment includes the standard shoulder arthroscopy equipment with a 30-degree, 4.5-mm arthroscope. Cannulas without trephinations are useful as trephinations can allow fluid to escape into soft tissues and limit working time due to swelling extravasation. A radiofrequency ablator is useful for bleeding control, capsular release, and synovectomy. Standard arthroscopic biters and graspers are useful, as are 4.5-mm burrs and shavers. Retractors, such as Howarth retractors, freer elevators, and blunt trocars, are helpful and can be used to gain visualization. This is preferred to using high flow, high pressure to gain a view as the elbow will quickly swell and eventually limit visualization.

Positioning and Portals

General anesthesia is preferred for optimal postoperative neurovascular evaluation. Block anesthesia can be used, but if a nerve injury occurs, it may be several hours or days later that the injury may be identified. Although lateral positioning is most effective, supine and prone positioning may also be used. The arm is secured in a dedicated arm holder (Figure 10-1) with the elbow positioned higher than the shoulder. Careful attention is made to ensure the holder is placed proximal enough to avoid pressure on the antecubital fossa while allowing full elbow flexion and extension to be maintained throughout the procedure.

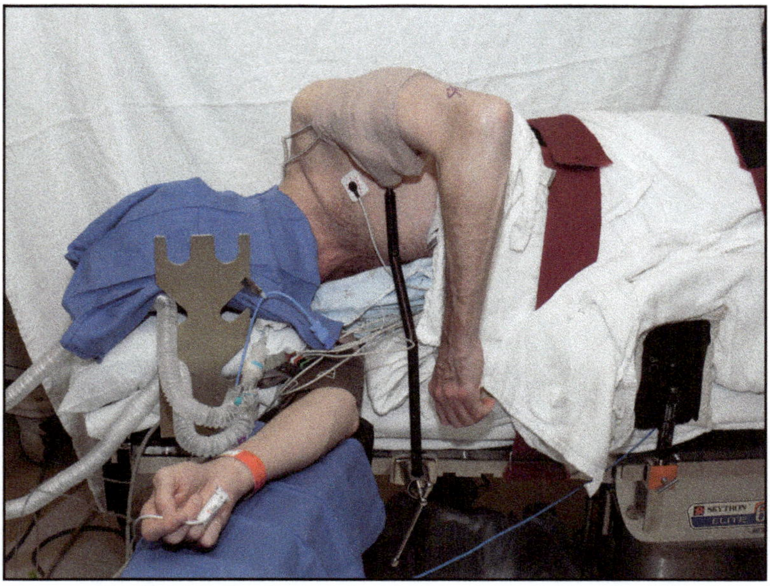

Figure 10-1. Patient placed in the lateral position with the arm placed in a low-profile elbow arm holder. The elbow should be placed higher than the body to limit arthroscope or shaver impingement against the body.

Step-by-Step Description of the Procedure

All bony and soft tissue landmarks, including the olecranon, radiocapitellar joint, medial epicondyle, and ulnar nerve, are marked out. The ulnar nerve should be palpated during flexion and extension of the elbow to be sure there is no subluxation. Standard portals, including the anteromedial, anterolateral, and direct posterior portals, are next marked out. Accessory portals, including the soft spot portal (direct lateral portal) and the distal ulnar portal, may also be marked and used for potential debridement of the posterior capitellum.

The tourniquet is inflated to 250 mm Hg after arm elevation. The joint is insufflated with normal saline (25 to 30 cc) via an 18-gauge needle and syringe through the direct lateral portal or direct posterior portal. Slight elbow extension following the injection confirms appropriate intra-articular insufflation. Following this, portals may be placed. An anteromedial or anterolateral portal is placed first. Preference depends on the surgeon. The authors prefer anterolateral placement first followed by anteromedial portal placement (Figure 10-2). The anterolateral portal is the closest portal to a major nerve (radial), and placement of this portal prior to any swelling of the joint when the surgical landmarks can be palpated is ideal.

The anterolateral portal is established just anterior to the radiocapitellar joint. The anterior aspect of the radiocapitellar joint is easily palpated prior to any swelling of the joint. Care should be made not to place the portal too distal as the posterior interosseous nerve may be at risk. Portals are placed with careful skin incision followed by blunt hemostat dissection down to the capsule to diminish cutaneous nerve injury. The anteromedial portal is approximately 1 to 2 cm distal and 1 to 2 cm anterior to the medial epicondyle. If the anterolateral portal is established first, the anteromedial portal can be made from an inside-out technique.

After medial and lateral portals are established, joint inspection can be performed. The coronoid process and fossa, as well as the anterior trochlea and radiocapitellar joint, are examined for articular cartilage lesions, osteophytes, or associated loose body pathology. The radial nerve is close to the anterolateral joint capsule; thus, debridement in this area requires caution. A fat pad is located just anterior to the radial head, and the radial nerve is located in this area. When this fat pad is visualized, further debridement should be stopped. If needed, proximal anterolateral or proximal anteromedial accessory portals may be established to assist in capsular retraction.

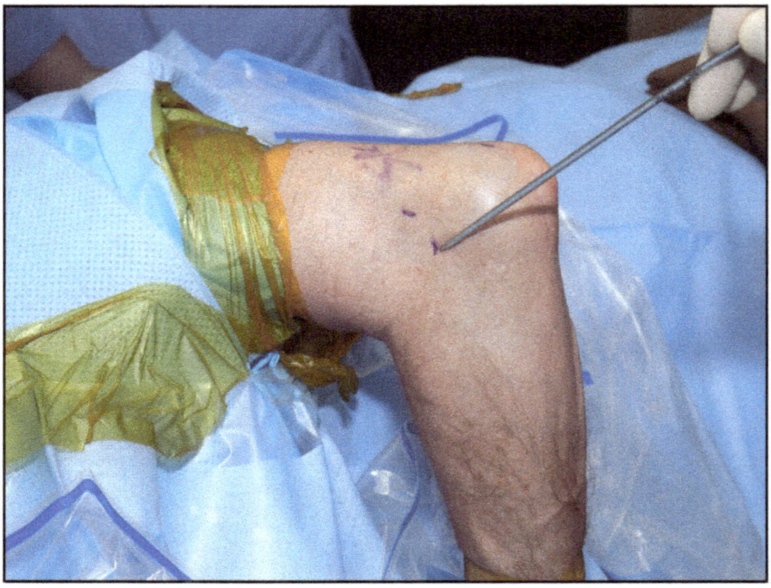

Figure 10-2. Anterolateral portal placed just anterior to the radiocapitellar joint.

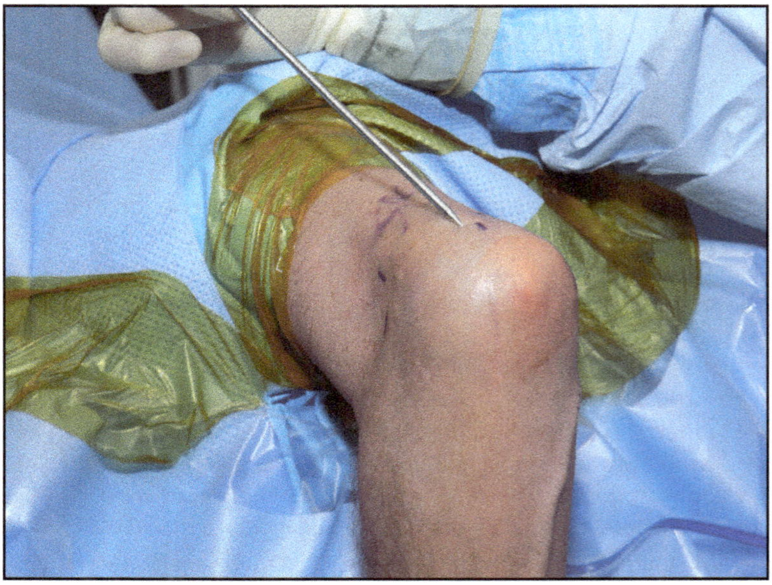

Figure 10-3. Direct posterior portal.

Following completion of the anterior arthroscopy, a direct posterior portal is established 2 to 3 cm directly proximal to the posterior olecranon (Figure 10-3). An incision is made through the skin and triceps and a blunt trochar may be used to create a viewing space. The posterolateral portal is made next and is a relatively safe portal considering its distance from any major nerve. The posterolateral portal is made level with the proximal edge of the olecranon near the lateral border of the triceps. It is an ideal viewing portal for the posterior aspect of the joint, with the direct posterior portal acting as the working portal. The olecranon fossa and medial and lateral gutters may all be successfully accessed from these 2 portals.

Postoperative Protocol

At the completion of the surgery, a compressive soft dressing is applied from wrist to mid-humerus. This is usually applied prior to letting the tourniquet down to limit bleeding into the joint. The dressing is left in place for 2 days postoperatively and is then removed as active motion is initiated. Splints can be used as an adjunct to stretch the elbow in flexion and extension.

Potential Complications

Published reports have identified injury to all major nerves about the elbow. The ulnar nerve is the most common major nerve involved followed by the radial nerve. Sensory cutaneous nerves can also be affected. Although most injuries are transient in nature, permanent nerve injury is a real and devastating complication.[3-16] In the setting of posttraumatic distorted anatomy or capsular thinning, such as in rheumatoid arthritis, the risk of nerve injury is higher.

Although heterotopic ossification may occur less frequently during arthroscopic treatment than open treatment, it can still occur. A short course of indomethacin postoperatively is recommended by some surgeons after an extensive debridement.

Elbow joint space infection is unusual following elbow arthroscopy; however, persistent portal drainage or fistulae formation is more common.[7]

Top Technical Pearls for the Procedure

1. A preoperative computed tomography scan is helpful for providing a roadmap for osteophyte excision and debridement.
2. Use of general anesthesia will allow for examination of median, ulnar, and radial nerve function immediately after surgery in the recovery room.
3. Joint insufflation prior to initial portal placement is important to allow for ease of joint access.
4. Use retractors to allow visualization instead of increased pump pressure, which can lead to overdistension of the joint
5. Compressive dressing and 2 days of rest to allow for resolution of edema prior to initiating early active and passive ROM.

References

1. Sahajpal DT, Blonna D, O'Driscoll SW. Anteromedial elbow arthroscopy portals in patients with prior ulnar nerve transposition or subluxation. *Arthroscopy.* 2010;26(8):1045-1052.
2. Cain EL Jr, Dugas JR, Wolf RS, Andrews JR. Elbow injuries in throwing athletes: a current concepts review. *Am J Sports Med.* 2003;31(4):621-635.
3. Steinmann SP. Elbow arthroscopy: where are we now? *Arthroscopy.* 2007;23(11):1231-1236.
4. Gay DM, Raphael BS, Weiland AJ. Revision arthroscopic contracture release in the elbow resulting in an ulnar nerve transection: a case report. *J Bone Joint Surg Am.* 2010;92(5):1246-1249.

5. Adams JE, Steinmann SP. Nerve injuries about the elbow. *J Hand Surg Am.* 2006;31(2):303-313.
6. Haapaniemi T, Berggren M, Adolfsson L. Complete transection of the median and radial nerves during arthroscopic release of posttraumatic elbow contracture. *Arthroscopy.* 1999;15(7):784-787.
7. Kelly EW, Morrey BF, O'Driscoll SW. Complications of elbow arthroscopy. *J Bone Joint Surg Am.* 2001;83(1):25-34.
8. Lynch GJ, Meyers JF, Whipple TL, Caspari RB. Neurovascular anatomy and elbow arthroscopy: inherent risks. *Arthroscopy.* 1986;2(3):190-197.
9. Marshall PD, Fairclough JA, Johnson SR, Evans EJ. Avoiding nerve damage during elbow arthroscopy. *J Bone Joint Surg Br.* 1993;75(1):129-131.
10. Miller CD, Jobe CM, Wright MH. Neuroanatomy in elbow arthroscopy. *J Shoulder Elbow Surg.* 1995;4(3):168-174.
11. O'Driscoll SW, Morrey BF. Arthroscopy of the elbow. Diagnostic and therapeutic benefits and hazards. *J Bone Joint Surg Am.* 1992;74(1):84-94.
12. Papilion JD, Neff RS, Shall LM. Compression neuropathy of the radial nerve as a complication of elbow arthroscopy: a case report and review of the literature. *Arthroscopy.* 1988;4(4):284-286.
13. Park JY, Cho CH, Choi JH, Lee ST, Kang CH. Radial nerve palsy after arthroscopic anterior capsular release for degenerative elbow contracture. *Arthroscopy.* 2007;23(12):1360.e1-1360.e3.
14. Ruch DS, Poehling GG. Anterior interosseus nerve injury following elbow arthroscopy. *Arthroscopy.* 1997;13(6):756-758.
15. Thomas MA, Fast A, Shapiro D. Radial nerve damage as a complication of elbow arthroscopy. *Clin Orthop Relat Res.* 1987;(215):130-131.
16. Verhaar J, van Mameren H, Brandsma A. Risks of neurovascular injury in elbow arthroscopy: starting anteromedially or anterolaterally? *Arthroscopy.* 1991;7(3):287-290.

Please see videos on the accompanying website at

www.routledge.com/9781630910013

11

Arthroscopic Synovectomy for Inflammatory Arthritis

Marc Prud'homme-Foster, MD, FRCSC and
Graham J. W. King, MD, MSc, FRCSC

Introduction

Arthroscopic elbow synovectomy is a well-established treatment for inflammatory synovitis by surgeons who have advanced technical skills in elbow arthroscopy. Synovectomy is advocated in patients with uncontrolled synovitis who remain symptomatic despite appropriate medical management. Although open synovectomy is still performed, several facets of arthroscopy make it appealing to surgeons and patients. An arthroscopic synovectomy is less invasive and can be conducted as an outpatient procedure with better postoperative pain control. Its smaller incisions allow more rapid recovery and earlier participation in rehabilitation with a lower risk of infection and wound complications. Finally, arthroscopy usually allows better visualization of intra-articular pathology. However, it remains a technically demanding procedure in this patient population and is associated with a higher risk of nerve injury than other routine arthroscopic procedures. Visualization can be challenging with decreased capsular volume, abundant synovitis, and thinning of the capsule, affording the surgeon less of a safeguard. Before performing arthroscopic synovectomy, one should be familiar with the indications, contraindications, and important technical considerations.

Indications

- Persistent synovitis in patients with inflammatory arthritis refractory to medical management, preserved articular cartilage, and mild deformity[1-5]
- Recurrent hemarthrosis with persistent synovitis after failed treatment with factor replacement for 3 to 6 months in patients with hemophilic arthritis[6-9]

Controversial Indications

- May be considered in younger patients with more deformity given concerns in this group about longevity of total elbow arthroplasty

Savoie FH III, Field LD, Steinmann SP, eds. *The Elbow and Wrist: AANA Advanced Arthroscopic Surgical Techniques* (pp 99-108).

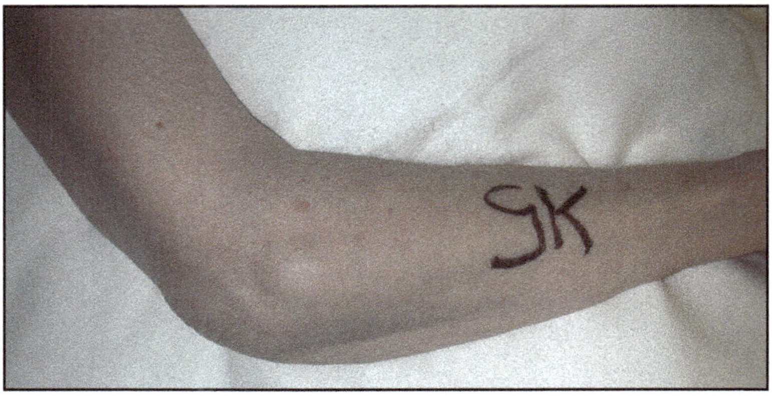

Figure 11-1. Lateral swelling indicative of extensive synovitis in a 65-year-old female with Mayo grade III rheumatoid arthritis of the right elbow.

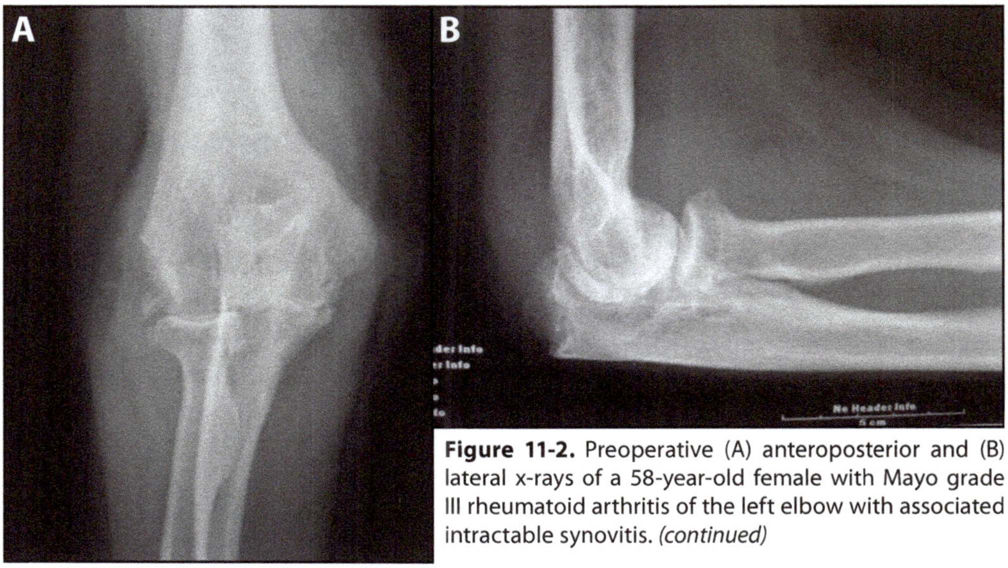

Figure 11-2. Preoperative (A) anteroposterior and (B) lateral x-rays of a 58-year-old female with Mayo grade III rheumatoid arthritis of the left elbow with associated intractable synovitis. *(continued)*

Pertinent Physical Findings

- Review of all joints to help identify joints involved
- Inspection of skin for lesions in psoriatic arthritis or sequelae of bleeding disorders
- Examination of the elbow for posterolateral swelling indicative of synovitis or effusion (Figure 11-1)
- Document range of motion (ROM) of elbow and forearm with goniometer and note if end points are soft or firm
- Rule out distal radioulnar joint involvement
- Neurovascular examination of major nerves crossing elbow joint
- Verification of ulnar nerve location and stability

Pertinent Imaging

- Plain radiographs to reveal the degree of joint destruction (Figures 11-2A and B)

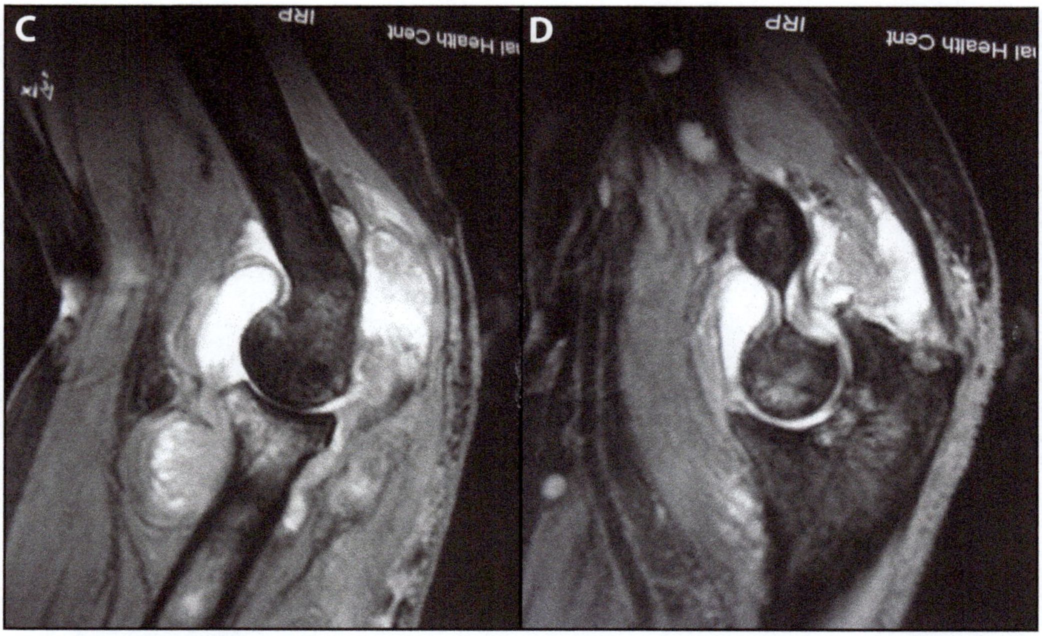

Figure 11-2 (continued). Preoperative sagittal magnetic resonance images of the (C) radiocapitellar and (D) ulnohumeral joints.

Table 11-1. Preoperative Radiographic and Pathological Changes

Grade	Description	Synovectomy Outcome
I	No radiographic changes other than periarticular osteopenia or soft tissue swelling	Good
II	Joint space narrowing	Good
III	Alteration of the subchondral architecture	Fair; reserved for young patients
IV	Gross joint destruction	Not recommended
V	Ankylosis	No role

- Mayo Clinic Classification of rheumatoid elbow[10] grades the severity of disease and can be useful in guiding treatment (Table 11-1)
- Computed tomography is useful to better define the osseous anatomy, including osteophytes and deformity of the radial head
- Magnetic resonance imaging is useful to determine the extent of synovitis and nonossified loose bodies (Figures 11-2C and D)

Equipment

- Arthroscope (4-mm, 30-degree with cannula and trocar)
- Cannulas and obturators (2 x 4.5-mm for scope and instruments, 5.5-mm outflow)

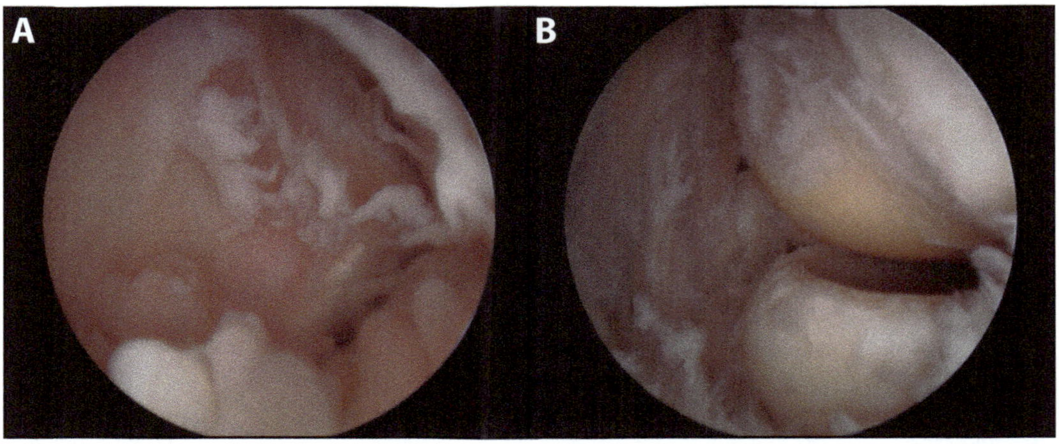

Figure 11-3. (A) Characteristic appearance of proliferative synovitis seen in inflammatory arthritis. (B) Improved visualization of the anterior radiocapitellar joint after synovectomy.

- Switching sticks with blunt and sharp tips
- Shaver (4.5-mm hooded with connection to cannula)
- Burr (5.5-mm hooded with connection to cannula)
- Pituitary rongeur for retrieval of loose bodies
- Howarth elevator for retraction
- Arm holder for positioning and sterile tourniquet maximum exposure
- Kelly forceps for establishing portals

Positioning and Portals

- Lateral decubitus position with the arm positioned over a well-padded support and axillary roll to protect the contralateral arm

Step-by-Step Description of the Procedure

General anesthesia is typically used. In patients with more severe stiffness, a continuous brachial plexus block is useful for postoperative pain control and to allow early mobilization. The authors prefer a lateral decubitus position with the arm positioned over a well-padded support. Standard elbow arthroscopic equipment and portals are used. Gravity inflow is used to maintain low inflow pressures to avoid excessive joint swelling. A 4.0-mm arthroscope is used for visualization and a 4.5-mm hooded shaver blade is used for the synovectomy. Avoiding more aggressive shavers and opening the outflow to the floor rather than to suction will help preserve the integrity of the capsule, thereby reducing the risk of nerve injury. Retractors can be used to retract the joint capsule or muscles if needed to improve visualization.

The extensive synovitis often makes the initial view very poor (Figure 11-3). The shaver should not be turned on until it is confirmed that the instruments are within the joint. The joint synovium is removed with the shaver while preserving the joint capsule. Visualization improves with the removal of synovium and the surgeon should proceed cautiously until a good view is obtained. The capsule is typically very thin in rheumatoid elbows, making it particularly easy to

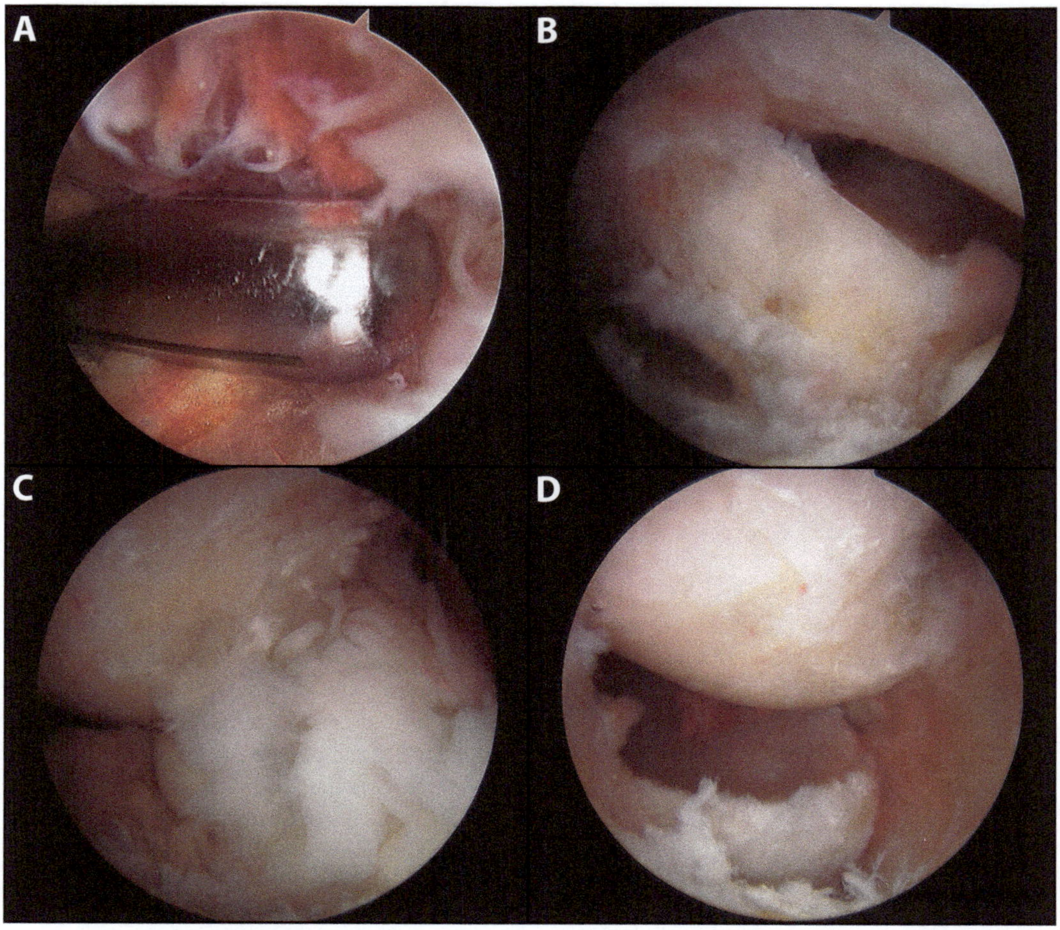

Figure 11-4. A 57-year-old female with Mayo grade III rheumatoid arthritis of the left elbow with associated intractable synovitis. (A) Initial view of the anterior joint from the proximal anterolateral portal reveals extensive synovitis. (B) View of the coronoid after anterior synovectomy. (C) Synovitis of the radiocapitellar joint while viewing from the proximal anteromedial portal. (D) View of the radiocapitellar joint after anterior synovectomy. *(continued)*

inadvertently penetrate or resect. Keep the tip of the shaver in view at all times and pointed away from the capsule. Use caution when removing synovium anterior to the radial head in the region of the posterior interosseous nerve and in the posteromedial gutter near the ulnar nerve.

The authors prefer to start the synovectomy in the anterior compartment (Figures 11-4A to D). The proximal anterolateral portal is the viewing portal and the proximal anteromedial portal is the working portal. A direct posterior portal is used as an outflow portal with a drainage cannula. The viewing and working portals are exchanged using a switching stick in order to complete the anterior synovectomy. If the view is insufficient, a mid-anterolateral or mid-anteromedial portal can be established, and a retractor (typically a Howarth elevator) is inserted to retract the capsule. Bone resection, if required, can be performed using the shaver alone or using a hooded arthroscopic burr. The posterior synovectomy is performed next, starting with a direct posterior viewing portal and a mid-posterolateral working portal. Debridement of the olecranon fossa with direct visualization of the shaver is performed first to establish a working space. A hooded burr should be used to remove osteophytes in the fossa and on the olecranon. Care is taken in the area of the medial recess due to the risk of injury to the ulnar nerve. The lateral compartment can be addressed by viewing from the mid-posterolateral portal and working through a mid-posterolateral (soft spot)

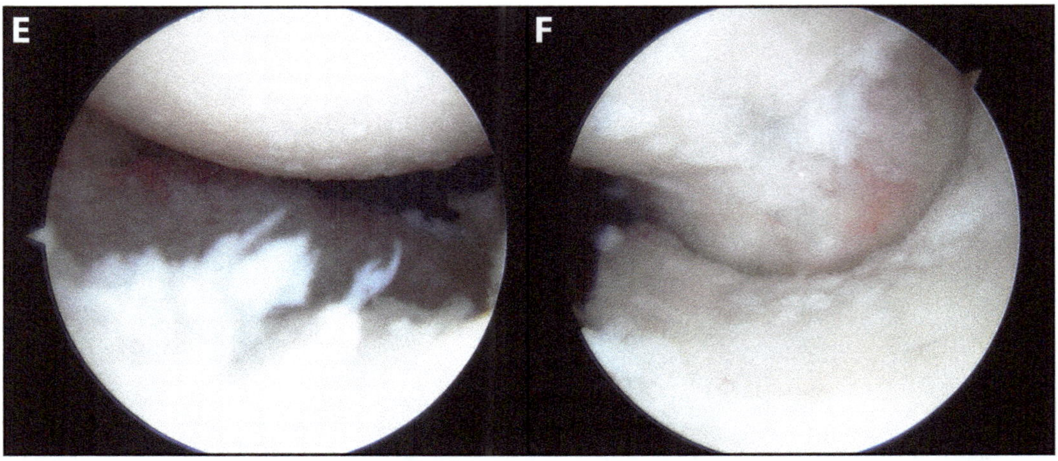

Figure 11-4 (continued). A 57-year-old female with with Mayo grade III rheumatoid arthritis of the left elbow with associated intractable synovitis. View of the (E) radiocapitellar and (F) ulnohumeral joints from the midlateral portal after synovectomy.

portal and vice versa (Figures 11-4E and F). Occasionally, a more distal posterolateral portal is needed for the synovectomy around the radial neck and for addressing bone deformities in the posterior radiocapitellar joint.[11]

Radial head excision should generally be reserved for patients with a stable elbow and a radial head deformity impeding rotation. Capsulectomy may be indicated in some cases and can also be performed arthroscopically concomitant with the synovectomy. An anterior or posterior capsulectomy is performed if there is significant restriction of elbow flexion or extension and the patient desires improved motion. The capsule directly anterior to the radiocapitellar joint should be preserved to reduce the risk of injury to the posterior interosseous nerve.

At the conclusion of the procedure, portal sites are sutured to prevent the formation of synovial fistulas. A bulky dressing is applied for comfort and to allow early elbow ROM.

Postoperative Protocol

Postoperative management depends on the extent of the surgery. Synovectomy alone is usually an outpatient procedure managed postoperatively with early active ROM. The bulky dressing is removed by the patient 48 hours postoperatively, and adhesive dressings are applied to the portal sites. Sutures are removed at 10 days and physical therapy is initiated if motion recovery is slow. If combined with a significant osseous debridement or capsulectomy, patients are admitted for 48 hours and placed in a continuous passive motion machine with a continuous brachial plexus block for postoperative analgesia. In these latter patients, a night-time static progressive extension splint for 12 weeks can be useful to retain extension.

Potential Complications

Open elbow synovectomy, with or without radial head excision, is an effective treatment for the rheumatoid elbow.[12-27] The best results are obtained in patients with some preserved articular cartilage and mild bony deformity (corresponding to grades I, II, and early III involvement).[28] Results vary, but studies indicate that 70% to 90% are considered to have satisfactory outcomes within the first 3 to 5 years, with these improvements deteriorating with time.[28] There is no evidence that open synovectomy arrests the progress of the disease process; however, further studies are needed using more potent disease remitative agents.

Current literature provides limited information about the results of arthroscopic synovectomy for rheumatoid arthritis and even less information for other conditions. Arthroscopic synovectomy offers theoretical advantages of being less invasive, which speeds recovery, limits postoperative pain, and allows the surgeon to better visualize and address intra-articular pathology in all areas of the elbow. Although there are no published randomized, clinical trials comparing the relative efficacy and risk of open vs arthroscopic synovectomy, reports in the literature suggest that the outcomes of arthroscopic synovectomy are comparable to open synovectomy (Table 11-2). As with open synovectomy, results deteriorate with time[1,2,4] and are dependent on the severity of arthritis, with better results expected in elbows without significant osseous destruction and some preserved articular cartilage.[1,2]

In 1997, Lee and Morrey[1] reported 93% good to excellent results initially; however, these results had deteriorated to 57% by 42 months postoperatively. In 2001, Horiuchi et al[2] reported 71% good to excellent results at 2 years, which deteriorated to 43% by 8 years. However, if elbows with advanced cartilage loss and bony deformity were excluded, the results were 100% and 71% good or excellent results at 2 and 8 years, respectively. Patients maintained on concomitant disease-modifying agents had a lower incidence of recurrent synovitis and a better long-term outcome. In 2006, Tanaka et al[4] reported on a prospective comparative study of arthroscopic vs open synovectomy with 23 elbows in each group. At a mean follow-up of 10 years, 48% of those treated arthroscopically and 70% of those treated openly had minimal or no pain. There were no significant differences found between the groups with respect to pain, function, or ROM. Improvements in each of these outcomes deteriorated with time. A subgroup of patients with a preoperative flexion arc of less than 90 degrees had significantly better function when treated arthroscopically vs openly.

Less is known about the results of arthroscopic synovectomy for hemophilic arthropathy of the elbow. Although studies are limited to small numbers and often combine results of synovectomy of other joints, there is evidence that arthroscopic synovectomy decreases the rate of recurrent hemarthrosis.[6-9,29]

Transient nerve paresthesias, recurrent synovitis, and persistent pain requiring repeated synovectomy or total elbow arthroplasty have been reported as complications of arthroscopic synovectomy.[1-4,30]

Top Technical Pearls for the Procedure

1. Use a 20-cc syringe of irrigating solution with a large-gauge needle to expand the joint capsule by injecting the posterior fossa.
2. Avoid debriding the capsule directly anterior to the radiocapitellar joint to minimize the risk of injury to the radial nerve and its branches.
3. Use switching sticks and cannulas to maintain the portals.
4. Establish an auxiliary portal for use of a Howarth or switching stick to serve as a retractor when required.
5. When ulnar nerve decompression is required, perform at the beginning of the procedure to minimize the risk of injury.

Table 11-2. Results of Arthroscopic Synovectomy

Study	No. of Elbows	Mean Age, y	Mean Follow-Up, mo	Results	Complications
Lee and Morrey[1]	14	N/A (<65)	42 (24 to 84)	Pain and function (MEPS) improved, but improvement decreased over time. Flexion and rotation improved slightly.	One radial and 1 transient ulnar nerve paresthesias; 4 patients converted to total elbow arthroplasty
Horiuchi et al[2]	21	51 (19 to 71)	97 (42 to 160)	Pain and function (MEPS) improved, but improvement decreased over time. Flexion improved, no change in rotation. Joint arthritic damage increased over time. Best results were in patients with preserved joint space and those on disease-modifying antirheumatic drugs.	Three transient ulnar nerve paresthesias 5 with recurrent synovitis, 2 of which went on to total elbow arthroplasty
Nemoto et al[3]	11	54 (38 to 68)	37 (15 to 39)	Pain and function improved. Flexion improved, no change in rotation. Joint arthritic damage increased over time.	One repeat synovectomy
Tanaka et al[4]	23	51 (31 to 64)	156 (120 to 216)	Pain and function improved, but improvement decreased over time. Flexion and rotation improved. Joint arthritic damage increased over time.	Transient neuropraxia of the radial nerve in 1 and ulnar nerve in 1; 5 with recurrent synovitis

MEPS, Mayo Elbow Performance Score.

References

1. Lee BP, Morrey BF. Arthroscopic synovectomy of the elbow for rheumatoid arthritis. A prospective study. *J Bone Joint Surg Br.* 1997;79(5):770-772.
2. Horiuchi K, Momohara S, Tomatsu T, Inoue K, Toyama Y. Arthroscopic synovectomy of the elbow in rheumatoid arthritis. *J Bone Joint Surg Am.* 2002;84(3):342-347.
3. Nemoto K, Arino H, Yoshihara Y, Fujikawa K. Arthroscopic synovectomy for the rheumatoid elbow: a short-term outcome. *J Shoulder Elbow Surg.* 2004;13(6):652-655.
4. Tanaka N, Sakahashi H, Hirose K, Ishima T, Ishii S. Arthroscopic and open synovectomy of the elbow in rheumatoid arthritis. *J Bone Joint Surg Am.* 2006;88(3):521-525.
5. Jerosch J, Hoffstetter I, Schröder M, Castro WH. Septic arthritis: arthroscopic management with local antibiotic treatment. *Acta Orthop Belg.* 1995;61(2):126-134.
6. Dunn AL, Busch MT, Wyly JB, Sullivan KM, Abshire TC. Arthroscopic synovectomy for hemophilic joint disease in a pediatric population. *J Pediatr Orthop.* 2004;24(4):414-426.
7. Tamurian RM, Spencer EE, Wojtys EM. The role of arthroscopic synovectomy in the management of hemarthrosis in hemophilia patients: financial perspectives. *Arthroscopy.* 2002;18(7):789-794.
8. Journeycake JM, Miller KL, Anderson AM, Buchanan GR, Finnegan M. Arthroscopic synovectomy in children and adolescents with hemophilia. *J Pediatr Hematol Oncol.* 2003;25(9):726-731.
9. Verma N, Valentino LA, Chawla A. Arthroscopic synovectomy in haemophilia: indications, technique and results. *Haemophilia.* 2007;13(suppl 3):38-44.
10. Morrey BF, Adams RA. Semiconstrained arthroplasty for the treatment of rheumatoid arthritis of the elbow. *J Bone Joint Surg Am.* 1992;74(4):479-490.
11. van den Ende KI, McIntosh AL, Adams JE, Steinmann SP. Osteochondritis dissecans of the capitellum: a review of the literature and a distal ulnar portal. *Arthroscopy.* 2011;27(1):122-128.
12. Woods DA, Williams JR, Gendi NS, Mowat AG, Burge PD, Carr AJ. Surgery for rheumatoid arthritis of the elbow: a comparison of radial-head excision and synovectomy with total elbow replacement. *J Shoulder Elbow Surg.* 1999;8(4):291-295.
13. Gendi NS, Axon JM, Carr AJ, Pile KD, Burge PD, Mowat AG. Synovectomy of the elbow and radial head excision in rheumatoid arthritis. Predictive factors and long-term outcome. *J Bone Joint Surg Br.* 1997;79(6):918-923.
14. Lonner JH, Stuchin SA. Synovectomy, radial head excision, and anterior capsular release in stage III inflammatory arthritis of the elbow. *J Hand Surg Am.* 1997;22(2):279-285.
15. Ferlic DC, Patchett CE, Clayton ML, Freemand AC. Elbow synovectomy in rheumatoid arthritis. Long-term results. *Clin Orthop Relat Res.* 1987;(220):119-125.
16. Mäenpää HM, Kuusela PP, Kaarela K, Kautiainen HJ, Lehtinen JT, Belt EA. Reoperation rate after elbow synovectomy in rheumatoid arthritis. *J Shoulder Elbow Surg.* 2003;12(5):480-483.
17. Makai F, Chudacek J. Long-term results of synovectomy of the elbow with excision of the radial head in rheumatoid arthritis. In: Hamalainen M, Hagena FW, eds. *Rheumatoid Surgery of the Elbow.* Vol 15. Basel, Switzerland: Karger; 1991:22-26.
18. Tulp NJ, Winia WP. Synovectomy of the elbow in rheumatoid arthritis. Long-term results. *J Bone Joint Surg Br.* 1989;71(4):664-666.
19. Taylor AR, Mukerjea SK, Rana NA. Excision of the head of the radius in rheumatoid arthritis. *J Bone Joint Surg Br.* 1976;58(4):485-487.
20. Rymaszewski LA, Mackay I, Amis AA, Miller JH. Long-term effects of excision of the radial head in rheumatoid arthritis. *J Bone Joint Surg Br.* 1984;66(1):109-113.
21. Wilson HDW, Arden GP, Ansell BM. Synovectomy of the elbow in rheumatoid arthritis. *J Bone Joint Surg Br.* 1973;55(1):106-111.
22. Eichenblat M, Hass A, and Kessler I. Synovectomy of the elbow in rheumatoid arthritis. *J Bone Joint Surg Am.* 1982;64(7):1074-1078.
23. Brumfield RH Jr, Resnick CT. Synovectomy of the elbow in rheumatoid arthritis. *J Bone Joint Surg Am.* 1985;67(1):16-20.
24. Herold N, Schrøder HA. Synovectomy and radial head excision in rheumatoid arthritis. 11 patients followed for 14 years. *Acta Orthop Scand.* 1995;66(3):252-254.
25. Rodríguez-Merchán EC, Magallón M, Galindo E, López-Cabarcos C. Hemophilic synovitis of the knee and the elbow. *Clin Orthop Relat Res.* 1997;(343):47-53.

26. Linclau LA, Winia WP, Korst JK. Synovectomy of the elbow in rheumatoid arthritis. *Acta Orthop Scand.* 1983;54(6):935-937.
27. Saito T, Koshino T, Okamoto R, Horiuchi S. Radical synovectomy with muscle release for the rheumatoid elbow. *Acta Orthop Scand.* 1986;57(1):71-73.
28. Lee BPH, Morrey BF. Synovectomy of the elbow. In: Morrey BF, ed. *The Elbow and Its Disorders.* 3rd ed. Philadelphia, PA: Saunders; 2000:708-717.
29. van den Ende KI, Steinmann SP. Arthroscopic treatment of septic arthritis of the elbow. *J Shoulder Elbow Surg.* 2012;21(8):1001-1005.
30. Kelly EW, Morrey BF, O'Driscoll SW. Complications of elbow arthroscopy. *J Bone Joint Surg Am.* 2001;83(1):25-34.

Please see videos on the accompanying website at
www.routledge.com/9781630910013

12

Arthroscopic Radial Head Resection and Open Radial Head Replacement

William Desloges, MD, FRCSC and Graham J. W. King, MD, MSc, FRCSC

Introduction

A comprehensive understanding of the role and function of the radial head is required when treating patients with radial head pathology. Biomechanically, the radial head is an important elbow stabilizer, especially in the setting of valgus instability secondary to medial collateral ligament (MCL) insufficiency. Furthermore, the radial head tensions the lateral collateral ligament (LCL) and posterolateral rotatory instability has been reported following radial head excision.[1-4] Using an in vitro forearm testing system, it was demonstrated that resection of the radial head nearly doubles the tension in the interosseous membrane.[5] Therefore, the common finding of proximal migration of the radius following radial head resection reflects the role of the radial head in the axial stability of the forearm, especially in the presence of an incompetent interosseous membrane.[6-10] Significant loads are carried across the radiocapitellar joint,[11] and excision of the radial head accelerates ulnohumeral wear secondary to the compensatory loads it must face.

Surgical treatment options for symptomatic degenerative or posttraumatic conditions of the radial head include open or arthroscopic synovectomy and debridement of the radial head, open or arthroscopic radial head resection, radial head replacement, unicompartmental radiocapitellar arthroplasty, or total elbow arthroplasty. In selecting the best treatment option, one must take into account patient factors, such as age and comorbidities, ulnohumeral joint involvement, collateral ligament integrity, and the status of the interosseous membrane. In the event that radial head resection is deemed the most appropriate treatment, arthroscopy is a useful means of excising the radial head. Although arthroscopic radial head excision has not been shown in the literature to be superior to open techniques, it offers the potential advantage of minimizing soft tissue dissection, which may reduce postoperative pain and stiffness. The improved intra-articular visualization with arthroscopy also allows concomitant pathologies to be addressed. Replacement of the radial head should be considered in the setting of a capitellum, which has relatively normal articular cartilage to prevent the late complications of radial resection, including long-term overload of the MCL with secondary valgus instability, posterolateral rotatory instability, proximal migration of the radius leading to ulnar impaction syndrome at the wrist, and ulnohumeral arthritis.[12,13]

Savoie FH III, Field LD, Steinmann SP, eds. *The Elbow and Wrist: AANA Advanced Arthroscopic Surgical Techniques* (pp 109-125).

Indications

Arthroscopic radial head resection is indicated for the following:

- Proximal radius articular deformity or arthritis resulting in pain and/or loss of motion in the presence of competent elbow collateral ligaments and an intact forearm interosseous membrane
- Rheumatoid arthritis[14-17] and posttraumatic arthritis[14-18] because capitellar disease often precludes treatment with radial head replacement
- Chronic hemophilic synovitis resulting in enlargement and irregularity of the radial head may also be treated with arthroscopic synovectomy and radial head resection, although reports in the literature are limited to open techniques.
- Selected patients with congenital or acquired radial head dislocations with symptoms refractory to nonoperative modalities may be candidates. Elbow arthroscopy may be relatively contraindicated in severe cases due to the distortion of anatomy.

Radial Head Replacement

- Most nonreconstructable radial head fractures warrant radial head replacement rather than excision because the incidence of concomitant injury to the interosseous membrane of the forearm or the collateral ligaments of the elbow is greater than 75% in the setting of comminuted radial head fractures.[19,20]
- Management of failed internal fixation, malunions, nonunions, or failed radial head resection, particularly in the presence of elbow or forearm instability
- Reasonable preservation of capitellar cartilage and alignment of the proximal radius with the capitellum are prerequisites for successful radial head replacement.

Pertinent Physical Findings

Following a thorough history, documenting pain, stiffness, mechanical symptoms, history of trauma, and prior surgical procedures, a detailed physical examination should be performed.

- Inspection of the bony contours of the elbow, the carrying angle, and documenting prior traumatic or surgical scars is performed.
- A goniometer is then used to obtain accurate measurements of elbow and forearm range of motion (ROM). Motion lost can be attributable to osseous or soft tissue deformities.
- In most cases, osseous impingement results in a firm end point. For example, in hemophilic arthropathy, although radial head dysmorphism often results in loss of motion, the hypertrophic and highly vascular synovial tissue can become impinged between the articular surfaces, producing loss of motion and a soft end point.[21]
- Elbow and forearm stability should be examined carefully because radial head excision is contraindicated in the setting of axial instability of the forearm and valgus or posterolateral rotatory instability of the elbow.
- Valgus instability, which suggests MCL insufficiency, can be detected using valgus stress testing,[22,23] the milking maneuver,[24] and the moving valgus stress test.[25]
- The pivot shift test,[1] the posterolateral drawer test,[26] the hypersupination test, and the supine and seated push-up tests[27,28] are used to detect posterolateral rotatory instability, which suggests lateral ulnar collateral ligament insufficiency.

- Longitudinal radioulnar instability is difficult to determine on physical examination and is easily missed. In the setting of an acute injury, pain to palpation at the mid-dorsal forearm, the distal radioulnar joint (DRUJ), and/or the fovea may indicate forearm axial instability.[29]
- Prominence of the ulnar head, DRUJ instability, wrist motion abnormalities, and weakness in grip strength may be seen with chronic radioulnar instability.

The location and function of the ulnar nerve should be documented, especially in preparation to perform an elbow arthroscopy. In the presence of a subluxating ulnar nerve or of a previous ulnar nerve subcutaneous transposition, open placement of medial portals is recommended in an effort to prevent iatrogenic nerve injury.

Pertinent Imaging

- Proximal radial deformity or arthritis can usually be visualized on plain x-rays with anteroposterior (AP), lateral, and radiocapitellar views.[30,31]
- In preparation for a radial head replacement in the setting of previous radial head excision or comminuted radial head fracture, contralateral elbow views should be performed to assist with implant sizing and templating.
- Bilateral wrist views are helpful to rule out conditions that may contribute to loss in forearm rotation, such as DRUJ pathology and radioulnar synostosis.
- Wrist views, including posteroanterior, lateral, and grip-loaded pronation posteroanterior views, may help identify static and/or dynamic ulnar-positive variance and DRUJ widening in the setting of longitudinal radioulnar dissociation.[29]
- Elbow stress views or a fluoroscopic examination to rule out valgus, varus, and axial instability should be considered when instability is suspected on clinical examination.
- When longitudinal radioulnar dissociation is suspected and x-rays are nondiagnostic, magnetic resonance imaging and ultrasound may be helpful in making the diagnosis.[32-36]
- Concomitant collateral ligament injuries can be identified using magnetic resonance imaging.[37]
- The articular congruity and joint space of the ulnohumeral, radiohumeral, and proximal radioulnar joints are best visualized using computed tomography scan.
- Furthermore, bony deformities, loose bodies, osteophytes, and heterotopic ossification can be defined more accurately and help to formulate the surgical plan.

Equipment for Arthroscopic Radial Head Resection

Elbow Arthroscopy

- Standard 4.0-mm, 30-degree offset arthroscope
- Arthroscope sheath with dull trocar
- Camera
- Light cord
- 18-gauge spinal needle along with a 20-cc, saline-filled syringe
- Hemostat

Figure 12-1. Recommended setup with the patient held in the lateral decubitus position using a bean bag with the arm on a bolster. An axillary roll is placed caudad to the axilla to prevent pressure on the contralateral brachial plexus. Careful padding of the contralateral ulnar nerve is ensured.

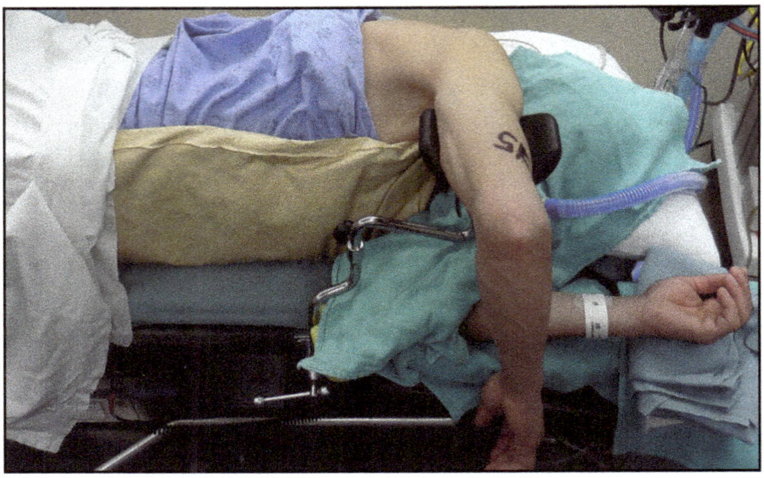

- Switching rods
- Inflow tubing
- Cannulas

Basic Instruments

- Diagnostic hook
- Standard mechanical shaver and a full-radius resector and burr attachments
- Curved and straight arthroscopic retractors
- Hand biters
- Pituitary graspers
- Osteotomes
- Bipolar electrocautery device

Positioning and Portals for Arthroscopic Radial Head Resection

General anesthesia is typically preferred. To assist with postoperative pain management and to initiate early motion, brachial plexus blockade with an indwelling catheter is useful. Although elbow arthroscopy has been described in the supine and prone positions, the authors prefer the lateral decubitus position with the arm positioned over a well-padded bolster (Figure 12-1). An axillary roll is placed caudad to the axilla to prevent pressure on the contralateral brachial plexus.

Step-by-Step Description of Arthroscopic Radial Head Resection

Use fluoroscopy to re-evaluate the stability of the elbow and forearm prior to proceeding with radial head excision. Apply a sterile tourniquet to the proximal arm and inflate it. Verify and mark the location of the ulnar nerve. Distend the joint with saline using an 18-gauge needle inserted through the location of the direct posterior portal into the olecranon fossa. After making a small skin incision, use a hemostat to enter the joint through the proximal anteromedial portal. Insert the arthroscope. Use gravity inflow or a pump on low pressure to avoid excessive joint swelling. Insert a drainage cannula in the posterior central portal for outflow. Under direct visualization, establish a mid-anterolateral portal using the inside-out or outside-in technique. Often, the initial view is poor due to extensive synovitis. Perform a careful synovectomy using a full-radius resector until adequate visualization of the radial head is obtained. Take care to preserve the anterolateral capsule due to the proximity of the posterior interosseous nerve (PIN). Evaluate the entire elbow anteriorly, posteriorly, and laterally to identify and manage cartilage defects, synovitis, osteophytic bony impingement, loose bodies, and capsular contracture.

Resect the radial head starting anteriorly and working posteriorly using a motorized burr in the mid-anterolateral portal. Ensure the cutting surface of the burr faces posteriorly at all times to avoid injury to the PIN. Place a retractor as required through a proximal anterolateral portal to facilitate visualization and further protect the PIN. The radial head should be resected to the level of the radial neck just distal to the sigmoid notch of the ulna to avoid impingement during forearm rotation. The annular ligament should be retained given its important contribution to varus and posterolateral rotatory elbow stability. Complete the posterior resection of the radial head using a burr placed through the posterolateral soft spot portal while maintaining the arthroscope in the proximal anteromedial portal (Figure 12-2). Remove residual cartilage fragments and debris using a full-radius resector and pituitary rongeur. Use an image intensifier to confirm an adequate radial head resection. Rotate the forearm under direct arthroscopic visualization to rule out mechanical blocks to rotation and ensure smooth tracking of the proximal radius. After removing the arthroscope, recheck elbow and forearm stability using an image intensifier. The radius pull test has been shown to be useful in detecting axial forearm instability after radial head resection. Three millimeters or more of proximal radial migration upon applying longitudinal traction on the proximal part of the radius is indicative of disruption of the interosseous membrane.[38] The steps of this procedure are summarized in Table 12-1.

Postoperative Protocol for Arthroscopic Radial Head Resection

Patients are usually discharged home on the same day of the operation, and active ROM as tolerated is encouraged (Figure 12-3). Patients who underwent concomitant contracture releases are admitted for a continuous brachial plexus block to allow for continuous passive motion for the first few days postoperatively. To reduce the incidence of heterotopic ossification, indomethacin 25 mg 3 times daily is administered for a duration of 3 weeks unless contraindicated.[39]

Potential Complications of Arthroscopic Radial Head Resection

The complications encountered with arthroscopic radial head resection are similar to the reported complications with open resection and include valgus instability, proximal radial migration, DRUJ symptoms, posterolateral rotatory instability, proximal radioulnar impingement, ulnohumeral degenerative osteoarthritis, heterotopic ossification, and nerve injury.[4,12,13] However, elbow arthroscopy is technically challenging, and the risk of neurovascular injury may be increased in the hands of an inexperienced surgeon, especially in the setting of inflammatory arthritis.[40] Careful portal placement and the use of retractors can minimize the risk of neurovascular injury.

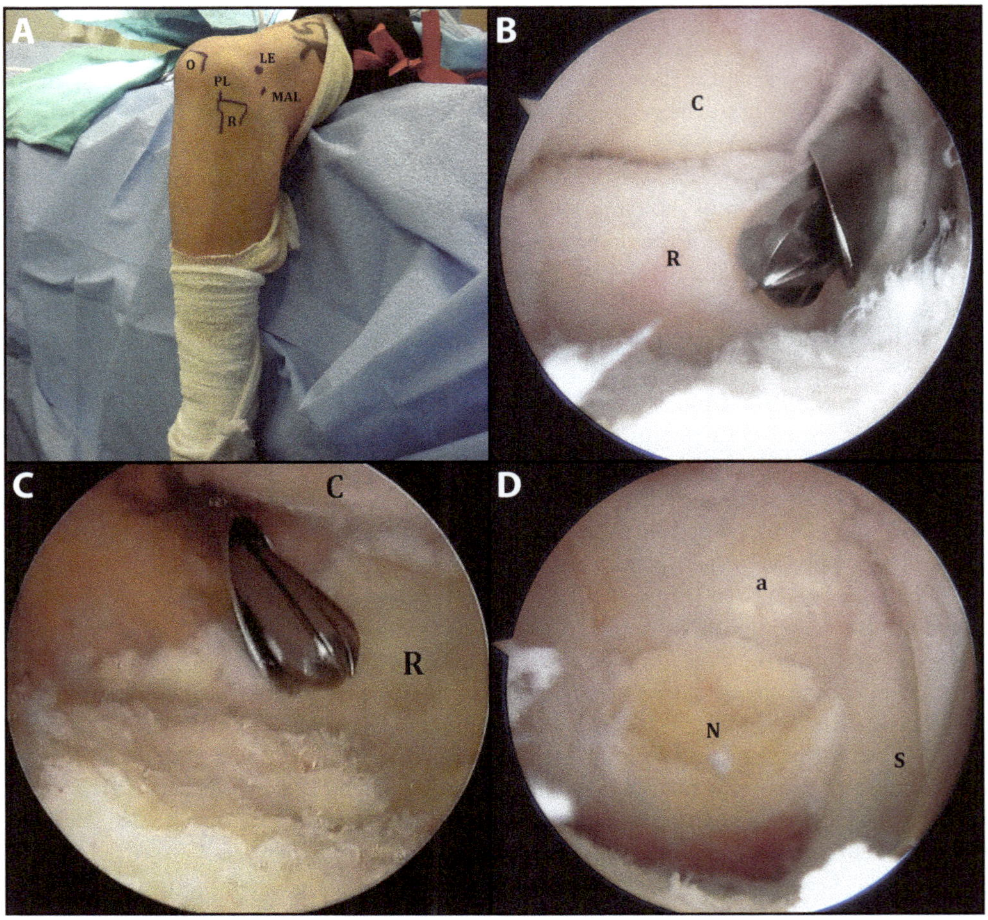

Figure 12-2. (A) Surgical setup with skin markings depicting anatomical landmarks, including the mid-anterolateral (MAL) portal and the posterolateral soft spot portal (PL). (B) Radial resection is initiated using a motorized burr in the mid-anterolateral portal. (C) While maintaining the arthroscope in the proximal anteromedial portal, resection of the posterior aspect of the radial head is completed by positioning the burr through the posterolateral soft spot portal. (D) Arthroscopic view from the mid-posterolateral portal of a completed radial head resection. The radial head should be resected to the level of the radial neck (N) just distal to the sigmoid notch(s). Abbreviations: a, annular ligament; C, capitellum; LE, lateral epicondyle; O, olecranon; R, radial head.

Results

Arthroscopic radial head resection is a relatively novel technique and, therefore, current understanding of its outcome is mostly extrapolated from the results of open radial head resection. Few studies in the literature look at the outcomes of arthroscopic radial head resection.[41-44] No studies compare the outcomes of open vs arthroscopic radial head resection.

Menth-Chiari et al[42] performed arthroscopic radial head excision for chronic mechanical pain in the presence of radiocapitellar arthritis in 10 patients with posttraumatic arthritis and 2 patients with rheumatoid arthritis. At a mean follow-up of 39 months, 11 of the 12 patients were satisfied with improved pain with motion and decreased mechanical symptoms. ROM improved in all patients. Although 2 patients were found to have 2 and 3 mm of proximal radial migration, no patient had elbow instability.

Table 12-1. Arthroscopic Radial Head Resection: Step-by-Step Procedure Summary

1. Use fluoroscopy to re-evaluate the stability of the elbow and forearm prior to proceeding with radial head excision.
2. Use the anteromedial portal as your viewing portal.
3. Establish a mid-anterolateral portal using the inside-out or outside-in technique.
4. Perform a careful synovectomy using a full-radius resector until adequate visualization of the radial head is obtained.
5. Resect the radial head starting anteriorly and working posteriorly using a motorized burr in the mid-anterolateral portal.
6. Complete the posterior resection of the radial head using a burr placed through the posterolateral soft spot portal while maintaining the arthroscope in the proximal anteromedial portal.
7. Use an image intensifier to confirm an adequate radial head resection.
8. Confirm elbow and forearm stability.

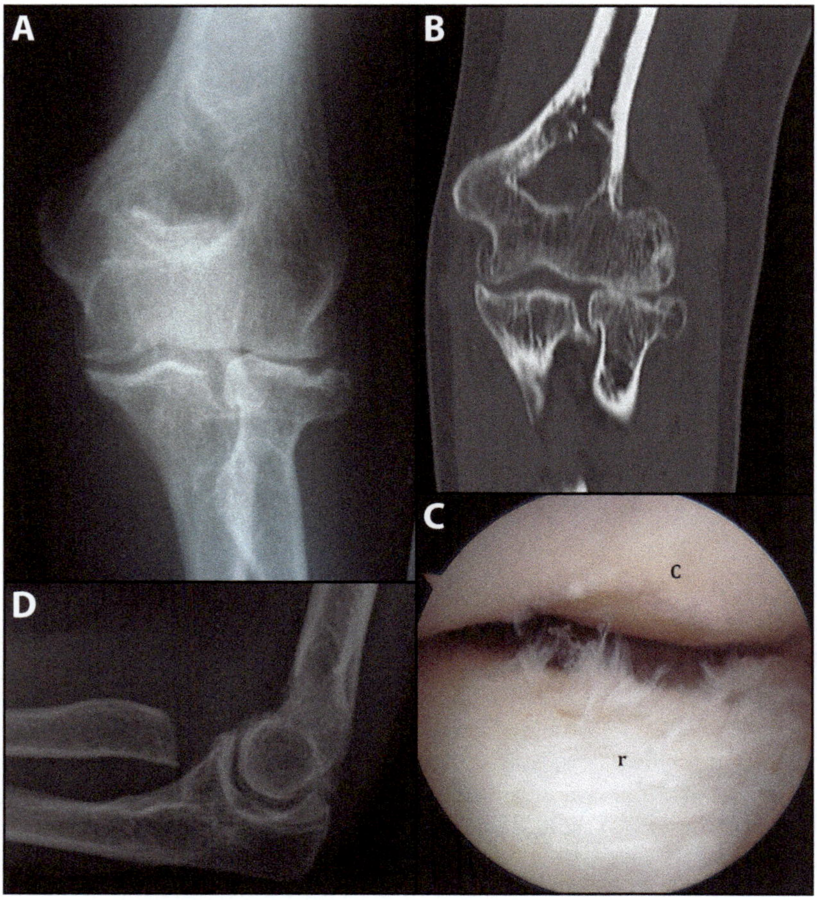

Figure 12-3. (A) Anteroposterior x-ray and (B) coronal CT scan of a 51-year-old female who sustained a radial head fracture ten years prior treated nonoperatively. The CT scan and intraoperative arthroscopic view of the radiocapitellar joint (C) demonstrate posttraumatic arthritis with capitellar pathology that precludes treatment with radial head replacement. This patient was treated with an arthroscopic radial head resection following adequate testing to rule out elbow and longitudinal forearm instability (D). Abbreviations: c, capitellum; r, radial head.

McLaughlin et al[43] reported on a series of 36 patients with radiocapitellar arthritis treated with arthroscopic debridement and radial head excision. Eight patients underwent arthroscopic radial head resection alone, whereas the remainder of the patients had concurrent arthroscopic modification of the Outerbridge-Kashiwagi procedure for ulnohumeral arthritis. Based on the Andrew and Carson score, 7 of the 8 patients who underwent arthroscopic radial head resection alone had good to excellent results, and no complications occurred. They reported an average increased flexion/extension ROM of 62 degrees, which is significantly better than that reported in the open procedure,[45,46] although most series on open radial head resection are in the setting of inflammatory arthritis. Decreased soft tissue injury achieved with arthroscopy may allow for earlier ROM postoperatively and decreased scarring. Twenty-six of the 28 patients who had concurrent arthroscopic modification of the Outerbridge-Kashiwagi procedure for ulnohumeral arthritis and radial head excision had significant pain relief with satisfactory outcomes. One patient required subsequent contracture release and another required a radial head replacement for pain.

Wijeratna et al[44] reported on a series of 4 patients with an unreconstructable comminuted radial head fracture treated early with an arthroscopic radial head resection and 11 patients with pain and loss of motion with an associated radial head fracture non- or malunion treated with late arthroscopic radial head resection at a mean of 27 weeks following the injury. At a mean of 20 months postoperatively, the average visual analog scale was 1.7 and the average Quick Disabilities of the Arm, Shoulder and Hand (DASH) score was 24.7. No patient experienced postoperative elbow instability or forearm axial instability clinically or radiographically.

Top Technical Pearls for the Procedure

1. Optimize visualization with an adequate synovectomy and debridement using a full-radius resector.
2. Address concomitant pathology following complete diagnostic arthroscopy.
3. Preserve the anterior capsule and use retractors to minimize the risk of neurovascular injury.
4. Carefully place the mid-anterolateral and posterolateral soft spot working portals to optimize the position of the burr.
5. Ensure adequate resection of the proximal radius to just distal to the sigmoid notch of the ulna.

Equipment for Radial Head Arthroplasty

Metallic radial head implants have become mainstay in radial head replacement. These are available as spacer implants, press-fit stems, and cemented stems. Furthermore, monoblock, modular, and bipolar designs exist. The senior author has been involved in the design of the EVOLVE Proline Radial Head System (Wright Medical Technology), which is a modular smooth stem spacer–type implant.

Positioning and Portals for Radial Head Arthroplasty

Regional or general anesthesia is used. Evaluate varus, valgus, and posterolateral stability as well as forearm axial stability clinically and fluoroscopically after induction of anesthesia. Position the patient supine with a bolster under the ipsilateral scapula to facilitate positioning of the arm across the chest. Alternatively, an arm table can be used. Use a sterile tourniquet and routine prophylactic antibiotics.

Step-by-Step Description of Radial Head Arthroplasty

Through a midline posterior elbow incision just lateral to the tip of the olecranon, elevate a full-thickness lateral fasciocutaneous flap. This incision allows access to the medial and lateral aspects of the elbow as required, albeit with an increased risk of seroma and hematoma. Alternatively, a more direct lateral skin incision may be used.

Use a Kocher interval between the extensor carpi ulnaris and anconeus in the presence of an injured or deficient LCL to facilitate its repair or reconstruction following radial head replacement. When the LCL is competent, use a common extensor tendon splitting approach to protect the lateral ulnar collateral ligament, a primary stabilizer to posterolateral instability.[47,48] Pronate the forearm to move the PIN medially and split the common extensor tendon longitudinally. Section the underlying radial collateral ligament and annular ligament at the equator of the radiocapitellar joint. Further exposure can be attained through proximal extension by detaching the radial collateral ligament from its humeral origin and elevation of the overlying extensor muscles anteriorly.

The decision to repair a radial head fracture or proceed to arthroplasty is often decided intraoperatively based on fracture pattern, patient factors, and surgeon experience. When radial head replacement is decided upon, remove all loose fragments and reassemble them in a sizing template to assist in component sizing. Remove remnants of the radial head perpendicular to the radial neck using a small oscillating saw. Following complete excision of the radial head, concomitant fractures of the coronoid or capitellum are optimally visualized and should be addressed.

The precise surgical procedure for radial head implant arthroplasty will depend on the system used. The following reflects the use of a smooth stem modular implant design. At least two-thirds of the circumference of the neck must be present to prevent subsidence or angulation of a smooth stem prosthesis. Shorten the radial neck as required when radial head fractures extend distally or reconstruct the radial neck with cerclage wires or small plates if substantial radial neck shortening is anticipated, which cannot be compensated with the implant system. Use a radial head planer to optimize radial neck contact with the implant.

The native radial head is typically elliptical. The minor diameter of the excised radial head is selected as the diameter of the axisymmetric implant (Figure 12-4). This is typically 2 mm smaller than the major diameter measured using the head sizer dish. Implant thickness is judged based on the thinnest portion of the fractured radial head because the implant will rest on the most proximal extent of the remaining radial neck.

When the radial head is too comminuted to function as a template, is dysmorphic, or has previously been excised, preoperative radiographic templating of the contralateral side is mandatory. Measurements of the ipsilateral capitellum have also been shown to correlate with the inner and outer diameters of the native radial head.[49] The distance from the stump of the radial neck to the proximal edge of the lesser sigmoid notch has been found to reliably correlate with radial head thickness in the setting of an intact interosseous membrane.[50]

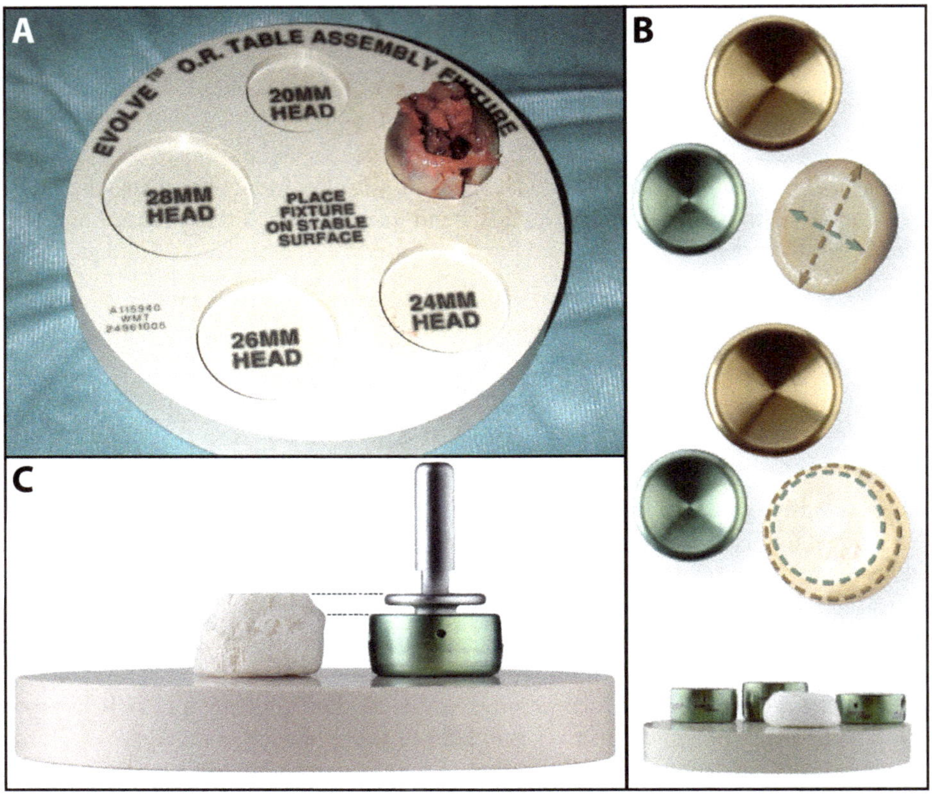

Figure 12-4. (A) Fragments from the resected radial head are reassembled for sizing. (B) The minor diameter (green) of the ellipsoidal radial head is selected, which is typically 2 mm smaller than the major diameter (gold) measured. Implant thickness is judged based on the thinnest portion of the fractured radial head. (C) Adjust the head and/or stem heights to achieve the desired implant height. (Figures B and C are reprinted with permission from Wright Medical Technology.)

Place a Hohman retractor around the posterior aspect of the radial neck and lever it laterally to facilitate broaching of the medullary canal and insertion of the prosthesis (Figure 12-5). Do not use anteriorly placed retractors because of the risk of injury to the PIN. Use sequential broaches until cortical contact is achieved. Use a stem 1 mm less than the largest broach when using a smooth stem implant to optimize articular tracking of the implant with the capitellum.

Insert trial components and evaluate the diameter, height, tracking, and congruency visually as well as using an image intensifier. Adjust the head and/or stem heights to achieve the desired implant height. Ensure that the proximal edge of the lesser sigmoid notch is even with the proximal articular surface of the implant and no gap is present in the lateral ulnohumeral joint surfaces.[51] The lateral ulnohumeral joint is most easily visualized anteriorly by extension of the approach proximally or with the help of a dental mirror. Although fluoroscopic incongruity of the normally parallel medial ulnohumeral articular surfaces is suggestive of overlengthening, such finding only becomes apparent when 6 mm or greater of radial overlengthening is present; therefore, it is not a reliable marker.[52] Downsize the stem to allow the implant to adapt to the annular ligament tension and contour of the capitellum if maltracking of the trial component is present during forearm rotation following provisional repair of the annular ligament. If maltracking persists, ensure anatomic reduction of concomitant ulnar fractures. Perform the push-pull test[38] while fluoroscopically visualizing the DRUJ to assess ulnar variance and forearm axial stability with and without the trial in place.

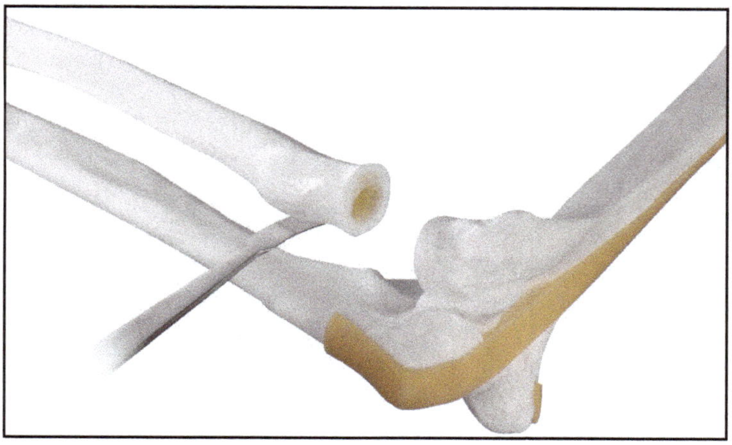

Figure 12-5. Adequate exposure of the medullary canal to facilitate broaching and insertion of the prosthesis is obtained through placement of a Hohmann retractor around the posterior aspect of the radial neck and levering it laterally. (Reprinted with permission from Wright Medical Technology.)

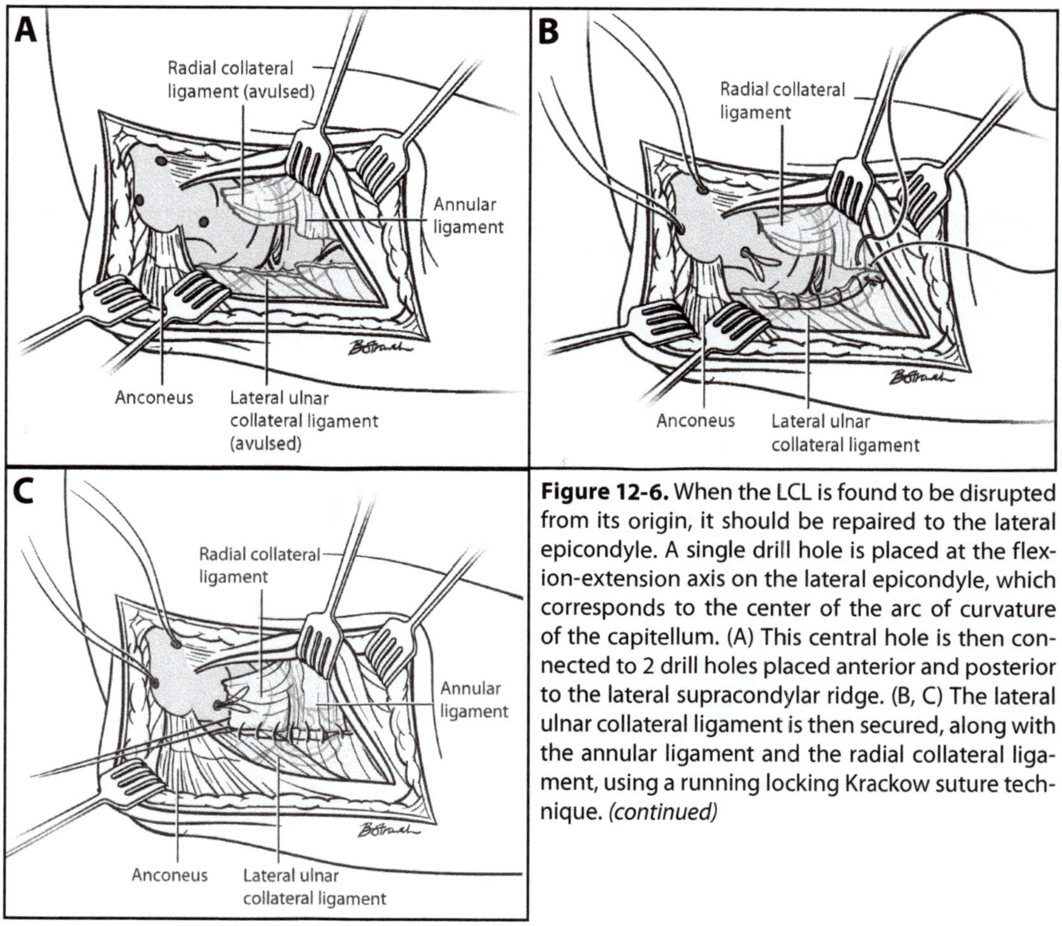

Figure 12-6. When the LCL is found to be disrupted from its origin, it should be repaired to the lateral epicondyle. A single drill hole is placed at the flexion-extension axis on the lateral epicondyle, which corresponds to the center of the arc of curvature of the capitellum. (A) This central hole is then connected to 2 drill holes placed anterior and posterior to the lateral supracondylar ridge. (B, C) The lateral ulnar collateral ligament is then secured, along with the annular ligament and the radial collateral ligament, using a running locking Krackow suture technique. *(continued)*

Insert the definitive component, then close the wound in layers. Repair the LCL if it is avulsed or detached from the lateral epicondyle using locking Krackow nonabsorbable sutures and transosseous bone tunnels or a suture anchor placed at the flexion-extension axis on the lateral epicondyle (Figure 12-6).[53] Repair the common extensor tendon split or Kocher interval and re-evaluate elbow stability. X-rays are taken postoperatively to confirm joint congruency and implant position (Figure 12-7).

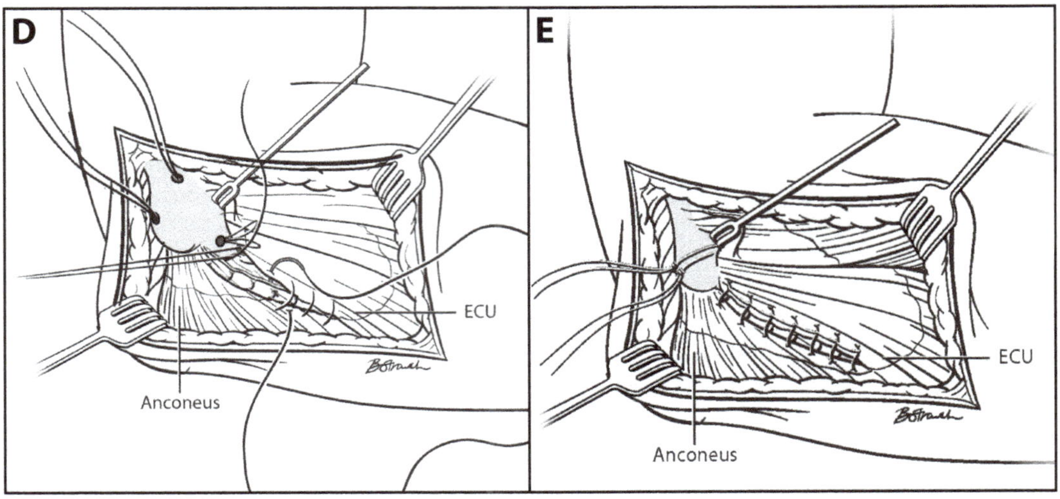

Figure 12-6 (continued). (D) Similarly, using a running locking suture technique, the common extensor muscle fascia is repaired. (E) The sutures are then pulled through the transosseous tunnels using a suture retriever, tensioned with the forearm in pronation and tied over the supracondylar ridge. Abbreviation: ECU, extensor carpi ulnaris. (Reprinted with permission from the American Society for Surgery of the Hand.)

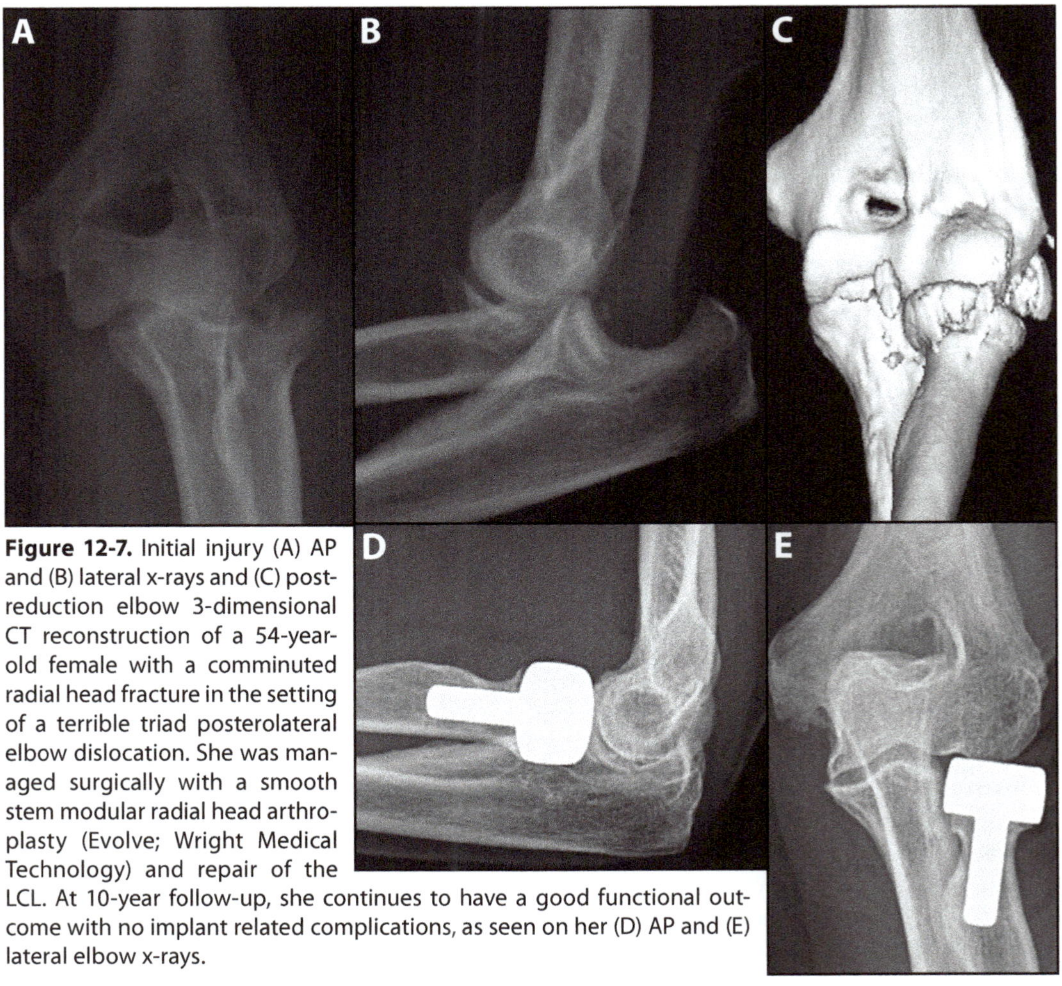

Figure 12-7. Initial injury (A) AP and (B) lateral x-rays and (C) post-reduction elbow 3-dimensional CT reconstruction of a 54-year-old female with a comminuted radial head fracture in the setting of a terrible triad posterolateral elbow dislocation. She was managed surgically with a smooth stem modular radial head arthroplasty (Evolve; Wright Medical Technology) and repair of the LCL. At 10-year follow-up, she continues to have a good functional outcome with no implant related complications, as seen on her (D) AP and (E) lateral elbow x-rays.

Postoperative Protocol for Radial Head Arthroplasty

The presence of concomitant injuries and intraoperative elbow stability will dictate the postoperative rehabilitation. In the setting of a stable joint with intact collateral ligaments, no limitations are prescribed. Patients are given a cuff and collar as required for comfort during the day and a static progressive extension splint at night.

Patients with associated fractures and ligamentous injuries are allowed to initiate active ROM within their safe zone in the first postoperative week. To minimize stress on injured or repaired collateral ligaments, active forearm rotation is only permitted past 90 degrees of elbow flexion for the first 6 weeks. Active elbow extension is performed in pronation when the LCL has been repaired,[54] in supination if the MCL is deficient,[55] and neutral if both collateral ligaments are injured. The elbow is maintained in a resting splint with the appropriate forearm rotation position for the first 6 weeks postoperatively. Nighttime static progressive extension splinting and daytime elbow flexion cuff may then be initiated. Passive stretching is not permitted until 6 weeks after surgery to protect concomitant fracture fixation, protect ligamentous repairs, and reduce the incidence of heterotopic ossification. Unless contraindicated, administration of indomethacin is considered to potentially lower the incidence of heterotopic ossification and help reduce postoperative pain and swelling.

Potential Complications of Radial Head Arthroplasty

Reported complications include infection, PIN injuries, loss of motion secondary to capsular contractures, heterotopic ossification, retained radial head fragments, prosthetic loosening or wear, elbow instability, and ulnar neuropathy.[56,57] Some of those complications can be attributed to concomitant injuries. Overstuffing of the radiocapitellar joint can lead to accelerated capitellar wear and pain,[58,59] as well as decrease in elbow flexion.[60] Although radiolucency around smooth-stemmed prostheses is common, it does not appear to correlate with forearm pain or the functional outcome.[61] Osteoarthritis of the capitellum can occur secondary to damage from the initial injury, from prosthesis maltracking, and altered contact mechanics from the metallic implant.

Results

Successful treatment of complex radial head fractures with associated elbow osseous and ligamentous injuries has been reported with metallic smooth-stem radial head implants.[56,59,61-63] The senior author reported on the outcomes of a cohort of patients with nonreconstructable radial head fractures and associated elbow injuries treated with modular smooth-stem radial head implants.[59] Despite slight-to-moderate deficits in ROM and strength in comparison to the unaffected side, patients were satisfied at 2-year follow-up, with an average DASH score of 24 and Mayo Elbow Performance Index of 83. No implants required revision and all elbows remained stable. Similarly, when using a smooth-stem bipolar implant, Zunkiewicz et al[64] reported a mean Mayo Elbow Performance Index of 92 at an average of 3 years and did not report lucent lines around the implant stems as being problematic. A high prevalence of periprosthetic osteolysis was reported at an average of 8 years by Popovic et al[65] when using a bipolar cemented prosthesis. Using a press-fit porous coated stem bipolar implant, Burkhart et al[66] reported good results, with a mean DASH score of 9.8 and a mean ROM of 124 degrees of flexion and 21 degrees of extension at an average of 8.8 years. Despite a high prevalence of radiographic degenerative changes, they did not report prosthetic loosening or osteolysis. In contrast, Flinkkilä et al[67] reported early stem loosening in 12 of 37 patients reviewed who had monopolar metallic press-fit prostheses at an average of 4 years. Nine patients required prosthetic removal due to symptomatic progressive osteolysis. The use of a loose-fitting, smooth-stemmed component or a bipolar head may allow better adaptation to the complex biomechanics of the radiocapitellar joint, preventing eccentric forces, stem loosening, and osteolysis. Pyrocarbon, which is thought to be biocompatible and mechanically similar to bone, is an alternative bearing surface to metal in radial head arthroplasty. Sarris et al[68] reported good clinical outcomes at a mean of 27 months postoperatively in 97% of patients treated with a radial head made of pyrocarbon, along with an anatomic neck angled at 15 degrees and a press-fit stem, both made of titanium. Despite these encouraging results, 6 patients developed asymptomatic osteolysis and 2 had dissociation at the head-neck junction.

When used to reconstruct elbows with a chronic posttraumatic disorder, Shore et al[69] reported satisfactory outcome scores and 100% implant survival at an average of 8 years postoperatively using metallic radial head arthroplasty. Further studies are required to assess the long-term results of radial head arthroplasty.

Top Technical Pearls for the Procedure

1. Perform an examination under anesthesia of the elbow to assess for concomitant ligamentous injuries and decide which deep interval is best to approach the radial head.
2. Use a Hohmann retractor placed around the posterior radial neck to bring the radial canal laterally into view and to minimize PIN injury.
3. The diameter of the implant chosen should match the minor diameter of the back table reassembly of the radial head fragments or, in the setting of secondary surgery, should be based on templating the size of the contralateral radial head.
4. Avoid overstuffing the radiocapitellar joint by ensuring appropriate implant height.
5. If maltracking of the implant is present following provisional repair of the annular ligament, ensure that ulnar fractures have been anatomically reduced; downsize the stem to allow greater degree of freedom of the implant in the shaft if required.

References

1. O'Driscoll SW, Bell DF, Morrey BF. Posterolateral rotatory instability of the elbow. *J Bone Joint Surg Am*. 1991;73(3):440-446.
2. Jensen SL, Olsen BS, Søjbjerg JO. Elbow joint kinematics after excision of the radial head. *J Shoulder Elbow Surg*. 1999;8(3):238-241.
3. Beingessner DM, Dunning CE, Gordon KE, Johnson JA, King GJ. The effect of radial head excision and arthroplasty on elbow kinematics and stability. *J Bone Joint Surg Am*. 2004;86(8):1730-1739.
4. Hall JA, McKee MD. Posterolateral rotatory instability of the elbow following radial head resection. *J Bone Joint Surg Am*. 2005;87(7):1571-1579.
5. Lanting BA, Ferreira LM, Johnson JA, Athwal GS, King GJ. The effect of excision of the radial head and metallic radial head replacement on the tension in the interosseous membrane. *Bone Joint J*. 2013;95(10):1383-1387.
6. Morrey BF, Chao EY, Hui FC. Biomechanical study of the elbow following excision of the radial head. *J Bone Joint Surg Am*. 1979;61(1):63-68.

7. Stephen IB. Excision of the radial head for closed fracture. *Acta Orthop Scand.* 1981;52(4):409-412.
8. Janssen RP, Vegter J. Resection of the radial head after Mason type-III fractures of the elbow: follow-up at 16 to 30 years. *J Bone Joint Surg Br.* 1998;80(2):231-233.
9. Ikeda M, Oka Y. Function after early radial head resection for fracture: a retrospective evaluation of 15 patients followed for 3-18 years. *Acta Orthop Scand.* 2000;71(2):191-194.
10. Leppilahti J, Jalovaara P. Early excision of the radial head for fracture. *Int Orthop.* 2000;24(3):160-162.
11. Johnson JA, Beingessner DM, Gordon KD, Dunning CE, Stacpoole RA, King GJ. Kinematics and stability of the fractured and implant-reconstructed radial head. *J Shoulder Elbow Surg.* 2005;14(1 suppl S):195S-201S.
12. Kauffman JI, Chen AL, Stuchin S, Di Cesare PE. Surgical management of the rheumatoid elbow. *J Am Acad Orthop Surg.* 2003;11(2):100-108.
13. Morrey BF. Radial head fracture. In: Morrey BF, ed. *The Elbow and Its Disorders.* 3rd ed. Philadelphia, PA: Saunders; 2000:341-364.
14. Menth-Chiari WA, Poehling GG, Ruch DS. Arthroscopic resection of the radial head. *Arthroscopy.* 1999;15(2):226-230.
15. Savoie FH III, Nunley PD, Field LD. Arthroscopic management of the arthritic elbow: indications, technique, and results. *J Shoulder Elbow Surg.* 1999;8(3):214-219.
16. Menth-Chiari WA, Ruch DS, Poehling GG. Arthroscopic excision of the radial head: clinical outcome in 12 patients with post-traumatic arthritis after fracture of the radial head or rheumatoid arthritis. *Arthroscopy.* 2001;17(9):918-923.
17. Steinmann SP, King GJ, Savoie FH III. Arthroscopic treatment of the arthritic elbow. *Instr Course Lect.* 2006;55:109-117.
18. Lo IK, King GJ. Arthroscopic radial head excision. *Arthroscopy.* 1994;10(6):689-692.
19. van Riet RP, Morrey BF. Documentation of associated injuries occurring with radial head fracture. *Clin Orthop Relat Res.* 2008;466(1):130-134.
20. Itamura J, Roidis N, Mirzayan R, Vaishnav S, Learch T, Shean C. Radial head fractures: MRI evaluation of associated injuries. *J Shoulder Elbow Surg.* 2005;14(4):421-424.
21. Silva M, Luck JV Jr. Radial head excision and synovectomy in patients with hemophilia. *J Bone Joint Surg Am.* 2007;89(10):2156-2162.
22. Jobe FW, Stark H, Lombardo SJ. Reconstruction of the ulnar collateral ligament in athletes. *J Bone Joint Surg Am.* 1986;68(8):1158-1163.
23. Chen FS, Rokito AS, Jobe FW. Medial elbow problems in the overhead-throwing athlete. *J Am Acad Orthop Surg.* 2001;9(2):99-113.
24. Veltri DM, O'Brien SJ, Field LD, Deutsch A, Altchek DW, Potter HG. The milking maneuver: a new test to evaluate the MCL of the elbow in the throwing athlete. In: Programs and Abstracts of the 10th Open Meeting of the American Shoulder and Elbow Surgeons. Rosemont, IL: American Academy of Orthopaedic Surgeons; 1994.
25. O'Driscoll SW, Lawton RL, Smith AM. The "moving valgus stress test" for medial collateral ligament tears of the elbow. *Am J Sports Med.* 2005;33(2):231-239.
26. O'Driscoll SW. Classification and spectrum of elbow instability: recurrent instability. In: Morrey BF, ed. *The Elbow and its Disorders.* 2nd ed. Philadelphia, PA: Saunders; 1993:453-463.
27. Regan WD, Morrey BF. The physical examination of the elbow. In Morrey BF, ed. *The Elbow and its Disorders.* 2nd ed. Philadelphia, PA: Saunders; 1993:73-85.
28. Regan W, Lapner PC. Prospective evaluation of two diagnostic apprehension signs for posterolateral instability of the elbow. *J Shoulder Elbow Surg.* 2006;15(3):344-346.
29. Loeffler BJ, Green JB, Zelouf DS. Forearm instability. *J Hand Surg Am.* 2014;39(1):156-167.
30. Greenspan A, Norman A. The radial head, capitellum view: useful technique in elbow trauma. *AJR Am J Roentgenol.* 1982;138(6):1186-1188.
31. Tomás FJ, Proubasta IR. Modified radial head—capitellum projection in elbow trauma. *Br J Radiol.* 1998;71(841):74-75.
32. Jaakkola JI, Riggans DH, Lourie GM, Lang CJ, Elhassan BT, Rosenthal SJ. Ultrasonography for the evaluation of forearm interosseous membrane disruption in a cadaver model. *J Hand Surg Am.* 2001;26(6):1053-1057.
33. Starch DW, Dabezies EJ. Magnetic resonance imaging of the interosseous membrane of the forearm. *J Bone Joint Surg Am.* 2001;83(2):235-238.

34. Fester EW, Murray PM, Sanders TG, Ingari JV, Leyendecker J, Leis HL. The efficacy of magnetic resonance imaging and ultrasound in detecting disruptions of the forearm interosseous membrane: a cadaver study. *J Hand Surg Am.* 2002;27(3):418-424.
35. Soubeyrand M, Lafont C, Oberlin C, France W, Maulat I, Degeorges R. The "muscular hernia sign": an original ultrasonographic sign to detect lesions of the forearm's interosseous membrane. *Surg Radiol Anat.* 2006;28(4):372-378.
36. Rodriguez-Martin J, Pretell-Mazzini J, Vidal-Bujanda C. Unusual pattern of Essex-Lopresti injury with negative plain radiographs of the wrist: a case report and literature review. *Hand Surg.* 2010;15(1):41-45.
37. Brunton LM, Anderson MW, Pannunzio ME, Khanna AJ, Chhabra AB. Magnetic resonance imaging of the elbow: update on current techniques and indications. *J Hand Surg Am.* 2006;31(6):1001-1011.
38. Smith AM, Urbanosky LR, Castle JA, Rushing JT, Ruch DS. Radius pull test: predictor of longitudinal forearm instability. *J Bone Joint Surg Am.* 2002;84(11):1970-1976.
39. Gofton WT, King GJ. Heterotopic ossification following elbow arthroscopy. Arthroscopy. 2001;17(1):E2.
40. Kelly EW, Morrey BF, O'Driscoll SW. Complications of elbow arthroscopy. *J Bone Joint Surg Am.* 2001;83(1):25-34.
41. Savoie FH III, Nunley PD, Field LD. Arthroscopic management of the arthritic elbow: indications, technique, and results. *J Shoulder Elbow Surg.* 1999;8(3):214-219.
42. Menth-Chiari WA, Ruch DS, Poehling GG. Arthroscopic excision of the radial head: clinical outcome in 12 patients with post-traumatic arthritis after fracture of the radial head or rheumatoid arthritis. *Arthroscopy.* 2001;17(9):918-923.
43. McLaughlin RE II, Savoie FH III, Field LD, Ramsey JR. Arthroscopic treatment of the arthritic elbow due to primary radiocapitellar arthritis. *Arthroscopy.* 2006;22(1):63-69.
44. Wijeratna M, Bailey KA, Pace A, Tytherleigh-Strong G, Van Rensburg L, Kent M. Arthroscopic radial head excision in managing elbow trauma. *Int Orthop.* 2012;36(12):2507-2512.
45. Taylor AR, Mukerjea SK, Rana NA. Excision of the head of the radius in rheumatoid arthritis. *J Bone Joint Surg Br.* 1976;58(4):485-487.
46. Gendi NS, Axon JM, Carr AJ, Pile KD, Burge PD, Mowat AG. Synovectomy of the elbow and radial head excision in rheumatoid arthritis. *J Bone Joint Surg Br.* 1997;79(6):918-923.
47. Morrey BF. Surgical exposures of the elbow. In: Morrey BF, ed. *The Elbow and Its Disorders.* Philadelphia, PA: Saunders; 2009:115-122.
48. Desloges W, Louati H, Papp SR, Pollock JW. Objective analysis of lateral elbow exposure with the extensor digitorum communis split compared with the Kocher interval. *J Bone Joint Surg Am.* 2014;96(5):387-393.
49. Leclerc AE, Deluce S, Ferreira L, Desai S, King GJ, Athwal GS. Measurements of the ispilateral capitellum can reliably predict the diameter of the radial head. *J Shoulder Elbow Surg.* 2013;22(12):1724-1728.
50. van Riet RP, van Glabbeek F, de Weerdt W, Oemar J, Bortier H. Validation of the lesser sigmoid notch of the ulna as a reference point for accurate placement of a prosthesis for the head of the radius: a cadaver study. *J Bone Joint Surg Br.* 2007;89(3):413-416.
51. Athwal GS, Frank SG, Grewal R, Faber KJ, Johnson J, King GJ. Determination of correct implant size in radial head arthroplasty to avoid overlengthening: surgical technique. *J Bone Joint Surg Am.* 2010;92(suppl 1 pt 2):250-257.
52. Frank SG, Grewal R, Johnson J, Faber KJ, King GJ, Athwal GS. Determination of correct implant size in radial head arthroplasty to avoid overlengthening. *J Bone Joint Surg Am.* 2009;91(7):1738-1746.
53. Fraser GS, Pichora JE, Ferreira LM, Brownhill JR, Johnson JA, King GJ. Lateral collateral ligament repair restores the initial varus stability of the elbow: an in vitro biomechanical study. *J Orthop Trauma.* 2008;22(9):615-623.
54. Dunning CE, Zarzour ZD, Patterson SD, Johnson JA, King GJ. Muscle forces and pronation stabilize the lateral ligament deficient elbow. *Clin Orthop Relat Res.* 2001;(388):118-124.
55. Armstrong AD, Dunning CE, Faber KJ, Duck TR, Johnson JA, King GJ. Rehabilitation of the medial collateral ligament-deficient elbow: an in vitro biomechanical study. *J Hand Surg Am.* 2000;25(6):1051-1057.
56. Moro JK, Werier J, MacDermid JC, Patterson SD, King GJ. Arthroplasty with a metal radial head for unreconstructible fractures of the radial head. *J Bone Joint Surg Am.* 2001;83(8):1201-1211.
57. Giannicola G, Sacchetti FM, Antonietti G, Piccioli A, Postacchini R, Cinotti G. Radial head, radiocapitellar and total elbow arthroplasties: a review of recent literature. *Injury.* 2014;45(2):428-436.

58. Van Glabbeek F, Van Riet RP, Baumfeld JA, et al. Detrimental effects of overstuffing or understuffing with a radial head replacement in the medial collateral-ligament deficient elbow. *J Bone Joint Surg Am.* 2004;86(12):2629-2635.
59. Grewal R, MacDermid JC, Faber KJ, Drosdowech DS, King GJ. Comminuted radial head fractures treated with a modular metallic radial head arthroplasty. Study of outcomes. *J Bone Joint Surg Am.* 2006;88(10):2192-2200.
60. Birkedal JP, Deal DN, Ruch DS. Loss of flexion after radial head replacement. *J Shoulder Elbow Surg.* 2004;13(2):208-213.
61. Fehringer EV, Burns EM, Knierim A, Sun J, Apker KA, Berg RE. Radiolucencies surrounding a smooth-stemmed radial head component may not correlate with forearm pain or poor elbow function. *J Shoulder Elbow Surg.* 2009;18(2):275-278.
62. Harrington IJ, Sekyi-Otu A, Barrington TW, Evans DC, Tuli V. The functional outcome with metallic radial head implants in the treatment of unstable elbow fractures: a long-term review. *J Trauma.* 2001;50(1):46-52.
63. Doornberg JN, Parisien R, van Duijn PJ, Ring D. Radial head arthroplasty with a modular metal spacer to treat acute traumatic elbow instability. *J Bone Joint Surg Am.* 2007;89(5):1075-1080.
64. Zunkiewicz MR, Clemente JS, Miller MC, Baratz ME, Wysocki RW, Cohen MS. Radial head replacement with a bipolar system: a minimum 2-year follow-up. *J Shoulder Elbow Surg.* 2012;21(1):98-104.
65. Popovic N, Lemaire R, Georis P, Gillet P. Midterm results with a bipolar radial head prosthesis: radiographic evidence of loosening at the bone-cement interface. *J Bone Joint Surg Am.* 2007;89(11):2469-2476.
66. Burkhart KJ, Mattyasovszky SG, Runkel M, et al. Mid- to long-term results after bipolar radial head arthroplasty. *J Shoulder Elbow Surg.* 2010;19(7):965-972.
67. Flinkkilä T1, Kaisto T, Sirniö K, Hyvönen P, Leppilahti J. Short- to mid-term results of metallic press-fit radial head arthroplasty in unstable injuries of the elbow. *J Bone Joint Surg Br.* 2012;94(6):805-810.
68. Sarris IK, Kyrkos MJ, Galanis NN, Papavasiliou KA, Sayegh FE, Kapetanos GA. Radial head replacement with the MoPyC pyrocarbon prosthesis. *J Shoulder Elbow Surg.* 2012;21(9):1222-1228.
69. Shore BJ, Mozzon JB, MacDermid JC, Faber KJ, King GJ. Chronic posttraumatic elbow disorders treated with metallic radial head arthroplasty. *J Bone Joint Surg Am.* 2008;90(2):271-280.

Please see videos on the accompanying website at

www.routledge.com/9781630910013

13

Arthroscopic Radial Head Resection

Stephanie C. Petterson, MPT, PhD; Sarah Stelma, MD;
and Kevin D. Plancher, MD, MS

Introduction

The radial head is the primary restraint to proximal migration of the radius and provides axial stability to the forearm. It transmits approximately 60% of the load across the radiocapitellar joint and 40% to the ulnohumeral joint with the elbow in extension; when the elbow is in flexion, the load is shared equally.[1,2] In addition, the radial head is a secondary restraint to valgus forces at the elbow. The radial head shifts the center of varus-valgus rotation laterally, decreasing the forces on the medial ligaments.[3]

Radial head fractures are one of the most common types of elbow fractures and account for up to 30% of all elbow injuries.[4,5] As high as 30% of radial head fractures also have concomitant soft tissue injuries, including distal radioulnar joint (DRUJ) injuries, interosseous membrane disruption, coronoid fractures, medial and lateral collateral ligament injuries, Essex-Lopresti lesion, and elbow dislocation.[6] The most common mechanism of injury is a fall on the outstretched hand with the forearm in a pronated position, resulting in pain and tenderness along the lateral aspect of the elbow and limited elbow and forearm motion.

Radial head fractures are classified according to the Mason classification.[7] A nondisplaced fracture is classified as a Mason type I fracture. Mason type II fractures are partial articular fractures with displacement of less than 2 mm. Comminuted fractures involving the entire radial head are classified as Mason type III. Mason type IV fractures are radial head fractures that are associated with elbow dislocation.

Radiocapitellar arthritis, whether primary or posttraumatic, is also an indication for radial head resection. Although uncommon, primary osteoarthritis of the elbow typically occurs in middle-aged men and heavy laborers. Posttraumatic arthritis, however, is typically the consequence of a radial head fracture malunion and occurs more commonly in women. These patients typically present with lateral-sided elbow pain and pain with forearm supination and pronation.

Radial head resection is indicated when conservative measures have failed to restore range of motion (ROM) and provide pain relief. Radial head resection allows for excellent restoration of elbow ROM contributing to pain-free return to activities for these patients. When the radial head fragments compose less than 25% of the surface area of the radial head or 25% to 33% of the

Savoie FH III, Field LD, Steinmann SP, eds. *The Elbow and Wrist: AANA Advanced Arthroscopic Surgical Techniques* (pp 127-136).

capitellar surface area, fragment excision can be performed; however, when the fracture is more extensive and comminuted, a complete radial head excision is indicated.

The radial head provides a secondary restraint to valgus force at the elbow; therefore, resection of the radial head is contraindicated when the fracture is associated with medial or lateral ligament injuries or DRUJ disruption. The proximal radius migrates up to 7 mm when an axial load is applied through the forearm following radial head excision.[8] However, if the triangular fibrocartilage complex or interosseous membrane, which also resists proximal migration, are compromised, radial migration increases and the load is shifted back to the radial column.[8]

The advantages of the arthroscopic approach compared to the traditional, open approach to radial head excision include accelerated postoperative recovery, decreased risk of injury to the annular ligament, lateral ligamentous complex, and the posterior interosseous nerve.

Indications

- Degenerative or posttraumatic elbow arthritis
- Isolated, type III radial head fracture (eg, comminuted, displaced fracture with a mechanical block to motion)[9,10]
- Radial head fracture with no associated ligamentous injury
- Rheumatoid arthritis[11,12]
- Arthrofibrosis of the elbow[13]

Controversial Indications

- Isolated Mason type II radial head fracture[14]
- Lateral epicondylitis secondary to radial head trauma

Pertinent Physical Findings

- Tenderness to palpation and crepitus along the lateral aspect of the elbow
- Decreased elbow ROM, most limited in forearm pronation and supination, followed by limited elbow extension and flexion
- Aspiration of joint hematoma and injection of local anesthetic to assess for mechanical block
- Diagnostic lidocaine injection: A lidocaine injection into the common extensor tendon origin or the radiocapitellar joint can aid in localizing symptoms and aid in the differential diagnosis.
- Varus and valgus elbow stress test: The elbow is positioned in approximately 20 degrees of flexion. For the valgus stress test, the examiner palpates the medial joint line and, while stabilizing the distal humerus, applies a valgus stress to the elbow. For the varus stress test, the examiner palpates the lateral joint line, and while stabilizing the distal humerus, applies a varus stress to the elbow. The test is positive if the patient reports pain or there is greater laxity compared to the noninjured side.
- Radial pull test[15]: This test is performed in the operating room to assess longitudinal radioulnar stability. The patient is supine with the shoulder abducted 90 degrees and internally rotated. The elbow is flexed to 90 degrees with the forearm in neutral. A bone-reduction tenaculum is used to grasp the proximal radius, and a manual pull of approximately 20 lb is applied longitudinally. Fluoroscopy is used to measure ulnar variance and proximal radial migration.

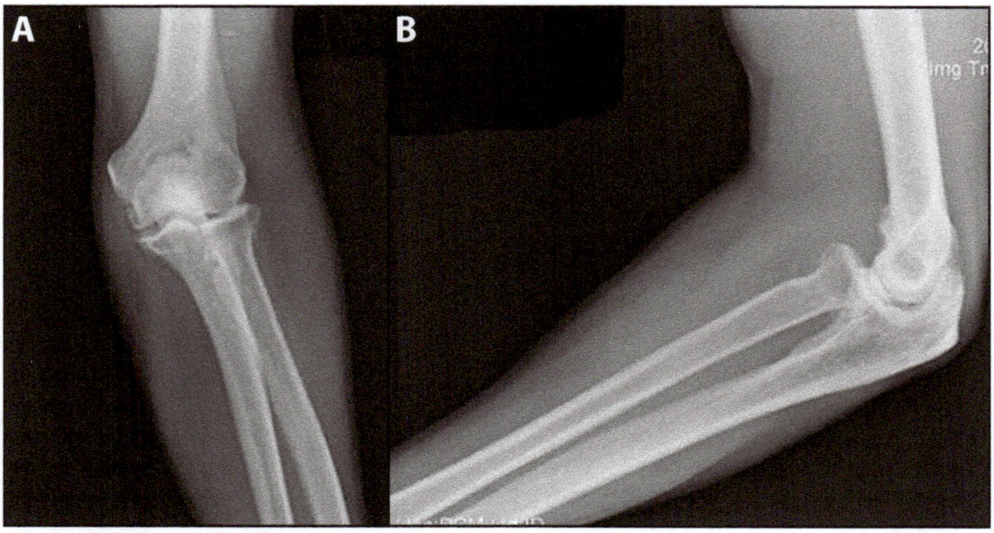

Figure 13-1. Plain (A) anteroposterior view and (B) lateral x-rays of a left elbow demonstrating degenerative arthritis in the same patient.

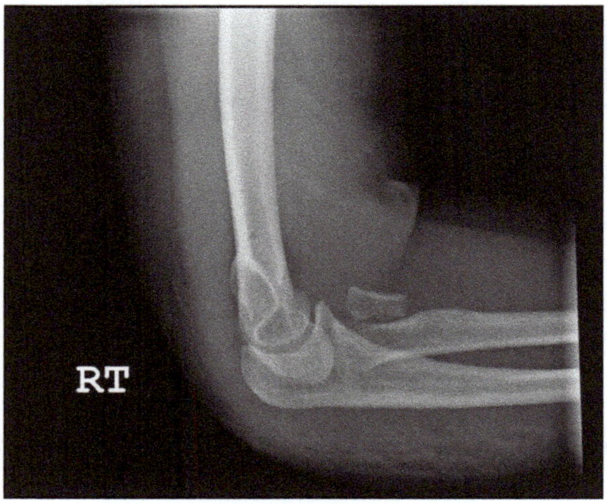

Figure 13-2. Plain lateral x-ray of a right elbow demonstrating a comminuted radial head fracture.

Pertinent Imaging

- Plain x-ray series of the elbow, including the following:
  - Anteroposterior view: The elbow is placed in full extension. This view assesses for a fat pad sign, which indicates possible minimally displaced fracture of the radial head (Figure 13-1A).
  - Lateral view: The elbow is placed in 90 degrees of flexion (Figures 13-1B and 13-2).
  - Radiocapitellar view (oblique lateral, Greenspan view): This is a lateral view of the elbow with the tube angled 45 degrees toward the shoulder and the forearm in neutral rotation. The elbow is placed in 90 degrees of flexion. This view can help detect subtle radial head fractures when suspected and not apparent on anteroposterior and lateral views.
- Computed tomography is recommended for comminuted fractures to identify the fracture segments (Figure 13-3).

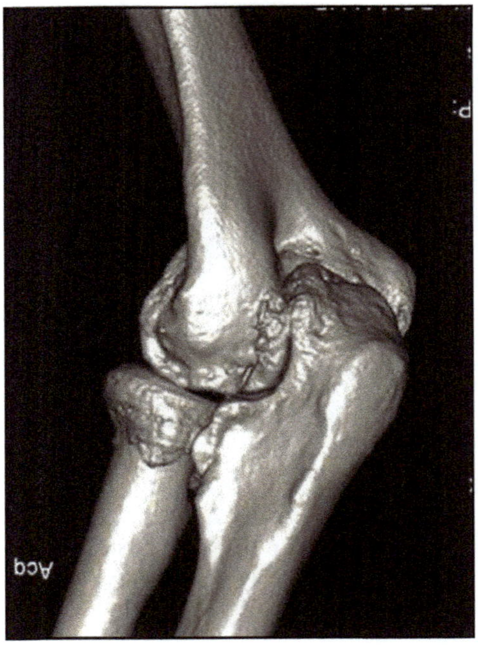

Figure 13-3. Computed tomography scan of a left elbow (same patient as in Figure 13-1) demonstrating grade IV changes of the radial head.

Equipment

A standard 2.7- or 4.0-mm, 30- or 70-degree arthroscope can be used to perform radial head resection. Blunt trocars are encouraged to minimize potential nerve damage. Nonfenestrated cannulas minimize extravasation of fluid and unnecessary tissue distension. Pump pressure, when used, should be maintained below 30 mm Hg to optimize the distance between important neurovascular structures and intra-articular cannulas without excessive pressure on the joint capsule. A hooded oscillating shaver and hooded burr are used for removal of tissues and bone.

Positioning and Portals

General anesthesia and a regional axillary block can be used for arthroscopic procedures of the elbow. A brachial plexus block can also be used to manage postoperative pain and promote early ROM; however, the ability to conduct a thorough postoperative neurovascular examination is limited.

Radial head resection is performed in the lateral decubitus position. The advantages of this position are that it provides stability to the upper arm, allows equal access to the anterior and posterior compartments, and allows the anesthesiologist to more readily manage the patient's airways compared to the prone position. The arm is draped over a well-padded bolster and stabilized with the elbow flexed to 90 degrees for ease of access to all elbow compartments (Figure 13-4A). A complete physical examination under anesthesia should be performed, including ROM (eg, flexion, extension, pronation, and supination) and stability testing (eg, varus/valgus, posterolateral, and axial stress) to identify structural damage or a mechanical block to motion. Evidence of lateral, medial, or rotary instability would preclude excision of the radial head. The arm is prepped with a tourniquet for exsanguination, and the forearm and hand are wrapped with a semicompressive dressing to minimize fluid extravasation to the distal compartments during the arthroscopy.

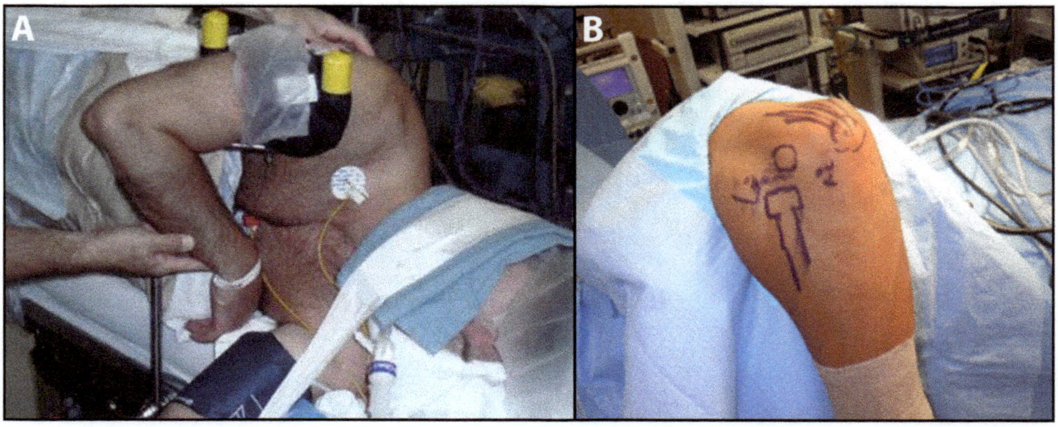

Figure 13-4. (A) Patient positioned in the lateral decubitus position for elbow arthroscopic radial head resection. (B) The patient is draped and landmarks are drawn out in preparation for radial head resection.

Step-by-Step Description of the Procedure

Step 1: Establishing Portals

Anatomic landmarks are drawn out, including location of epicondyles, olecranon tip, radial head, and ulnar nerve (Figure 13-4B). Portal locations are drawn for a proximal anteromedial, proximal anterolateral, and direct lateral portal. Although other arthroscopic portals have been described, these are most useful for this procedure and are safer anatomically. Twenty to 30 mL of saline are injected into the anconeus triangle (soft spot; direct lateral) bordered by the lateral epicondyle, tip of the olecranon, and radial head to distend joint.

A proximal anteromedial portal is established using an 18-gauge spinal needle approximately 2 cm proximal to the medial epicondyle just anterior to the intermuscular septum.[16] This proximal anteromedial portal is used as a viewing portal to aid in the placement of other portals under arthroscopic visualization. A blunt trocar in a nonfenestrated cannula is then advanced along the anterior humeral cortex, ensuring to stay anterior to the medial supracondylar ridge. With the arthroscope in the proximal anteromedial portal, the anterior capsule, trochlea, capitellum, radial head, and medial and lateral gutters can be inspected. Caution must be taken to avoid injury to the medial antebrachial cutaneous nerve, located 2.3 mm from the cannula, and the ulnar nerve, 3 to 4 mm away, by staying anterior to intermuscular septum.[17] The median nerve, while also at risk, is less of a concern as it is approximately 12 mm away at 90 degrees of elbow flexion and 22 mm away with the elbow distended.[17]

The proximal anterolateral portal is created 2 cm proximal and 1 cm anterior to the lateral epicondyle.[18] This proximal anterolateral portal is used as a working portal for radial head resection and allows access to the lateral gutter, capitellum, coronoid, trochlea, and anterior and lateral radial head. Under arthroscopic visualization, an 18-gauge spinal needle is directed toward the center of the joint. Then, the skin is incised and a trocar is inserted. Care must be taken to avoid injury to the posterior branch of the antebrachial cutaneous nerve, which is located 0 to 14 mm from the cannula, and the posterior interosseous nerve, which is adjacent to the anterior joint capsule overlying the radial head.[17] Retractors can be placed in the proximal anterolateral portal to decrease the risk to the posterior interosseous nerve. The radial nerve is farthest from the portal—7.9 mm away when the elbow is in extension and 13.7 mm away when the elbow is in 90 degrees of flexion.[19]

A direct lateral portal can be used as a second working portal, established in the anconeus triangle (soft spot) in a similar fashion. This direct lateral portal gives access to the posterior radial

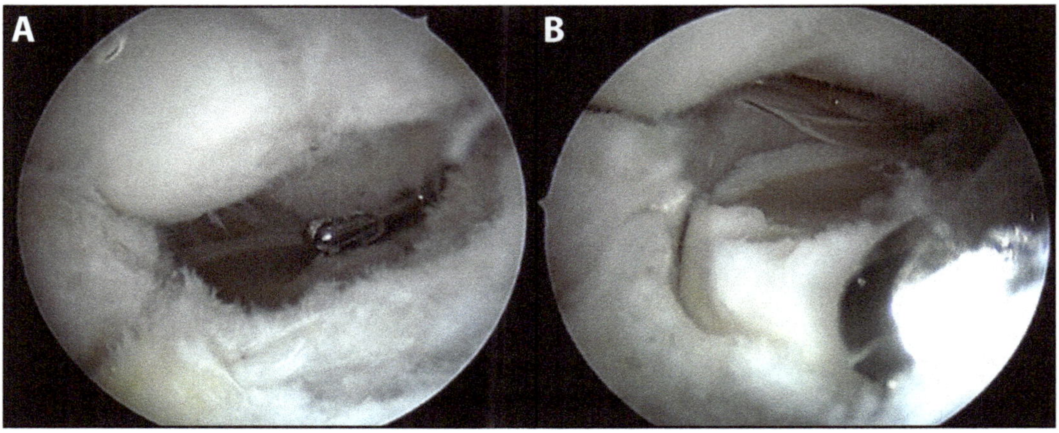

Figure 13-5. (A) Intraoperative photo of an arthritic radial head viewing from the anteromedial portal with the shaver placed in the anterolateral portal. A synovectomy is performed to allow for adequate visualization. (B) Synovectomy nearly complete with adequate visualization. Note the grade IV changes of the radial head.

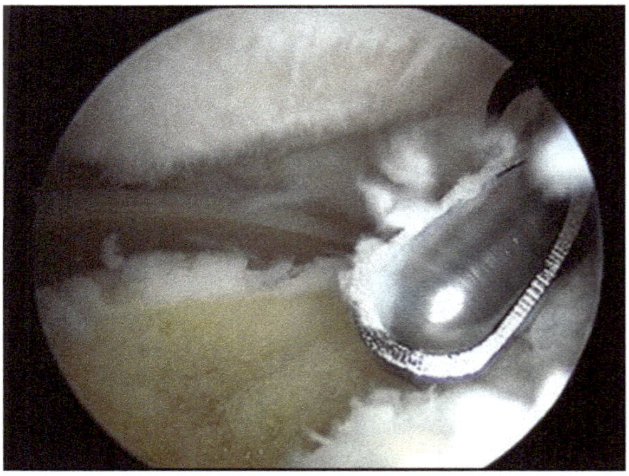

Figure 13-6. Close arthroscopic view of noted grade IV changes of the radial head in the same patient. The shaver is in the anterolateral portal.

head, capitellum, and radioulnar joint to achieve posterolateral plicae excision or debridement of any posterolateral osteophytes.

Step 2: Arthroscopic Assessment/Synovectomy

A 2.7- or 4.0-mm, 30- or 70-degree arthroscope is first introduced and a standard arthroscopic elbow examination is completed to determine the extent of bone and associated soft tissue injury. Debridement and synovectomy are performed with the arthroscope in the proximal anteromedial portal and the full radius shaver in the proximal anterolateral and, in rare occasions, direct lateral working portal (Figure 13-5). If treatment is selected for an acute fracture and excision has been decided, evacuation of the fracture hematoma must be performed.

Step 3: Resection of the Anterior Radial Head

Resection of the anterior one-half radial head is performed first with the arthroscope in the proximal superior medial portal and a 3.5-mm mini-mounted shaver and 3.0-mm burr in the proximal anterolateral portal (Figure 13-6). In order to protect the posterior interosseous nerve, which lies adjacent to the anterior capsule, the cutting surface of the shaver should always be

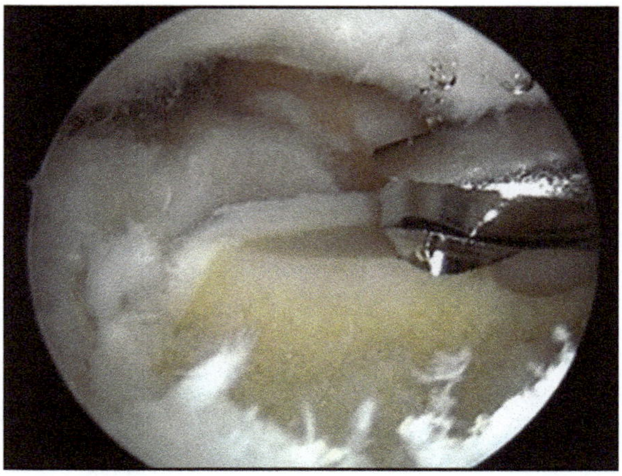

Figure 13-7. Arthroscopic view of the radial head with the hooded burr in the anterolateral portal removing the anterior one-half of the radial head. Pronating and supinating the forearm will allow the surgeon to gain access to the entire radial head.

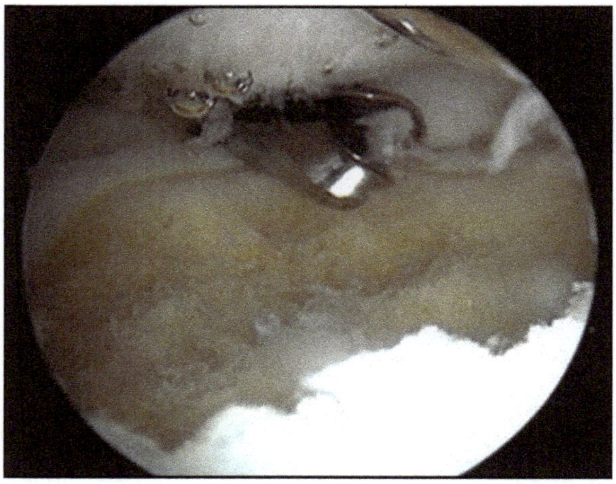

Figure 13-8. Arthroscopic view of the radial head resection. The burr has been removed and placed in the direct lateral portal for easy access to the posterior one-half of the radial head to ensure a smooth resection.

directed posteriorly. A cutting block technique may be used, similar to that described by Sampson et al[20] for acromioplasty (Figure 13-7).

Step 4: Resection of the Posterior Radial Head

Resection of the posterior one-half of the radial head will complete the radial head resection. Using switching sticks to transfer instruments, the burr needs to be placed in the direct lateral portal and posterior portals to complete the resection (Figure 13-8). Again, a cutting block technique is used for the posterior resection. As more of the radial head is removed, a more aggressive, larger burr can be used if necessary. Supination and pronation of the forearm throughout the procedure can help to ensure complete and adequate resection of the radial head. Caution must be taken to avoid compromising the annular ligament and subsequent instability of the proximal radioulnar joint. The goal of radial head resection is to excise 5 to 7 mm of the proximal radius to allow for adequate space between the proximal radius and the capitellum and to prevent impingement. The cancellous bone of the proximal radius should appear smooth.

Step 5: Assessment of Resection

After completion of the procedure, a thorough washout should be performed to remove any remaining debris. Under arthroscopic visualization, repeat assessment of ROM (particularly pronation and supination) and varus, valgus, posterolateral, and axial stress stability should be

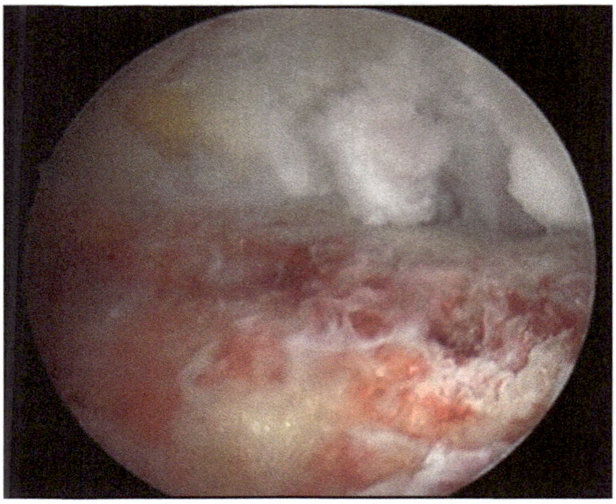

Figure 13-9. Arthroscopic radial head resection with the tourniquet down and testing supination and pronation to ensure no cartilage was left behind.

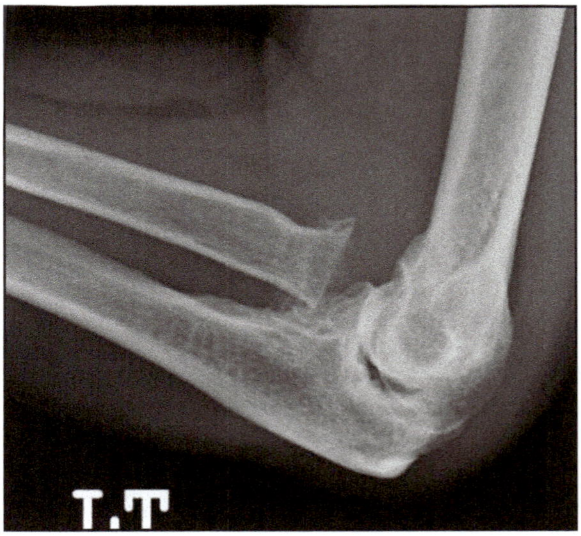

Figure 13-10. Plain lateral x-ray of the left elbow demonstrating adequate radial head resection postoperatively.

performed to identify any limitations (Figure 13-9). If there is a capsular contracture or other constraint to motion, additional procedures may be warranted, including anterior capsular release, olecranon osteophyte excision, or fossa debridement (Figure 13-10).

Postoperative Protocol

All portals are sutured closed to prevent synovial-cutaneous fistulas in standard fashion. A bulky dressing is applied to control swelling, and the arm is placed in a sling for comfort. Elbow ROM exercises are initiated under the supervision of a licensed occupational hand therapist within the first 1 to 2 days to promote early ROM in elbow flexion and extension. When edema is controlled, gentle, active assisted ROM in supination and pronation are commenced. The goal is to achieve full passive ROM by 2 weeks. In addition, wrist ROM and gripping exercises are commenced to maintain distal strength and ROM. Depending on swelling, resistive, strengthening exercises of the muscles around the elbow are begun around weeks 4 to 6 postoperatively. Full return to activities is allowed around 6 to 8 weeks as long as no other concomitant procedures (eg, Essex Lopresti) were performed.

Potential Complications

Complications following radial head resection include wrist pain, weakness, valgus elbow instability, arthrofibrosis, heterotopic ossification, and arthritis. Initiation of early ROM in a controlled environment can minimize the incidence of arthrofibrosis. In addition, indomethacin can be administered prophylactically in select situations to reduce the incidence of heterotopic ossification.[21] Neurological damage can be a transient neuropraxia, transaction, or neuroma; these are prevented by limiting surgical time, careful anatomic placement of portals, and using blunt trocars after incising only skin, respectively. Limiting surgical time also prevents infarction leading to compartment syndrome.

Conclusion

Radial head resection is a viable option to eliminate pain and improve elbow ROM for patients with radial head fractures or elbow arthritis. Patients with radial head fractures and radiocapitellar arthritis typically present with lateral-sided elbow pain and limited pain and ROM, primarily in supination and pronation. Radial head resection alleviates symptoms without resultant instability and yields excellent patient satisfaction.

Top Technical Pearls for the Procedure

1. Usage of appropriately sized instruments makes radial head resection a simple procedure.
2. A cutting block technique, similar to acromioplasty, can be used to ensure adequate radial head resection without compromising stability.
3. The cutting surface of the shaver should be directed posteriorly when resecting the anterior one-half of the radial head to protect the posterior interosseous nerve.
4. Move the forearm through supination and pronation throughout the procedure to ensure complete and adequate resection of the radial head.
5. Excision of 5 to 7 mm of the proximal radius is optimal to prevent impingement.

References

1. Morrey BF, An KN. Stability of the elbow: osseous constraints. *J Shoulder Elbow Surg.* 2005;14(1 suppl S):174S-178S.
2. Halls AA, Travill A. Transmission of pressures across the elbow joint. *Anat Rec.* 1964;150:243-247.
3. Egol KA, Koval KJ, Zuckerman JD. *Radial Head. Handbook of Fractures.* 4th ed. Philadelphia, PA: Wolters Kluwer/Lippincott Williams & Wilkins Health; 2010:800.
4. Herbertsson P, Josefsson PO, Hasserius R, Besjakov J, Nyqvist F, Karlsson MK. Fractures of the radial head and neck treated with radial head excision. *J Bone Joint Surg Am.* 2004;86(9):1925-1930.
5. Ditsios KT, Stavridis SI, Christodoulou AG. The effect of haematoma aspiration on intra-articular pressure and pain relief following Mason I radial head fractures. *Injury.* 2011;42(4):362-365.
6. van Riet RP, Morrey BF, O'Driscoll SW, Van Glabbeek F. Associated injuries complicating radial head fractures: a demographic study. *Clin Orthop Relat Res.* 2005;(441):351-355.
7. Mason ML. Some observations on fractures of the head of the radius with a review of one hundred cases. *Br J Surg.* 1954;42(172):123-132.

8. Rabinowitz RS, Light TR, Havey RM, et al. The role of the interosseous membrane and triangular fibrocartilage complex in forearm stability. *J Hand Surg.* 1994;19(3):385-393.
9. Faldini C, Nanni M, Leonetti D, et al. Early radial head excision for displaced and comminuted radial head fractures: considerations and concerns at long-term follow-up. *J Orthop Trauma.* 2012;26(4):236-240.
10. Wijeratna M, Bailey KA, Pace A, Tytherleigh-Strong G, Van Rensburg L, Kent M. Arthroscopic radial head excision in managing elbow trauma. *Int Orthop.* 2012;36(12):2507-2512.
11. Smilowicz M. Surgical treatment of the elbow joint in rheumaid arthritis, with particular attention to resection arthroplasty. *Ortop Traumatol Rehabil.* 2000;2(4):36-40.
12. Yeoh KM, King GJ, Faber KJ, Glazebrook MA, Athwal GS. Evidence-based indications for elbow arthroscopy. *Arthroscopy.* 2012;28(2):272-282.
13. Kim SJ, Kim HK, Lee JW. Arthroscopy for limitation of motion of the elbow. *Arthroscopy.* 1995;11(6):680-683.
14. Zarattini G, Galli S, Marchese M, Mascio LD, Pazzaglia UE. The surgical treatment of isolated mason type 2 fractures of the radial head in adults: comparison between radial head resection and open reduction and internal fixation. *J Orthop Trauma.* 2012;26(4):229-235.
15. Smith AM, Urbanosky LR, Castle JA, Rushing JT, Ruch DS. Radius pull test: predictor of longitudinal forearm instability. *J Bone Joint Surg Am.* 2002;84(11):1970-1976.
16. Poehling GG WT, Whipple TL, Sisco L, Goldman B. Elbow arthroscopy: a new technique. *Arthroscopy.* 1989;5(3):222-224.
17. Tashjian R KH, Galatz LM, Yamaguchi K. Elbow arthroscopy portals and techniques. In: Trumble TE, Budoff J, eds. *Wrist and Elbow Reconstruction and Arthroscopy.* Chicago, IL: American Society for Surgery of the Hand; 2006:367-375.
18. Stothers K, Day B, Regan WR. Arthroscopy of the elbow: anatomy, portal sites, and a description of the proximal lateral portal. *Arthroscopy.* 1995;11(4):449-457.
19. Field LD, Altcheck DW, Warren RF, O'Brien SJ, Skyhar MJ, Wickiewicz TL. Arthroscopic anatomy of the lateral elbow: a comparison of three portals. *Arthroscopy.* 1994;10(6):602-607.
20. Sampson TG, Nisbet JK, Glick JM. Precision acromioplasty in arthroscopic subacromial decompression of the shoulder. *Arthroscopy.* 1991;7(3):301-307.
21. Baird EO, Kang QK. Prophylaxis of heterotopic ossification - an updated review. *J Orthop Surg Res.* 2009;4:12.

Please see videos on the accompanying website at

www.routledge.com/9781630910013

14

Arthroscopic and Open Radial Ulnohumeral Ligament Reconstruction for Posterolateral Rotatory Instability of the Elbow

Michael J. O'Brien, MD and Felix H. Savoie III, MD

Introduction

Posterolateral rotatory instability (PLRI) of the elbow, as originally described by O'Driscoll et al in 1991,[1] is a diagnosis of lateral-sided instability that results from an incompetent radial ulnohumeral ligament (RUHL), also known as the *lateral ulnar collateral ligament* (LUCL). When the RUHL is nonfunctional, the radial head rolls off of the capitellum during forearm supination. As the radial head subluxates posterolaterally, the ulnohumeral joint begins to gap and, as the pattern of instability continues, the entire elbow joint may dislocate.[1] Lateral-sided elbow instability can be debilitating. Simple activities of daily living, such as pushing up from a chair or lifting objects with the elbow extended, become painful and difficult.[2,3]

Anatomy

The RUHL complex is composed of 3 separate ligaments that may have a variable expression (Figure 14-1).[1] The radial collateral ligament is adjacent to the capsule and courses from the lateral epicondyle to the annular ligament and then down to the ulna. The LUCL begins on the posterolateral aspect of the lateral epicondyle and courses distally to the supinator crest of the ulna while sending fibers to the annular ligament and blending with radial collateral ligament near the humeral origin. The annual ligament originates and inserts on the ulna following a course around the radial neck.

Patient History

Patients with PLRI will complain of lateral-sided elbow pain and discomfort with activities. They frequently report mechanical symptoms of locking, catching, and clicking, or a palpable clunk with certain activities.[1] This is typically noted at midflexion as the elbow goes into extension, especially with the forearm supinated, such as opening doors or lifting objects in front of them with the elbow extended. Pushing up from a chair or a seated position can cause pain and feelings of instability because the combination of supination, valgus force, and axial load causes the radial head to subluxate posterolaterally. The treating physician should inquire about prior trauma because

Savoie FH III, Field LD, Steinmann SP, eds. *The Elbow and Wrist: AANA Advanced Arthroscopic Surgical Techniques* (pp 137-146).

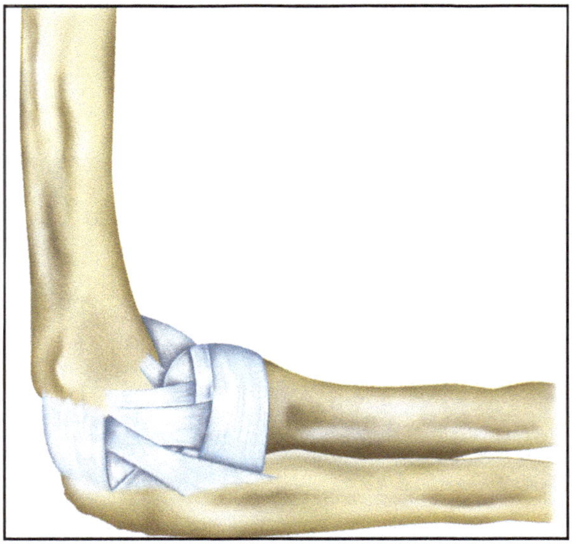

Figure 14-1. The LCL complex of the elbow.

the injury usually results from a fall onto the outstretched hand or a frank elbow dislocation. Elbow dislocations are the second most common dislocation of the upper extremity after the glenohumeral joint.[3] It is also important to inquire about previous treatment for concomitant conditions because PLRI resulting from cortisone injections or surgery for lateral epicondylitis has been described.[4]

Indications

- PLRI
- Chronic elbow instability
- Chronic elbow subluxation

Controversial Indications

- Acute elbow dislocation
- Acute lateral-sided ligament avulsion

Pertinent Physical Findings

- PLRI of the elbow is best demonstrated clinically with the lateral pivot shift test of the elbow.[1] This test can be performed in the supine or prone position and will elicit gross instability or pain and apprehension.
- Two additional tests described by Regan and Lapner[5] are also useful.
  - The chair push-up test is performed with the patient pushing up from an arm chair with the palms facing inward and forearms supinated.[5]
  - The table-top relocation test requires the patient to push up from a prone or wall-leaning position first with the forearms maximally pronated and then repeat the test with the forearms maximally supinated.[5]
  - These tests are considered positive when they reproduce the patient's pain, instability, or both.

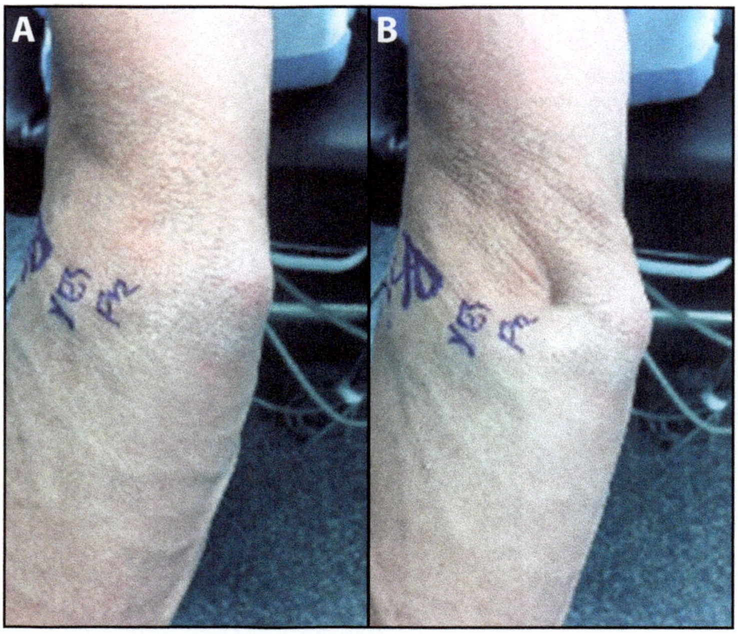

Figure 14-2. Clinical photographs of PLRI while performing the prone lateral pivot shift test. (A) Beginning with the elbow reduced and flexed to 90 degrees, the forearm is supinated while applying an axial load and valgus force across the elbow. (B) As the elbow is brought into extension, the radial head subluxates posterolaterally at approximately 40 degrees of flexion, with a dimple demonstrating the dislocated radiocapitellar joint.

- In the authors' experience, they prefer to examine the elbow with the patient in the prone position and use the table as a base to stabilize the humerus. Begin by manually rotating the forearm with the elbow in 90 degrees of flexion, palpating the radiocapitellar joint, and using the wrist to supinate the forearm. This movement reproduces the radial column subluxation as the forearm rotates away from the humerus. The radial head movement on the capitellum is more easily seen and felt in this position and the elbow can be flexed and extended while maintaining the subluxation force (Figure 14-2).

Pertinent Imaging

- Routine elbow x-rays, including anteroposterior (AP), lateral, and oblique projections are routinely obtained. X-rays are often normal, but, in acute cases, may reveal a lateral avulsion fragment from the posterior aspect of the lateral epicondyle of the humerus.
- Stress x-rays or fluoroscopy while performing the lateral pivot shift test may show the radial head and proximal ulna subluxate in a posterolateral position.
- Magnetic resonance imaging (MRI) of the elbow has been described to identify a lesion in the RUHL (Figure 14-3).[6] MR arthrography is the best modality to identify lesions to the medial and lateral collateral ligaments (LCLs). A formal arthrogram, with injection of contrast dye into the elbow joint prior to the scan, can greatly enhance the effectiveness of the test.

Equipment

Arthroscopic Ligament Repair

- Standard arthroscopic equipment
- 4-mm arthroscope (A smaller caliber arthroscope can be used but is usually not necessary.)

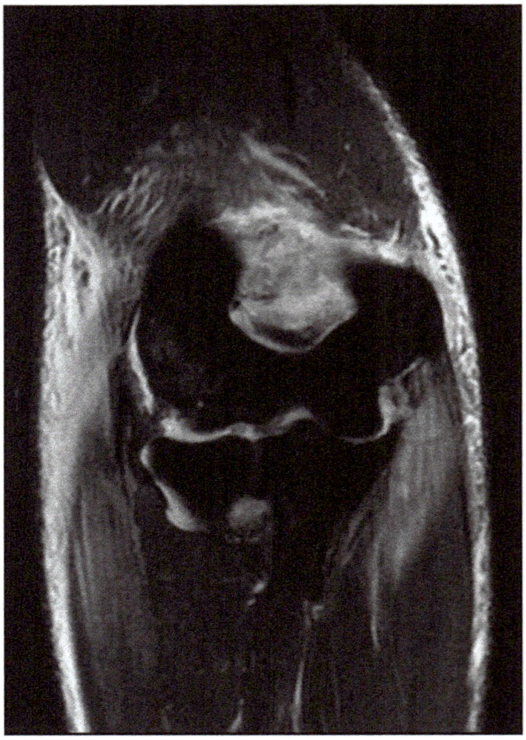

Figure 14-3. Coronal T2-weighted MRI demonstrating avulsion of the LCL complex off the posterior aspect of the lateral epicondyle of the humerus, with edema in the surrounding musculature. Also note the complete midsubstance rupture of the media ulnar collateral ligament on the medial side of the elbow.

- Small double-loaded glenoid suture anchors (1.9-mm, all-suture anchors or 2.9-mm solid anchors)
- Retrograde suture passer, suture retriever, crochet hook, and arthroscopic knot pusher

Open Ligament Reconstruction

- Standard arthroscopic equipment if arthroscopy is to be performed
- Graft of choice (palmaris longus autograft, gracilis autograft, gracilis allograft)
- 4-mm drill bit, power drill
- Ulnar fixation: small interference screw (5 or 6 mm) or EndoButton device (Smith & Nephew)
- Humeral fixation: small interference screw (5 or 6 mm) or bone tunnels

Positioning and Portals

Arthroscopic surgery can be performed in the supine, prone, or lateral decubitus position. In ligament repair or reconstructive procedures, the authors prefer the prone position with the arm on a bolster, which stabilizes the humerus and provides excellent access to the posterior compartment of the elbow. Standard arthroscopic portals are used. The anterior compartment is accessed through proximal anteromedial and proximal anterolateral portals. The posterior compartment is accessed with a posterior central viewing portal and a posterolateral working portal. It is paramount not to stray medial to the midline when making the posterior transtendon portal due to risk of injury to the ulnar nerve. A posterolateral soft spot portal and accessory distal soft spot portal are used for suture passage and suture tying.

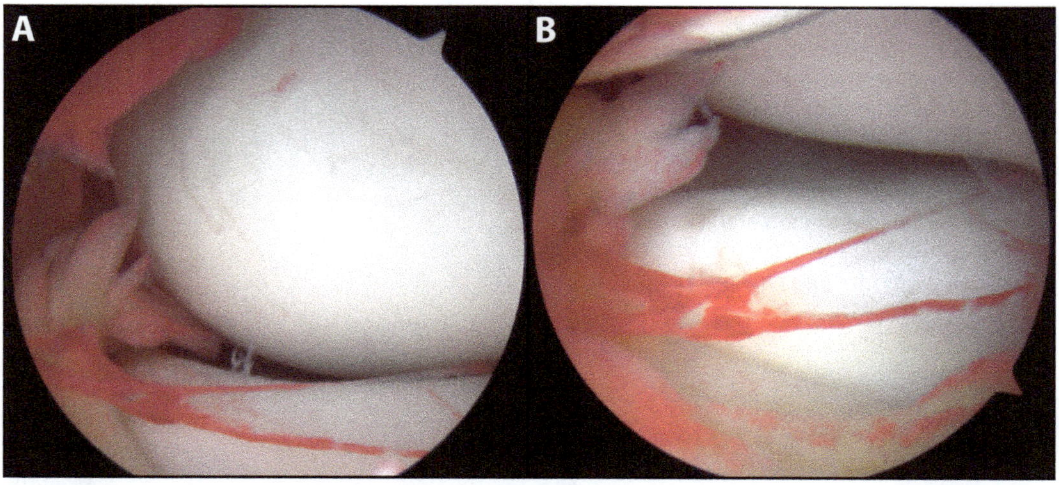

Figure 14-4. (A) View of the radiocapitellar joint in the anterior compartment from a proximal anteromedial viewing portal in a right elbow. The image demonstrates laxity of the annular ligament and tearing of the anterior capsule with hematoma, indicative of recent trauma. (B) The annular ligament droops down to the radial neck with gapping between the ligament and radial head, signifying incompetence of the RUHL complex. Forearm supination and valgus force cause the radiocapitellar joint to gap with posterolateral subluxation of the radial head. Tightening of the annular ligament following repair is one sign of an adequate repair.

Step-by-Step Description of the Procedure

Arthroscopic Repair

Arthroscopy of the acutely injured elbow demands efficiency and precision because tearing of the capsule will allow fluid extravasation and swelling. A concrete preoperative plan must be formulated and followed with adjustment made for arthroscopic findings.

The anterior compartment is accessed through a proximal anteromedial portal and a diagnostic arthroscopy is performed. Fractures of the radial head or coronoid can be identified. In the acute setting, abundant hematoma will be encountered in the joint with tearing of the anterior capsule and exposed muscle fibers of the brachialis. A proximal anterolateral portal can be established for the shaver to clean out the associated hematoma.

On the lateral side, laxity of the annular ligament and LCL complex will be evident in every case (Figure 14-4). It is important to assess the annular ligament for damage and gapping from the radial head. Valgus load and forearm supination demonstrates PLRI with the radial head subluxating off the capitellum, indicative of injury to the RUHL. On the medial side, an arthroscopic valgus stress test can be performed to evaluate for incompetence of the medial ulnar collateral ligament.[7] During evacuation of the hematoma, great care is taken not to resect or damage the LCL complex.

The arthroscope is then placed into the posterior compartment through a posterior central portal, and the hematoma in the posterior compartment is evacuated via a posterolateral portal. Both of these portals need to be relatively proximal to allow for the later repair of the ligament, usually at least 3 cm above the olecranon tip. A view of the medial gutter will show hemorrhage and occasional tearing of the capsule near the posterior aspect of the medial epicondyle.

One common finding is the ability to move an arthroscope placed down the posterolateral gutter straight across the ulnohumeral articulation into the medial gutter. This maneuver is not possible in a stable elbow and is termed the *drive-through sign of the elbow* (Figure 14-5). It is

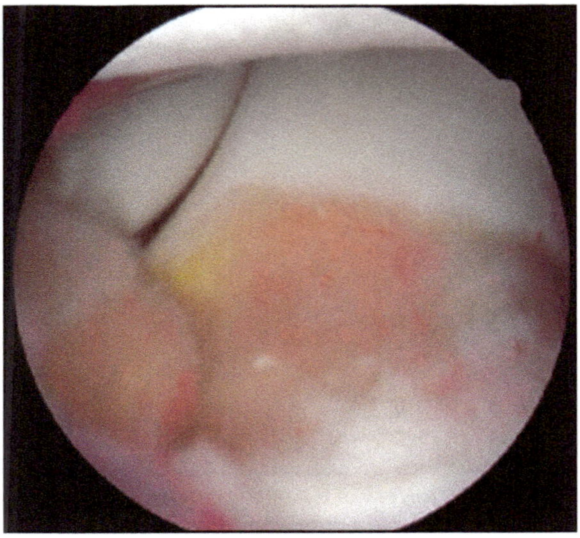

Figure 14-5. The drive-through sign of the elbow is performed by placing the arthroscope into the posterolateral gutter and moving it straight across the ulnohumeral articulation into the medial gutter. In this view, the arthroscope is in the ulnohumeral articulation from a posterior central portal in a left elbow with the distal humerus at the top of the image, the articular cartilage of the olecranon at the bottom of the image, and the proximal radioulnar joint in the upper left corner.

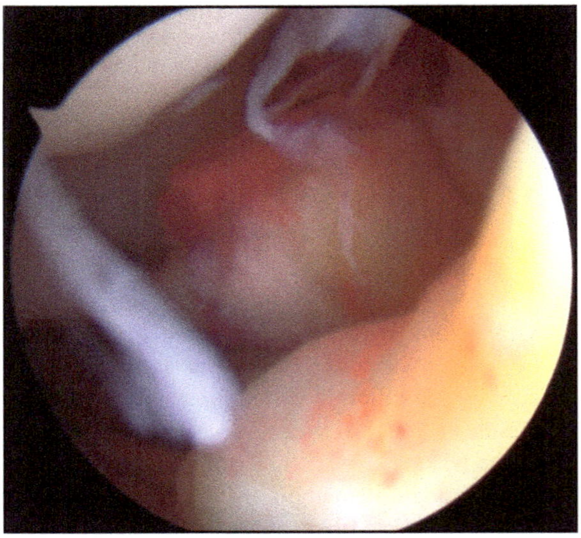

Figure 14-6. View of the posterolateral gutter from a posterior central portal in a right elbow, demonstrating the RUHL avulsed from the lateral epicondyle of the humerus and sitting posterior to the radiocapitellar joint. The avulsed ligament is in the center of the image. Great care must be taken when using the shaver in order to not damage or resect the RUHL.

somewhat analogous to the drive-through sign in shoulder instability. The elimination of the laxity that allows this maneuver is one of the key aspects of confirming an adequate arthroscopic reconstruction in patients with PLRI.

The lateral gutter and capsule are evaluated next. The arthroscope is easily advanced down the lateral gutter due to incompetence of the LCL complex. It is important to stay close to the ulna as the lateral gutter is evaluated and the hematoma debrided because the avulsed ligament and bone fragments are displaced distally and may inadvertently be removed by the shaver (Figure 14-6). The origin of the LCL complex on the posterior aspect of the lateral epicondyle can be visualized as a bare area where the ligament has avulsed off of the humerus. It is usually directly lateral and slightly inferior to the center of the olecranon fossa. This area on the posterior humerus should be lightly debrided with a motorized shaver.

Once the area of damage has been defined, a suture anchor may be placed percutaneously into the humerus at the site of origin of the RUHL. A percutaneous suture passer is placed through a soft spot portal to retrieve the sutures. The limbs of the suture are retrieved to place 2 horizontal mattress sutures through the noninjured part of the ligament (Figure 14-7). In the case of a bony

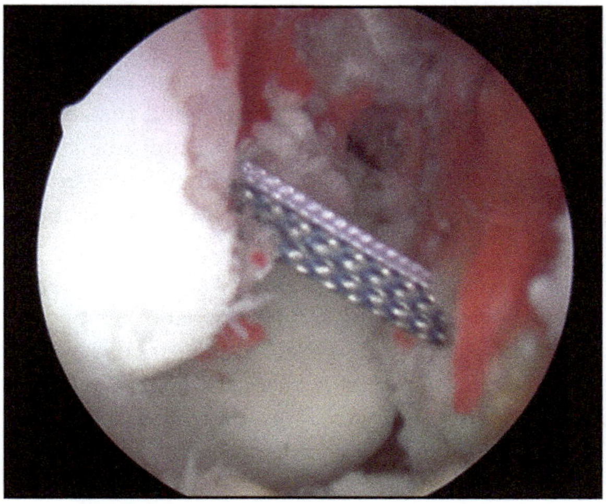

Figure 14-7. A suture anchor is placed percutaneously at the avulsion site of the RUHL on the posterior aspect of the lateral epicondyle of the humerus. The humeral origin of the RUHL is just lateral and distal to the olecranon fossa of the humerus. Two mattress sutures have been placed through the healthy portion of the ligament. The arthroscope is in a posterior central viewing portal in a right elbow.

avulsion, place one set of sutures around the bone fragment and the other distal to the fragment. The elbow is extended to approximately 30 degrees and the sutures are tied beneath the anconeus muscle, tightening the ligament. The sutures are tensioned while viewing with the arthroscope down the lateral gutter, which should have the effect of pushing the arthroscope out of the lateral gutter as tension is restored to the LCL complex. Motion and stability are evaluated with the arthroscope back in the anterior compartment, confirming that tension has been restored to the annular ligament.

Arthroscopic Plication

The development of an arthroscopic technique for the treatment of chronic PLRI was described by Smith et al in 2001.[8] The arthroscopic technique for chronic instability has the following 2 key features: plication of the 2 major components of the complex and repair of the complex to the humerus.[9,10] Both components can be managed via arthroscopic techniques if there is enough ligamentous and capsular tissue. This assessment is, in part, determined by the preoperative evaluation, including palpation of the structures in the area to be reconstructed, the amount of prior surgery, and the tissue present on MR arthrography.

If adequate lateral tissue is present in the posterolateral gutter, 4 to 7 absorbable sutures are placed in oblique fashion beginning at the most distal extent of the RUHL complex attached to the ulna. The sutures are placed into the lateral gutter via an 18-gauge spinal needle that slides along the radial border of the ulna. The first suture is delivered into the joint through the mid-portion of the annular ligament. Subsequent sutures are brought into the joint in a progressively more proximal position. Each suture is immediately retrieved with a retrograde suture retriever that passes into the joint from the posterior lateral aspect of the lateral epicondyle. It is important that the retrograde retriever comes under the entire RUHL near its proximal attachment to the humerus.

Once all of the sutures have been placed, they are retrieved one at a time percutaneously through the existing skin portals. The sutures are pulled to tension the ligament and evaluate the plication. If the plication has been properly performed, the arthroscope is driven out of the lateral gutter as this tensioning occurs. The arthroscope is removed, the elbow is extended, and the sutures are tied individually from distal to proximal. If laxity persists after the sutures are pretensioned, an anchor can be placed at the isometric point of the lateral epicondyle to further tension the LCL complex to the humerus. One limb of suture is passed under all of the plication sutures and one limb is placed over the plicated sutures to pull the entire plicated complex back to the humerus. This is usually noted as part of the preoperative planning and is accomplished before the plication sutures are tied.

Open Technique

The open technique for plication and repair is similar to that described by O'Driscoll et al.[1] A diagnostic arthroscopy may be performed to confirm the presence of instability and the absence of associated pathology, such as loose osteochondral fragments. A posterolateral approach is used and the anconeus muscle is split and retracted anteriorly to access the RUHL complex. If adequate tissue is found to allow repair, the ligaments are plicated and repaired back to the humerus as described in the section on arthroscopic repair.

In revision surgery or in patients with inadequate tissue for repair, a palmaris autograft or gracilis allograft may be used to reconstruct the lateral ligament complex. The supinator crest of the ulna, just posterior to the radial neck, is dissected free and the insertion site is identified. A 4-mm bone tunnel is created at the supinator crest and at the ulnar attachment of the RUHL, and the mid-portion of the graft is secured into the ulna using an interference screw technique. The 2 free graft limbs are then brought proximally, pulling one under the annular ligament and one over the ligament, and are attached to the isometric point on the posterior aspect of the lateral epicondyle. Bringing one limb of the graft under the annular ligament creates a more anatomic reconstruction with the added benefit of increasing stability of the proximal radioulnar joint. The graft should be slightly lax in extension and should tighten with flexion.

Postoperative Protocol

Following acute repair and chronic reconstruction, patients are immediately placed into a splint or hinged brace with the elbow in approximately 30 degrees of extension to relax tension on the repair. Fluoroscopy or x-rays should be obtained to check the reduction after the splint or brace is applied because additional flexion may be necessary to tighten the reconstruction and keep the joint reduced. The first postoperative visit usually takes place within 3 to 5 days of the surgery and the patient is placed into a hinged elbow brace that allows comfortable movement, usually 0 to 45 degrees. Shoulder, periscapular, wrist, and hand exercises are allowed as long as they do not produce pain in the elbow.

The patient is seen at 2-week intervals and motion is slowly increased 10 to 20 degrees per week as pain and swelling allow. Physical therapy is initiated at 6 to 8 weeks postoperatively to include upper extremity and core strengthening exercises with the elbow brace in place. Full elbow range of motion should be obtained by 8 weeks, if not sooner. Depending on individual progression, patients are allowed to start strengthening exercises out of the brace at 10 to 12 weeks. They must be able to perform all strengthening exercises pain free in the brace prior to progression out of the brace.

Potential Complications

Nerve injury is a potential complication of any elbow arthroscopic procedure. Thorough knowledge of the 3-dimensional anatomy of the neurovascular structures is crucial to avoid iatrogenic injury. Use great caution when working in the posteromedial compartment and medial gutter to avoid injury to the ulnar nerve. Use limited suction on the shaver in the lateral gutter to avoid damage or inadvertent resection of the torn RUHL. When tying the sutures during ligament repair, hold the elbow in approximately 30 degrees of flexion; tying the sutures with the elbow flexed 90 degrees will not adequately tension the ligament and may result in residual lateral instability.

Results

Smith et al[8] reported satisfactory outcomes in more than 20 patients following arthroscopic plication of the RUHL complex for chronic PLRI. Savoie et al[9,10] reported a retrospective review on 54 patients with PLRI who underwent open or arthroscopic surgical repair. The average follow-up was 41 months, and Andrews-Carson scores for all repairs improved from 145 to 180 ($P < 0.0001$). Acute repairs performed the best, with 9 of 10 returning to normal activities. There was no statistically significance difference between the results of open vs arthroscopic repair.

The authors recently reported on 14 consecutive patients who underwent all-arthroscopic RUHL repair using the same surgical technique in the acute (< 3 weeks) or subacute (< 3 months) period following elbow dislocation.[11] All patients were in-season athletes or high-demand professionals who could not afford to miss a significant amount of time away from their respective sports or professions. Mayo Elbow Performance scores were excellent in all 14 patients. The 7 patients in the acute repair group returned to full activities at a mean 2.7 weeks in a brace and 6.6 weeks out of a brace. The 7 patients in the subacute repair group returned to full activities at a mean 4.6 weeks in a brace and 8.9 weeks out of a brace. All patients returned to their sport or profession at the same level, and none experienced residual instability.

Acute open repair of the RUHL complex for the unstable elbow has very good results. Kim et al[12] recently reported on 19 patients who underwent acute open repair of the LCL complex for persistent instability following reduction of an elbow dislocation. The mean time to surgery was 8 days and the mean follow-up was 6.6 months. The mean Mayo Elbow Performance score was 86.9 points (range, 65 to 100 points), with 13 excellent cases, 5 good cases, and 1 fair case.

Numerous studies have shown favorable results for open RUHL reconstruction with a local tissue, autograft, or allograft tendon for chronic PLRI.[13-19] Although the patient cohorts are small (Sanchez-Sotelo et al[17] had the largest series of 32 patients published in 2005), results are promising, with recurrent instability rates ranging from 0% to 25%.

Top Technical Pearls for the Procedure

1. When working in the posterior compartment, keep the inflow in the anterior compartment. The flow of arthroscopy fluid from the anterior compartment will help to expand the posterolateral gutter, creating space and facilitating visualization.
2. The anatomic humeral origin of the RUHL is lateral and distal to the olecranon fossa on the posterior aspect of the lateral epicondyle of the humerus.
3. During suture passage, use an arthroscopic retriever to preplace the sutures down the lateral gutter. This will make retrieving the sutures easier after placing the suture passer through the healthy portion of the ligament.
4. Use a retrograde suture passer through a distal soft spot portal to penetrate the healthy ligament at the level of the radiocapitellar joint and retrieve the sutures from the anchor.
5. Use a crochet hook to retrieve the sutures subcutaneously out of the soft spot portal and tie the sutures with an arthroscopic knot pusher.

References

1. O' Driscoll SW, Bell DF, Morrey BF. Posterolateral rotatory instability of the elbow. *J Bone Joint Surg Am.* 1991;73(3):440-446.
2. Mehlhoff TL, Noble PC, Bennett JB, Tullos HS. Simple dislocation of the elbow in the adult. Results after closed treatment. *J Bone Joint Surg Am.* 1988;70(2):244-249.
3. Stoneback JW, Owens BD, Sykes J, Athwal GS, Pointer L, Wolf JM. Incidence of elbow dislocations in the United States population. *J Bone Joint Surg Am.* 2012;94(3):240-245.
4. Kalainov DM, Cohen MS. Posterolateral rotatory instability of the elbow in association with lateral epicondylitis. A report of three cases. *J Bone Joint Surg Am.* 2005;87(5):1120-1125.
5. Regan W, Lapner PC. Prospective evaluation of two diagnostic apprehension signs for posterolateral instability of the elbow. *J Shoulder Elbow Surg.* 2006;15(3):344-346.
6. Potter HG, Weiland AJ, Schatz JA, Paletta GA, Hotchkiss RN. Posterolateral rotator instability of the elbow: usefulness of MR imaging in diagnosis. *Radiology.* 1997;204(1):185-189.
7. O' Driscoll SW, Lawton RL, Smith AM. The "moving valgus stress test" for medial collateral ligament tears of the elbow. *Am J Sports Med.* 2005;33(2):231-239.
8. Smith JP III, Savoie FH III, Field LD. Posterolateral rotatory instability of the elbow. *Clin Sports Med.* 2001;20(1):47-58.
9. Savoie FH III, Field LD, Gurley DJ. Arthroscopic and open radial ulnohumeral ligament reconstruction for posterolateral rotatory instability of the elbow. *Hand Clin.* 2009;25(3):323-329.
10. Savoie FH III, O'Brien MJ, Field LD, Gurley DJ. Arthroscopic and open radial ulnohumeral ligament reconstruction for posterolateral rotatory instability of the elbow. *Clin Sports Med.* 2010;29(4):611-618.
11. O'Brien MJ, Lee Murphy R, Savoie FH III. A preliminary report of acute and sub-acute arthroscopic repair of the radial ulnohumeral ligament in the high-demand patient. *Arthroscopy.* 2014;30(6):679-687.
12. Kim BS, Park KH, Song HS, Park SY. Ligamentous repair of acute lateral collateral ligament rupture of the elbow. *J Shoulder Elbow Surg.* 2013;22(11):1469-1473.
13. DeLaMora SN, Hausman M. Lateral ulnar collateral ligament reconstruction using the lateral triceps fascia. *Orthopedics.* 2002;25(9):909-912.
14. Olsen BS, Søjbjerg JO. The treatment of recurrent posterolateral instability of the elbow. *J Bone Joint Surg Br.* 2003;85(3):342-346.
15. Lee BP, Teo LH. Surgical reconstruction for posterolateral rotatory instability of the elbow. *J Shoulder Elbow Surg.* 2003;12(5):476-479.
16. Eygendaal D. Ligamentous reconstruction around the elbow using triceps tendon. *Acta Orthop Scand.* 2004;75(5):516-523.
17. Sanchez-Sotelo J, Morrey BF, O'Driscoll SW. Ligamentous repair and reconstruction for posterolateral rotatory instability of the elbow. *J Bone Joint Surg Br.* 2005;87(1):54-61.
18. Jones KJ, Dodson CC, Osbahr DC, et al. The docking technique for lateral ulnar collateral ligament reconstruction: surgical technique and clinical outcomes. *J Shoulder Elbow Surg.* 2012;21(3):389-395.
19. Lin KY, Shen PH, Lee CH, Pan RY, Lin LC, Shen HC. Functional outcomes of surgical reconstruction for posterolateral rotatory instability of the elbow. *Injury.* 2012;43(10):1657-1661.

Please see videos on the accompanying website at

www.routledge.com/9781630910013

15

Arthroscopic and Open Treatment of the Throwing Elbow
The Docking Technique

Timothy Griffith, MD; Joshua S. Dines, MD; and David W. Altchek, MD

Introduction

As the primary restraint of the elbow to valgus load, the anterior band of the medial ulnar collateral ligament (MUCL) withstands significant force during the late cocking and early acceleration phases of throwing. Repetitive microtrauma and overloading may eventually lead to ligament injury.[1,2] After injury, symptomatic valgus instability frequently prompts surgical intervention. Initially described by Jobe et al,[3] surgical reconstruction of the MUCL led to the return to sport of 68% of elite throwers at their prior activity levels, with a notable 21% rate of ulnar nerve complications. Multiple concerns with the early UCL reconstruction as described by Jobe et al,[3] including lack of adequate tensioning and fixation, routine ulnar nerve transposition, detachment of the flexor mass origin, and creation of 3 large humeral drill holes, led to the development of the docking technique for MUCL reconstruction by the senior author. First described in 2002, this technique features the avoidance of routine ulnar nerve transposition, a muscle-splitting approach, reduction to one large humeral drill hole, simplification of graft tension and fixation, and placement of the graft into bone tunnels. In addition, as originally described, systematic arthroscopy was part of the procedure.[4] Multiple published series from the authors' institution demonstrate reliable clinical results with minimal complications in adult and adolescent overhead-throwing athletes with symptomatic UCL insufficiency. Specifically, 90% to 92% of athletes attained excellent results and returned to play at the same or higher activity level, with 0% to 7% complications.[2,4-6] A recent systematic review revealed the docking technique to result in a significantly higher return to play and lower complication rate relative to Jobe and modified Jobe techniques.[7]

Indications

Nonoperative treatment of MUCL injuries in throwing athletes frequently leads to a poor return to previous level of competition.[8]

Savoie FH III, Field LD, Steinmann SP, eds. *The Elbow and Wrist: AANA Advanced Arthroscopic Surgical Techniques* (pp 147-153).

- Subjective symptoms and the inability to perform in sport due to medial elbow pain often serve as indications for surgery.
- For throwing athletes with complete, isolated tears of the MUCL resulting in symptomatic pain and instability, the authors recommend operative reconstruction.
- Athletes with partial tears are often treated with rest, strengthening, nonsteroidal anti-inflammatory drugs, and potentially platelet-rich plasma; however, failure of that treatment further prompts recommendations for surgical intervention.[9]

Pertinent Physical Findings

Physical examination of the athlete's elbow involves inspection, palpation, range of motion (ROM) evaluation, and stability testing.

- Inspection for elbow swelling and fullness, especially medially, is the initial aspect of the authors' examination.
- The clinician should then palpate the medial elbow, starting at the medial epicondyle and flexor pronator mass.
  - The MUCL, which originates from the anteroinferior surface of the medial epicondyle and inserts at the sublime tubercle at the medial aspect of the coronoid, can be palpated with the elbow flexed at 90 or greater degrees of flexion under the flexor pronator mass.[10,11] Although no physical examination test is definitive, tenderness may suggest an MUCL injury.
- The ulnar nerve should be evaluated with provocative, sensory, and motor testing for signs of ulnar neuritis.
- ROM, including flexion, extension, and pronosupination, should then be evaluated. Pain and lack of extension may indicate posteromedial olecranon impingement.
- Stability testing is performed. The manual valgus stress test is performed by creating a valgus stress with the elbow in 30 degrees of flexion and maximal pronation.
  - Both elbows should be examined and compared. A positive test involves increased elbow opening or recreation of the patient's pain.
  - The moving valgus stress test, the authors' best test, is 100% sensitive and 75% specific for MUCL injury.[12] This test involves placing a valgus stress on the athlete's elbow from flexion to extension in an arc of 70 to 120 degrees of flexion. A positive test is indicated by apprehension, pain, or subjective instability during this maneuver.

Pertinent Imaging

- Anteroposterior, lateral, and oblique x-rays are obtained to evaluate for osteoarthritis, osteophytes, osteochondral lesions, loose bodies, and malalignment.
- Olecranon axial views may be obtained to reveal the characteristic posteromedial osteophyte in valgus extension overload.
- Contralateral comparison x-rays may be helpful, especially in the pediatric population.
- The authors do not routinely use stress x-rays in adults.
- MRI, as the primary means of assessing soft tissue and articular cartilage, is helpful to assess for full- and partial-thickness MUCL tears, osteochondral lesions not detected by plain x-rays, and flexor-pronator mass injury.

The aforementioned combined preoperative imaging is important for planning a successful surgery involving MUCL reconstruction and treatment of associated pathology.

Equipment

- 30- and 70-degree, 4-mm arthroscopes
- Appropriate shavers and microfracture awls
- Appropriate arthroscopic cannulas
- Tendon stripper, closed mouth, small
- Micro burr (1.5 mm)
- Burr (3.0 mm)
- Burr (4.0 mm)
- Acufex Graftmaster II (Smith & Nephew) for graft preparation
- #1 Ethibond suture (Ethicon) for graft
- 4-0 surgical steel for placement of shuttling sutures
- Bipolar electrocautery device

Positioning and Portals

Typically, regional anesthesia is used for this procedure. A tourniquet is placed once anesthesia has been administered. If arthroscopy is required for confirmation of the diagnosis or treatment of intra-articular pathology, this is performed initially. In this case, the patient is placed supine on the operating room table. The elbow arthroscopy is performed with the surgical extremity positioned across the patient's chest and supported on the contralateral side of the bed with an arm holder. The open graft harvest and MUCL reconstruction are performed with the patient supine and the arm on a hand table.

Step-by-Step Description of the Procedure

If present, the ipsilateral palmaris longus tendon is harvested. A 1-cm incision is made over the tendon in the volar wrist crease. Retractors are not used for this portion of the procedure because the tendon is superficial. A #1 Ethibond suture suture is placed in the tendon at the level of the volar wrist crease in a Krackow fashion (Figure 15-1). The tendon is incised distal to the suture previously placed, and the tendon stripper is used to harvest the tendon (Figure 15-2). This incision is closed with nylon suture immediately. If a palmaris is not present, gracilis autograft is the authors' second choice.

The arm is exsanguinated and the tourniquet is inflated. An approximately 8-cm incision is made in line with the intermuscular septum proximal to the medial epicondyle to a point approximately 2 cm distal to the sublime tubercle. The medial antebrachial nerve is exposed and protected throughout the procedure. In order to perform the muscle-splitting approach, the raphe between the flexor carpi ulnaris and anterior flexor bundle, indicating an internervous plane, is identified and incised. The anterior bundle of the MUCL is then exposed and longitudinally incised in line with its fibers from the anterior half of the medial epicondyle to the insertion on the sublime tubercle. Tagging sutures of 0-vicryl are placed for repair of the native ligament later in the procedure.

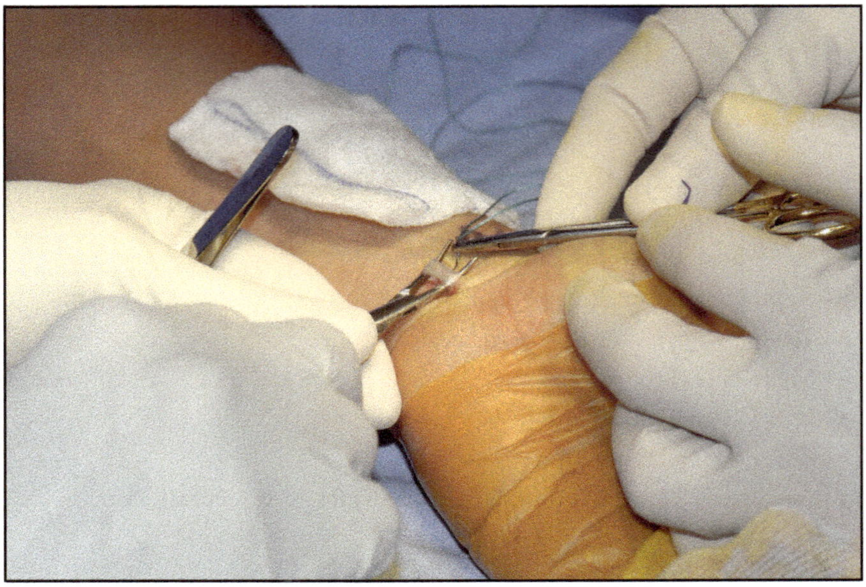

Figure 15-1. A Krackow suture is placed in the palmaris longus tendon.

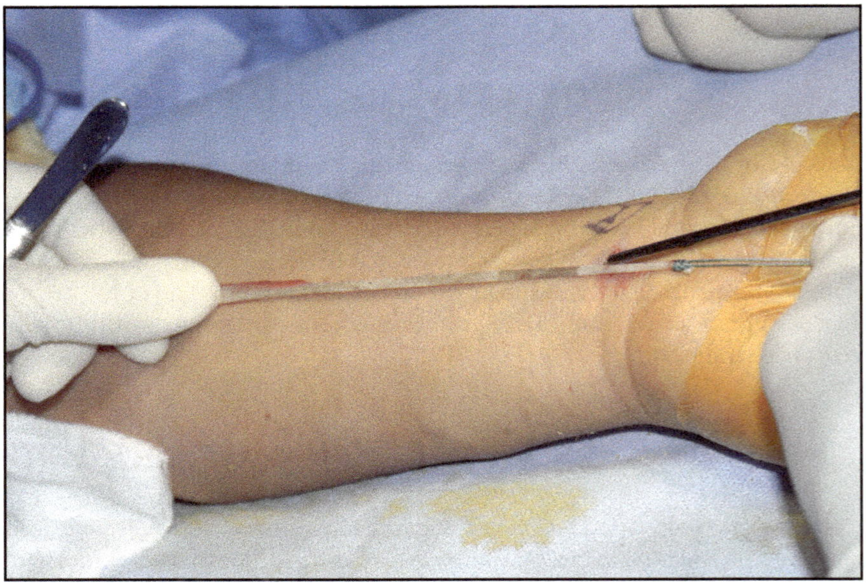

Figure 15-2. The palmaris longus tendon has been harvested with a tendon stripper.

The sublime tubercle is exposed in a subperiosteal fashion. An elevator is used during this portion of the procedure to protect the ulnar nerve as the posterior portion of the sublime tubercle is exposed. Anterior and posterior to the sublime tubercle, 2 tunnels are created with a 3-mm burr with at least a 1.5-cm bone bridge between the 2. A curette is used to connect the tunnels carefully. Attention is then turned to the medial epicondyle. Along the anatomic axis of the anterior half of the medial epicondyle, a 4-mm burr is used to create a longitudinal tunnel. Care is taken to not violate the posterior cortex of the medial epicondyle. Separated by a distance of approximately 1 cm in a proximal-distal fashion, 2 punctuate burr holes are created with a 1.5-mm burr at the anterior aspect of the medial epicondyle, anterior to the intermuscular septum, in line with the proximal aspect of the humeral tunnel, keeping the ulnar nerve carefully protected at all times.

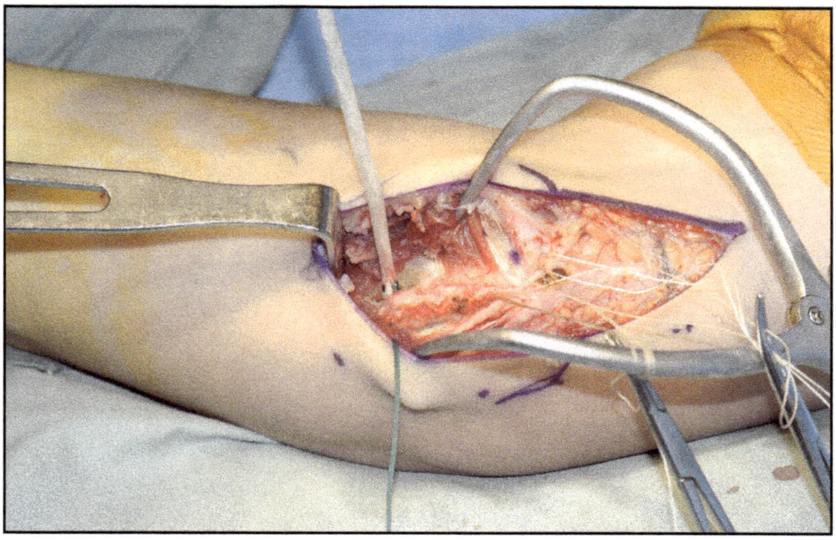

Figure 15-3. The graft is passed from anterior to posterior through the 3-mm sublime tubercle drill holes.

The graft is brought into the surgical field. From anterior to posterior, the graft is passed through the 3-mm burr holes previously created adjacent to the sublime tubercle (Figure 15-3). The native ligament is first repaired with the elbow in slight flexion and varus with the forearm supinated with the previously placed tagging sutures. At this point, the posterior limb of the graft is docked into the 4-mm humeral tunnel, and the sutures placed at the time of the harvest are retrieved through the proximal 1.5-mm tunnel created previously in the anteromedial epicondyle exiting the humeral tunnel. While tensioning these sutures and with the elbow in slight flexion with varus stress and the forearm supinated, the elbow is taken through ROM. The ideal length of the anterior arm of the graft is determined under these conditions and referenced to the entrance of the 4-mm humeral tunnel. This point is marked and a Krackow suture is placed again. By referencing the proximal entrance of the humeral tunnel, the authors ensure that the graft will be of sufficient length to enter the tunnel without bottoming out. After the suture is placed, the excess graft is sharply excised and the newly placed suture is retrieved from the relatively distal 1.5-mm humeral exit hole (Figure 15-4). The sutures from the anterior and posterior limbs of the graft are tied over the 1-cm bone bridge of the medial epicondyle in 30 degrees of flexion, with varus stress and the forearm supinated. The tourniquet is released, hemostasis obtained, and copious irrigation performed. The fascia of the flexor pronator mass is closed and the wound is closed in layers. A plaster splint is fashioned with the elbow in 45 degrees of flexion and the forearm in supination.[2,13]

Postoperative Protocol

The operative extremity remains in the plaster splint for 1 week. The elbow is then placed in a hinged brace, and motion from 30 to 90 degrees of flexion is initiated. Starting on week 3, motion is progressed to a range from 15 to 105 degrees of flexion. Removal of the brace and physical therapy, aimed at shoulder and elbow ROM and scapula and forearm strengthening, occurs at 6 weeks. Tossing is allowed starting at 16 weeks, every other day, at a distance of 45 feet. This distance is increased at regular intervals and decreased if any pain is experienced. If the patient can throw in a pain-free manner from 180 feet 9 months postoperatively, he or she may begin pitching from the mound. The authors do not recommend returning to competition until at least 1 year postoperatively.[2,13]

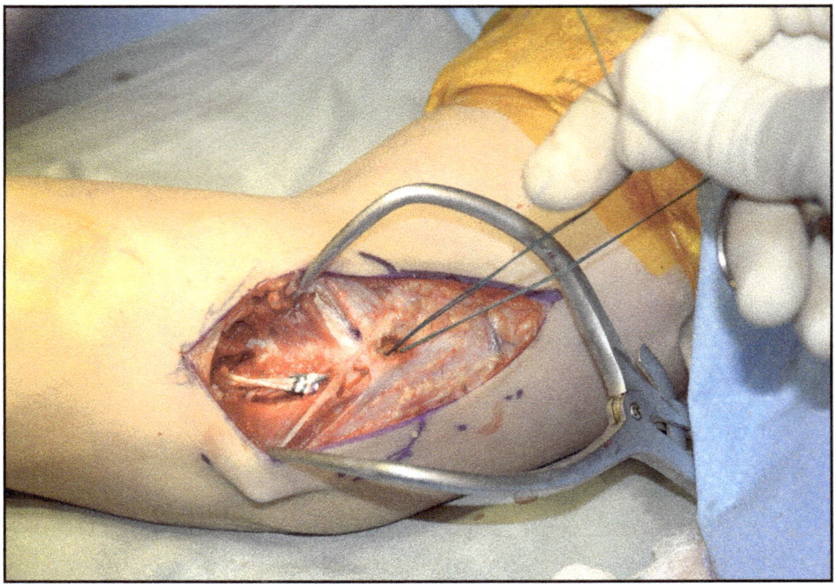

Figure 15-4. The anterior and posterior limbs of the palmaris longus graft have been docked in the 4-mm humeral tunnel.

Potential Complications

The most common complication, reported between 0% and 7%, include ulnar and medial antebrachial cutaneous neuritis and resulting paresthesias. These symptoms typically resolve without surgical intervention and do not typically influence outcomes.[1,2,4,6,13] Humeral or ulnar tunnel drilling complications, such as fractures, have not been demonstrated in recent series from the authors' institution reporting on clinical outcomes of the docking technique, including results in adult competitive baseball players, tennis players, adolescents, and javelin throwers.[2,5,6]

Top Technical Pearls for the Procedure

1. Although not done routinely, transposition of the ulnar nerve for motor sysmptoms or persistent sensory symptoms is critical for obtaining a good result. When indicated, the authors prefer an anterior subcutaneous transfer.
2. Use a muscle-splitting approach to avoid detachment of the flexor mass.
3. Preserve at least a 1.5-cm bone bridge between the ulnar tunnels on the sublime tubercle to prevent tunnel fracture.
4. Close the native ligament to strengthen the repair and keep the graft extra-articular.
5. Keep the humeral connecting holes anterior to the intermuscular septum while preserving adequate bone bridge.

References

1. Cain EL Jr, Andrews JR, Dugas JR, et al. Outcome of ulnar collateral ligament reconstruction of the elbow in 1281 athletes: results in 743 athletes with minimum 2-year follow-up. *Am J Sports Med.* 2010;38(12):2426-2434.
2. Dodson CC, Thomas A, Dines JS, Nho SJ, Williams RJ III, Altchek DW. Medial ulnar collateral ligament reconstruction of the elbow in throwing athletes. *Am J Sports Med.* 2006;34(12):1926-1932.
3. Jobe FW, Stark H, Lombardo SJ. Reconstruction of the ulnar collateral ligament in athletes. *J Bone Joint Surg Am.* 1986;68(8):1158-1163.
4. Rohrbough JT, Altchek DW, Hyman J, Williams RJ III, Botts JD. Medial collateral ligament reconstruction of the elbow using the docking technique. *Am J Sports Med.* 2002;30(4):541-548.
5. Dines JS, Jones KJ, Kahlenberg C, Rosenbaum A, Osbahr DC, Altchek DW. Elbow ulnar collateral ligament reconstruction in javelin throwers at a minimum 2-year follow-up. *Am J Sports Med.* 2012;40(1):148-151.
6. Jones KJ, Dines JS, Rebolledo BJ, et al. Operative management of ulnar collateral ligament insufficiency in adolescent athletes. *Am J Sports Med.* 2014;42(1):117-121.
7. Watson JN, Mcqueen P, Hutchinson MR. A systematic review of ulnar collateral ligament reconstruction techniques. *Am J Sports Med.* 2014;42(10):2510-2516.
8. Rettig AC, Sherrill C, Snead DS, Mendler JC, Mieling P. Nonoperative treatment of ulnar collateral ligament injuries in throwing athletes. *Am J Sports Med.* 2001;29(1):15-17.
9. Podesta L, Crow SA, Volkmer D, Bert T, Yocum LA. Treatment of partial ulnar collateral ligament tears in the elbow with platelet-rich plasma. *Am J Sports Med.* 2013;41(7):1689-1694.
10. Hyman J, Breazeale NM, Altchek DW. Valgus instability of the elbow in athletes. *Clin Sports Med.* 2001;20(1):25-45.
11. O'Driscoll SW, Jaloszynski R, Morrey BF, An KN. Origin of the medial ulnar collateral ligament. *J Hand Surg Am.* 1992;17(1):164-168.
12. O'Driscoll SW, Lawton RL, Smith AM. The "moving valgus stress test" for medial collateral ligament tears of the elbow. *Am J Sports Med.* 2005;33(2):231-239.
13. Dodson CC, Altchek DW. Ulnar collateral ligament reconstruction revisited: the procedure I use and why. *Sports Health.* 2012;4(5):433-437.

Please see videos on the accompanying website at

www.routledge.com/9781630910013

16

Open Ulnar Collateral Ligament Reconstruction
The Andrews Technique

Chris S. Warrell, MD; Daryl C. Osbahr, MD;
and James R. Andrews, MD

Introduction

The ulnar collateral ligament (UCL) is the primary static contributor to valgus elbow stability.[1-3] Injuries to the UCL are common in athletes participating in overhead throwing sports, secondary to the significant valgus forces placed upon the elbow. Insufficiency of the UCL most commonly presents with valgus instability and medial elbow pain, and UCL reconstruction is generally recommended for high-level overhead athletes who wish to return to competition. The Andrews technique for UCL reconstruction is a modification of the original figure-8 technique first described by Jobe and it uses a flexor-pronator mass elevation approach between the 2 heads of the flexor carpi ulnaris with obligatory ulnar nerve transposition.[4]

Indications

- Reconstruction is recommended for a complete rupture of the UCL in a high-level throwing athlete who wishes to return to throwing sports.
- Ligament reconstruction is also considered in throwing athletes who sustain a partial tear and continue to have pain and/or instability despite an appropriate course of nonoperative treatment, including a comprehensive rehabilitation program.

Controversial Indications

The decision to proceed with surgery often needs to be tailored to the individual athlete.

- High-level throwing athletes with UCL sprains may be considered candidates for UCL reconstruction once they fail nonoperative treatment.
- The concept for ligament attenuation and injury with no frank tear may lead the surgeon to recommend this treatment option.
- With valgus stress x-rays and dynamic ultrasound, subclinical valgus instability may be recognized despite a normal-appearing UCL on magnetic resonance imaging (MRI) evaluation.

Savoie FH III, Field LD, Steinmann SP, eds. *The Elbow and Wrist: AANA Advanced Arthroscopic Surgical Techniques* (pp 155-165).

Pertinent Physical Findings

The physical examination involves a standardized approach to evaluation of the elbow, shoulder, and kinetic chain to recognize and improve the entire pathological process involving the injured throwing athlete. When evaluating the UCL in particular, pertinent physical examination findings often relate to defining the presence or absence of functional medial elbow instability as well as ruling out any other concomitant or isolated pathology.

- Functional medial elbow instability is assessed through provocative maneuvers, including the valgus stress test, the milking maneuver, and the moving valgus stress test.[5-9]

Pertinent Imaging

- Diagnostic imaging should begin with standard anteroposterior, lateral, and oblique x-rays.
- An oblique axial view with the elbow in 110 degrees of flexion may be obtained to visualize posteromedial olecranon osteophytes, and anteroposterior valgus stress views can reveal excessive medial joint line opening.[10]
- Advanced imaging options include ultrasound, bone scan, and computed tomography with or without arthrography.
- MRI has become the gold standard in the radiographic confirmation of a UCL injury. Standard MRI without contrast has been reported to have a sensitivity of 57% to 79% and a specificity of 100% for diagnosing UCL tears; however, enhancement of the MRI with intra-articular saline or contrast may increase the sensitivity to greater than 90% and improves the diagnosis of partial tears.[6,11-13]

Equipment

The majority of the equipment required for UCL reconstruction may be found in a basic orthopedic instrument tray. Additional necessary equipment includes a power drill with a 3.2- or 3.5-mm drill bit for palmaris or gracilis graft, respectively; a Hewson suture passer (Smith & Nephew) for graft passage; a basic curette tray; and a basic retractor tray. If a gracilis autograft is used, a tendon harvester should be available and mineral oil may be needed to help with graft passage. Other essential items to have available include Metzenbaum scissors to decompress the ulnar nerve and create the medial intermuscular septum leash for ulnar nerve transposition, electrocautery to obtain hemostasis, and a small burr or osteotome to perform optional posteromedial olecranon osteophyte excision. In addition to routine suture for closure, the authors also routinely utilize 0-Ticron (Covidien) suture to tie the graft reconstruction limbs together, and 3-0 Ticron (Covidien) to suture the sling of the intermuscular septum for the ulnar nerve transposition.

Positioning and Portals

The patient is placed supine on the operating room table with a radiolucent hand table on the side of the injured arm. The authors prefer to use the ipsilateral palmaris longus tendon for autograft; however, they will use gracilis autograft when palmaris is not present or the UCL tissue is deficient or infiltrated with calcification, which requires excision. If autologous graft tissue is to be obtained from the contralateral arm or either lower extremity, the surgeons must anticipate prepping and draping the appropriate extremities.

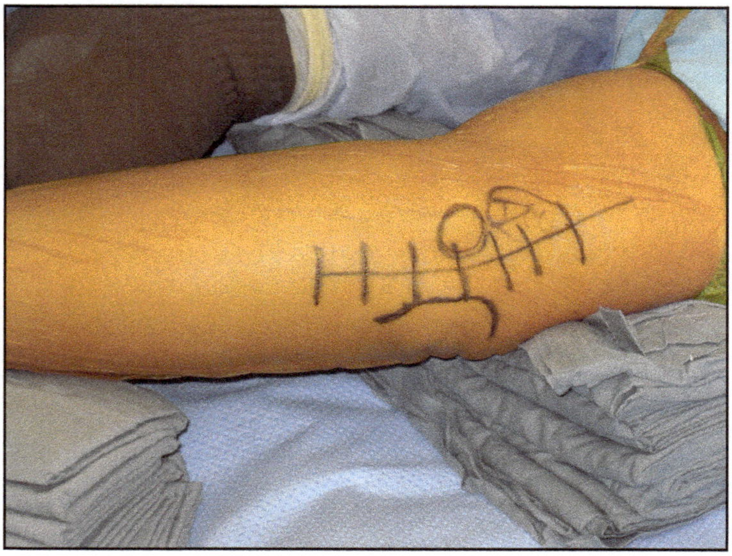

Figure 16-1. A curvilinear incision is made over the medial elbow, extending approximately 4 cm proximal and 6 cm distal to the medial epicondyle. (Copyright Daryl C. Osbahr.)

Step-by-Step Description of the Procedure

For a complete list of steps, please see Table 16-1.

Following induction of general anesthesia, the elbow is examined for range of motion (ROM) and valgus laxity. Next, a well-padded, nonsterile tourniquet is applied to the upper arm. The arm is then prepped and draped in sterile fashion, the limb is exsanguinated using an Esmarch bandage, and the tourniquet is inflated to 250 mm Hg.

The surgical procedure typically begins with harvest of the ipsilateral palmaris longus tendon, contralateral palmaris longus tendon, or contralateral gracilis tendon. For the palmaris longus tendon, the authors use a 3-incision technique to ensure that the correct structure is harvested and that the nearby median nerve and adjacent flexor tendons are not injured.[14,15] For the gracilis tendon, the authors use a standard harvesting technique with an incision placed over the pes anserinus with care not to injure the medial collateral ligament or saphenous nerve.[16]

Attention is then directed to the elbow to perform the UCL reconstruction. The incision is made directly over the medial epicondyle, extending approximately 4 cm proximal and 6 cm distal to the medial epicondyle (Figure 16-1). Blunt dissection is carried down through the subcutaneous tissue with care taken to identify and protect the medial antebrachial cutaneous nerve, which is variable in its course and can have multiple branches at this location. Once the nerve is identified, it may be protected with a vessel loop and dissection may proceed to expose the flexor-pronator mass, the medial epicondyle, and the cubital tunnel.

Because the Andrews modification involves a flexor-pronator elevation approach, the cubital tunnel is entered and obligatory ulnar nerve transposition is performed. The cubital tunnel is opened with Metzenbaum scissors and the ulnar nerve is identified, released, and mobilized. Proximally, the nerve should be decompressed at the arcade of Struthers. The medial intermuscular septum of the upper arm is divided at the most proximal portion of the incision and released from the medial humerus, but the authors save its distal attachment to the medial epicondyle to create a strip of fascial tissue that will be used as a sling at the end of procedure to hold the ulnar nerve in its transposed position. Distally, the ulnar nerve is released by splitting the fascia of the flexor carpi ulnaris (FCU) in line with its muscular fibers between the humeral and ulnar heads of the FCU. Care must be taken to identify and protect the first motor branch to the FCU. At this point, a vessel loop is used to protect and mobilize the ulnar nerve.

Table 16-1. Step-by-Step Description of the Procedure

Step	Description
1. Autograft harvest	Obtain palmaris longus tendon via 3-incision technique or gracilis tendon with use of a standard tendon harvester. Whipstitch the free ends of the graft.
2. Incision	Incise the skin and subcutaneous tissue over the medial epicondyle, extending approximately 4 cm proximal and 6 cm distal.
3. Dissection	Protect and mobilize branches of the medial antebrachial cutaneous nerve. Expose the medial epicondyle, flexor-pronator mass (FPM), and cubital tunnel.
4. Ulnar nerve release	Open the cubital tunnel with Metzenbaum scissors. Release the nerve proximally from the arcade of Struthers and distally from the fascia of the FCU.
5. Creation of ulnar nerve sling	Divide the medial intermuscular septum at the proximal extent of the incision and release it from the humerus, saving its distal attachment to the medial epicondyle.
6. Posterior elbow arthrotomy	Make a small, vertically oriented incision at the posteromedial joint.
7. Olecranon osteophyte removal	Remove osteophytic overgrowth with use of a quarter-inch osteotome, rongeur, and/or burr while preserving the native olecranon process.
8. UCL exposure	Sharply elevate the flexor digitorum superficialis off of the native UCL with a #15 blade scalpel. Begin distally at the sublime tubercle and continue proximally to the medial epicondyle of the humerus. Preserve the origin of the FPM.
9. UCL split	Split the native UCL in line with its fibers. Observe for undersurface tearing and ulnohumeral joint pathology.
10. Ulnar tunnel creation	Drill 2 converging tunnels starting at the posterior and anterior edge of the sublime tubercle. Connect and clear the tunnels with aid of a curette.
11. Humeral tunnel creation	Drill 2 tunnels to create a Y-shaped tunnel configuration. Use a curette to connect and clear the tunnels.
12. Native UCL closure	Close the native UCL split in a side-to-side fashion.
13. Graft passage	Pass the graft through the ulnar tunnel, leaving equal lengths of tendon on each side. Cross free limbs of the graft and pass through the humeral tunnels. Use a Hewson suture passer and mineral oil to aid passage.
14. Graft fixation	Tension the graft with the elbow flexed to 30 degrees and a slight varus stress applied to the elbow, and suture the 2 limbs together at the medial epicondyle. Suture the portion of the graft that spans the joint.
15. Ulnar nerve transposition	Transpose the nerve anteriorly to overlie the FPM. Lay the sling of the medial intermuscular septum loosely over the nerve and suture to the fascia of the FPM. Take the elbow through a gentle range of motion to ensure that the ulnar nerve moves freely.
16. Wound closure	Irrigate the wound and close in a layered fashion over a Hemovac drain.
17. Immobilization	Place a well-padded, long-arm splint with the elbow in approximately 90 degrees of flexion.

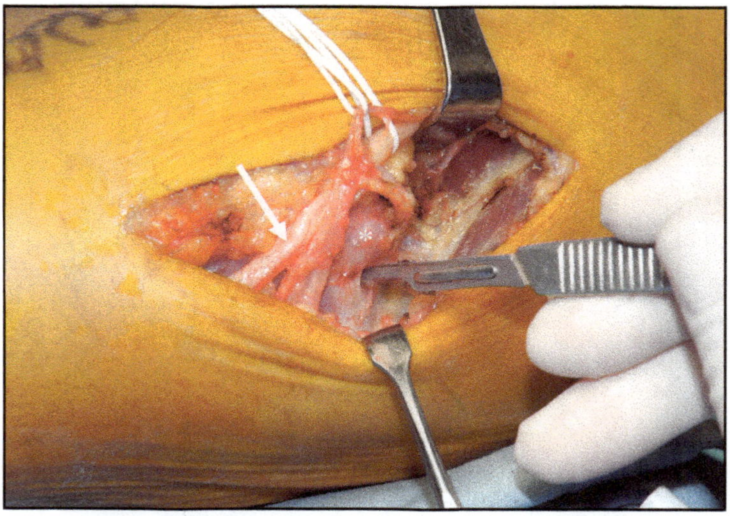

Figure 16-2. Posteromedial olecranon osteophytes are removed through a vertically oriented posterior elbow arthrotomy. The ulnar nerve (arrow) is retracted anterior to the medial epicondyle (*) to allow access to the joint. (Copyright Daryl C. Osbahr.)

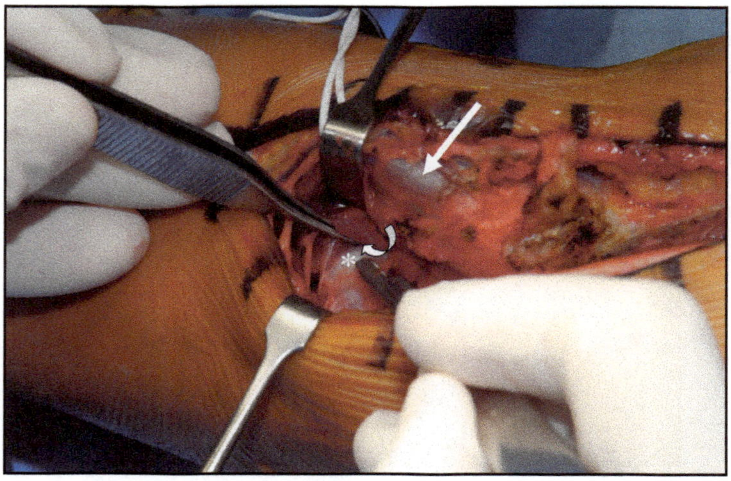

Figure 16-3. Elevation of the flexor digitorum superficialis (curved arrow) begins distally at the sublime tubercle and continues proximally toward the medial epicondyle to reveal the underlying UCL (*). The remainder of the flexor-pronator mass is retracted anteriorly (arrow). (Copyright Daryl C. Osbahr.)

If imaging reveals posteromedial olecranon osteophytes, these are removed through a small, vertically oriented posterior arthrotomy (Figure 16-2). Osteophyte removal is achieved with use of a quarter-inch osteotome, rongeur, and/or burr. Approximately 5 to 10 mm of osteophytic overgrowth is removed, whereas the native olecranon is left intact to ensure proper postoperative kinematics of the elbow. The capsule is closed side-to-side following osteophyte removal, with care not to overtighten.

The dissection is continued to expose the injured UCL. A #15 blade is used to sharply elevate the flexor digitorum superficialis muscle, which lies just superficial to the anterior fibers of the UCL. Elevation of the flexor digitorum superficialis begins distally at the sublime tubercle of the ulna and continues proximally to the origin of the UCL on the medial humeral epicondyle (Figure 16-3). The origin of the flexor-pronator mass is left intact. With small Hohmann retractors, the flexor-pronator mass is retracted anteriorly, allowing visualization of the anterior bundle of the UCL (Figure 16-4). During the exposure, great care is taken in cauterizing any small vascular channels to prevent postoperative bleeding. The UCL is then examined for any defects, including a tear, avulsion fracture, calcification, or abnormal laxity. A longitudinal incision is then made in the ligament in line with the fibers to evaluate if there is undersurface tearing consistent with a partial rupture. The ulnohumeral joint is also examined for pathology at this time (Figure 16-5).

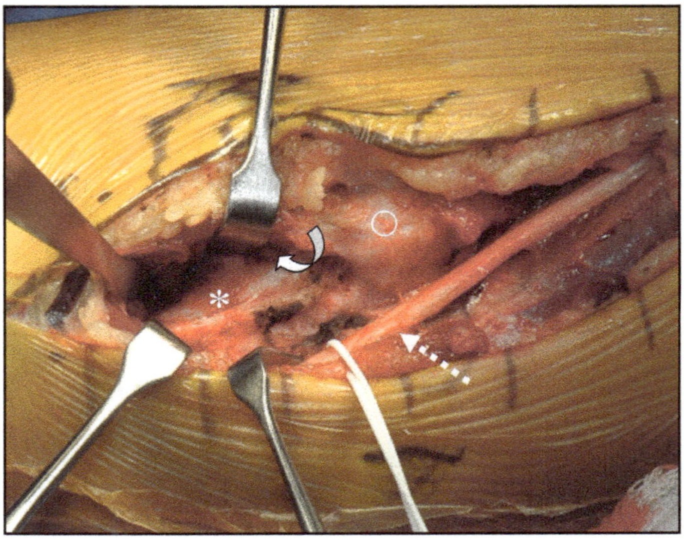

Figure 16-4. The curved arrow demonstrates elevation of the flexor-pronator mass near its origin on the medial epicondyle (circle). This allows exposure of the UCL (*). The ulnar nerve (dashed arrow) has been completely released and is safely mobilized with a large vessel loop. (Copyright Daryl C. Osbahr.)

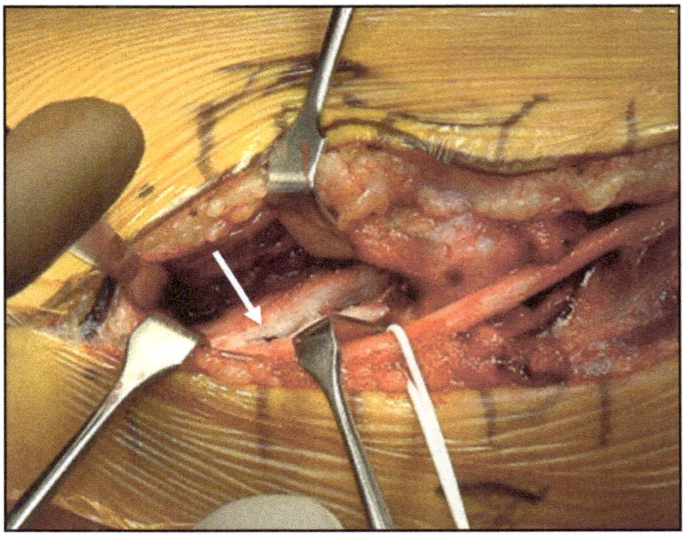

Figure 16-5. A longitudinal incision is made in the native UCL to access the ulnohumeral joint (arrow) and evaluate for undersurface ligament tearing and intra-articular pathology. The incision is closed prior to ligament reconstruction. (Copyright Daryl C. Osbahr.)

The authors then proceed with bone tunnel preparation using a 3.2- or 3.5-mm drill, depending on the diameter of the graft to be used. The first ulnar drill hole is made at the posterior edge of the sublime tubercle, aiming anterior and parallel to the ulnohumeral joint line (Figure 16-6A). The second drill hole is started at the anterior edge of the sublime tubercle and is aimed posterior to converge with the first drill hole at a right angle (Figure 16-6B). On the humeral side, 2 tunnels are drilled to create a Y-shaped tunnel configuration. The first tunnel is started at the origin of the UCL and is aimed proximal and lateral to exit the posterosuperior border of the medial epicondyle (Figure 16-7A). The second tunnel is drilled in an antegrade fashion starting at the medial prominence of the medial epicondyle and pointed to converge with the first tunnel at the origin of the UCL (Figure 16-7B).

With the bone tunnels complete, the graft may now be passed and fixated. Using a Hewson suture passer, the graft is first passed through the ulnar tunnel, leaving equal lengths of tendon on each side. Next, the free limbs of the graft are crossed and passed in a retrograde direction through the humeral tunnels (Figure 16-8). The forearm is supinated, the elbow is flexed to approximately

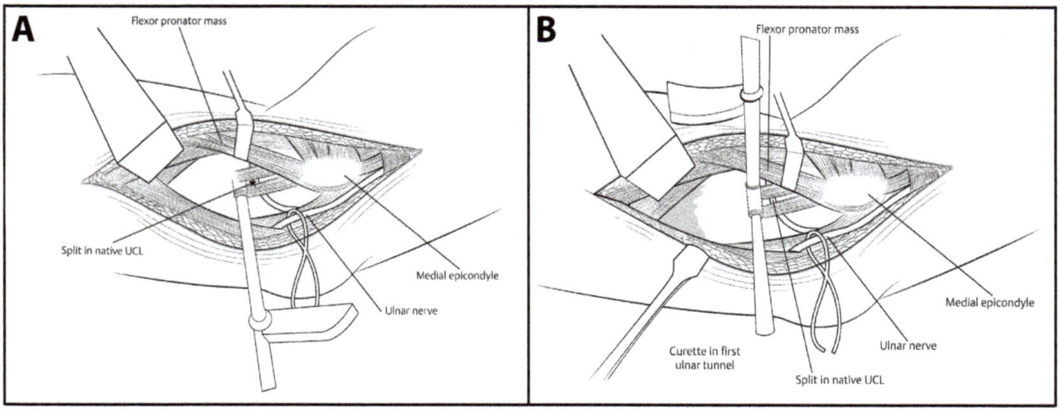

Figure 16-6. (A) The first ulnar drill hole is made at the posterior edge of the sublime tubercle, aiming anterior and parallel to the ulnohumeral joint line. The ulnohumeral joint is seen through the split in the native UCL. (B) The second drill hole is started at the anterior edge of the sublime tubercle and is aimed posterior to converge with the first drill hole at a right angle. The ulnohumeral joint is seen through the split in the native UCL.

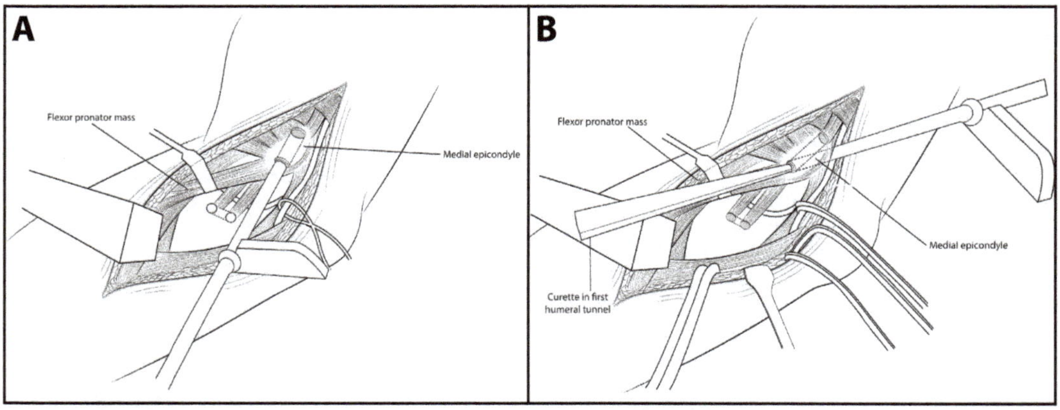

Figure 16-7. (A) The first humeral tunnel is started at the origin of the UCL and is aimed proximal and laterally to exit the posterosuperior border of the medial epicondyle. The flexor-pronator mass is retracted anteriorly to reveal the starting point. Medial epicondyle. (B) The second tunnel is drilled in an antegrade fashion starting at the medial prominence of the medial epicondyle and pointed to converge with the first tunnel at the origin of the UCL. A curette may be used to aid in triangulation. Flexor-pronator mass. Medial epicondyle.

30 degrees, and slight varus stress is applied so that the articular surfaces of the ulnohumeral joint are in contact. Prior to graft fixation, the native UCL split is closed and imbricated in a side-to-side fashion. The graft is then tensioned and the 2 limbs are overlapped and sutured together at the medial epicondyle, as well as to the periosteum of the medial epicondyle. The portion of the graft that spans the joint is also sutured together so that the graft better recreates the course of the anterior bundle of the native UCL (Figure 16-9). For both of these steps, a large, braided, size 0 nonabsorbable suture is used.

Once the UCL reconstruction is complete, the ulnar nerve is transposed anteriorly to overlie the flexor-pronator mass. The sling of the medial intermuscular septum is laid loosely over the nerve and sutured to the fascia of the flexor-pronator mass using a size 3-0 nonabsorbable, braided suture (Figure 16-10). At this time, the elbow is taken through a gentle ROM to ensure that the ulnar nerve is able to move freely without compression or tethering.

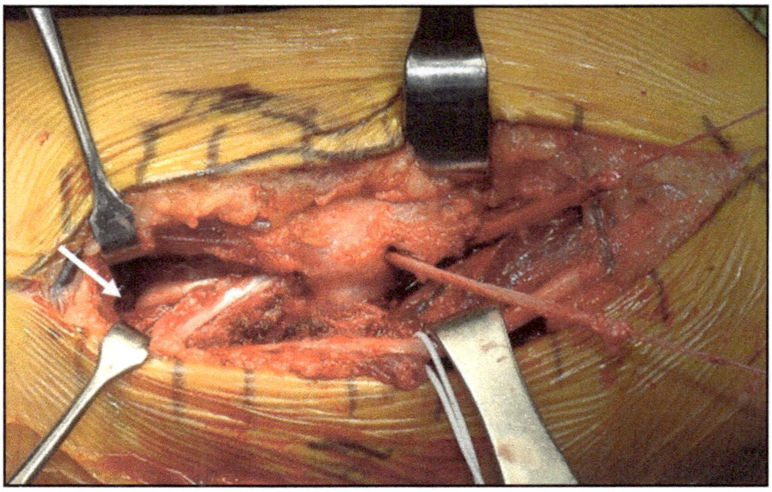

Figure 16-8. The graft is first placed through the ulnar tunnel (arrow), leaving equal lengths of tendon on either side. The free limbs of the graft are then crossed and passed through the Y-shaped humeral tunnels. (Copyright Daryl C. Osbahr.)

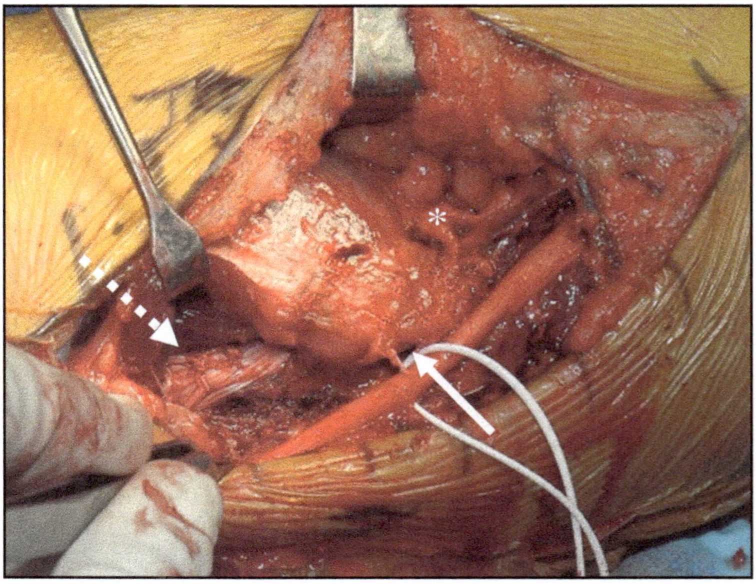

Figure 16-9. With the graft properly tensioned, the free limbs are sutured together at the medial epicondyle (solid arrow), and the portion of the graft spanning the joint is also sutured together (dashed arrow). Note the strip of the medial intramuscular septum set aside for later ulnar nerve transposition (*). (Copyright Daryl C. Osbahr.)

The tourniquet is deflated and hemostasis is achieved using electrocautery. The wound is thoroughly irrigated with sterile normal saline. The cubital tunnel and fascia of the FCU are closed loosely with a size 0 absorbable suture, with care taken to make sure that the ulnar nerve is not compressed or tethered. A small Hemovac (Zimmer) drain is placed with plans for removal before discharging the patient the same day. The subcutaneous tissue and skin are closed using size 2-0 and 3-0 absorbable suture, respectively, and Steri-strips (3M) are placed. The incision is dressed with sterile gauze and a well-padded long-arm splint is applied and molded with the elbow in 90 degrees of flexion.

Postoperative Protocol

The postoperative rehabilitation program consists of a standardized 4-phase approach as described by Wilk et al.[17-20] This program transitions to an interval throwing program around

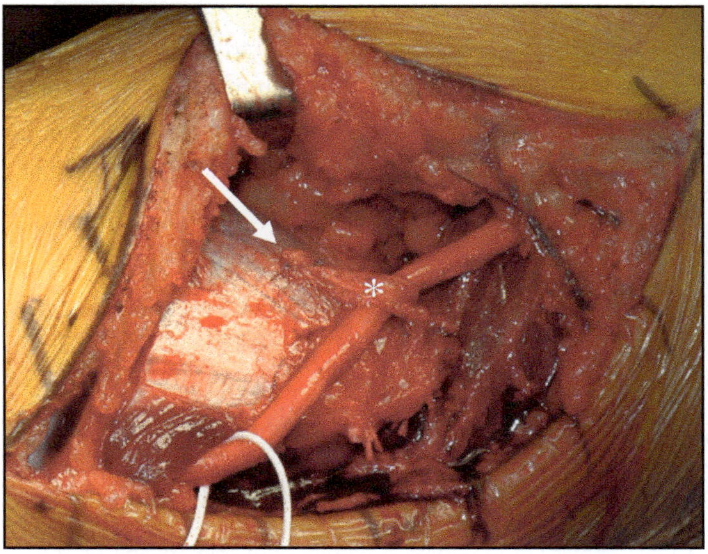

Figure 16-10. The ulnar nerve is transposed anteriorly, and the sling of the medial intermuscular septum (*) is laid loosely over the nerve and sutured to the fascia of the flexor-pronator mass (arrow). The nerve should move freely without compression or tethering when the elbow is taken through a ROM. (Copyright Daryl C. Osbahr.)

16 weeks after surgery, and return to competitive throwing can be expected around 12 months after surgery.

Potential Complications

The Andrews technique has reported complications commensurate to other techniques. The most common complication, seen in approximately 20% of patients, is transient ulnar nerve neurapraxia, which presents as sensory paresthesias in the ring and small fingers and typically resolves within 6 weeks. Rare complications include persistent (> 3 months) ulnar nerve symptoms (3%), arthrofibrosis (3%), and medial epicondyle avulsion fractures (0.5%).[21,22]

Top Technical Pearls for the Procedure

1. Nerve management: Identify, protect, and isolate the multiple branches of the medial antebrachial cutaneous nerve. Carefully dissect the ulnar nerve and protect it posteriorly. Proximal and distal ulnar nerve decompression is essential. Suture the edge of the triceps back to the medial epicondyle and septum to prevent subluxation of its edge. The medial septum (sling) should be placed loosely over the transposed ulnar nerve; otherwise, the septum will contract during the healing process and potentially cause compression.
2. Native UCL considerations: If bony calcification is present within the ligament, excise the calcification, repair the ligament, and use a larger graft (ie, hamstring) for reconstruction.
3. Tunnel preparation: Do not use excessively large drill holes for tunnel preparation for fear of graft breakage through the sublime tubercle and/or medial epicondyle.

(continued)

4. Graft tension: Tension the graft by applying a varus load at about 30 degrees of elbow flexion, and secure the graft in side-to-side fashion over the top (proximal side) of the medial epicondyle.
5. Closure: Release the tourniquet, use copious irrigation, obtain thorough hemostasis, and place a Hemovac drain before closure.

References

1. Schwab GH, Bennett JB, Woods GW, Tullos HS. Biomechanics of elbow instability: the role of the medial collateral ligament. *Clin Orthop Relat Res.* 1980;(146):42-52.
2. Morrey BF, An KN. Articular and ligamentous contributions to the stability of the elbow joint. *Am J Sports Med.* 1983;11(5):315-319.
3. Morrey BF, Tanaka S, An KN. Valgus stability of the elbow. A definition of primary and secondary constraints. *Clin Orthop Relat Res.* 1991;(265):187-195.
4. Andrews JR, Timmerman LA. Outcome of elbow surgery in professional baseball players. *Am J Sports Med.* 1995;23(4):407-413.
5. Jones KJ, Osbahr DO, Schrumpf MA, Dines JS, Altcheck DW. Ulnar collateral ligament reconstruction in throwing athletes: a review of current concepts. AAOS exhibit selection. *J Bone Joint Surg Am.* 2012;94:e49.
6. Timmerman LA, Schwartz ML, Andrews JR. Preoperative evaluation of the ulnar collateral ligament by magnetic resonance imaging and computed tomography arthrography. Evaluation in 25 baseball players with surgical confirmation. *Am J Sports Med.* 1994;22(1):26-31.
7. Chen FS, Rokito AS, Jobe FW. Medial elbow problems in the overhead-throwing athlete. *J Am Acad Orthop Surg.* 2001;9(2):99-113.
8. Thompson WH, Jobe FW, Yocum LA, Pink MM. Ulnar collateral ligament reconstruction in athletes: muscle-splitting approach without transposition of the ulnar nerve. *J Shoulder Elbow Surg.* 2001;10(2):152-157.
9. O'Driscoll SW, Lawton RL, Smith AM. The "moving valgus stress test" for medial collateral ligament tears of the elbow. *Am J Sports Med.* 2005;33(2):231-239.
10. Wilson FD, Andrews JR, Blackburn TA, McCluskey G. Valgus extension overload in the pitching elbow. *Am J Sports Med.* 1983;11(2):83-88.
11. Schwartz ML, al-Zahrani S, Morwessel RM, Andrews JR. Ulnar collateral ligament injury in the throwing athlete: evaluation with saline-enhanced MR arthrography. *Radiology.* 1995;197(1):297-299.
12. Hill NB Jr, Bucchieri JS, Shon F, Miller TT, Rosenwasser MP. Magnetic resonance imaging of injury to the medial collateral ligament of the elbow: a cadaver model. *J Shoulder Elbow Surg.* 2000;9(5):418-422.
13. Ouellette H, Bredella M, Labis J, Palmer WE, Torriani M. MR imaging of the elbow in baseball pitchers. *Skeletal Radiol.* 2008;37(2):115-121.
14. Azar FM, Andrews JR, Wilk KE, Groh D. Operative treatment of ulnar collateral ligament injuries of the elbow in athletes. *Am J Sports Med.* 2000;28(1):16-23.
15. Bruce JR, Andrews JR. Ulnar collateral ligament injuries in the throwing athlete. *J Am Acad Orthop Surg.* 2014;22(5):315-325.
16. Pagnani MJ, Warner JJ, O'Brien SJ, Warren RF. Anatomic considerations in harvesting the semitendinosus and gracilis tendons and a technique of harvest. *Am J Sports Med.* 1993;21(4):565-571.
17. Wilk KE, Arrigo C, Andrews JR. Rehabilitation of the elbow in the throwing athlete. *J Orthop Sports Phys Ther.* 1993;17(6):305-317.
18. Wilk KE, Azar FM, Andrews JR. Conservative and operative rehabilitation of the elbow in sports. *Sports Med Arthrosc Rev.* 1995;3(3):237-258.
19. Wilk KE, Arrigo C, Andrews JR, Azar FM. Rehabilitation following elbow surgery in the throwing athlete. *Oper Tech Sports Med.* 1996;4:114-132.

20. Wilk KE, Arrigo C, Andrews JR, et al. *Preventive and Rehabilitation Exercises for the Shoulder and Elbow.* 4th ed. Birmingham, AL: American Sports Medicine Institute; 1996.
21. Cain EL Jr, Andrews JR, Dugas JR, et al. Outcome of ulnar collateral ligament reconstruction of the elbow in 1281 athletes: results in 743 athletes with minimum 2-year follow-up. *Am J Sports Med.* 2010;38:2426-2434.
22. Osbahr DC, Cain EL Jr, Raines BT, Fortenbaugh D, Dugas JR, Andrews JR. Long-term outcomes after ulnar collateral ligament reconstruction in competitive baseball players: minimum 10-year follow-up. *Am J Sports Med.* 2014;42(6):1333-1342.

Please see videos on the accompanying website at
www.routledge.com/9781630910013

17

Endoscopic Distal Biceps Repair

Lucas H. B. Walschot, MD, PhD;
Joideep Phadnis, MBChB, MRCS, Dip Sports Med, FRCS (Tr&Orth);
and Gregory Bain, MBBS, FRACS, FA (Ortho)A, PhD

Introduction

Distal biceps tendon rupture results in significant flexion, supination strength, and endurance deficit. It occurs almost exclusively in men, typically older than 40 years or involved in weight training. There is an association with anabolic steroid use. The distal biceps has short and long heads. Their footprint is on the ulnar surface of the radial tuberosity where they attach to the periosteum of the radial tuberosity. Hence, in full supination, the tendon drapes around the radial tuberosity. Distal biceps repair reliably restores function regardless of technique and approach, although debate remains regarding whether to use a single- or double-incision technique and which technique is most effective. Cortical EndoButtons (Smith & Nephew), suture anchors, transosseous tunnels, and interference screws have all been used with satisfactory results. Partial distal biceps tears are less common and cause considerable anterior elbow pain during activity. They may go undiagnosed for some time.[1] There is a paucity of evidence regarding their optimal treatment; however, endoscopy is especially useful for these tears as an accurate diagnosis of the degree of tearing, tendinosis, and footprint coverage can be made. Chronic tears pose a surgical challenge due to tendon retraction but have been successfully treated with grafts and by fixation in extreme flexion. The authors have found endoscopy valuable in treating all varieties of distal biceps pathology, and it has improved their understanding and refined their management of these conditions.

Surgical Anatomy

The distal biceps tendon can be divided into the following 3 zones: pre-aponeurosis; aponeurosis, in which the lacertus fibrosus arises; and post-aponeurosis, in which the tendons of the short head and the long head are connected by loose connective tissue.[1] The tendon externally rotates around 90 degrees as it travels from its musculotendinous junction to its insertion at the radial tuberosity. The short head curves anterior to the long head to insert in a fanlike manner into the distal portion of the radial tuberosity. The long head has an oval footprint and inserts proximal to the short head occupying most of the tuberosity.[2] This makes it more important as a supinator

Savoie FH III, Field LD, Steinmann SP, eds. *The Elbow and Wrist: AANA Advanced Arthroscopic Surgical Techniques* (pp 167-175).

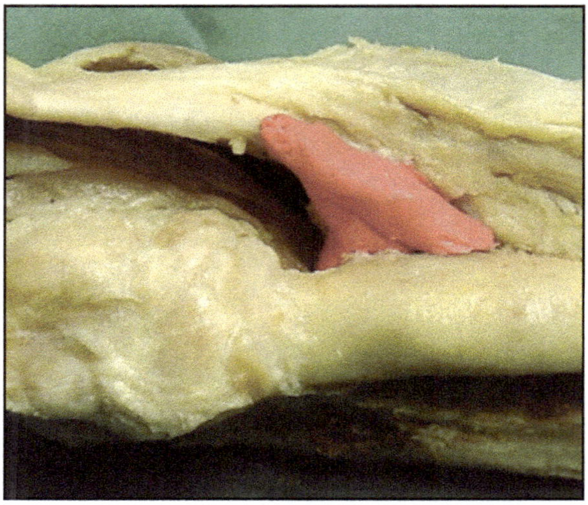

Figure 17-1. Location of the bicipitoradial bursa between the distal biceps tendon and the radius (proximal: left; distal: right).[2]

than the short head, which is a more important flexor. The bicipitoradial bursa completely drapes over both parts of the tendon and is teardrop shaped. It is more adherent to the ulnar aspect of the distal biceps than the radial aspect. It lies between the groove in the brachialis muscle and the distal biceps tendon with the elbow extended and between the proximal radius and the biceps tendon during pronation (Figure 17-1). The tendon footprint measures 2 x 14 mm and is located at the posteromedial margin of the radial tuberosity, 25 to 30 degrees posterior to the frontal plane. Partial and complete ruptures occur at the tendon-bone interface. The long head inserts more posteriorly than the short head and becomes more important in a supinated forearm.[3] Considering that the biceps tendon insertion has a lever of approximately 1 cm relative to the rotational axis of the radius, at least 3 to 3.5 cm of distal biceps tendon is needed to wrap around the proximal radius during its rotation from 90 degrees supination to 90 degrees pronation.[4]

Indications

- Diagnosis and debridement of distal biceps tendinopathy
- Debridement of bicipitoradial bursitis
- Evaluation of the painful biceps tendon
- Assessment of suspected partial head tears
- Assessment of suspected complete tears
- Repair of acute tears
- Retrieval of chronic retracted tendon stump
- Identification and debridement of chronic pseudotendon

Diagnostic Indications

Distal Biceps Tendinitis/Tendinosis or Bicipitoradial Bursitis

This often presents as deep-seated anterior elbow pain generally exacerbated by repetitive use. The condition may go undiagnosed for some time as imaging is unreliable. Endoscopy is useful to confirm either condition and rule out a partial tendon tear.

Table 17-1. Interpretation of the Hook Test

Hook Test Finding	Grade	Features of Tendon
Normal	N	Taut, unyielding and symmetric with contralateral arm
Abnormal	A1	Taut but yielding and asymmetric with contralateral arm
Abnormal	A2	Lax and asymmetric
Abnormal	A3	Absent cord

Suspected Partial Tendon Rupture

Confirming the diagnosis of a partial tear is difficult. Clinical examination is unreliable, as is imaging. Magnetic resonance imaging has a sensitivity of 59% for partial ruptures and cannot distinguish between partial ruptures that do or do not need repair.[5] The role of ultrasonography remains undefined. Given these issues, endoscopic evaluation is, in the authors' practice, the current gold standard to establish a definitive diagnosis. The extent of the tear and quality of the residual tendon can be assessed, as can the short and long head attachments.

Suspected Complete Tear

Complete tears can usually be diagnosed on clinical examination. The hook test[6] is thought to be the most useful test in making the diagnosis. However, it can be unclear on occasion. This happens when the biceps tendon sheath remains attached distally despite retraction of the tendon or a pseudotendon develops to bridge the gap in a chronic tear. The hook test is also unclear in partial- or single-head ruptures. The authors have categorized the features found on examination when performing the hook test (Table 17-1) and outlined in which pathologies these features may be found (Table 17-2). Any abnormality on the hook test should be interpreted as pathological and should be investigated further. Endoscopy is particularly useful for cases in which the diagnosis is unclear.

Painful Biceps Tendon Repair

Repair of complete tears are usually successful. However, patients occasionally have persistent pain or develop pain later on. Endoscopy can be used to assess whether there is impingement, fraying, or partial rerupture without having to reopen the whole wound.

Therapeutic Indications

The authors graded distal biceps tendon pathology on a scale from 0 to 4 (see Table 17-2). Each grade has distinct clinical, radiologic, and operative findings. The hook test should be interpreted carefully in certain grades.

Grade 0: Tendinosis, Bursitis

These patients present with deep-seated anterior elbow pain. The condition is atraumatic, but patients often relate their symptoms to a vague inciting event. Uncommonly for distal biceps pathology, many patients are female and often have comorbidities that predispose them to tendon degeneration, such as diabetes mellitus, renal disease, and immunosuppressive therapy. Management should be nonoperatively focused, using splinting, rest, nonsteroidal anti-inflammatory drugs, and corticosteroid injections. Endoscopic debridement may be used in resistant cases, but the results are less predictable, and biopsy should be performed to ensure that an unusual etiology is not overlooked.

Table 17-2. Classification and Management of Distal Biceps Pathologies

Grade	Injury	Clinical	Hook Test	Magnetic Resonance Imaging	Recommended Management
0	Tendinosis, bursitis	Atraumatic, tender, swollen, often older, female with comorbidities	N	Bursitis, effusion, tendinosis	Nonoperative, bursectomy, biopsy
1A	Low-grade partial tear (< 50%)	Pain and weakness against resistance	N, A1	Bursitis, effusion, footprint irregularity	Debridement
1B	Isolated head rupture	Weakness against resistance	A1	Isolated head avulsion	Repair isolated head
1C	High-grade partial tear (> 50%)	Pain and weakness against resistance	A1	Incomplete footprint detachment	Complete and repair
2	Complete tendon rupture, lacertus intact	Tendon medialized by intact lacertus, marked weakness	A2	Complete footprint detachment, tendon within sheath	Repair
3	Complete tendon and lacertus rupture with retraction	Retracted muscle, marked weakness	A3	Complete footprint detachment, retracted tendon and muscle	Repair
4A	Chronic rupture	Tendon medialized by intact lacertus, marked weakness	A1, A2	Complete footprint detachment and contracted tendon within sheath (A2), a pseudotendon may bridge the native tendon to the footprint (A1)	Repair
4B	Chronic retracted rupture	Retracted muscle, marked weakness	A3	Complete footprint detachment, retracted tendon within fibrous cocoon	Repair in flexion or use tendon graft

Grades 1 A Through C: Partial Tears

Partial tears have a traumatic history and tend to be more painful than complete tears. They also tend to remain symptomatic or progress despite nonsurgical treatment.[2,7] Partial tears are subclassified according to the size of footprint detachment (< 50% or > 50%). On occasion, 1 of the 2 biceps heads can be ruptured in isolation. Low-grade tears, if symptomatic, tend to be treated with endoscopic debridement, whereas larger tears are completed and reattached. In the case of an isolated head rupture, the individual head can be reattached.

Grades 2 and 3: Complete Tears

The differentiating feature between grade 2 and 3 tears is the integrity of the lacertus fibrosus. When the lacertus remains intact, it limits the retraction of the ruptured tendon but also medializes it compared to its normal course, which can be seen on careful clinical inspection. When the lacertus is intact, the hook test is often not completely abnormal, although there will be asymmetry and marked weakness with an appropriate history.

Grades 4A and 4B: Chronic Tears

Chronic complete tears can be challenging to treat because tendon retraction and scarring can encase the tendon and form a cocoon around it. Normal tendon length is 7 cm from the musculotendinous junction. Reattachment may not be possible with retraction greater than 4 cm, although good results have been reported for repair in extreme flexion.[8] In severe cases, the authors use a tendon graft, such as a semitendinosus autograft or tendon allograft to bridge the deficient tendon. Endoscopy can be used to identify the level of the retracted tendon and to circumferentially release it without making multiple incisions up the arm. A common finding on exploration in chronic cases is the presence of a pseudotendon still attached to the tuberosity. At first glance, it appears to be normal tendon extending to the footprint, but on closer inspection, it is only thinned scar tissue that lacks tendon fibers. The true tendon can be identified at the proximal extent of the pseudotendon as a rolled up ball. It can lie within a cocoon of fibrous tissue and even be invaginated within the muscle substance.

Contraindications

Distal biceps endoscopy is relatively contraindicated in patients with preexisting abnormal anatomy, such as from previous injury or surgery at the elbow and antecubital fossa. The authors also recommend only attempting repairs endoscopically after a considerable number of open repairs have been performed and the surgeon has developed familiarity with diagnostic endoscopy.

Pertinent Physical Findings

Partial Tears

- Deep-seated anterior elbow pain
- Crepitus on forearm rotation

Complete Tears

- Proximal bunching of the tendon
- Asymmetric rise and fall of the tendon with forearm rotation
- Positive hook test (see Table 17-1)

Pertinent Imaging

- Plain anteroposterior and lateral elbow x-rays
- If the diagnosis is in doubt, obtain the following:
  - Ultrasound scan
  - Magnetic resonance imaging in the flexed abducted supinated position

Equipment

- Tourniquet, sterile syringe with 10 mL of NaCl 0.9%, size 10 or 15 scalpel
- 4.0-mm, 30-degree arthroscope (70-degree scope can be used)
- Hook probe, nylon tape, and small artery clip
- Full-radius resector without teeth, hooked monopolar cautery device
- EndoButton CL Ultra 20 mm (no loop required), 2.4-mm drill tip guide wire (30-cm length), #2 FiberWire (Arthrex), and #1-0 Prolene suture (Ethicon/Johnson & Johnson)

Positioning and Portals

The patient is positioned supine with the arm on an arm table under general anesthesia. The whole arm is prepared with alcoholic chlorhexidine, and a sterile tourniquet is applied. The arm should be free to allow full elbow range of motion. The operating surgeon sits in the patient's axilla, with the assistant opposite and scrub nurse at the end of the arm table. The arthroscopic stack is placed on the opposite side of the patient.

A 2.5-cm longitudinal incision is made over the palpable biceps tendon, 2 cm distal to the anterior elbow crease. This is the standard viewing portal for the arthroscope and instruments. A posterior accessory portal can be made with an inside-out technique by passing a Wissinger rod between the radius and ulna exiting in the posterior forearm. This is similar to advancing the curved clamp with the Boyd Anderson technique.[9]

Step-by-Step Description of the Procedure

An examination under anesthesia is performed, including assessment of motion and elbow stability. A 2-cm longitudinal incision is made distal to the anterior elbow crease. The lateral cutaneous nerve of the forearm must be identified and protected. The distal biceps tendon and its bicipitoradial bursa are identified by digital dissection. A small transverse portal is made on the radial side at the apex of the bursa for introduction of the scope (Figure 17-2). It is important to stay lateral to the biceps tendon to avoid the median nerve and the brachial artery. The authors use a dry endoscopy because this allows clear identification of tissue planes and avoids fluid extravasation into the soft tissues. The bursa, proximal radius, and distal biceps tendon are inspected. The tendon is inspected dynamically through forearm rotation and with traction applied to a nylon tape placed around the tendon. A hook probe or trocar may be introduced through the same portal to examine at the axilla of insertion. The tendon is inspected for evidence of fraying, delamination, synovitis, and partial tear (Figure 17-3). If present, tenosynovitis and low-grade fraying is debrided. The authors do this without suction, using a full-radius resector without teeth, which minimizes the risk of the soft tissue being caught in the aperture. The aperture should be in full

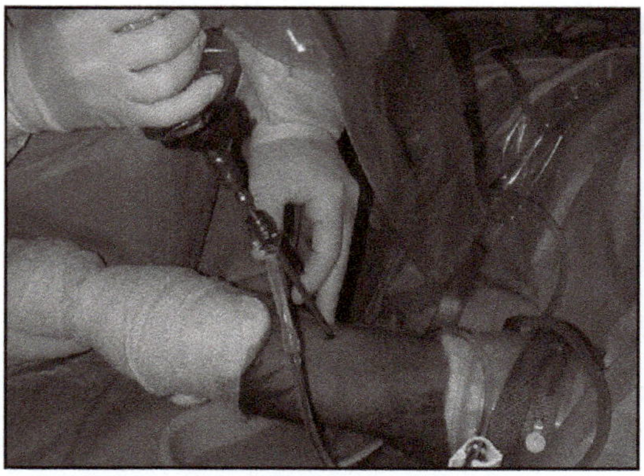

Figure 17-2. Orientation of the surgeon and the arthroscope during distal biceps tendon endoscopy in a left elbow.[1]

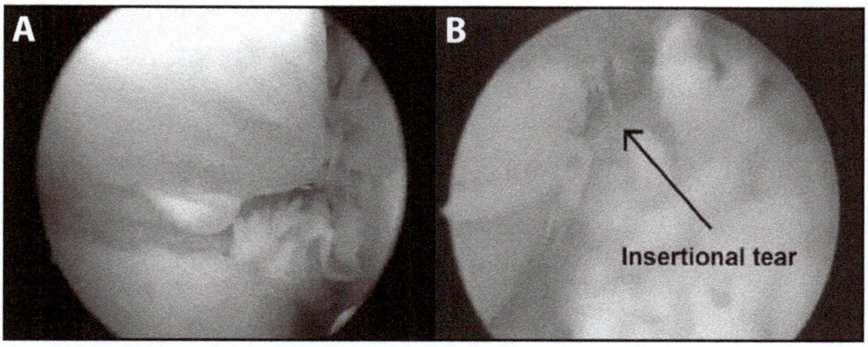

Figure 17-3. Picture of (A) an intact tendon insertion and (B) a grade 1A (< 50%) partial distal biceps tendon rupture.

view whenever the resector is active. If the partial tendon rupture is to be completed, a hooked monopolar cautery device is used for division of the remaining tendon insertion.[7]

If the tendon is completely torn from the radial tuberosity, the chondrotome is used to debride the natural footprint. A 2.5-mm drill is advanced from the anterior cortex of the radius, exiting just posterior to the footprint. A suture on a straight needle is advanced backward through this drill hole, and the loop is retrieved. This is used to shuttle the preplaced whipstitch in the distal biceps tendon. The sutures are threaded through an EndoButton and are tied firmly to the anterior aspect of the proximal radius. This accurately recreates the biceps footprint and provides transosseous EndoButton fixation (Figure 17-4).

An alternative method was described by Sharma and MacKay.[10] The ruptured distal biceps tendon is delivered out of the wound, freshened, and sutured to an EndoButton. The endoscope is inserted along the tract of the avulsed tendon and positioned on the tuberosity. The camera is removed and a 2.4-mm guide wire is advanced across the radius under fluoroscopic guidance to the posterior aspect of the forearm. Over the guide wire, a 4.5-mm cannulated drill creates a bicortical hole in the radius, followed by a 6.0-mm drill of the near cortex. The guide wire is used to advance the sutures and the EndoButton, which is then toggled using leading and trailing sutures. The endoscope and fluoroscopy are used to confirm the position of the tendon and EndoButton.

Despite being endoscopic, this cannulated technique replicates the open method and does not reproduce the native footprint of the biceps tendon, which is important to create full supination strength. The authors feel the aim should be anatomic restoration of the tendon to the ulnar aspect of the radial tuberosity.

Both described endoscopic methods are initially challenging; hence, the authors recommend that if other surgeons wish to embrace endoscopic techniques, they should initially develop their skills in a cadaveric model before introduction into clinical practice in a graduated manner.

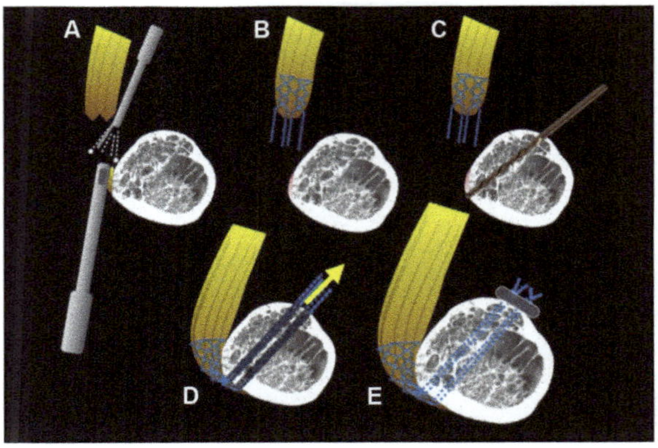

Figure 17-4. (A) Endoscopic debridement of the torn biceps tendon stump. (B) Whipstitch of the torn tendon with nonabsorbable suture. (C) Two oblique drill holes made in the radial tuberosity aiming to exit on the dorsal ulnar surface. (D) Sutures shuttled through drill holes. (E) Sutures tied over the EndoButton restoring the tendon to its footprint on the ulnar aspect of the tuberosity.

Postoperative Protocol

For a grade 0 injury (no rupture) and grade 1A (rupture < 50%), the patient is encouraged to mobilize and strengthen the arm with a physiotherapist. In some cases, prodromal symptoms remain.

For grade 1B to 4 injuries, the patient is provided with a sling and is encouraged to mobilize as tolerated. Patients are advised not to perform any heavy lifting or grasping for 3 months.

Potential Complications

- Lateral cutaneous nerve of the forearm injury
- Posterior interosseous nerve injury
- Radioulnar synostosis
- Radial neck fracture
- Heterotopic ossification
- Hematoma formation

Top Technical Pearls for the Procedure

1. Pre- and intraoperatively, ensure that the patient is accurately classified because this will direct treatment.
2. Enter the bicipitoradial bursa on the radial side under direct vision to avoid damage to neurovascular structures.
3. Use dry endoscopy to improve visualization and prevent soft tissue swelling.
4. Use a full-radius resector without teeth or suction to avoid entrapping soft tissues.
5. Reinsert the tendon onto its anatomic footprint on the posterior rim of the tuberosity.

References

1. Bain GI, Johnson LJ, Turner PC. Treatment of partial distal biceps tendon tears. *Sports Med Arthrosc.* 2008;16(3):154-161.
2. Eames MH, Bain GI, Fogg QA, van Riet RP. Distal biceps tendon anatomy: a cadaveric study. *J Bone Joint Surg Am.* 2007;89(5):1044-1049.
3. Jarrett CD, Weir DM, Stuffmann ES, Jain S, Miller MC, Schmidt CC. Anatomic and biomechanical analysis of the short and long head components of the distal biceps tendon. *J Shoulder Elbow Surg.* 2012;21(7):942-948.
4. Nesterenko S, Domire ZJ, Morrey BF, Sanchez-Sotelo J. Elbow strength and endurance in patients with a ruptured distal biceps tendon. *J Shoulder Elbow Surg.* 2010;19(2):184-189.
5. Festa A, Mulieri PJ, Newman JS, Spitz DJ, Leslie BM. Effectiveness of magnetic resonance imaging in detecting partial and complete distal biceps tendon rupture. *J Hand Surg Am.* 2010;35(1):77-83.
6. O'Driscoll SW, Goncalves LB, Dietz P. The hook test for distal biceps tendon avulsion. *Am J Sports Med.* 2007;35(11):1865-1869.
7. Dürr HR, Stäbler A, Pfahler M, Matzko M, Refior HJ. Partial rupture of the distal biceps tendon. *Clin Orthop Relat Res.* 2000;(374):195-200.
8. Morrey ME, Abdel MP, Sanchez-Sotelo J, Morrey BF. Primary repair of retracted distal biceps tendon ruptures in extreme flexion. *J Shoulder Elbow Surg.* 2014;23(5):679-685.
9. Boyd HB, Anderson LD. A method for reinsertion of the distal biceps brachii tendon. *J Bone Joint Surg Am.* 1961;43(7):1041-1043.
10. Sharma S, MacKay G. Endoscopic repair of distal biceps tendon using an EndoButton. *Arthroscopy.* 2005;21(7):897.

Please see videos on the accompanying website at

www.routledge.com/9781630910013

18

Open Medial Ulnar Collateral Ligament Repair

Murphy P. Martin III, MD; Michael J. O'Brien, MD; and Felix H. Savoie III, MD

Introduction

The anterior bundle of the ulnar collateral ligament (UCL) complex is the primary stabilizer of the elbow to valgus stress from 20 to 120 degrees of flexion,[1-8] the primary arc of motion used in overhead throwing. Isolated UCL deficiency was first identified in javelin throwers by Waris[9] in 1946 and was once thought to be a career-ending injury. The initial operative intervention for the condition involved repair of the native ligament, which was supported by Barnes and Tullos,[10] who noted that athletes with UCL injury had better clinical outcomes after repair than nonoperative treatment. Much of the current operative management of UCL deficiency is focused upon symptomatic valgus instability in high-level throwing athletes and usually requires some variation of the reconstructive procedure pioneered by Jobe in 1974 for return to play.[11-15] However, there has been a substantial increase in the number of patients sustaining a more acute form of this injury at younger ages,[16,17] for which a reconstruction may not be warranted. In contrast to elite athletes who have sustained repetitive microtrauma over years of high-level competition with resultant ligament damage through its length and secondary pathologic changes in the elbow from chronic valgus extension overload syndrome,[11,13] younger or acutely injured athletes can be expected to have a ligament of better quality, with isolated damage to specific areas and a more biomechanically stable joint.[18-23] In patients with a single area of injury at the proximal or distal end of the ligament or both, primary repair of the UCL has proven to be a viable option, with reliable results and a quicker return to sports than with standard reconstruction.[24]

Indications

- Injuries to the proximal or distal end of an otherwise normal ligament in athletes who would like to continue to play and are unable to do so due to the injury to the medial ulnar collateral ligament (MUCL) of the elbow

Savoie FH III, Field LD, Steinmann SP, eds. *The Elbow and Wrist: AANA Advanced Arthroscopic Surgical Techniques* (pp 177-185).

Contraindications

- Ligaments with midsubstance injuries
- Evidence of damage over an extended length of the ligament
- Generally poor-quality ligament with calcifications or defects (In the aforementioned cases, a standard graft reconstruction procedure is required.)
- Lack of desire to continue to play the affected sport

Pertinent Physical Findings

A general physical examination of the throwing athlete includes an evaluation of hip and core strength, scapular position, and tracking patterns, as well as the shoulder and elbow. Specifically in the elbow, the following are noted:

- Active and passive motion are documented.
- Inspection is usually normal but may reveal subluxation of the ulnar nerve during motion.
- Palpation often reveals mild edema on the medial side of the elbow, with tenderness over the injured area of the MUCL.
- Medial and lateral stability testing is then accomplished, with the most benefit noted with positive findings with the moving valgus stress test to be the most specific. As described by O'Driscoll et al,[25] the moving valgus stress test is performed on a patient in the upright position with the shoulder abducted to 90 degrees, in maximal external rotation with the elbow fully flexed. The examiner then extends the elbow while applying a constant valgus load. A positive test will reproduce medial elbow pain that the patient experiences with provocative activities and should be maximal between the positions of 120 and 70 degrees of elbow extension, correlating to the late cocking and early acceleration phases of throwing.
- Other physical examination findings that are usually positive include the milk test and the moving valgus extension overload test.

Pertinent Imaging

- Standard radiographic evaluation of the elbow begins with anteroposterior, lateral, and oblique x-rays.
- A true lateral view of the hyperflexed elbow or an axial olecranon view in 110 degrees of flexion may identify posteromedial osteophytes, suggestive of a chronic valgus extension overload syndrome.
- Comparative stress x-rays may help identify ligamentous laxity, and a greater than 5-mm side-to-side difference may be sufficient as a diagnostic study.
- In younger patients, contralateral comparison views may be helpful to identify growth disturbances and variant ossification centers.
- When advanced imaging is needed, magnetic resonance imaging with contrast can identify ligament injury and provide excellent visualization of the articular cartilage (Figure 18-1).[26]

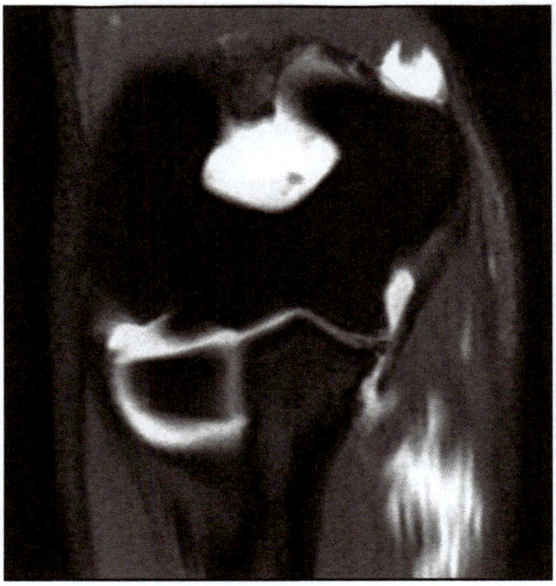

Figure 18-1. Postcontrast coronal T1-weighted real-time magnetic resonance imaging sequence demonstrating avulsion of the distal attachment of the UCL at the sublime tubercle of the ulna.

Equipment

- Room setup should allow the surgeon ample space to access the operative extremity with a scrub assistant and surgical instruments behind the surgeon and arthroscopy monitor and tower positioned on the opposite side of the operating table.
- Gravity or pulsed irrigation system with a pump, based on surgeon preference (will be needed and placed appropriately)
- One arm board will need to be positioned on the operative side at the patient's hip along with a bolster to hold the elbow in 90 degrees of flexion during the arthroscopic portion of the case.
- Spinal needle and 2.7- or 4.0-mm arthroscope with a 30- or 70-viewing angle, cannula system, switching stick, and blunt-tipped trocars based on surgeon preference
- Arthroscopic shavers and standard arthroscopic instruments (probes, graspers, and biters)
- Bioabsorbable double-loaded suture anchors with semiabsorbable suture
- Standard instrument tray for open portion of the procedure and MUCL reconstruction set should repair be abandoned
- Splinting material

Positioning and Portals

For the authors' UCL repair protocol, they prefer to place their patients in the standard prone arthroscopy position with the shoulder abducted to 90 degrees and the elbow flexed to 90 degrees over a block. This position eliminates the need for traction, allows for easier intraoperative manipulation of the elbow, permits access to the posterior aspect of the joint, and affords a more stable position to the elbow.[27] Following the arthroscopic portion of the case, this position allows the surgeon to convert to an open procedure by internally rotating the shoulder and placing the hand on an arm board near the patient's hip, exposing the medial side of the elbow while providing a constant varus stress for the repair (Figure 18-2).

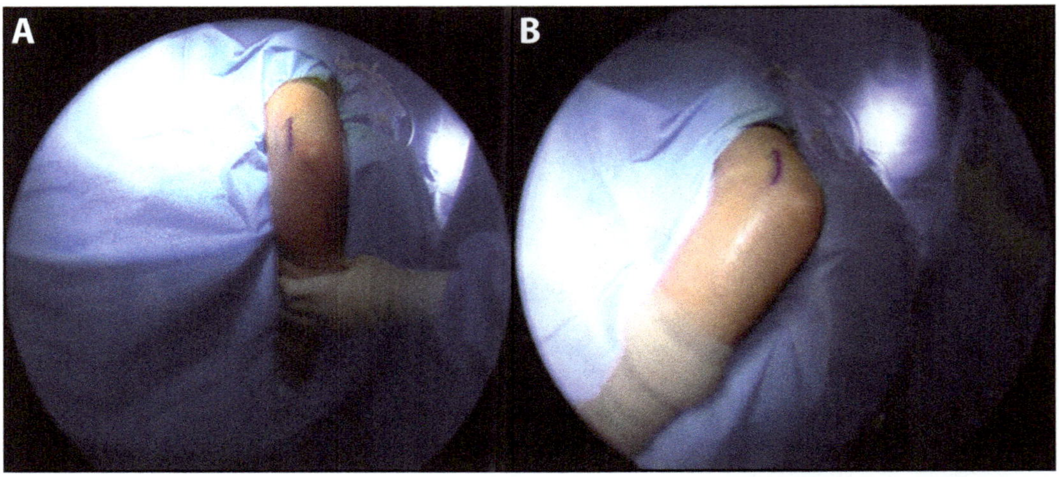

Figure 18-2. (A) The prone arthroscopy position with the patient's elbow flexed over a block, which provides excellent stability, eliminates the need for traction, and allows conversion to an open procedure (B) by fully internally rotating the arm and placing it on an arm board positioned at the patients hip.

Step-by-Step Description of the Procedure

With the patient in the prone arthroscopy position as previously described, a thorough examination under anesthesia is performed to evaluate the elbow for instability and motion, comparing the injured elbow to the opposite, uninjured side. A standard diagnostic arthroscopy is then performed to evaluate the articular cartilage, specifically of the capitellum and the posterolateral plica. Although rare in young athletes, additional pathology, including loose bodies and ulnohumeral spurs, can be addressed if present. The arthroscopic stress test of Field and Altchek[28] can also be performed at this time, which produced positive findings of medial opening 3 mm or greater in all of the authors' 60 patients investigated in a previously reported case series on MUCL repair.[24]

With the arthroscopic portion of the case complete, the surgery is converted to an open procedure with the arm positioning change as previously stated. A skin incision is made on the tip of the medial epicondyle and extended distally 5 cm. A pronator muscle-splitting approach as described by Smith et al[15] is then used to expose the UCL (Figure 18-3). The outer surface of the UCL is evaluated for tissue quality and the location of the tear (Figure 18-4). An incision is then made along the anterior border of the MUCL, and the undersurface of the ligament is inspected (Figure 18-5).

If a humeral avulsion is encountered, the bone in the area of the origin of the UCL from the distal, lateral aspect of the medial epicondyle and adjacent trochlea is lightly debrided and rasped. Angling toward the olecranon fossa, a double-loaded suture anchor is then placed at the apex of the "V" formed by the junction of the trochlea and medial epicondyle. The sutures are then passed in horizontal mattress configuration through the most proximal area of the undamaged ligament in a mattress fashion, one set at the proximal end of the normal ligamentous tissue and one set 5 mm distal to the first mattress stitch. Each set of mattress sutures is placed at the anterior and posterior aspect of the ligament (Figure 18-6). One should be aware of the position of the ulnar nerve adjacent to the posterior edge of the MUCL. In most cases, it is safe to expose the nerve and retract it at the level of the suture passage to prevent inadvertent injury. Alternatively, direct suture repair without anchors can be accomplished proximally by placing convergent drill holes from the medial tip of the epicondyle and the origin site of the UCL. The drill holes are then connected with a curved Keith needle, and the suture is shuttled from the origin site through the medial hole. Care must be taken to be cognizant of the location of the ulnar nerve along the posterior aspect of the ligament to avoid tethering it with sutures.

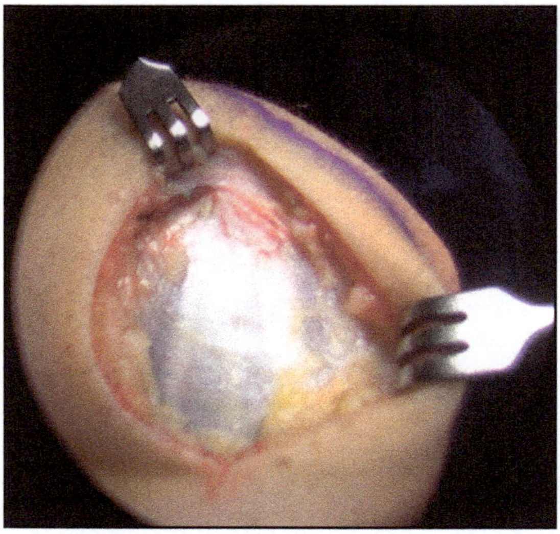

Figure 18-3. Intraoperative photograph demonstrating the appearance of the flexor pronator mass. An incision is made over the medial epicondyle and the mass is split to gain exposure of the UCL while identifying and protecting the ulnar nerve.

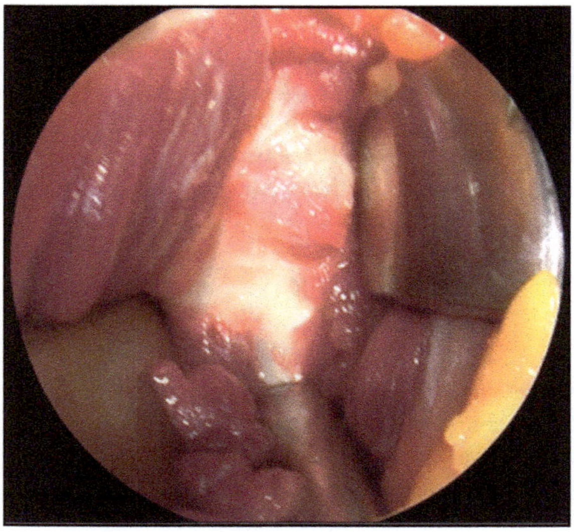

Figure 18-4. With the flexor pronator mass split, the UCL is encountered. A ligament of good quality is demonstrated with complete avulsion of its humeral attachment.

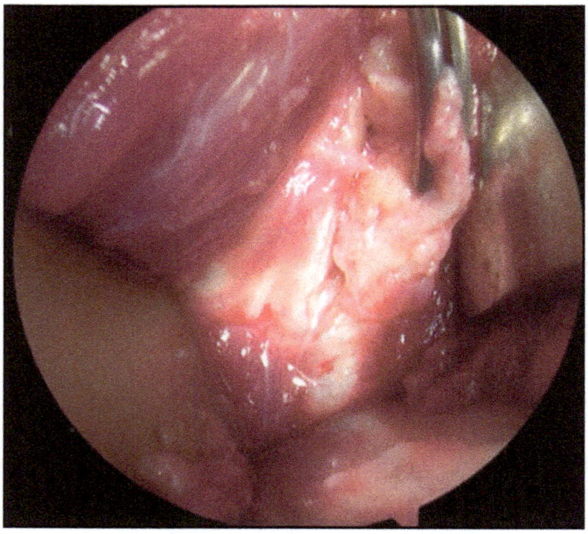

Figure 18-5. With the UCL exposed, an incision is made along the anterior aspect of the ligament, allowing its undersurface to be inspected.

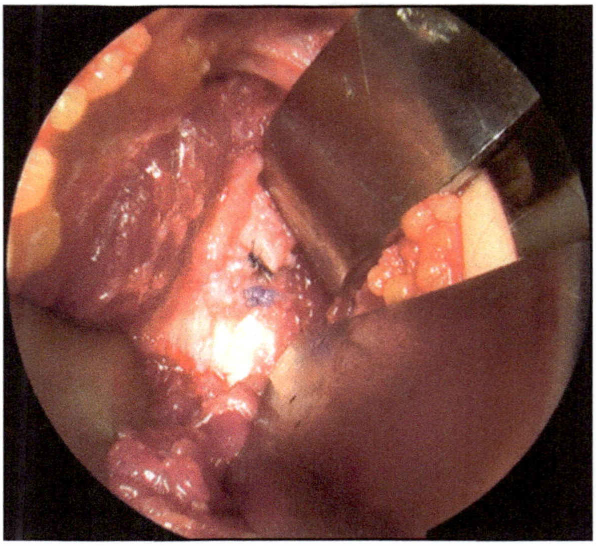

Figure 18-6. After preparation of the humeral insertion site of the UCL, a double-loaded suture anchor is placed and sutures are passed in a double horizontal mattress fashion through the most proximal undamaged portion of the ligament and another set 5 mm distal in the anterior and posterior aspects of the ligament.

In the case of distal avulsions, the suture anchor is placed directly into the sublime tubercle and angled distally to avoid violating the ulnohumeral joint. The sutures are passed through the most distal aspect of the undamaged ligament in a way similar to the proximal sutures, with the same precautions about the ulnar nerve. The ligament is then tensioned and tied. The elbow is taken through a complete range of motion to evaluate the isometrics of the repair.[24]

Postoperative Protocol

The elbow is immobilized in a posterior slab splint at 90 degrees of flexion for 1 week. Active range of motion is started at 1 week in a hinged brace set at 30 to 90 degrees and increased 10 degrees in each direction until full motion is achieved. Physical therapy focused on the hip, core, and scapula are started at this time. At 3 to 4 weeks, strengthening exercises for the wrist, forearm, and rotator cuff are added to the core program, while maintaining the brace on the elbow at all times. Patients are started on an activity-specific program at 6 weeks. At this time, plyometrics are incorporated, along with sport-specific activity in the brace. Throwing and hitting are initiated between 8 and 12 weeks in the brace depending on shoulder posture, scapular position, and core strength and are progressed as tolerated provided there is no pain over the repaired UCL. The sport-specific rehabilitation is continued without the brace beginning at 12 weeks and continued until full activity is achieved, usually by 16 to 24 weeks.[24]

Results

Historically, surgical repair of the UCL after failed nonoperative management has produced varied results. However, in appropriately selected patients, repair of the ligament in the absence of secondary pathologic changes can produce a reliable result and allow a more rapid return to sports than standard reconstruction. In a recent case series, 60 patients younger than 22 years with symptomatic valgus instability of the elbow underwent MUCL repair after failing nonoperative management. Overall, 93% of the patients achieved good to excellent results according to the Andrews-Carson elbow outcome score, and 56 of the 60 patients returned to sports within 6 months at the same or higher level of competition. Four patients were considered to have failures based on their functional results and Andrews-Carson rating scale.[24] In a similar study by Richard et al,[29] the investigators reported comparable success.

Potential Complications

Ulnar nerve neuropraxia has been shown to be a common complication following UCL repair and reconstruction, and ulnar nerve symptoms should be evaluated if discovered preoperatively. Most often, the symptoms are transient and related to sensory disturbances in the distribution of the ulnar nerve. Rarely, this complication may necessitate a neurolysis or transposition procedure, and postoperative ulnar nerve symptoms are not likely to affect outcome.[13,24,30] Postoperative arthrofibrosis has shown to occur and may require prolonged therapy and/or additional arthroscopic capsular release.[24]

Conclusion

- Position patient prone on operating table, flex operative extremity over bump with arm board at hip (see Figure 18-2). Perform exam under anesthesia.
- Perform diagnostic elbow arthroscopy and address any concomitant pathology as indicated. Perform arthroscopic stress test of Field and Altchek.
- Convert to open procedure by abducting and internally rotating the operative arm to be placed on an arm board at hip (see Figure 18-2).
- Incise skin from tip of medial epicondyle, extending 5 cm distally. Pronator muscle splitting approach is used to expose the UCL (see Figure 18-3).
- Assess UCL for size of tear, location, and overall quality of ligament from both superficial and deep surfaces (see Figures 18-4 and 18-5). (If any of the above preclude repair and necessitate reconstruction, the conversion is made at this point.)
- With the tear identified and the decision to repair made, bioabsorbable double-loaded suture anchors are inserted at the origin and/or insertion of the damaged UCL (ie, at the apex of the "V" formed by the junction of the trochlea and medial epicondyle for proximal repair or in the sublime tubercle for distal repair).
- Pass sutures in a horizontal mattress configuration through the most proximal end of undamaged ligamentous tissue, then another set 5 mm distal to the first mattress stitch (see Figure 18-6).
- Tension and tie ligament, and the elbow is then taken through a complete range of motion to evaluate isometry of repair.
- Perform layered closure, apply sterile dressing, and immobilize elbow in posterior slab splint, which will remain in place for 1 week.

Top Technical Pearls for the Procedure

1. Do not operate too soon. These patients may respond well to conservative management of bracing, rest, periscapular and core strengthening, and improved throwing mechanics.
2. Carefully examine the ligament on preoperative imaging and on direct inspection to ensure that it is adequate for repair. If there is any doubt, reconstruction should be performed.

(continued)

3. Absorbable, double-loaded anchors with semiabsorbable sutures using a double-mattress repair of the ligament into the anatomic origin or insertion seems to provide the best results. Bioabsorbable anchors will limit the distortion of surgical site anatomy if a future reconstruction procedure is needed, and double-mattress suture repair affords a broader surface area, 2-point fixation to the damaged ligament to bone.
4. Careful attention must be paid to the location of the ulnar nerve to avoid vigorous retraction or tethering with sutures. In patients with a preoperative Tinel's sign or ulnar nerve subluxation, many authors recommend a transposition, which may be warranted in these cases.

References

1. An K, Morrey BF, Chao EYS. The effect of partial removal of proximal ulna on elbow constraint. *Clin Orthop Relat Res.* 1986;(209):270-279.
2. Andrews JR, Heggland EJ, Fleisig GS, Zheng N. Relationship of ulnar collateral ligament strain to amount of medial olecranon osteotomy. *Am J Sports Med.* 2001;29(6):716-721.
3. Morrey BF, An KN. Articular and ligamentous contributions to the stability of the elbow joint. *Am J Sports Med.* 1983;11(5):315-319.
4. Morrey BF, An KN. Functional anatomy of the ligaments of the elbow. *Clin Orthop Relat Res.* 1985;(201):84-90.
5. Morrey BF, Tanaka S, An K. Valgus stability of the elbow. A definition of primary and secondary constraints. *Clin Orthop Relat Res.* 1991;(265):187-195.
6. Regan WD, Korinek SL, Morrey BF, An KN. Biomechanical study of ligaments around the elbow joint. *Clin Orthop Relat Res.* 1991;(271):170-179.
7. Schwab GH, Bennett JB, Woods GW, Tullos HS. Biomechanics of elbow instability: the role of the medial collateral ligament. *Clin Orthop Relat Res.* 1980;(146):42-52.
8. Søjbjerg JO, Ovesen J, Nielsen S. Experimental elbow instability after transaction of the medial collateral ligament. *Clin Orthop Relat Res.* 1987;(218):186-190.
9. Waris W. Elbow injuries of javelin-throwers. *Acta Chir Scand.* 1946;93(6):563-575.
10. Barnes DA, Tullos HS. An analysis of 100 symptomatic baseball players. *Am J Sports Med.* 1978;6(2):62-67.
11. Jobe FW, Stark H, Lombardo SJ. Reconstruction of the ulnar collateral ligament in athletes. *J Bone Joint Surg Am.* 1986;68(8):1158-1163.
12. Azar FM, Andrews JR, Wilk KE, Groh D. Operative treatment of ulnar collateral ligament injuries of the elbow in athletes. *Am J Sports Med.* 200;28(1):16-23.
13. Conway JE, Jobe FW, Glousman RE, Pink M. Medial instability of the elbow in throwing athletes. Treatment by repair or reconstruction of the ulnar collateral ligament. *J Bone Joint Surg Am.* 1992;74(1):67-83.
14. Thompson WH, Jobe FW, Yocum LA, Pink MM. Ulnar collateral ligament reconstruction in athletes: muscle-splitting approach without transposition of the ulnar nerve. *J Shoulder Elbow Surg.* 2001;10(2):152-157.
15. Smith GR, Altchek DW, Pagnani MJ, Keeley JR. A muscle-splitting approach to the ulnar collateral ligament of the elbow. Neuroanatomy and operative technique. *Am J Sports Med.* 1996;24(5):575-580.
16. Petty DH, Andrews JR, Fleisig GS, Cain EL. Ulnar collateral ligament reconstruction in high school baseball players: clinical results and injury risk factors. *Am J Sports Med.* 2004;32(5):1158-1164.
17. Olsen SJ II, Fleisig GS, Dun S, Loftice J, Andrews JR. Risk factors for shoulder and elbow injuries in adolescent baseball pitchers. *Am J Sports Med.* 2006;34(6):905-912.
18. Fleisig GS, Barrentine SW. Biomechanical aspects of the elbow in sports. *Sports Med Arthrosc Rev.* 1995;3(3):149-159.

19. Fleisig GS, Andrews JR, Dillman CJ, Escamilla RF. Kinetics of baseball pitching with implications about injury mechanisms. *Am J Sports Med.* 1995;23(2):233-239.
20. Gainor BJ, Piotrowski G, Puhl J, Allen WC, Hagen R. The throw: biomechanics and acute injury. *Am J Sports Med.* 1980;8(2):114-118.
21. Kenter K, Behr CT, Warren RF, O'Brien SJ, Barnes R. Acute elbow injuries in the National Football League. *J Shoulder Elbow Surg.* 2000;9(1):1-5.
22. Mirabello SC, Loeb PE, Andrews JR. The wrist: field evaluation and treatment. *Clin Sports Med.* 1992;11(1):1-25.
23. Norwood LA, Shook JA, Andrews JR. Acute medial elbow ruptures. *Am J Sports Med.* 1981;9(1):16-19.
24. Savoie FH III, Trenhaile SW, Roberts J, Field LD, Ramsey JR. Primary repair of ulnar collateral ligament injuries of the elbow in young athletes: a case series of injuries to the proximal and distal ends of the ligament. *Am J Sports Med.* 2008;36(6):1066-1072.
25. O'Driscoll SW, Lawton RL, Smith AM. The "moving valgus stress test" for medial collateral ligament tears of the elbow. *Am J Sports Med.* 2005;33(2):231-239.
26. Glajchen N, Schwartz ML, Andrews JR, Gladstone J. Avulsion fracture of the sublime tubercle of the ulna: a newly recognized injury in the throwing athlete. *AJR Am J Roentgenol.* 1998;170(3):627-628.
27. Poehling GG, Whipple TL, Sisco L, Goldman B. Elbow arthroscopy: a new technique. *Arthroscopy.* 1989;5(3):222-224.
28. Field LD, Altchek DW. Evaluation of the arthroscopic valgus instability test of the elbow. *Am J Sports Med.* 1996;24(2):177-181.
29. Richard MJ, Aldridge JM III, Wiesler ER, Ruch DS. Traumatic valgus instability of the elbow: patho-anatomy and results of direct repair. Surgical technique. *J Bone Joint Surg Am.* 2009;91(suppl 2):191-199.
30. Cain EL Jr, Andrews JR, Dugas JR, et al. Outcome of ulnar collateral ligament reconstruction of the elbow in 1281 athletes: results in 743 athletes with minimum 2-year follow-up. *Am J Sports Med.* 2010;38(12):2426-2434.

Please see videos on the accompanying website at

www.routledge.com/9781630910013

19

Arthroscopic Triceps Repair

Jonathan D. Brown, MD; Michael J. O'Brien, MD; and Felix H. Savoie III, MD

Introduction

The triceps brachii muscle is the major extensor of the forearm. The long head arises from the infraglenoid tubercle and the medial and lateral heads from the posterior humerus inferior and superior to the radial groove, respectively. The muscle coalesces to form a single tendinous insertion on the posterior aspect of the olecranon. The triceps is innervated by the radial nerve and receives its blood supply from perforating branches of the profunda brachii artery.[1]

Ruptures of the triceps tendon are rare injuries.[2] Traumatic events, including direct trauma and motor vehicle accidents, have been implicated in triceps ruptures.[3-5] They commonly occur during heavy weight lifting or fall with eccentric contraction of the muscle.[6] Often, the patient will report a pop with pain and swelling at the time of injury. The patient may complain of pain with active extension or complete loss of active extension at the time of presentation. The mean age at the time of injury is 33 years, and men are more affected than women.[7] Triceps ruptures encompass complete tendon ruptures, partial tears, and bony avulsions. There is an increased risk for triceps tendon ruptures in patients with renal osteodystrophy, metabolic bone diseases, corticosteroid injections, and anabolic steroid use.[8-10] Open physes may pose an additional risk for rupture as well.[11]

Indications

- Symptomatic partial or complete ruptures of the triceps tendon

Controversial Indications

Partial tendon avulsions or tears. In a recent review of the literature, Tom et al[12] reported that nonoperative management may result in full range of motion (ROM) and subjective strength within 3 to 9 months. Repair was reported to result in full ROM and subjective strength within

Savoie FH III, Field LD, Steinmann SP, eds. *The Elbow and Wrist: AANA Advanced Arthroscopic Surgical Techniques* (pp 187-196).

3 to 6 months. Strauch[10] recommended operative treatment for partial tears involving greater than 50% of the tendon width. Mair et al[13] reported a series of 10 professional football players with tendon injuries ranging from 30% to 75% of the tendon width. All were initially treated nonoperatively, and 6 recovered with no residual symptoms. Three required surgery after the season secondary to pain and weakness. Nonoperative treatment may be considered initially for partial repairs, but evidence exists for early repair. Patients undergoing delayed surgical repair are at increased risk for a more extensive grafting procedure. Reconstruction has been reported to lead to decreased ROM and increased recovery times of up to 1 year.[14]

The decision for operative intervention of partial tears must be patient specific. Overall health, activity level, and comorbidities are considered. In addition, time from initial injury to presentation is an important consideration. Ideally, primary repair is performed within 2 weeks of injury. Although primary repair has been successful several months after injury,[6] Van riet et al[14] reported primary repair was only possible in 6 of 15 patients presenting greater than 25 days. The surgeon must consider multiple factors to determine if operative intervention is recommended.

Pertinent Physical Findings

- Inspect the elbow for swelling and ecchymosis.
- Palpation of the tendon may demonstrate a defect or tenderness.
- Neurovascular status is assessed and documented.
- Active and passive ROM of the injured extremity is compared to the contralateral extremity.
- Weakness of active extension against resistance may be seen with partial or complete tears but is not diagnostic.[12]
- Triceps stress test will produce pain directly over the site of injury, indicating a more subtle tear.
  - Have the patient try to extend the elbow from a fully flexed position.
- A modified Thompson test may be used. No elbow motion is seen in complete rupture.[15] Partial tendon tears are more difficult to diagnose, and the surgeon must have a high clinical suspicion.
  - The examiner supports the injured arm parallel to the ground. The elbow is allowed to hang and flex to 90 degrees. The triceps muscle belly is gently squeezed.

Advanced imaging is recommended for definitive diagnosis.

Pertinent Imaging

- X-rays are the initial imaging of choice when triceps tendon rupture is suspected.
  - Orthogonal views of the elbow are obtained and examined.
  - The lateral view may demonstrate a flake of bone avulsed from the olecranon. The flake sign is pathognomonic for triceps rupture.[12,16]
  - X-rays may be nondiagnostic for partial, musculotendinous junction, and intramuscular substance tears, and advanced imaging is warranted.
- Ultrasound is reported to correlate tendon injury with surgical and magnetic resonance imaging (MRI) findings. Patient discomfort is minimal. Complete rupture, partial rupture, and tendinosis may be differentiated. Currently, specificity and sensitivity are not reported and the examination is operator-dependent. Ultrasound provides a useful imaging modality for diagnosis, especially in the setting of partial tears.[17-20]

- MRI is the gold standard for definitive diagnosis and differentiation of complete and partial tendon injuries. In addition, MRI may detect associated ligamentous injuries[21] and correlates well with surgical findings.
- Ultrasonography and MRI can provide valuable information for surgical planning, especially in the setting of partial tears.

Equipment

- Standard operating table
- Tourniquet
- Bolster (to be used if the patient is placed prone)
- Standard 4-mm, 30-degree arthroscope
- Standard arthroscopic blue cannula
- Arthroscopic burr and shaver
- Arthroscopic graspers
- Arthroscopic suture retriever
- Double-loaded suture anchors
- Retrograde suture passer
- Power drill
- Drill bit for anchors
- Bone awl and bone tap

Positioning and Portals

The patient is placed in the prone or lateral decubitus position. All bony prominences are padded. The authors prefer prone. An unsterile tourniquet is applied and an arm board is placed parallel to the operative bed. A bolster is used to position the operative extremity. The glenohumeral joint is abducted 90 degrees to the ground, and the elbow is allowed to flex to 90 degrees. The patient is sterilely prepped and draped according to surgeon preference.

Step-by-Step Description of the Procedure

The course of the ulnar nerve is identified and marked on the skin. A standard anteromedial or anterolateral portal is established for diagnostic arthroscopy. Additional pathology, including loose bodies or coronoid spurring, are identified and treated before tendon repair.

Once the anterior compartment has been fully evaluated, the posterior compartment can be evaluated. Make a standard posterior central portal. The entry point is located in the midline approximately 3 cm proximal to the tip of the olecranon. This portal typically traverses the triceps tendon tear. The arthroscope is inserted into the posterior portal and a posterior lateral portal is made under direct visualization. The arthroscope is then placed in the posterior lateral portal and a shaver is introduced into the posterior central portal. The ulnohumeral joint is inspected and debrided. The triceps tendon is identified, freed, and debrided with a shaver (Figures 19-1 through 19-3). The ulnar insertion of the triceps tendon is identified. The soft tissue overlying the footprint is debrided with a shaver. A burr is introduced and is used to prepare the tendon insertion site (Figures 19-4 through 19-6).

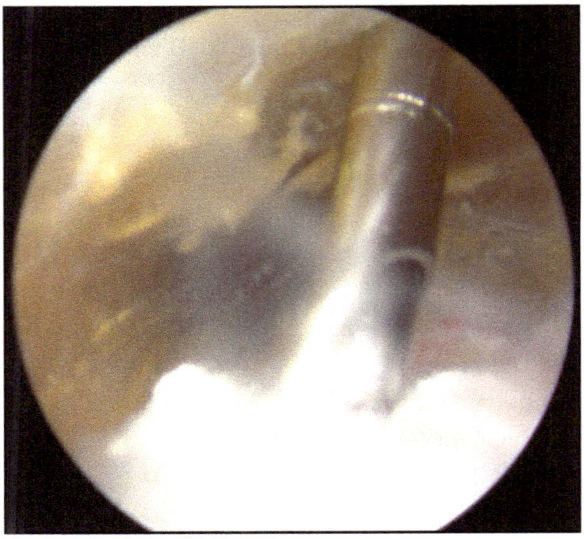

Figure 19-1. Bursectomy is performed.

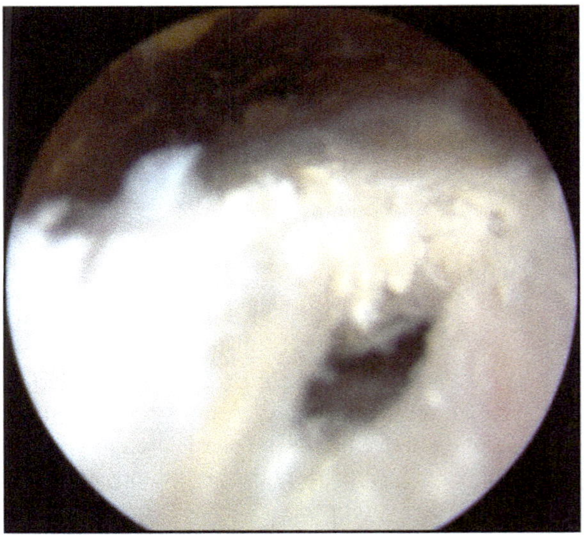

Figure 19-2. Debridement of the tendon.

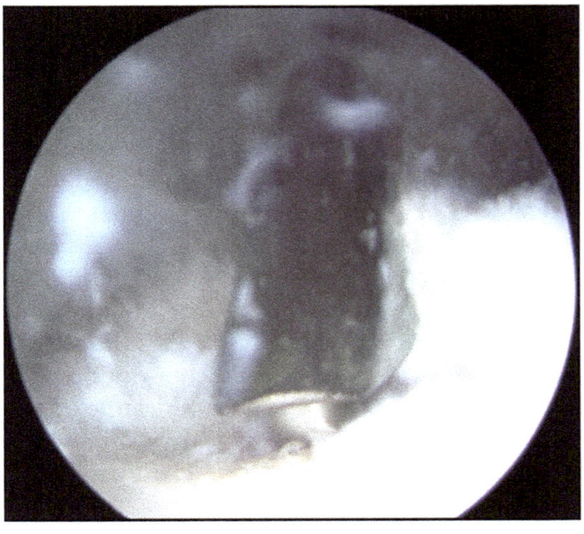

Figure 19-3. Debridement of the tendon and footprint.

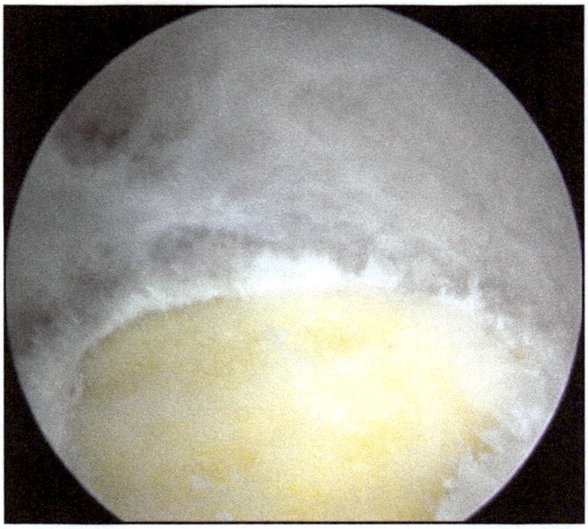

Figure 19-4. Prepared footprint.

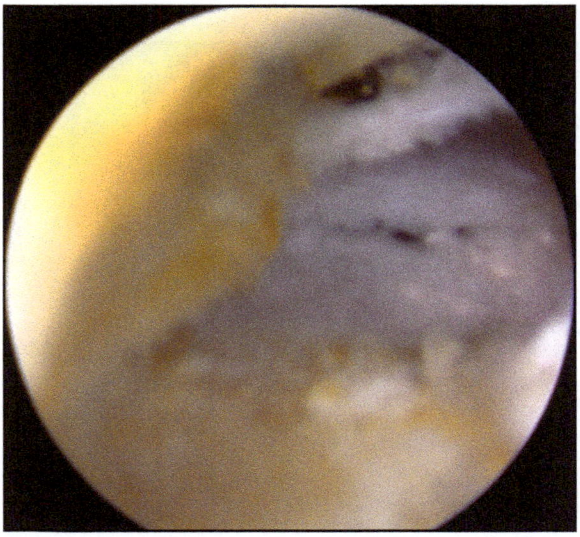

Figure 19-5. Prepared tendon and footprint.

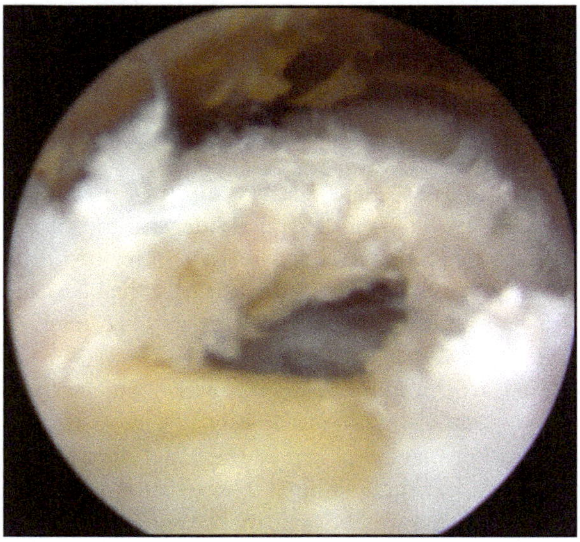

Figure 19-6. Tendon and footprint ready to accept the anchor.

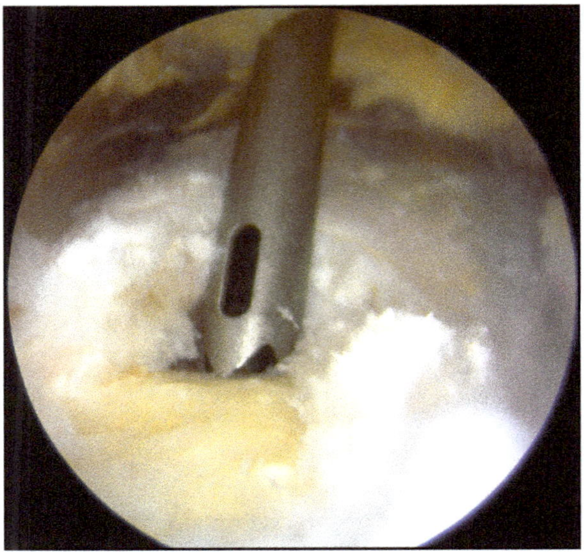

Figure 19-7. The awl is positioned.

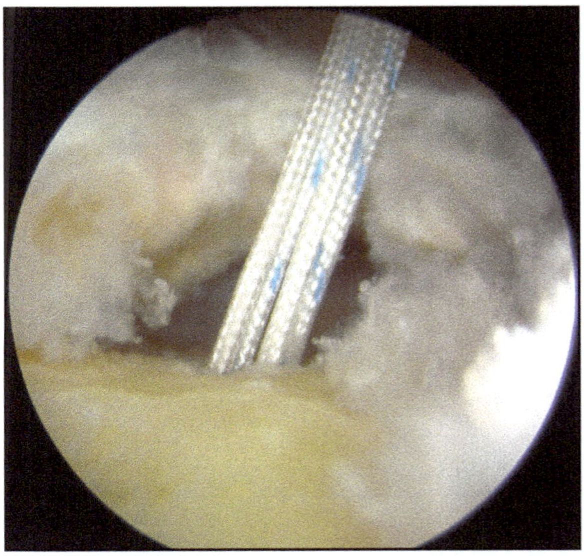

Figure 19-8. The suture anchor is placed.

A double-loaded suture anchor is introduced through the posterior central portal. It is placed at the proximal footprint angling toward the coronoid base to prevent penetration of the ulnohumeral joint (Figures 19-7 and 19-8).

A retrograde suture passer is used percutaneously to pass a single mattress suture in the medial aspect of the musculotendinous junction. This step is repeated on the lateral side with the second set of sutures. The instruments are withdrawn into the bursa. A blue cannula is inserted in the posterior central (bursal) portal above the triceps. The sutures are retrieved through the blue cannula. Sliding knots are tied, compressing the triceps against the proximal olecranon (Figures 19-9 and 19-10).

The sutures from the proximal anchor, once tied, are placed into a second anchor, which can be inserted into the more distal olecranon to create a suture bridge repair (Figure 19-11).

Alternatively, a second double-loaded suture anchor may be placed in the distal ulna. These sutures are passed through the distal tendon and tied in simple fashion. The repair is complete. The arthroscope is placed in the posterior central (bursal) portal to evaluate the repair.

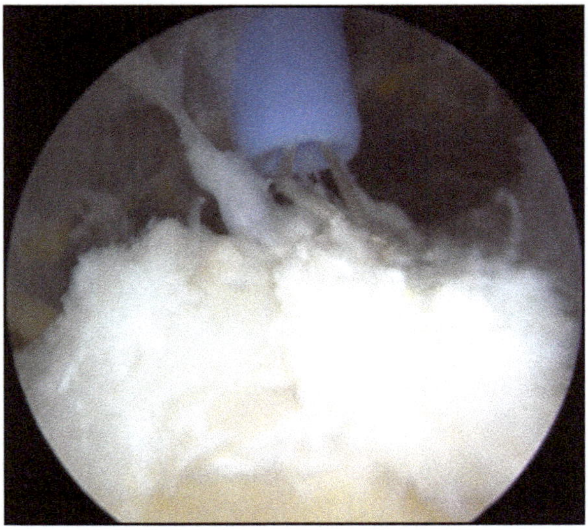

Figure 19-9. Sutures are passed and retrieved through the blue cannula.

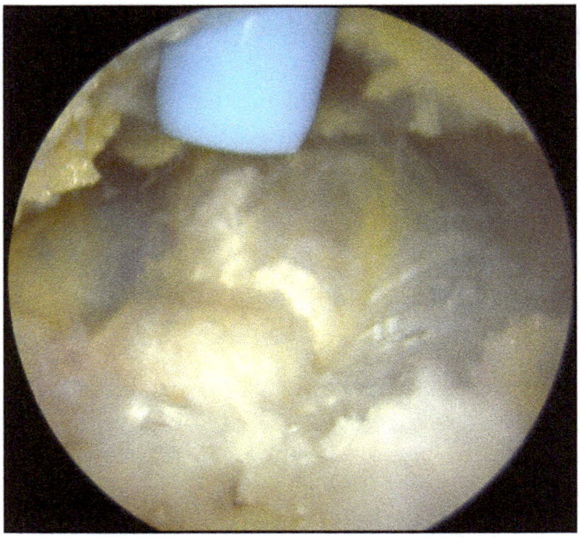

Figure 19-10. Sutures are tied, securing the tendon.

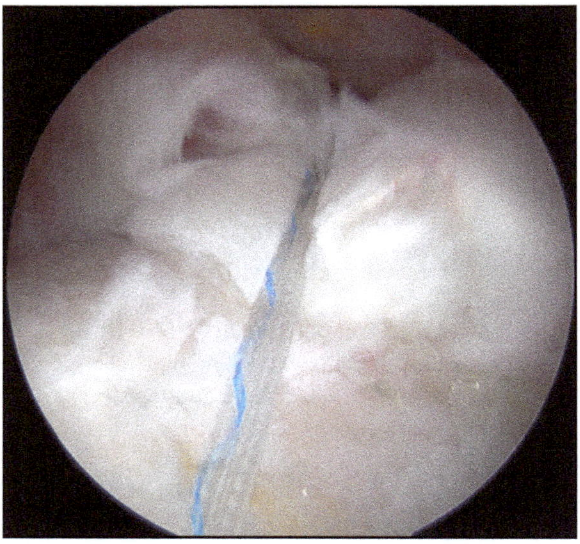

Figure 19-11. Suture bridge repair.

A complete list of steps is as follows:

1. Mark out the ulnar nerve.
2. Make a standard anteromedial or anterolateral portal and evaluate anterior compartment.
3. Establish a posterior central portal.
4. Make a posterior lateral portal under direct visualization and evaluate the posterior compartment.
5. Place the camera in the posterolateral portal, and introduce the shaver into the posterior central working portal.
6. Debride the posterior compartment.
7. Free the triceps tendon and debride to healthy tissue with the shaver.
8. Debride the triceps footprint.
9. Use a burr from the posterior central working portal to prepare the footprint.
10. Identify the location of the first suture anchor and place the double-loaded anchor through the posterior central portal.
11. Use a retrograde suture passer to pass sutures through the medial and lateral aspects of the tendon in a horizontal mattress fashion.
12. Withdraw the instruments into the bursa, and place a blue cannula into the posterior central bursal portal.
13. Retrieve sutures into the blue cannula.
14. Tie the sutures with a sliding knot.
15. Place a second drill hole in the distal footprint.
16. Insert the tied suture ends into an anchor and insert the anchor to create a suture bridge.
17. Cut the suture ends.
18. Remove the blue cannula, place the camera into the posterior central bursal portal, and evaluate the repair.

Postoperative Protocol

The extremity is placed in anterior and posterior splints with the elbow in near full extension. At the first postoperative visit 7 to 10 days postoperatively, the patient is placed in a hinged elbow brace that allows 0 to 30 degrees of motion. Weekly advances of 10 degrees of motion are allowed until 6 to 8 weeks postoperatively. The brace is discontinued at 8 weeks and a strengthening program is initiated.

Potential Complications

In the acute setting, swelling may obscure the anatomy. It is imperative to identify the course of the ulnar nerve and protect it. The bone of the olecranon may be extremely hard. To prevent breaking of anchors during insertion, the surgeon can oversize the pilot hole and tap deeper into the bone. An expansion anchor may also be used. Fluid extravasation may interfere with satisfactory repair. The surgeon must be prepared to abandon arthroscopic technique for open repair.

Top Technical Pearls for the Procedure

1. Mark out the ulnar nerve to avoid injuring it.
2. Free the tendon and muscle from the underlying humerus to obtain length.
3. Oversize the anchor pilot hole; use an expansion anchor or tap past the usual endpoint because the olecranon bone is usually hard and may fracture a screw-in anchor.
4. Separate anchors to get adequate footprint coverage.
5. Be prepared to abandon arthroscopic technique if the anatomy becomes distorted.

References

1. Moore KL, Dalley AF. *Clinically Oriented Anatomy.* 4th ed. Philadelphia, PA: Lippincott Williams & Wilkins; 1999.
2. Anzel SH, Covey KW, Weiner AD, Lipscomb PR. Disruption of muscles and tendons; an analysis of 1,014 cases. *Surgery.* 1959;45(3):406-414.
3. Bach BR Jr, Warren RF, Wickiewicz TL. Triceps rupture. A case report and literature review. *Am J Sports Med.* 1987;15(3):285-289.
4. Tarsney FF. Rupture and avulsion of the triceps. *Clin Orthop Relat Res.* 1972;83:177-83.
5. Farrar EL III, Lippert FG III. Avulsion of the triceps tendon. *Clin Orthop Relat Res.* 1981;(161):242-246.
6. Vidal AF, Drakos MC, Allen AA. Biceps tendon and triceps tendon injuries. *Clin Sports Med.* 2004;23(4):707-722.
7. Kandemir U, Fu FH, McMahon PJ. Elbow injuries. *Curr Opin Rheumatol.* 2002;14(2):160-167.
8. Johnson DC, Allen AA. Biceps and triceps tendon injury. In: Altchek DW, Andrews JR, eds. *The Athlete's Elbow.* Philadelphia, PA: Lippincott Williams & Willkins; 2001:105-120.
9. Morrey BF. Rupture of the triceps tendon. In: Morrey BF, ed. *The Elbow and Its Disorders.* 3rd ed. Philadelphia, PA: Saunders; 2000:479-484.
10. Strauch RJ. Biceps and triceps injuries of the elbow. *Orthop Clin North Am.* 1999;30(1):95-107.
11. Pina A, Garcia I, Sabater M. Traumatic avulsion of the triceps brachii. *J Orthop Trauma.* 2002;16(4): 273-276.
12. Tom JA, Kumar NS, Cerynik DL, Mashru R, Parrella MS. Diagnosis and treatment of triceps tendon injuries: a review of the literature. *Clin J Sport Med.* 2014;24(3):197-204.
13. Mair SD, Isbell WM, Gill TJ, Schlegel TF, Hawkins RJ. Triceps tendon ruptures in professional football players. *Am J Sports Med.* 2004;32(2):431-434.
14. Van riet RP, Morrey BF, Ho E, O'Driscoll SW. Surgical treatment of distal triceps ruptures. *J Bone Joint Surg Am.* 2003;85(10):1961-1967.
15. Viegas SF. Avulsion of the triceps tendon. *Orthop Rev.* 1990;19(6):533-536.
16. McCulloch PC, Spellman J, Bach BR Jr. Familial triceps tendon ruptures. *Orthopedics.* 2008;31(6): 600-602.
17. Tagliafico A, Gandolfo N, Michaud J, Perez MM, Palmieri F, Martinoli C. Ultrasound demonstration of distal triceps tendon tears. *Eur J Radiol.* 2012;81(6):1207-1210.
18. Sisson C, Nagdev A, Tirado A, Murphy M, Suner S. Ultrasound diagnosis of traumatic partial triceps tendon tear in the emergency department. *J Emerg Med.* 2011;40(4):436-438.
19. Konin GP, Nazarian LN, Walz DM. US of the elbow: indications, technique, normal anatomy, and pathologic conditions. *Radiographics.* 2013;33(4):E125-E147.

20. Kaempffe FA, Lerner RM. Ultrasound diagnosis of triceps tendon rupture. A report of 2 cases. *Clin Orthop Relat Res.* 1996;(332):138-142.
21. Simonson S, Lott K, Major NM. Magnetic resonance imaging of the elbow. *Semin Roentgenol.* 2010;45(3):180-193.

Please see videos on the accompanying website at
www.routledge.com/9781630910013

20

Arthroscopic Management of Elbow Fractures

Brent V. McCarty, MD; Michael J. O'Brien, MD; and Felix H. Savoie III, MD

Introduction

Increasingly, arthroscopic techniques are being used in elbow trauma and intra- and periarticular fracture management. Although relatively uncommon, elbow fractures are difficult to treat due to notorious wound complications, postoperative stiffness, heterotopic ossification, and instability often exacerbated by open approaches. The arthroscope allows for direct visualization of fracture patterns and reductions with no open exposure. Arthroscopic debridement of fracture debris may increase postoperative elbow range of motion. Superior visualization of fracture fragments and chondral injuries may decrease the need for intraoperative fluoroscopy. Depending on the personality and location of the fracture, elbow arthroscopy can be used in combination with indirect reduction techniques to ensure articular congruity or for direct arthroscopic reduction internal fixation (ARIF) with devices passed directly into the joint.

If there is any concern regarding the anatomy of neurovascular structures, an open or arthroscopic exposure and protection should be accomplished as the initial part of the procedure. The use of retractors to protect essential structures should be considered mandatory in elbow arthroscopy for fractures. Identification of pathology not evident on preoperative imaging allows for appropriate treatment measures and a more accurate prognosis. Adherence to basic principles of arthroscopy and fracture management should allow this tool to be used to maximum effectiveness: speeding recovery and improving results.

Indications

- Radial head fractures
    - Mason type II fracture ARIF[1-3]
    - Radial head malunion resection[4-6]
    - Acute resection of comminuted radial head fracture[7]

Savoie FH III, Field LD, Steinmann SP, eds. *The Elbow and Wrist: AANA Advanced Arthroscopic Surgical Techniques* (pp 197-205).

- Coronoid fractures[8]
  - Regan and Morrey type II and III fracture ARIF[9,10]
  - Type I fracture/fibrous nonunion excision[11]
- Anterior coronal shear capitellar fractures[12,13]
  - Type I fracture ARIF[14]
  - Type II osteochondral excision and microfracture[15,16]
  - Type II fracture suture fixation[17,18]
- Radial neck fractures: arthroscopic reduction and percutaneous fixation[19]
- Lateral condyle fractures: arthroscopic reduction and percutaneous fixation[20,21]
- Inter- and supracondylar fractures: ARIF
- Combination injuries (eg, terrible triad injuries)

Controversial Indications

Relative Contraindications

- Severe soft tissue swelling
- Severely displaced intra-articular fractures
- Altered anatomic landmarks in patients with previous ulnar nerve transposition (open nerve exploration may be necessary) or open fractures (may aid irrigation and debridement and minimize further soft tissue injury)

Absolute Contraindications

- Infection
- Neurovascular injuries
- Polytrauma
- Severely osteoporotic bone is recommended for radial head fractures with anterior capsular or brachialis penetration (requires open exploration of the posterior interosseous nerve).[22]

Pertinent Physical Findings

- History of the injury helps determine the extent of soft tissue damage.
- History of prior injuries, surgical interventions, and associated medical conditions
- Observation of deformity, skin integrity, and neurovascular status
- Evaluation of motion and stability (Aspiration of the hemarthrosis and infusion of lidocaine will provide analgesia for motion and stability examination.)

Pertinent Imaging

- Anteroposterior, lateral, and oblique elbow x-rays (Aspiration and infiltration of the joint may facilitate optimal positioning.)
- Magnetic resonance imaging provides further detail regarding ligament integrity in the setting of elbow fracture dislocations.

- Computed tomography scan with 3-dimensional reconstruction can further define intra-articular fracture patterns and may be used to determine screw length preoperatively.

Equipment

- 4.0-mm, 30-degree arthroscope (for visualization in the majority of cases)
- 4.0-mm, 70-degree arthroscope (to visualize the capitellum or radial head from a posterior portal when instrumentation is required from the soft spot portal)
- Retractors (Switching sticks, interchangeable cannulas, or blunt freer-type dissectors may be used to protect neurovascular structures.)
- 3.5-mm, full-radius shaver (for removal of fracture hematoma and debris)
- Fracture fixation implants (K-wires may be used to assist with reduction and allows for placement of a cannulated screw. Absorbable suture and suture anchors made of polylactic acid should be available.)
- Fluoroscopy device (for intraoperative imaging of reduction and fixation)
- Skin suture (Portals along the lateral side should be closed to minimize prolonged drainage.)
- Wound care (small drain or incisional negative-pressure wound therapy dressing to reduce swelling and improve healing[22])

Positioning and Portals

The authors prefer the prone position for fracture management with a small bump under the upper arm.[23-26] The shoulder can be internally or externally rotated to allow open access to either side of the elbow. The forearm and hand should be wrapped with compressive wrapping material to restrict swelling and fluid extravasation. The location of the nerves and vessels should be carefully marked with allowances for displacement prior to beginning the arthroscopy.

Step-by-Step Description of the Procedure

Radial Head Fractures

Displaced, 2-part radial head fractures[27] can be visualized through a proximal anteromedial or posterolateral portal to assess the degree of articular incongruity, fracture fragment stability, and any impingement to forearm rotation. Instrumentation is usually best achieved via direct lateral and soft spot portals. The fracture is visualized from the proximal anteromedial portal (Figure 20-1A). The fragments are debrided and then reduced using a probe/grasper in the anterior lateral portal. A spinal needle may be placed over the radial head to determine the best angle for instrumentation, and a K-wire can then be placed across the fracture site (Figure 20-1B) from the soft spot portal.

Definitive fixation can be performed using absorbable pins or cannulated screws (Figure 20-1C). Herbert-Whipple screws (Zimmer) and headless variable pitch screws (Acutrak screws; Acumed) are advantageous in providing secure fixation with compression to allow early motion while being buried beneath the articular surface to avoid impingement. A potential advantage of the arthroscopic technique is that a single screw is often sufficient to obtain stability, whereas the capsular dissection required in an open technique may increase fracture fragment instability, resulting

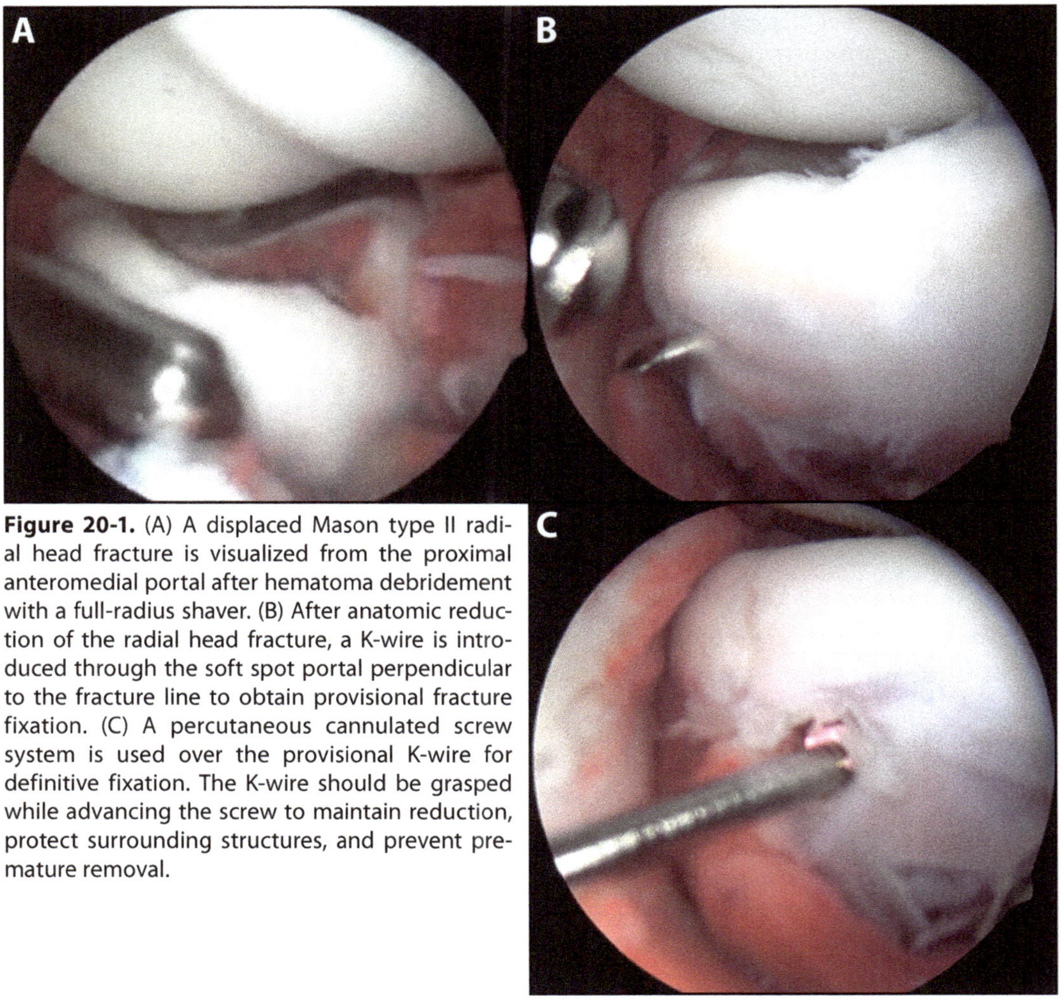

Figure 20-1. (A) A displaced Mason type II radial head fracture is visualized from the proximal anteromedial portal after hematoma debridement with a full-radius shaver. (B) After anatomic reduction of the radial head fracture, a K-wire is introduced through the soft spot portal perpendicular to the fracture line to obtain provisional fracture fixation. (C) A percutaneous cannulated screw system is used over the provisional K-wire for definitive fixation. The K-wire should be grasped while advancing the screw to maintain reduction, protect surrounding structures, and prevent premature removal.

in the requirement of additional fixation.[2] Reduction and stability of the fixation can be directly assessed during full rotation of the elbow.

Coronoid Fractures

Visualization of the fragment is achieved via a proximal anterolateral portal (Figure 20-2A). After the fracture bed is debrided of debris with the shaver (Figure 20-2B), the fragment is then manipulated by a probe placed via an anteromedial portal into anatomic reduction. A K-wire is inserted into the fracture bed posteriorly. Use of an anterior cruciate ligament guide system for placement of this K-wire has been described.[10] The fracture fragment is reduced to the fracture bed, and the K-wire is advanced through the fragment. As with the radial head, the wire should be held by a grasper to prevent accidental withdrawal while the fixation screw is inserted (Figure 20-2C). Fragments too small for screw fixation can be stabilized with the application of suture anchors placed within the base of the fracture or by the umbrella suture cerclage configuration described by Hausman et al.[28] A hinged brace or external fixator may be necessary to maintain joint stability and offload the repair until adequate healing has occurred.

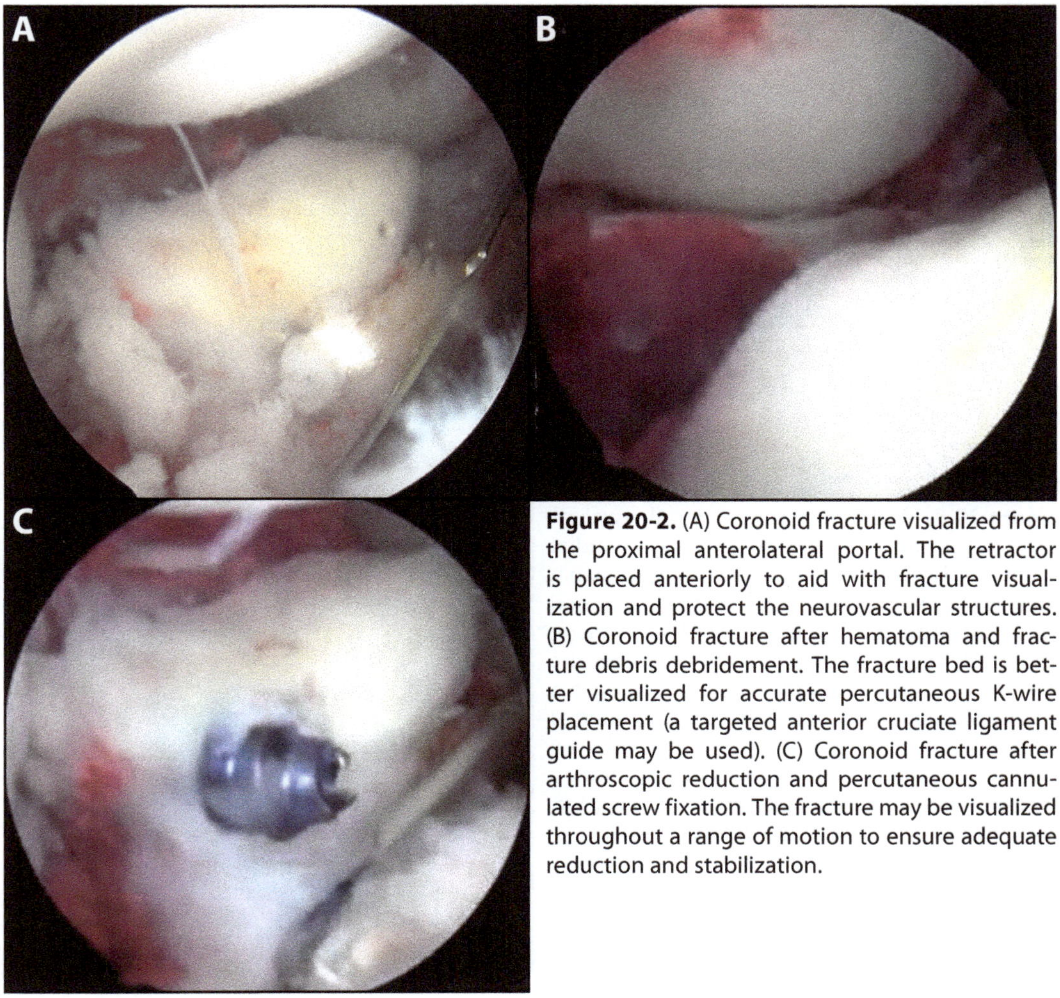

Figure 20-2. (A) Coronoid fracture visualized from the proximal anterolateral portal. The retractor is placed anteriorly to aid with fracture visualization and protect the neurovascular structures. (B) Coronoid fracture after hematoma and fracture debris debridement. The fracture bed is better visualized for accurate percutaneous K-wire placement (a targeted anterior cruciate ligament guide may be used). (C) Coronoid fracture after arthroscopic reduction and percutaneous cannulated screw fixation. The fracture may be visualized throughout a range of motion to ensure adequate reduction and stabilization.

Capitellar Coronal Shear Fractures

Type I fractures can be visualized with the arthroscope in the proximal anteromedial portal. An anterolateral portal is established, and with a varus stress test, the fragment is manipulated using a probe or grasper into an anatomic reduction. A K-wire is then inserted to stabilize the fragment. As with coronoid fractures, a guide may be used to assist with direction of the wire over which a screw may be placed. Mitani et al[29] demonstrated that, after arthroscopic reduction, screws may be placed percutaneously from posterior to anterior, perpendicular to the fracture line. This technique avoids violating the articular surface and maintains the vital posterior blood supply.

Type II fractures may undergo a diagnostic arthroscopy to evaluate for fixation indications. After removal of any fragments anteriorly, a posterior central portal can be established to look at the olecranon fossa and the medial and lateral gutters. If there is a positive drive-through sign on the lateral side, there is no question of lateral instability. Osteochondral fragments in the lateral gutter may have ligaments attached that would benefit from suture fixation. A spinal needle may be used to move the piece back into position carefully. The fracture bed is cleaned off and microfractured to enhance healing (Figure 20-3A). A suture anchor made of polylactic acid may be inserted into the fracture base (Figure 20-3B) and sewn through the fragment back down to its normal bed (Figure 20-3C). Hsu et al[18] used a bone tunnel created posteriorly to pass and tie mattress sutures though the osteochondral fragment in a patient with osteochondritis dissecans;

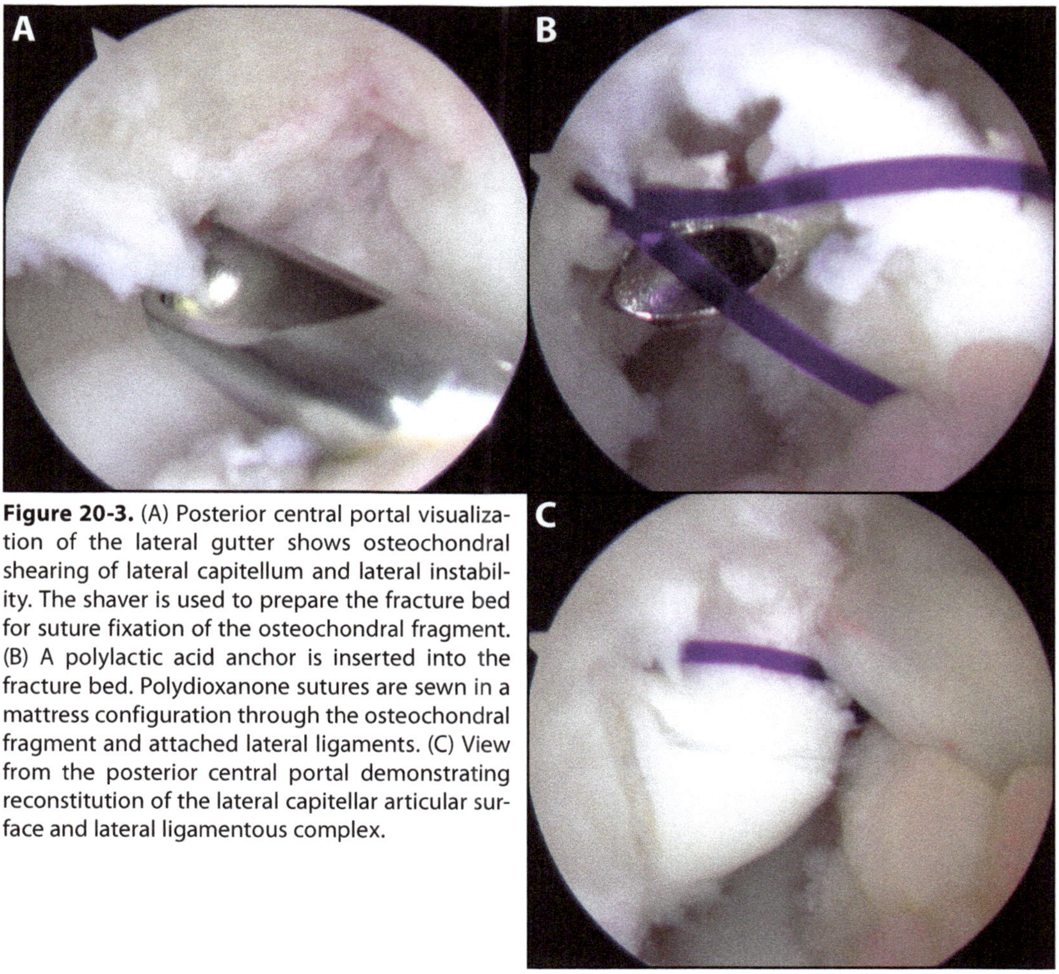

Figure 20-3. (A) Posterior central portal visualization of the lateral gutter shows osteochondral shearing of lateral capitellum and lateral instability. The shaver is used to prepare the fracture bed for suture fixation of the osteochondral fragment. (B) A polylactic acid anchor is inserted into the fracture bed. Polydioxanone sutures are sewn in a mattress configuration through the osteochondral fragment and attached lateral ligaments. (C) View from the posterior central portal demonstrating reconstitution of the lateral capitellar articular surface and lateral ligamentous complex.

this bone tunnel was additionally used to bone graft the osteochondritis dissecans lesion. Polydioxanone suture (Johnson & Johnson, Ethicon) is preferred so that this would dissolve and not cause any articular cartilage damage.

Radial Neck Fractures

In a case report, Dawson and Inostroza[19] described a technique of arthroscopic reduction and percutaneous pinning to treat an angulated radial neck fracture. The fracture is reduced through an anterolateral portal with hemostatic forceps while a K-wire is percutaneously inserted to obtain fixation of the radial head to the diaphysis. A cast is applied for 3 weeks, and the K-wire is then removed.

Lateral Condyle Fractures

Hausman et al[20] and Perez Carro et al[21] described their techniques for arthroscopically assisted treatment of pediatric lateral condyle fractures.[30] Standard anteromedial and anterolateral portals were used. The fracture fragment was reduced under direct visualization with the assistance of percutaneous 0.062 K-wire joysticks, including a K-wire placed transversely through the axis of the capitellum to facilitate rotational control of the reduction. The K-wire fixation was maintained for 4 weeks postoperatively in a long-arm cast.

Intercondylar and Supracondylar Fractures

Intercondylar and supracondylar fractures generally require open reduction with plate fixation. Of the 3 AO Group C classification subtypes, only the C1 type is amenable to arthroscopically assisted reduction with percutaneous fixation.[22] K-wires are drilled from a medial to lateral direction to reduce and provisionally secure each condyle together. Wires are then drilled proximally into each column to secure this construct to the distal humerus. Arthroscopic evaluation must confirm anatomic reduction anteriorly and posteriorly prior to definitive screw fixation. Single-column screw fixation limits this technique to individuals with bone quality sufficient enough to allow for early protected motion. Visualization can be augmented with an arthroscopic triceps reflection, if necessary. A retractor strategically placed through a superior portal can be used to lift the triceps to facilitate the exposure.

Combination Injuries

In some cases of fracture-dislocation, arthroscopy may be used for some or all of the procedure. In these cases, the entire team has to be prepared to work efficiently to prevent complications. The initial x-ray will only reveal a small part of the damage. The pattern of fixation is usually diagnostic, with hematoma clean-up followed by radial head fixation, coronoid fixation, and then lateral ligament repair.[22]

Postoperative Protocol

A balance of stability and stiffness is the most important aspect postoperatively. The majority of elbow fractures fixed arthroscopically will need to be immobilized postoperatively to maintain fracture stability. However, immobilization should be discontinued at the first postoperative follow-up 1 week after surgery. Progression from splint to hinged elbow brace with increased range of motion weekly is encouraged to limit postoperative stiffness.

The degree of immobilization is also determined by the injury. Isolated radial head fractures with stable fixation may only require sling immobilization with early active or active-assisted flexion-extension and supination-pronation exercises. Posterior long-arm splint immobilization at 90 degrees is routine with more unstable fracture dislocation injuries, but external fixation may be required to ensure stability and off load coronoid fixation. A capitellar shear fracture should be placed in a posterior long-arm splint in full extension to help maintain reduction and off load osteochondral repair.

A frank preoperative discussion about postoperative therapy is encouraged because dedication is required for excellent results. Finally, risk of repeat arthroscopy for arthrofibrosis debridement should be explained prior to operative intervention.

Potential Complications

Results of arthroscopic fracture management have generally been satisfactory, with few reported complications. However, the majority of articles have been written by experienced arthroscopists who have taken extraordinary precautions to prevent problems. Elbow arthroscopy has a higher reported complication rate than other joints, with an overall rate of major and minor complications approximating 10% in the reported literature. Moreover, the wound complication rate is substantial in the acutely traumatized elbow. It is essential to be familiar with the deformed anatomy inherent in the fractures and to use retractors to protect the soft tissues. Each case should have a time limit set preoperatively, after which the elbow must be opened or the procedure halted.

Top Technical Pearls for the Procedure

1. Have a preoperative plan and set up the back table and operating room personnel in sequence before starting the procedure. The goal is to maximize the efficiency and minimize swelling. These are difficult cases and require meticulous technique and timing.
2. Protection of neurovascular structures should be paramount because posttraumatic swelling and altered anatomy may increase the risk of iatrogenic injury.
3. Use fluoroscopy to place a small K-wire into the mobile fracture fragment before beginning arthroscopy at the beginning of the case. This will help you to understand the nature of the fracture and aid with reduction.
4. Grasp the end of the K-wire when advancing a screw to maintain fracture reduction, prevent premature withdrawal, and protect the undamaged articular surfaces.
5. One should be adept at multiple fracture fixation techniques, and the necessary instrumentation should be available because preoperative plans may change after direct visualization of the fracture.

References

1. Rolla PR, Surace MF, Bini A, Pilato G. Arthroscopic treatment of fractures of the radial head. *Arthroscopy.* 2006;22(2):233.e1-233.e6.
2. Michels F, Pouliart N, Handlelberg F. Arthroscopic management of Mason type 2 radial head fractures. *Knee Surg Sports Traumatol Arthrosc.* 2007;15(10):1244-1250.
3. Mason, ML. Some observations on fractures of the head of the radius with a review of one hundred cases. *Br J Surg.* 1954;42(172):123-132.
4. Broberg MA, Morrey BF. Results of delayed excision of the radial head after fracture. *J Bone Joint Surg Am.* 1986;68(5):669-674.
5. Menth-Chiari WA, Poehling GG, Ruch DS. Arthroscopic resection of the radial head. *Arthroscopy.* 1999;15(2):226-230.
6. Menth-Chiari WA, Ruch DS, Poehling GG. Arthroscopic excision of the radial head: clinical outcome of 12 patients with post-traumatic arthritis after fracture of the radial head or rheumatoid arthritis. *Arthroscopy.* 2001;17(9):918-923.
7. Wijeratna M, Bailey KA, Pace A, Tytherleigh-Strong G, Van Rensburg L, Kent M. Arthroscopic radial head excision in managing elbow trauma. *Int Orthop.* 2012;36(12):2507-2512.
8. Closkey RF, Goode JR, Kirchenbaum D, Cody RP. The role of the coronoid process in elbow stability. A biomechanical analysis of axial loading. *J Bone Joint Surg Am.* 2000;82(12):1749-1753.
9. Regan W, Morrey B. Fractures of the coronoid process of the ulna. *J Bone Joint Surg Am.* 1989;71(9):1348-1354.
10. Adams JE, Merten SM, Steinmann SP. Arthroscopic-assisted treatment of coronoid fractures. *Arthroscopy.* 2007;23(10):1060-1065.
11. Liu SH, Henry M, Bowen R. Complications of Type I coronoid fractures in competitive atheletes: report of two cases and review of the literature. *J Shoulder Elbow Surg.* 1996;5(3):223-227.
12. Bryan RS, Morrey BF. Fractures of the distal humerus. In: Morrey BF, ed. *The Elbow and Its Disorders.* Philadelphia, PA: Saunders; 1985:302-309.
13. McKee MD, Jupiter JB, Bamberger HB. Coronal shear fractures of the distal end of the humerus. *J Bone Joint Surg Am.* 1996;78(1):49-54.
14. Hardy P, Menguy F, Guillot S. Arthroscopic treatment of capitellum fracture of the humerus. *Arthroscopy.* 2002;18(4):422-426.

15. Feldman MD. Arthroscopic excision of type II capitellar fractures. *Arthroscopy.* 1997;13(6):743-748.
16. Steadman JR, Rodkey WG, Singleton SB, Briggs KK. Microfracture technique for full-thickness chondral defects: technique and clinical results. *Oper Tech Orthop.* 1997;7:300-304.
17. Sodl JF, Ricchetti ET, Huffman GR. Acute osteochondral shear fracture of the capitellum in a twelve-year-old patient. A case report. *J Bone Joint Surg Am.* 2008;90(3):629-633.
18. Hsu JW, Gould JL, Fonseca-Sabune H, Hausman MH. The emerging role of elbow arthroscopy in chronic use injuries and fracture care. *Hand Clin.* 2009;25(3):305-321.
19. Dawson FA, Inostroza F. Arthroscopic reduction and percutaneous fixation of a radial neck fracture in a child. *Arthroscopy.* 2004;20(suppl 2):90-93.
20. Hausman MR, Qureshi S, Goldstien R, et al. Arthroscopically-assisted treatment of pediatric lateral humeral condyle fractures. *J Pediatr Orthop.* 2007;27(7):739-742.
21. Perez Carro L, Golano P, Vega J. Arthroscopic-assisted reduction and percutaneous external fixation of lateral condyle fractures of the humerus. *Arthroscopy.* 2007;23(10):1131.e1-1131.e4.
22. Savoie FH III, O'Brien M. Arthroscopic management of elbow fractures and dislocations. *Oper Tech Sports Med.* 2014;22:169-176.
23. Brown TD, Peden JP, Savoie FH III, Field LD. Arthroscopic reduction internal fixation of elbow fractures. In: Levine WN, Blaine TA, Ahmad CS, eds. *Minimally Invasive Shoulder and Elbow Surgery.* London, UK: Informa Healthcare USA; 2007:375-383.
24. Holt MS, Savoie FH III, Field LD, Ramsey JR. Arthroscopic management of elbow trauma. *Hand Clin.* 2004;20(4):485-495.
25. Moskal MJ, Savoie FH III, Field LD. Elbow arthroscopy in trauma and reconstruction. *Orthop Clin North Am.* 1999;30(1):163-177.
26. Savoie FH III, Peden JP, Field LD. Arthroscopic reduction and internal fixation of elbow fractures. In: Yamaguchi K, King GJW, McKee MD, O'Driscoll SW, eds. *Advanced Reconstruction Elbow.* Chicago, IL: American Academy of Orthopaedic Surgeons; 2007:85-92.
27. Khalfayan EE, Culp RW, Alexander AH. Mason type II radial head fractures: operative versus nonoperative treatment. *J Orthop Trauma.* 1992:6(3):283-289.
28. Hausman MR, Klug RA, Qureshi S, Goldstein R, Parsons BO. Arthroscopically assisted coronoid fracture fixation: a preliminary report. *Clin Orthop Relat Res.* 2008;466(12):3147-3152.
29. Mitani M, Nabeshima Y, Ozaki A, et al. Arthroscopic reduction and percutaneous cannulated screw fixation of a capitellar fracture of the humerus: a case report. *J Shoulder Elbow Surg.* 2009;18(2):e6-e9.
30. Milch H. Fractures and fracture dislocations of the humeral condyles. *J Trauma.* 1964;4:592-607.

Please see videos on the accompanying website at

www.routledge.com/9781630910013

21

Rehabilitation of the Overhead Athlete's Elbow

Kevin E. Wilk, PT, DPT, FAPTA and Leonard C. Macrina, MSPT, SCS, CSCS

Introduction

The repetitive overhead motion required of these athletes, in particular with throwing, is responsible for unique and sport-specific patterns of injuries to the elbow. Injuries to the elbow are common in overhead athletes. Approximately 22% to 26% of all injuries to Major League Baseball pitchers involve the elbow joint.[1,2] Wilk et al[3] recently reported that bilateral differences in shoulder total rotation and flexion had a significant effect on the risk of elbow injuries in pitchers. Chronic stress overload or repetitive microtraumatic stress is observed during the overhead pitching motion as the elbow extends at over 2300 degrees, producing a medial shear force of 300 N and compressive force of 900 N.[4] In addition, the valgus stress applied to the elbow during the acceleration phase of throwing is 64 Nm,[4] exceeding the ultimate tensile strength of the ulnar collateral ligament (UCL).[5] Thus, the medial aspect of the elbow undergoes tremendous tension (distraction) forces, and the lateral aspect is forcefully compressed during the throw. These forces may cause a variety of specific elbow injuries in this athletic population.

Several forces act on the elbow during the act of throwing.[4] These forces are maximal during the acceleration phase of throwing.[4] Valgus stress, in particular, creates tensile forces across the medial aspect of the elbow, which may eventually cause tissue breakdown and the inability to throw. Compression forces are also applied to the lateral aspect of the elbow during the throwing motion. The posterior compartment is subject to tensile, compressive, and torsional forces during the acceleration and deceleration phases, which may result in valgus extension overload within the posterior compartment, potentially leading to osteophyte formation, stress fractures of the olecranon, or physeal injury.[6,7]

This chapter provides an overview of specific rehabilitation principles of common elbow injuries sustained by overhead athletes. Furthermore, postoperative UCL reconstruction treatment guidelines for the thrower's elbow are discussed.

Medial Epicondylitis and Flexor-Pronator Tendinitis

Medial epicondylitis occurs due to changes within the flexor-pronator musculotendinous unit. Nirschl[8] reported 4 stages of epicondylitis, beginning with an early inflammatory reaction

Savoie FH III, Field LD, Steinmann SP, eds. *The Elbow and Wrist: AANA Advanced Arthroscopic Surgical Techniques* (pp 207-219).

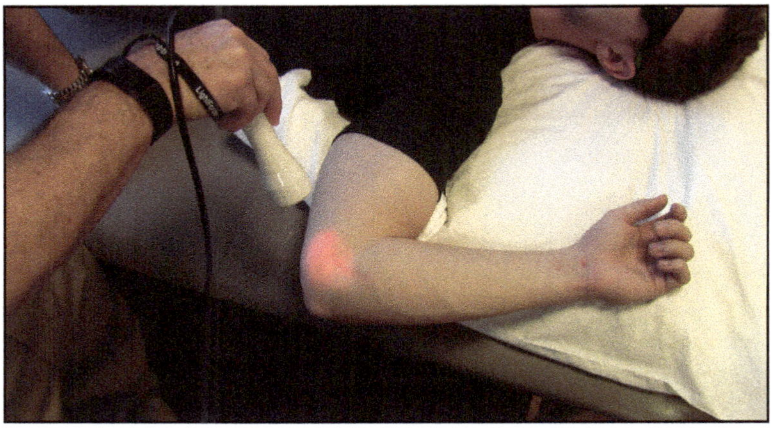

Figure 21-1. Low-level laser therapy used to stimulate a healing response to the soft tissue.

followed by angiofibroblastic degeneration and leading to structural failure and, ultimately, fibrosis or calcification. It is critical to identify the condition of the tendon because the stage of the injury will dictate the treatment.

The treatment of tendinopathy is based on a careful examination to determine the exact pathology present.[9] The treatment for tendonitis is typically targeted at reducing inflammation and pain. This is accomplished through reducing activities, steroid injections, anti-inflammatory drugs, cryotherapy, iontophoresis, light exercise, and stretching.

The nonoperative approach for treatment of epicondylitis (ie, tendinitis and/or paratendinitis) focuses on diminishing pain and inflammation associated with tendinitis and then gradually improving muscular strength. The initial treatment consists of modalities to control any underlying inflammation or promote improved circulation, stretching exercises to enhance flexibility, and light strengthening exercises to stimulate a repair response. Common modalities may include massage, cold laser therapy, iontophoresis (Hybresis DJO Global), ultrasound, nitric oxide, and extra corporeal shockwave therapy. When used in combination with exercise or with other modalities, studies have shown improved tissue quality and outcomes.[10,11]

Once the patient's symptoms have subsided, an aggressive stretching and (high load, low repetitions) strengthening program with emphasis on eccentric contractions are initiated. Wrist flexion and extension activities should be performed initially with the elbow flexed 30 to 45 degrees to decrease stress on the medial elbow structures. A gradual progression through plyometric and throwing activities precedes initiating the interval-throwing program.

Conversely, the treatment for tendinosis[12] focuses on increasing circulation to promote collagen synthesis and collagen organization. The treatment would include heat, stretching, eccentrics, laser therapy, transverse massage, and soft tissue mobilization. All of this is performed to increase circulation and promote tissue healing. Some authors have advocated dry needling for the pathology or other techniques to promote tendon healing.[13]

Tendon loading by eccentric exercise and strength training has been shown to improve results in this patient population by increasing collagen synthesis[14] and realigning fiber orientation.[15] Other modalities, such as laser therapy (Figure 21-1)[10,11] and extracorporeal shockwave therapy,[16,17] have also shown promising results.

Other emerging treatments have shown some promise in treating chronic tendinopathy. The goal of these treatments is to stimulate a regenerative response that has otherwise been difficult thus far. Platelet-rich plasma (PRP) is a promising intervention in which a small sample of the patient's own blood is separated out and the platelet-rich layer is injected into the sight of injury. The proposed mechanism delivers humoral mediators and growth factors locally to induce a healing response. Early research on the clinical application of PRP to promote healing and adaptive responses is promising.[18-26] Mishra and Pavelko[27] showed significant benefits to PRP in patients with chronic lateral epicondylitis. Thanasas et al[28] showed improved visual analog scale scores in ultrasound-guided PRP injections vs a single injection of autologous blood in patients with chronic lateral epicondylitis. In a randomized, controlled, double-blind study, Gosens et al[29] showed improved visual analog scale scores and Disabilities of the Arm, Shoulder, and Hand scores in the PRP group compared to a corticosteroid group even at a 2-year follow-up in patients with chronic lateral epicondylitis. Basic science and controlled studies have yet to truly surmise the efficacy of such a treatment.

Ulnar Collateral Ligament Injury

Injuries to the UCL are becoming increasingly more common in overhead throwing athletes, although the higher incidence of injury may be due to increased ability to diagnose these injuries.[30] The elbow experiences a tremendous amount of valgus stress during overhead throwing.[31] The repetitive nature of overhead throwing activities, such as baseball pitching, javelin throwing, and football passing, further increase the susceptibility of UCL injury by exposing the ligament to repetitive microtraumatic forces.

Valgus Extension Overload

Valgus extension overload occurs in sporting activities requiring repetitive, forceful extension, such as during the acceleration or deceleration phases of throwing as the olecranon wedges up against the medial olecranon fossa during elbow extension.[7] This mechanism may result in osteophyte formation and potentially loose bodies. Repetitive extension stress from the triceps may further contribute to this injury. There is often a certain degree of underlying valgus laxity of the elbow in these athletes, further facilitating osteophyte formation through compression of the radiocapitellar joint and the posteromedial elbow.[32] Overhead athletes typically present with pain at the posteromedial aspect of the elbow that is exacerbated with forced extension and valgus stress.

Postoperative Protocol

Ulnar Collateral Ligament Reconstruction

Surgical reconstruction of the UCL attempts to restore the stabilizing functions of the anterior bundle of the UCL.[33] Several surgical procedures exist, including the Jobe procedure,[34] the docking procedure,[35] and the DANE procedure.[36] At the authors' center, the procedure that has been used is the modified Jobe procedure in which the palmaris longus or gracilis graft source is taken and passed in a figure-8 pattern through drill holes in the sublime tubercle of the ulna and the medial epicondyle.[7] A subcutaneous ulnar nerve transposition is performed at the time of reconstruction.

The rehabilitation program following UCL reconstruction is based on the specific surgical procedure.[37] This chapter describes both programs briefly.

The rehabilitation program the authors currently use following UCL reconstruction is outlined in Table 21-1 and is based on the figure-8 surgical procedure. For an overview of the goals and specific exercises when performing rehabilitation of the overhead athlete's elbow, see Table 21-2. The athlete is placed in a posterior splint with the elbow immobilized at 90 degrees of flexion for the first 7 days postoperatively. This allows early healing of the UCL graft and fascial slings involved in the nerve transposition. The patient is allowed to perform wrist range of motion (ROM) and gripping and submaximal isometrics for the wrist and elbow. The patient is progressed from the posterior splint to a hinged elbow ROM brace (Figure 21-2) to protect the healing tissues from valgus stresses that may be detrimental. The brace is discontinued at the beginning of week 5.

Table 21-1. Postoperative Rehabilitation Protocol Following Ulnar Collateral Ligament Reconstruction Using Autogenous Palmaris Longus Graft

I. Immediate Postoperative Phase (0 to 3 weeks)

Goals: Protect healing tissue
Decrease pain/inflammation
Retard muscular atrophy
Protect graft site (allow healing)

A. Postoperative Week 1
Brace: Posterior splint at 90 degrees of elbow flexion
ROM: Wrist active ROM extension/flexion immediately postoperatively
Elbow postoperative compression dressing (3 to 5 days)
Wrist (graft site) compression dressing 7 to 10 days as needed
Exercises: Gripping exercises
Wrist ROM
Shoulder isometrics (no shoulder external rotation)
Biceps isometrics
Cryotherapy: To elbow joint and graft site at wrist

B. Postoperative Week 2
Brace: Elbow ROM at 25 to 100 degrees
Gradually increase ROM (5 degrees of extension/10 degrees of flexion per week)
Exercises: Continue all exercises listed above
Elbow ROM in brace (30 to 105 degrees)
Initiate elbow extension isometrics
Continue wrist ROM exercises
Initiate light scar mobilization over distal incision (graft)
Cryotherapy: Continue ice to elbow and graft site

C. Postoperative Week 3
Brace: Elbow ROM 15 to 115 degrees
Exercises: Continue all exercises listed above
Elbow ROM in brace
Initiate active wrist and elbow ROM (no resistance)
Initiate light wrist flexion stretching
Initiate active shoulder ROM
- Full can
- Lateral raises
- External/internal rotation tubing
- Elbow flexion/extension
Initiate light scapular strengthening exercises
May incorporate bicycle for lower extremity strength and endurance

II. Intermediate Phase (Weeks 4 to 7)

Goals: Gradual increase to full ROM
Promote healing of repaired tissue
Regain and improve muscular strength
Restore full function of graft site

A. Week 4
Brace: Elbow ROM 0 to 125 degrees
Exercises: Begin light resistance exercises for arm (1 lb)
- Wrist curls, extensions, pronation, supination
- Elbow extension/flexion
Progress shoulder program to emphasize rotator cuff and scapular strengthening
Initiate shoulder strengthening with light dumbbells

(continued)

Table 21-1 (continued). Postoperative Rehabilitation Protocol Following Ulnar Collateral Ligament Reconstruction Using Autogenous Palmaris Longus Graft

B. Week 5
- ROM: Elbow ROM 0 to 135 degrees
- Discontinue brace
- Continue all exercises: Progress all shoulder and upper extremity exercises (progress weight 1 lb)

C. Week 6
- Active ROM: 0 to 145 degrees without brace or full ROM
- Exercises: Initiate Thrower's Ten program
  - Progress elbow strengthening exercises
  - Initiate shoulder external rotation strengthening
  - Progress shoulder program

D. Week 7
- Progress Thrower's Ten program (progress weights)
- Initiate proprioceptive neuromuscular facilitation diagonal patterns (light)

III. Advanced Strengthening Phase (Weeks 8 to 14)

Goals: Increase strength, power, endurance
- Maintain full elbow ROM
- Gradually initiate sporting activities

A. Week 8
- Exercises: Initiate eccentric elbow flexion/extension
  - Continue isotonic program: forearm and wrist
  - Continue shoulder program (Thrower's Ten program)
  - Manual resistance diagonal patterns
  - Initiate plyometric exercise program (2-hand plyometrics close to body only)
    - Chest pass
    - Side throw close to body
  - Continue stretching calf and hamstrings

B. Week 10
- Exercises: Continue all exercises listed above
  - Program plyometrics to 2 hand drills away from body
    - Side-to-side throws
    - Soccer throws
    - Side throws

C. Weeks 12 to 14
- Continue all exercises
- Initiate isotonic machines strengthening exercises (if desired)
  - Bench press (seated)
  - Lateral pull down
- Initiate golf, swimming
- Initiate interval-hitting program

IV. Return to Activity Phase (Week 14-32)

Goals: Continue to increase strength, power, and endurance of upper extremity musculature
- Gradual return to sport activities

A. Week 14
- Exercises: Continue strengthening program
  - Emphasis on elbow and wrist strengthening and flexibility exercises
  - Maintain full elbow ROM
  - Initiate one-hand plyometric throwing (stationary throws)
  - Initiate one-hand wall dribble
  - Initiate one-hand baseball throws into wall

(continued)

Table 21-1 (continued). Postoperative Rehabilitation Protocol Following Ulnar Collateral Ligament Reconstruction Using Autogenous Palmaris Longus Graft

B. Week 16
   Exercises: Initiate interval-throwing program (Phase I; long toss program)
   Continue Thrower's Ten program and plyometrics
   Continue to stretch before and after throwing

C. Weeks 22 to 24
   Exercises: Progress to Phase II throwing (once successfully completed Phase I)

D. Weeks 30 to 32
   Exercises: Gradually progress to competitive throwing/sports

Table 21-2. Rehabilitation Guidelines for the Overhead Athlete's Elbow

Phase I: Acute

Goals

- Diminish pain and inflammation
- Normalize motion
- Re-establish dynamic stability (muscular balance)
- Strengthen shoulder musculature that presents with weakness (usually external rotation, scapular muscles [lower trapezius, middle trapezius, rhomboid])
- Control functional stresses/strains

Treatment Modalities

- Cryotherapy to elbow
- Iontophoresis patch
- Electrical muscle stimulation to shoulder musculature
- Low-level laser

Flexibility

- Improve shoulder ROM if appropriate
- Elbow and wrist ROM/stretching

Exercises

- Neuromuscular electrical stimulation to posterior cuff with exercises
- Rotator cuff strengthening (especially external rotation muscles)
- Scapular strengthening exercises
  - Retractors
  - Depressors
  - Protractors
- Dynamic stabilization exercises (rhythmic stabilization [RS])
- Proprioception training
- Elbow, wrist, and forearm strengthening exercises

Avoidance

- Abstain from throwing (advised by physician)

Phase II: Intermediate Phase

Goals

- Progress strengthening exercises
- Restore muscular balance (external/internal rotation), scapular area, and total arm
- Enhance dynamic stability
- Maintain flexibility and mobility
- Improve core stabilization

(continued)

Table 21-2 (continued). Rehabilitation Guidelines for the Overhead Athlete's Elbow

Flexibility

- Control stretches and flexibility exercises
  - Especially for internal rotation and horizontal adduction

Exercises

- Progress strengthening exercises
- Thrower's Ten exercise program
- Initiate core stabilization program
- Implement lower extremity training
- Initiate dynamic stabilization program
  - External rotation tubing with end-range stabilization
  - Wall stabilization onto ball

PHASE III: ADVANCED STRENGTHENING PHASE

Goals

- Aggressive strengthening program
- Progress neuromuscular control
- Improve strength, power, and endurance drills
- Initiate light throwing activities

Exercises

- Advanced Thrower's Ten program
- Stretch prior to exercise program
- Proprioceptive neuromuscular facilitation D2 flexion/extension with RS
- Sidelying external rotation manual resistance end-range stabs
- Dynamic stabilization drills
  - External rotation tubing with end-range stab at 90 degrees abduction
  - Push-ups on ball RS
  - Wall stabs
  - Ball throws into wall with RS
- May initiate plyometric activities
  - Two-hand drills
  - One-hand drills (baseball throws)
- Initiate light throwing activities
- Stretch post-exercise
- Ice after rehabilitation

PHASE IV: RETURN TO ACTIVITY PHASE

Goals

- Progress to throwing program
- Continue strengthening and flexibility exercises
- Return to competitive throwing

Exercises

- Stretching and flexibility drills
- Thrower's Ten program
- Plyometric program
- Dynamic stabilization drills
- Progress to long toss interval-throwing program Phase I
- Pitchers progress to Phase interval-throwing program
- Gradually progress to competitive throwing

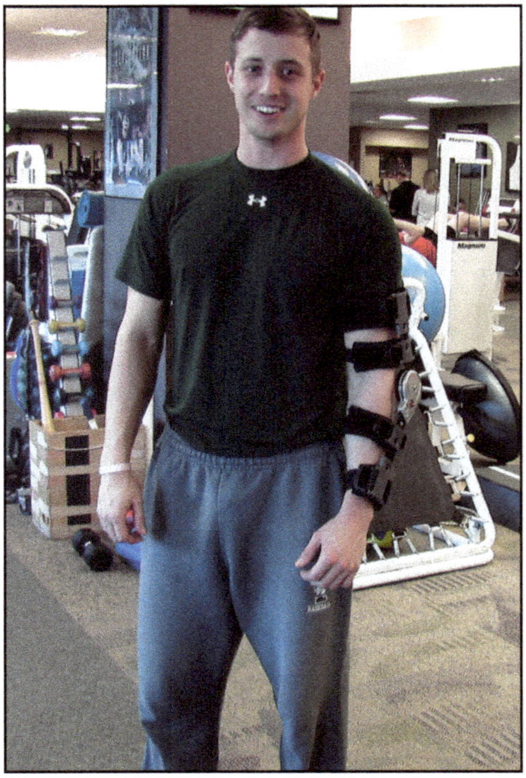

Figure 21-2. Hinged elbow brace used postoperatively to protect the healing tissues, particularly from excessive valgus stresses.

Passive ROM activities are initiated immediately to decrease pain and slowly stress the healing tissues. Initially, the focus of the rehabilitation is obtaining full elbow extension while gradually progressing flexion. Elbow extension is encouraged early on to at least 15 degrees, but if the patient can comfortably obtain full extension, it is allowed as long as there is no discomfort. A recent study by Bernas et al[38] produced 3% or less strain in both bands of the reconstructed ligament and approximately 1% strain for the anterior band of the UCL during passive ROM of the elbow joint. The authors determined that, in the immediate postoperative period, full elbow extension is safe and does not place excessive stress on the healing graft. Conversely, elbow flexion to 100 degrees is allowed and should be brought along at about 10 degrees per week until full ROM is achieved by 4 to 6 weeks postoperatively.

The exercise program is progressed to include light resistance isotonic exercises at weeks 3 to 4, whereas the Thrower's Ten program is initiated by week 6. Progressive resistance exercises are incorporated at weeks 8 to 9. Focus is again placed on developing dynamic stabilization of the medial elbow. Due to the anatomical orientation of the flexor carpi ulnaris and flexor digitorum superficialis overlying the UCL, isotonic and stabilization activities for these muscles may assist the UCL in stabilizing valgus stress at the medial elbow.[39] Thus, concentric and eccentric strengthening of these muscles is performed.

Aggressive exercises involving eccentric and plyometric contractions are included in the advanced phase, usually weeks 12 through 16. The advanced Thrower's Ten program is initiated at week 12 after surgery. Two-hand plyometric drills are performed at week 12 and one-hand drills are performed week 14. An interval-throwing program is allowed at week 16 postoperatively (Table 21-3). In most cases, throwing from a mound is progressed within 6 to 8 weeks following the initiation of an interval-throwing program and a return to competitive throwing at approximately 9 months following surgery.

Table 21-3. Interval-Throwing Program

45-Foot Phase	*60-Foot Phase*	*90-Foot Phase*	*120-Foot Phase*
Step 1	Step 3	Step 5	Step 7
A. Warm-up throwing	A. Warm-up throwing	A. 60 ft (10 throws)	A. 60 ft (5 to 7 throws)
B. 45 ft (25 throws)	B. 60 ft (25 throws)	B. 90 ft (20 throws)	B. 90 ft (5 to 7 throws)
C. Rest 3 to 5 minutes	C. Rest 3 to 5 minutes	C. Rest 3 to 5 minutes	C. 120 ft (15 throws)
D. Warm-up throwing	D. Warm-up throwing	D. 60 ft (10 throws)	D. Rest 3 to 5 minutes
E. 45 ft (25 throws)	E. 60 ft (25 throws)	E. 90 ft (20 throws)	E. 60 ft (5 to 7 throws)
Step 2	Step 4	Step 6	F. 90 ft (5 to 7 throws)
A. Warm-up throwing	A. Warm-up throwing	A. 60 ft (7 throws)	G. 120 ft (15 throws)
B. 45 ft (25 throws)	B. 60 ft (25 throws)	B. 90 ft (18 throws)	Step 8
C. Rest 3 to 5 minutes	C. Rest 3 to 5 minutes	C. Rest 3 to 5 minutes	A. 60 ft (5 throws)
D. Warm-up throwing	D. Warm-up throwing	D. 60 ft (7 throws)	B. 90 ft (10 throws)
E. 45 ft (25 throws)	E. 60 ft (25 throws)	E. 90 ft (18 throws)	C. 120 ft (15 throws)
F. Rest 3 to 5 minutes	F. Rest 3 to 5 minutes	F. Rest 3 to 5 minutes	D. Rest 3 to 5 minutes
G. Warm-up throwing	G. Warm-up throwing	G. 60 ft (7 throws)	E. 60 ft (5 throws)
H. 45 ft (25 throws)	H. 60 ft (25 throws)	H. 90 ft (18 throws)	F. 90 ft (10 throws)
			G. 120 ft (15 throws)
			H. Rest 3 to 5 minutes
			I. 60 ft (5 throws)
			J. 90 ft (10 throws)
			K. 120 ft (15 throws)

Flat Throwing

A. Throw 60 ft (10 to 15 throws)
B. Throw 90 ft (10 throws)
C. Throw 120 ft (10 throws)
D. Throw 60 ft (flat ground) using pitching mechanics (20 to 30 throws)
E. Rest 3 to 5 minutes
F. Throw 60 to 90 ft (10 to 15 throws)
G. Throw 60 ft (flat ground) using pitching mechanics (20 throws)

Throwing program should be performed every other day, with 1 day of rest between steps, unless otherwise specified by your physician.

Perform each step 2 times before progressing to the next step.

Interval-Throwing Program: Throwing Off the Mound (Phase II)

After the completion of Phase I of the Interval-Throwing program and the athlete can throw to the prescribed distance without pain, the athlete will be ready for throwing off the mound or return to his or her respective position. At this point, full strength and confidence should be restored in the athlete's arm. Just as the advancement to this point has been gradual and progressive, the return to unrestricted throwing must follow the same principles. A pitcher should first throw only fast balls at 50%, progressing to 75% and 100%. At this time, the athlete may start more stressful pitches, such as breaking balls. The position player should simulate a game situation, again progressing at 50% to 75% to 100%. Once again, if an athlete has increased pain, particularly at the joint, the throwing program should be backed off and re-advanced as tolerated, under the direction of the rehabilitation team.

(continued)

Table 21-3 (continued). Interval-Throwing Program

Summary: In using the Interval-Throwing program in conjunction with a structured rehabilitation program, the athlete should be able to return to full competition status, minimizing any chance of reinjury. The program and its progression should be modified to meet the specific needs of each individual athlete. A comprehensive program consisting of a maintenance strength and flexibility program, appropriate warm-up and cool-down procedures, proper pitching mechanics, and progressive throwing and batting will assist the baseball player in returning safely to competition.

Stage I: Fastballs Only		
Step 1:	Interval Throwing 15 throws off mound 50%	
Step 2:	Interval Throwing 30 throws off mound 50%	
Step 3:	Interval Throwing 45 Throws off mound 50%	
Step 4:	Interval Throwing 60 throws off mound 50%	
Step 5:	Interval Throwing 70 throws off mound 50%	
Step 6:	45 throws off mound 50% 30 throws off mound 75%	Use interval-throwing 120-ft phase as warm-up except Steps 12, 13, and 14
Step 7:	30 throws off mound 50% 45 throws off mound 75%	
Step 8:	65 throws off mound 75% 10 throws off mound 50%	ALL THROWING OFF THE MOUND SHOULD BE DONE IN THE PRESENCE OF YOUR PITCHING COACH TO STRESS PROPER THROWING MECHANICS.
Stage II: Fastballs Only		
Step 9:	60 throws off mound 75% 15 throws in batting practice	
Step 10:	50 to 60 throws off mound 75% 30 throws in batting practice	
Step 11:	45 to 50 throws off mound 75% 45 throws in batting practice	
Stage III		(use speed gun to aid in effort control)
Step 12:	30 throws off mound 75% (warm-up) 15 throws off mound 50% (breaking balls) 45 to 60 throws in batting practice (fastball only)	
Step 13:	30 throws off mound 75% (warm-up) 30 breaking balls 75% 30 throws in batting practice	
Step 14:	30 throws off mound 75% (warm-up) 60 to 90 throws in batting practice (gradually increase breaking balls)	
Step 15:	Simulated game: progressing by 15 throws per workout (pitch count)	

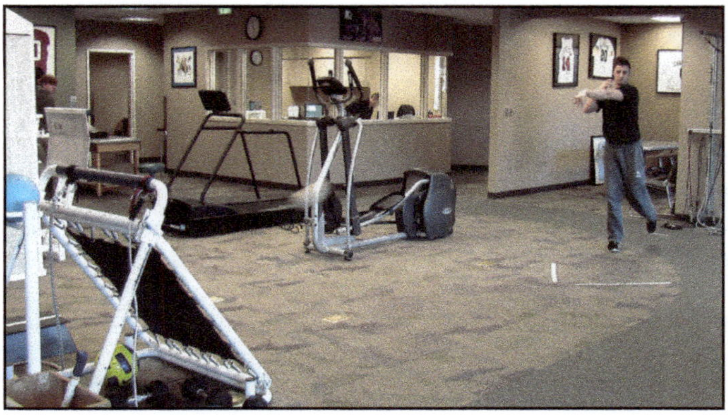

Figure 21-3. One-handed plyometrics to simulate the throwing motion initiated just prior to the interval-throwing program.

Cain et al[30] reported on the outcome of UCL reconstruction of the elbow in 743 athletes during a 2-year minimum follow-up. The authors went on to report that UCL reconstruction with subcutaneous ulnar nerve transposition was found to be effective in correcting valgus elbow instability in overhead athletes and allowed most athletes (83%) to return to previous or higher level of competition in less than 1 year. Major complications were noted in 4% of the patients.

The rehabilitation program following UCL reconstruction using the docking procedure is slightly different. Dodson et al[35] advocated an elbow brace with ROM from 30 to 60 degrees for the first 3 weeks then 15 to 90 degrees at week 4 postoperatively. The athlete should obtain full ROM by 6 weeks after surgery. Isotonic strengthening exercises are also initiated at week 6 to improve glenohumeral and scapulothoracic strength. Two-handed plyometric activities may be performed at approximately 10 to 12 weeks after the surgery to further stress the healing tissues in preparation for the interval-throwing program. The athlete may also incorporate heavier strengthening exercise using machine weights at this time. A positional player may begin a hitting program at 12 weeks postoperatively, which includes first hitting off of a tee, progressing to soft toss throws, and, finally, formal batting practice. One-handed plyometrics (Figure 21-3) are incorporated at 12 to 14 weeks postoperatively in an attempt to further stress the tissues in preparation for the interval-throwing program. The interval-throwing program is permitted at 4 months postoperatively and formal pitching is typically accomplished at 9 months after the surgery, although Cain et al[30] reported that the average time to full competition was 11.6 months (range, 3 to 72 months) after reconstruction.

Conclusion

The elbow joint is a common site of injury in athletes, especially in the overhead athlete. In the overhead throwing athlete, the injury is usually due to the repetitive microtraumatic injuries observed during the act of throwing. In other athletes, including collision sports such as football, wrestling, soccer, gymnastics, etc, the elbow injury is often due to macrotraumatic forces to the elbow, as seen in fractures, dislocations, and ligamentous injuries. Rehabilitation of the elbow, whether postinjury or postoperatively, must follow a progressive and sequential order to ensure that healing tissues are not overstressed but also provide appropriate stress at appropriate times to promote proper collagen alignment to withstand forces. The rehabilitation program should limit immobilization and achieve full ROM early, especially elbow extension. Furthermore, it is essential that the rehabilitation program progressively restore strength and neuromuscular control while gradually incorporating sports-specific activities in order to successfully return the athlete to their previous level of function as quickly and safely as possible. The rehabilitation of the elbow must include the entire kinetic chain (scapula, shoulder, hand, core/hips, and legs) to ensure the athlete's return to high-level sport participation.

References

1. Conte S, Requa RK, Garrick JG. Disability days in major league baseball. *Am J Sports Med.* 2001;29(4):431-436.
2. Posner M, Cameron KL, Wolf JM, Belmont PJ Jr, Owens BD. Epidemiology of Major League Baseball injuries. *Am J Sports Med.* 2011;39(8):1676-1680.
3. Wilk KE, Macrina LC, Fleisig GS, et al. Deficits in glenohumeral passive range of motion increase risk of elbow injury in professional baseball pitchers: a prospective study. *Am J Sports Med.* 2014;42(9):2075-2081.
4. Fleisig GS, Escamilla RF. Biomechanics of the elbow in the throwing athlete. *Op Tech Sports Med.* 1996;4(2):62-68.
5. Dillman CJ, Smutz P, Werner S. Valgus extension overload in baseball pitching. *Med Sci Sports Exerc.* 1991;23(suppl 4):S135.
6. Andrews JR, Craven WM. Lesions of the posterior compartment of the elbow. *Clin Sports Med.* 1991;10(3):637-652.
7. Wilson FD, Andrews JR, Blackburn TA, McCluskey G. Valgus extension overload in the pitching elbow. *Am J Sports Med.* 1983;11(2):83-88.
8. Nirschl RP. Prevention and treatment of elbow and shoulder injuries in the tennis player. *Clin Sports Med.* 1988;7(2):289-308.
9. Ellenbecker TS, Nirschl R, Renstrom P. Current concepts in examination and treatment of elbow tendon injury. *Sports Health.* 2013;5(2):186-194.
10. Bjordal JM, Lopes-Martins RA, Iversen VV. A randomised, placebo controlled trial of low level laser therapy for activated Achilles tendinitis with microdialysis measurement of peritendinous prostaglandin E2 concentrations. *Br J Sports Med.* 2006;40(1):76-80.
11. Lam LK, Cheing GL. Effects of 904-nm low-level laser therapy in the management of lateral epicondylitis: a randomized controlled trial. *Photomed Laser Surg.* 2007;25(2):65-71.
12. Nirschl RP, Ashman ES. Tennis elbow tendinosis (epicondylitis). *Instr Course Lect.* 2004;53:587-598.
13. James SL, Ali K, Pocock C, et al. Ultrasound guided dry needling and autologous blood injection for patellar tendinosis. *Br J Sports Med.* 2007;41(8):518-521.
14. Langberg H, Ellingsgaard H, Madsen T, et al. Eccentric rehabilitation exercise increases peritendinous type I collagen synthesis in humans with Achilles tendinosis. *Scand J Med Sci Sports.* 2007;17(1):61-66.
15. Shalabi A, Kristoffersen-Wilberg M, Svensson L, Aspelin P, Movin T. Eccentric training of the gastrocnemius-soleus complex in chronic Achilles tendinopathy results in decreased tendon volume and intratendinous signal as evaluated by MRI. *Am J Sports Med.* 2004;32(5):1286-1296.
16. Ko JY, Chen HS, Chen LM. Treatment of lateral epicondylitis of the elbow with shock waves. *Clin Orthop Relat Res.* 2001;(387):60-67.
17. Wang CJ, Chen HS. Shock wave therapy for patients with lateral epicondylitis of the elbow: a one- to two-year follow-up study. *Am J Sports Med.* 2002;30(3):422-425.
18. Creaney L, Hamilton B. Growth factor delivery methods in the management of sports injuries: the state of play. *Br J Sports Med.* 2008;42(5):314-320.
19. de Mos M, Koevoet W, van Schie HT, et al. In vitro model to study chondrogenic differentiation in tendinopathy. *Am J Sports Med.* 2009;37(6):1214-1222.
20. de Mos M, van der Windt AE, Jahr H, et al. Can platelet-rich plasma enhance tendon repair? A cell culture study. *Am J Sports Med.* 2008;36(6):1171-1178.
21. Kajikawa Y, Morihara T, Sakamoto H, et al. Platelet-rich plasma enhances the initial mobilization of circulation-derived cells for tendon healing. *J Cell Physiol.* 2008;215(3):837-845.
22. Lyras D, Kazakos K, Verettas D, et al. Immunohistochemical study of angiogenesis after local administration of platelet-rich plasma in a patellar tendon defect. *Int Orthop.* 2009;34(1):143-148.
23. Mishra A, Woodall J Jr, Vieira A. Treatment of tendon and muscle using platelet-rich plasma. *Clin Sports Med.* 2009;28(1):113-125.
24. Podesta L, Crow SA, Volkmer D, Bert T, Yocum LA. Treatment of partial ulnar collateral ligament tears in the elbow with platelet-rich plasma. *Am J Sports Med.* 2013;41(7):1689-1694.
25. Sampson S, Gerhardt M, Mandelbaum B. Platelet rich plasma injection grafts for musculoskeletal injuries: a review. *Curr Rev Musculoskelet Med.* 2008;1(3-4):165-174.

26. Sánchez M, Anitua E, Orive G, Mujika I, Andia I. Platelet-rich therapies in the treatment of orthopaedic sport injuries. *Sports Med.* 2009;39(5):345-354.
27. Mishra A, Pavelko T. Treatment of chronic elbow tendinosis with buffered platelet-rich plasma. *Am J Sports Med.* 2006;34(11):1774-1778.
28. Thanasas C, Papadimitriou G, Charalambidis C, Paraskevopoulos I, Papanikolaou A. Platelet-rich plasma versus autologous whole blood for the treatment of chronic lateral elbow epicondylitis: a randomized controlled clinical trial. *Am J Sports Med.* 2011;39(10):2130-2134.
29. Gosens T, Peerbooms JC, van Laar W, den Oudsten BL. Ongoing positive effect of platelet-rich plasma versus corticosteroid injection in lateral epicondylitis: a double-blind randomized controlled trial with 2-year follow-up. *Am J Sports Med.* 2011;39(6):1200-1208.
30. Cain EL Jr, Andrews JR, Dugas JR, et al. Outcome of ulnar collateral ligament reconstruction of the elbow in 1281 athletes: results in 743 athletes with minimum 2-year follow-up. *Am J Sports Med.* 2010;38(12):2426-2434.
31. Fleisig GS, Barrentine SW, Escamilla RF, Andrews JR. Biomechanics of overhand throwing with implications for injuries. *Sports Med.* 1996;21(6):421-437.
32. Azar FM, Andrews JR, Wilk KE, Groh D. Operative treatment of ulnar collateral ligament injuries of the elbow in athletes. *Am J Sports Med.* 2000;28(1):16-23.
33. Andrews JR, Jelsma RD, Joyse ME, Timmerman LA. Open surgical procedures for injuries of the elbow in throwers. *Op Tech Sports Med.* 1996;4(2):109-113.
34. Jobe FW, Stark H, Lombardo SJ. Reconstruction of the ulnar collateral ligament in athletes. *J Bone Joint Surg Am.* 1986;68(8):1158-1163.
35. Dodson CC, Thomas A, Dines JS, Nho SJ, Williams RJ III, Altchek DW. Medial ulnar collateral ligament reconstruction of the elbow in throwing athletes. *Am J Sports Med.* 2006;34(12):1926-1932.
36. Dines JS, ElAttrache NS, Conway JE, Smith W, Ahmad CS. Clinical outcomes of the DANE TJ technique to treat ulnar collateral ligament insufficiency of the elbow. *Am J Sports Med.* 2007;35(12):2039-2044.
37. Ellenbecker TS, Wilk KE, Altchek DW, Andrews JR. Current concepts in rehabilitation following ulnar collateral ligament reconstruction. *Sports Health.* 2009;1(4):301-313.
38. Bernas GA, Ruberte Thiele RA, Kinnaman KA, Hughes RE, Miller BS, Carpenter JE. Defining safe rehabilitation for ulnar collateral ligament reconstruction of the elbow: a biomechanical study. *Am J Sports Med.* 2009;37(12):2392-2400.
39. Davidson PA, Pink M, Perry J, Jobe FW. Functional anatomy of the flexor pronator muscle group in relation to the medial collateral ligament of the elbow. *Am J Sports Med.* 1995;23(2):245-250.

22

Arthroscopic Ulnar Nerve Release

Scott P. Steinmann, MD and Rudy Kovachevich, MD

Introduction

Cubital tunnel syndrome is a common entity and is the second most common peripheral compressive neuropathy in incidence behind carpal tunnel syndrome. Compression of the ulnar nerve within the cubital tunnel of the elbow typically occurs secondary to mechanical compression by repeated elbow flexion, posttraumatic scarring, nerve subluxation, anomalous musculature such as an anconeus epitrochlearis, or by direct compression. The superficial position of the nerve within the cubital tunnel, combined with increased intraneural pressure and decreased cubital tunnel volume with elbow flexion, makes the nerve within this region susceptible to irritation and compression.[1,2]

Controversy exists over the optimal technique for decompression of the ulnar nerve. Standard surgical approaches include open in situ decompression,[3] medial epicondylectomy,[4] subcutaneous transposition,[5] intramuscular transposition,[6] submuscular transposition,[7] and endoscopic techniques.[8-12] More recently, arthroscopic decompression has been described in the setting of underlying osteoarthritis.[13] Secondary to an increase in understanding of elbow anatomy and with refinements of arthroscopic techniques, an expanded interest in elbow arthroscopic management of elbow pathology has emerged.

Indications

The indications for arthroscopic decompression of the ulnar nerve at the elbow are currently limited to the following:

- Concomitant elbow osteoarthritis
- Concomitant plica or loose body excision

Savoie FH III, Field LD, Steinmann SP, eds. *The Elbow and Wrist: AANA Advanced Arthroscopic Surgical Techniques* (pp 221-226).

Pertinent Physical Findings

The ulnar nerve arises from the medial cord of the brachial plexus and contains nerve root fibers from C8 to T1. It provides motor function to numerous muscles within the forearm and hand, including the flexor carpi ulnaris, ring and small finger flexor digitorum profundi, hypothenar musculature, the 2 ulnar lumbricals, all interosseous muscles, and the adductor pollicis. The sensory distribution includes the palmar aspect of the small finger, ulnar portion of the ring finger, and the dorsoulnar carpus. The ulnar nerve may be compressed within a length of 10 cm proximal to 5 cm distal to the medial epicondyle. Major sites of compression include the arcade of Struthers, intermuscular septum, the 2 heads of the flexor carpi ulnaris fascia, an anconeus epitrochlearis if present, Osborne's ligament, and distal fascial bands within the flexor carpi ulnaris.

- Complaints clinically include numbness and paresthesias within the ring and small fingers with aching in the medial elbow and forearm.
- In more chronic cases, patients may experience loss of dexterity with fine manipulatory skills and overt weakness in the hand.
- Physical examination findings include a positive Tinel's sign over the nerve itself within the cubital tunnel proper.
- Provocative maneuvers include elbow flexion testing and direct ulnar nerve compression testing.
- With severe compression, patients may exhibit ring and small finger clawing, intrinsic muscle atrophy, or positive signs of ulnarly innervated muscular weakness, including Froment (flexion of the thumb interphalangeal joint with side pinching), Earle (difficulty crossing fingers or digital abduction/adduction), Jeanne (hyperextension of the thumb metacarpophalangeal joint), or Wartenberg (paradoxical abduction of small finger) signs.

Pertinent Imaging

- The gold standard for diagnosis of cubital tunnel syndrome is clinical because electrodiagnostic studies are frequently negative. However, electrodiagnostic study can be used to confirm the diagnosis.
- Nerve conduction studies and electromyography are beneficial in assisting with localization of the nerve compression level in addition to identifying other sites of peripheral nerve compression or other disease processes that could be present concomitantly.

Equipment

The following standard arthroscopic equipment is necessary for the procedure:

- 30-degree, 4.5-mm arthroscope
- Cannulas without trephinations (can be used at the surgeon's discretion)
- Arthroscopic radiofrequency ablation probe and a 4.0-mm nonaggressive shaver (useful to debride synovitis and capsular tissue during the procedure)
- A variety of standard arthroscopic biter instruments are also useful.
- Retractor instruments such as a Howarth, freer elevator, or blunt trocar can be used to assist with visualization.

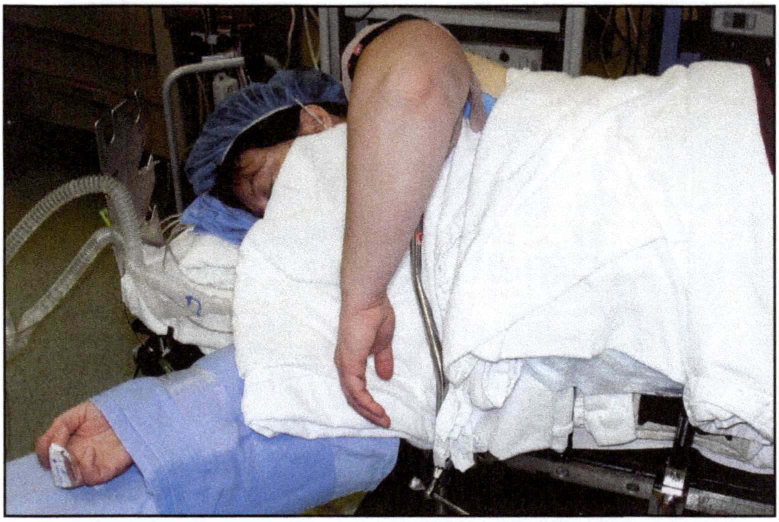

Figure 22-1. Patient placed in the lateral decubitus position for elbow arthroscopy.

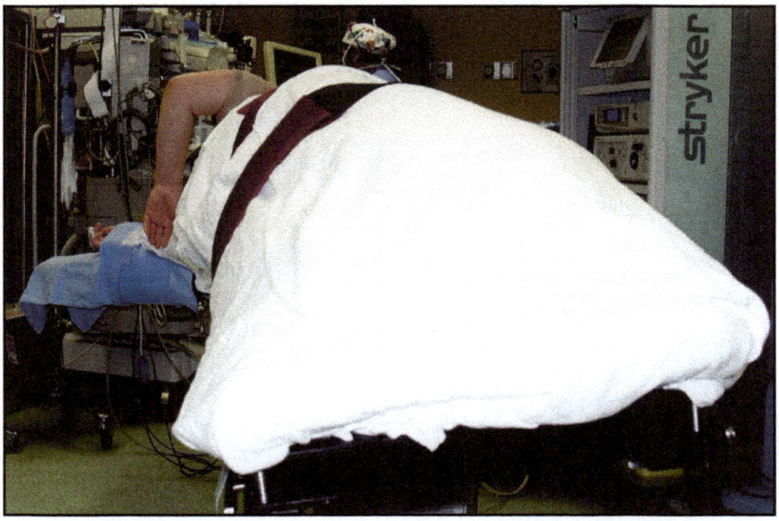

Figure 22-2. Patient in the lateral decubitus position tilted toward the surgeon.

Positioning and Portals

The patient is placed in the lateral decubitus position for standard elbow arthroscopy with all bony prominences well padded (Figure 22-1). The extremity is carefully placed within an elbow arm holder and an upper brachium tourniquet is used and insufflated prior to the start of the procedure. The patient is also tilted slightly toward the surgeon to facilitate operative exposure of the elbow (Figure 22-2). The arthroscopic equipment is positioned to allow the surgeon to see the monitor directly across the patient with instruments within close reach (Figure 22-3).

Step-by-Step Description of the Procedure

A standard posterolateral elbow arthroscopic portal is created as the viewing portal during the procedure. From this position, one is able to gain access to the olecranon fossa. A direct posterior elbow portal is then created though the triceps tendon, and an arthroscopic shaver is introduced

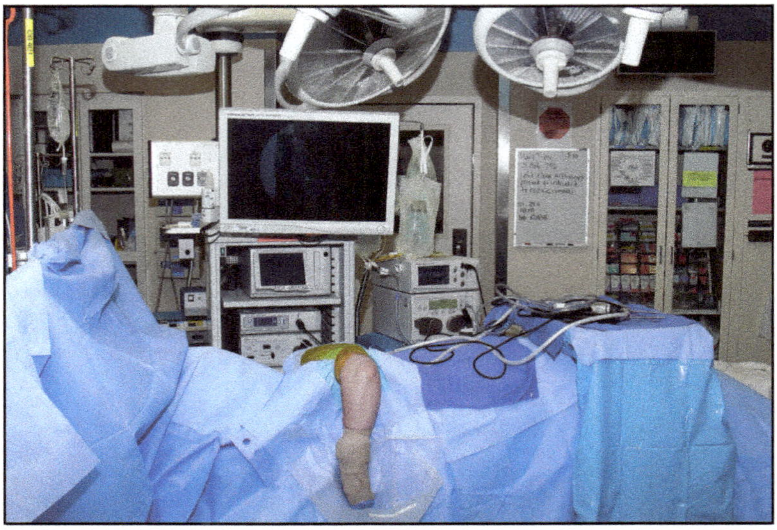

Figure 22-3. Standard operating room setup for elbow arthroscopy.

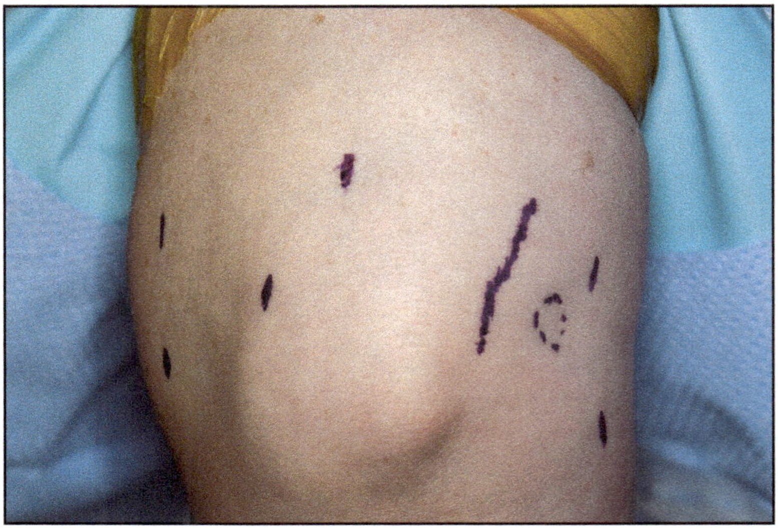

Figure 22-4. Portals used in elbow arthroscopy. The posterolateral portal is the standard viewing portal and the direct posterior portal is the standard working portal. Other portals marked are for visualization of the anterior joint.

and used to debride the posterior fat pad and gain a view of the posteromedial aspect of the joint (Figure 22-4). The arthroscope is then brought down the medial gutter and further debridement of the elbow joint synovium is then performed with a radiofrequency ablation probe. The goal of debridement in this initial portion of the procedure is to gain access to the posteromedial joint capsule. Once visualization is obtained and adequate space is established in which to work, a smooth arthroscopic biter instrument is introduced through the direct posterior working portal and the posteromedial joint capsule is carefully resected. Care is taken during this portion of the procedure to stay close to the humerus at all times. An accessory proximal posterior portal may be created to facilitate introduction of a retractor if visualization remains inadequate.

The ulnar nerve should now be visualized just anterior to the posteromedial joint capsule. Further resection of capsular tissue is then performed from proximal to distal, starting 3 to 4 cm proximal to the medial epicondyle and taken down distal to the level of the anterior band of the medial collateral ligament. This portion of the procedure should be performed with the arthroscopic biter instrument because use of the shaver is not advised. The ulnar nerve is sequentially further visualized. As the elbow is flexed, this allows increased visualization of the more superficial structures, including the Osborne ligament. With flexion, the nerve should now be free enough to move away laterally toward the joint, which also facilitates release of these compressive structures (see Video). Once the nerve is deemed adequately released, all arthroscopic equipment is removed and portal sites are closed per surgeon preference.

Postoperative Protocol

At the completion of surgery, a standard bulky long-arm sterile dressing with a posterior fiberglass splint is applied. The splint is removed on the second postoperative day and the patient is then encouraged to begin full active and active-assisted range of motion exercises. A compressive sleeve/elbow pad may be applied for support and protection for 1 to 2 weeks.

Potential Complications

As with all arthroscopic elbow procedures, the risk of complications average about 10%, which is markedly higher when compared to knee arthroscopy at 1% to 2%.[14] These risks include nerve palsy, persistent drainage from portal incision sites, and persistent joint contracture. The most concerning complication that can occur is nerve injury. Published series have documented injury to all major peripheral nerves around the elbow. The most commonly injured nerve within elbow arthroscopy is the ulnar nerve. This is followed by the superficial radial nerve, posterior interosseous nerve, anterior interosseous nerve, and medial antebrachial cutaneous nerve.[14] Although the majority of nerve injuries during elbow arthroscopy are transient, permanent injury has been documented.[14-27] In the only arthroscopic decompression study to date,[13] there were no transient or permanent nerve injuries or other complications when 15 elbows were studied.

Top Technical Pearls for the Procedure

1. Intra-articular release of the ulnar nerve can be performed as part of a planned elbow arthroscopy.
2. Safe exposure is paramount to a successful procedure.
3. Do not use the shaver near the ulnar nerve.
4. Blunt dissection for exposure of the ulnar nerve is best.
5. If visualization of the ulnar nerve is poor, convert to an open procedure.

References

1. Gelberman RH, Yamaguchi K, Hollstien SB, et al. Changes in interstitial pressure and cross-sectional area of the cubital tunnel and of the ulnar nerve with flexion of the elbow. An experimental study in human cadavera. *J Bone Joint Surg Am.* 1998;80(4):492-501.
2. Apfelberg DB, Larson SJ. Dynamic anatomy of the ulnar nerve at the elbow. *Plast Reconstr Surg.* 1973;51(1):79-81.
3. Osborne G. Compression neuritis of the ulnar nerve at the elbow. *Hand.* 1970;2(1):10-13.

4. King T, Morgan FP. Late results of removing the medial humeral epicondyle for traumatic ulnar neuritis. *J Bone Joint Surg Br.* 1959;41(1):51-55.
5. Eaton RG, Crowe JF, Parkes JC III. Anterior transposition of the ulnar nerve using a non-compressing fasciodermal sling. *J Bone Joint Surg Am.* 1980;62(5):820-825.
6. Taleisnik J, Szabo RM. Compression neuropathies of the upper extremity. In: Chapman MW, Madison W, eds. *Operative Orthopaedics.* 2nd ed. Philadelphia, PA: JB Lippincott; 1993:1419-1465.
7. Leffert RD. Anterior submuscular transposition of the ulnar nerves by the Learmonth technique. *J Hand Surg.* 1982;7(2):147-155.
8. Tsai TM, Chen IC, Majd ME, Lim BH. Cubital tunnel release with endoscopic assistance: results of a new technique. *J Hand Surg.* 1999;24(1):21-29.
9. Bain GI, Bajhau A. Endoscopic release of the ulnar nerve at the elbow using the Agee device: a cadaveric study. *Arthroscopy.* 2005;21(6):691-695.
10. Nakao Y, Takayama S, Toyama Y. Cubital tunnel release with lift-type endoscopic surgery. *Hand Surg.* 2001;6(2):199-203.
11. Mariani PP, Golanò P, Adriani E, Llusà M, Camilleri G. A cadaveric study of endoscopic decompression of the cubital tunnel. *Arthroscopy.* 1999;15(2):215-222.
12. Hoffmann R, Siemionow M. The endoscopic management of cubital tunnel syndrome. *J Hand Surg.* 2006;31(1):23-29.
13. Kovachevich R, Steinmann SP. Arthroscopic ulnar nerve decompression in the setting of elbow osteoarthritis. *J Hand Surg.* 2012;37(4):663-668.
14. Kelly EW, Morrey BF, O'Driscoll SW. Complications of elbow arthroscopy. *J Bone Joint Surg Am.* 2001;83(1):25-34.
15. Steinmann SP. Elbow arthroscopy: where are we now? *Arthroscopy.* 2007;23(11):1231-1236.
16. Gay DM, Raphael BS, Weiland AJ. Revision arthroscopic contracture release in the elbow resulting in an ulnar nerve transection: a case report. *J Bone Joint Surg Am.* 2010;92(5):1246-1249.
17. Adams JE, Steinmann SP. Nerve injuries about the elbow. *J Hand Surg.* 2006;31(2):303-313.
18. Haapaniemi T, Berggren M, Adolfsson L. Complete transection of the median and radial nerves during arthroscopic release of post-traumatic elbow contracture. *Arthroscopy.* 1999;15(7):784-787.
19. Lynch GJ, Meyers JF, Whipple TL, Caspari RB. Neurovascular anatomy and elbow arthroscopy: inherent risks. *Arthroscopy.* 1986;2(3):190-197.
20. Marshall PD, Fairclough JA, Johnson SR, Evans EJ. Avoiding nerve damage during elbow arthroscopy. *J Bone Joint Surg Br.* 1993;75(1):129-131.
21. Miller CD, Jobe CM, Wright MH. Neuroanatomy in elbow arthroscopy. *J Shoulder Elbow Surg.* 1995;4(3):168-174.
22. O'Driscoll SW, Morrey BF. Arthroscopy of the elbow. Diagnostic and therapeutic benefits and hazards. *J Bone Joint Surg Am.* 1992;74(1):84-94.
23. Papilion JD, Neff RS, Shall LM. Compression neuropathy of the radial nerve as a complication of elbow arthroscopy: a case report and review of the literature. *Arthroscopy.* 1988;4(4):284-286.
24. Park JY, Cho CH, Choi JH, Lee ST, Kang CH. Radial nerve palsy after arthroscopic anterior capsular release for degenerative elbow contracture. *Arthroscopy.* 2007;23(12):1360.e1-1360.e3.
25. Ruch DS, Poehling GG. Anterior interosseous nerve injury following elbow arthroscopy. *Arthroscopy.* 1997;13(6):756-758.
26. Thomas MA, Fast A, Shapiro D. Radial nerve damage as a complication of elbow arthroscopy. *Clin Orthop Relat Res.* 1987;(215):130-131.
27. Verhaar J, van Mameren H, Brandsma A. Risks of neurovascular injury in elbow arthroscopy: starting anteromedially and anterolaterally? *Arthroscopy.* 1991;7(3):287-290.

Please see videos on the accompanying website at

www.routledge.com/9781630910013

23

New Techniques
The Future of Elbow Arthroscopy

Akash Sabharwal, MBBS, MS, M.Ch Orthopedics;
Joideep Phadnis, MBChB, MRCS, Dip Sports Med, FRCS (Tr&Orth);
and Gregory Bain, MBBS, FRACS, FA (Ortho)A, PhD

Introduction

Fluid inflow is the established method of providing distension, visualization, and irrigation of the joint. The fluid also has a cooling effect to the joint if cautery is used. However, the surgeon must be wary of excessive swelling and extravasation, which can also hinder conversion to open surgery because of edematous tissue planes.[1]

Dry endoscopic procedures are commonplace for lapraoscopy and thoracoscopy and have been advocated for wrist arthroscopy by del Piñal et al.[2] The authors of this chapter have also used it for soft tissue endoscopy, such as endoscopic ulnar nerve release and transposition.[3,4]

In the elbow, the authors' experience has been that dry arthroscopy affords superior clarity and better understanding of subtle findings of the soft tissues and articular surface. If the joint is distended with air, the synovial and articular surfaces reflect the light and make the subtle details more obvious. The addition of fluid removes the air-water interface, which is required to reflect the light (Figures 23-1 and 23-2). Synovitis is better appreciated with dry arthroscopy because fluid tends to compress the soft tissues, change the shape of the synovium, and reduce its vascularity (Figure 23-3). Fluid distension also alters the laxity of the capsule, which is important when evaluating for instability.

Indications

The indications for dry arthroscopy are the same as for standard arthroscopy.

Contraindications

Radiofrequency Ablation

The wet technique is recommended when a radiofrequency probe or similar device is used to cool the joint and prevent risk of chondrocyte damage.

Savoie FH III, Field LD, Steinmann SP, eds. *The Elbow and Wrist: AANA Advanced Arthroscopic Surgical Techniques* (pp 227-235).

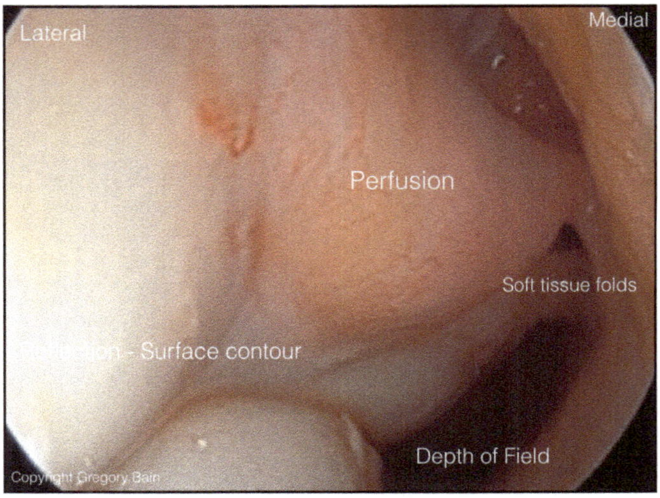

Figure 23-1. Dry arthroscopic appearance of the anteromedial gutter. Note the definition and clarity of the capsule and articular surfaces—a better appreciation of the surface contour, depth of field, and perfusion of the soft tissues.

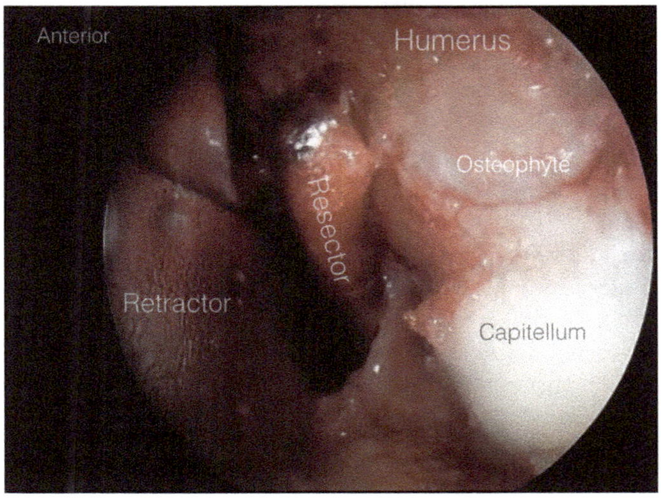

Figure 23-2. Dry arthroscopic resection of osteophytes over the radial fossa. Note the quality of the image and the depth of field. The anterior capsule is retracted while the resector abrades the osteophyte. Intermittent irrigation clears the debris.

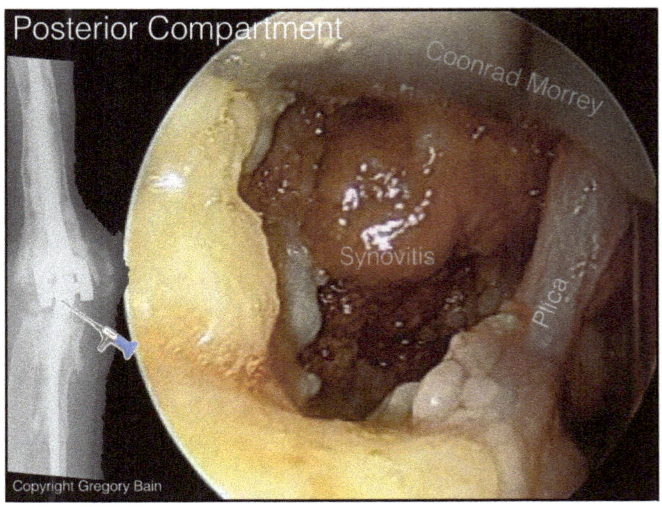

Figure 23-3. Dry arthroscopy of the posterior compartment of a total elbow arthroplasty. Multiple matched (histo- and micro-) biopsies are harvested from the synovitis, plica, and prosthesis-bone interfaces.

Air Pumps

There is a theoretical risk of air embolus with dry arthroscopy and endoscopy. If the arthroscopy is performed under air pump pressure with exposed subchondral or medullary bone and the tourniquet is not inflated, there is a real risk of air embolus. The authors caution against the use of this technique with an air pump until further research has been performed on the risk of air embolus.

Step-by-Step Description of the Procedure

The patient is placed in a lateral position and the arm is flexed to 90 degrees over a fixed bolster. Under tourniquet control, the joint is inflated with air through the soft spot. A standard 4.0-mm cannula is introduced using a trocar. Room air is used to insufflate the joint using a sterile syringe attached to the inlet of the cannula, which is then closed to reduce escape. With the dry technique, a standard arthroscopic trocar and cannula are used. The working and instrument portals are created. Skin incisions are kept small to minimize air leaks. Any bleeding can be managed with adding fluid into the joint and then aspirating the fluid and blood with suction attached to the inlet. The authors use an arthroscopic cannula with low-pressure suction attached as a probe. This enables any excess synovial fluid or bleeding to be removed.

Chondrotomes and burrs can be used in a similar way to the wet technique but with minimal suction to avoid collapse of the space (see Figure 23-2). It is not uncommon for the authors to revert to the standard wet technique if a considerable amount of bony resection is required. Fluid should be temporarily used if working with thermal probes to better dissipate the heat they generate, although this is only necessary during their use.

The following tricks and tips are used to maintain visualization during the procedure:

1. If blood, debris, or fog at the tip of the scope blurs vision, dabbing the tip on the surrounding fat usually cleans the scope and avoids removing the scope and wiping the lens with an alcohol wipe. The soft fat tends to prevent further condensation on the lens.
2. In case of blood obstructing the field of vision, washing with 20 mL of saline through the side valve of the scope and then aspirating with the probe or chondrotome is helpful.
3. When using a chondrotome or burr, direct its rotation so that the debris does not splash onto the lens.
4. Vision can sometimes be poor at the start of the procedure but usually improves as the surgery progresses. This occurs due to the temperature difference between the joint and the arthroscope. This can be minimized by wiping the lens with an alcohol swab or immersing the scope tip in warm saline before starting the procedure.
5. When using cautery, the joint may fill with smoke. This can be evacuated by leaving the valve on the trocar open and balloting the subcutaneous tissues, which acts as a bellows to pump out the smoke. Table 23-1 summarizes the advantages of dry and wet arthroscopy of the elbow.

Arthroscopic Management of Elbow Arthroplasty

The overall revision rate for total elbow arthroplasty is approximately 5% to 7%.[5-7] Common causes of total elbow arthroplasty failure are infection, periprosthetic fracture, instability (unlinked implants), loosening, and wear-induced osteolysis. Arthroscopy can be used in the management of many of these problems.

Table 23-1. Advantages of Dry and Wet Arthroscopy

DRY ARTHROSCOPY	WET ARTHROSCOPY
Decreased fluid extravasation and risk of compartment syndrome	Sustained distension of the joint
Conversion to open surgery is easier	Washes away blood and debris
Better quality of visualization	Cooling effect to the joint
	Irrigates chondrotome and burr

Infection

Up to 30% of revisions are due to infection.[5-7] Low-virulence organisms are often responsible for chronic infections and can be difficult to diagnose. Inflammatory markers, radiology, nuclear medicine, and aspiration are unreliable in this setting. Culture of biopsied tissue specimens remains the gold standard diagnostic investigation. Cultures may require up to 2 weeks to become positive, especially in low-virulent organisms such as *Propionibacterium acnes*.[8,9]

Arthroscopy allows collection of targeted biopsies for microbiological diagnosis. In addition, mechanical factors can be assessed, such as bushing wear, component wear, component dissociation, intervening soft tissue, cement loose bodies, and prosthesis loosening. This information allows for accurate planning based on the microbiological and mechanical factors of the definitive revision surgery.

The main advantage the authors have observed with arthroscopy of arthroplasty is to obtain a microbiological diagnosis. The patient is reviewed in the clinic 2 weeks after the arthroscopy, with the results of the microbiology and histology. The authors assess the delayed cultures and the polymorph neutrophil (PMN) count per high power field. The specimens are matched so that the histology can be correlated if there is any doubt regarding possible contamination. Therefore, an informed decision regarding the definitive management is made in consultation with the clinical microbiologist and the patient.

Preoperative Planning

The authors enforce an antibiotic holiday for 2 weeks prior to biopsy in which all antimicrobial drugs are withheld. All available prior operation records should be reviewed, with particular note made of the position of the ulnar nerve and whether an anterior transposition has been performed.

Procedure

The patient is set up as described previously. A standard superior medial viewing portal is created, followed by a superior lateral working portal under direct vision. Further accessory portals are made as necessary.

Once the first portal has been established, a sample of any fluid present in the joint is taken for microbiological analysis. The authors use dry arthroscopy initially to minimize contamination of the specimens. This also prevents extravasation of fluid, which may dilute the bacterial load. Once the initial specimens have been harvested, saline is introduced for further evaluation of the joint.

The presence or absence of the following features is noted (see Figure 23-3):

1. Capsule: areas of inflammation, wear debris
2. Prosthesis: worn bushings, metal wear

Table 23-2. Benefits and Limitations of Arthroscopy for Arthroplasty

Benefits	*Limitations*
Targeted tissue sample microbiological approach	Limited access (eg, implant-bone interface at tip of prosthesis)
More definitive planning of the revision arthroplasty	Inability to dislodge the biofilm
Reduced rate of inappropriate or unnecessary antibiotics	

3. Prosthesis-host interface: fibrous tissue, loose cement/other debris
4. The elbow is pistoned to elicit any loosening at the bone-cement or cement-prosthesis interface. Table 23-2 outlines the benefits and limitations of arthroscopy in the presence of a total elbow arthroplasty.

Biopsy

When the trocar is introduced into the joint, any joint fluid is collected in a sterile jar and sent to microbiology. A plastic arthroscopic cannula is inserted to assist in collecting specimens to minimize the chance of contamination. Clean biopsy forceps are introduced through the portal. A no-touch technique is used during handling of the samples. Matched microbiology and histology samples are harvested and labeled for later correlation. Specimens are harvested from any area of inflammation or synovitis, the bone-cement interface, and any bare bone within the joint. Pistoning of the articulation allows sampling of any loose debris from the humeral or ulnar canals. If the prosthesis is loose, specimens can be harvested from the medullary canal by gently inserting basket forceps past the cement interface.

Patients usually fall into one of the following categories:

- Mechanical symptoms improve: Some patients who have had a mechanical issue have symptomatic improvement from the debridement and have not required further surgery.
- Mechanical symptoms persist: In these cases, a single-stage revision arthroplasty is required.
- Specimen contamination: Only one specimen has a culture growth but has no PMN and, therefore, is likely to be a contaminant. However, if only one specimen had a culture growth but there are PMNs, it is likely to be a true infection.
- Infection, older patient with comorbidities: Suppression antibiotics may be appropriate. Fortunately, the antibiotic sensitivities are known, so this has a better chance of symptomatic improvement. Unfortunately, some of these patients require revision arthroplasty.
- Infection: In this case, an informed decision is made regarding the specific antibiotics. In most cases, it is the authors' practice to perform a 2-stage revision arthroplasty. In the first stage, they remove the prosthesis, all of the cement, and granulation tissue. If the prosthesis is loose, we insert the scope into the intramedullary canal to assess if there is any retained cement or debris. This can be removed endoscopically. If the authors are unable to remove the cement, an osteotomy is performed to ensure a complete debridement is performed. The authors then insert a linked prostalac, antibiotic cement arthroplasty, for 3 to 6 months. The specific antibiotics are use intravenously and within the cement.

Once the joint has settled, the second-stage arthroplasty can be performed. The prostalac is removed and the definitive prosthesis is inserted. If the joint is slow to settle, the authors perform a repeat arthroscopy to again obtain microbiological and histology specimens.

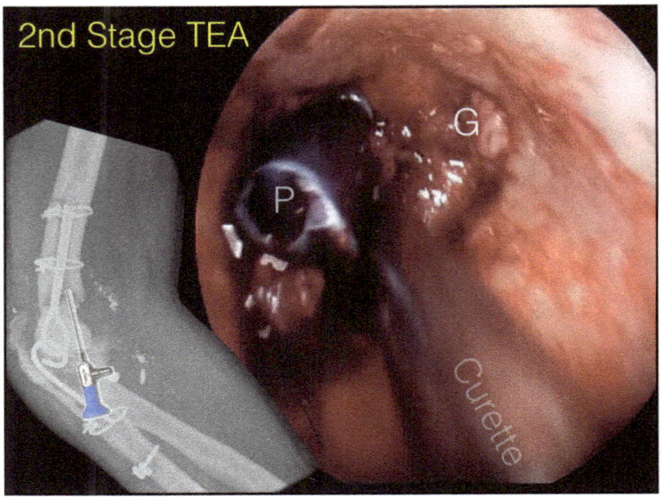

Figure 23-4. Endoscopy of the humeral shaft during the second stage of a revision elbow arthroplasty. A curette is being used to remove a prostalac (P) cement fragment stained with methylene blue. Granulation (G) tissue is also observed and removed with endoscopic assistance.

Difficulties due to the Presence of the Implant

Arthroscopy of a prosthetic joint presents challenges compared to that of native joint. Scarring and contracture of the joint pseudocapsule can result in difficulty entering the joint and a limited working space. If difficult, the trocar is introduced under fluoroscopic guidance.

Some areas of the joint can be difficult to access with conventional portals; however, development of alternate portals for access to these areas is underway. Nevertheless, there should be no hesitation to perform an open arthrotomy if sampling may be compromised.

Other Uses of Arthroscopy After Elbow Arthroplasty

Acute Septic Joint

In cases of acute septic joint, arthroscopy can be used to obtain samples and to irrigate the joint. Close observation of these patients is required, and revision arthroscopic or open surgery may be needed.

Instability

Arthroscopy can be used to assess instability of a symptomatic unlinked implant in a similar way to in a native joint. Dry arthroscopy with stress testing of the joint is performed while directly visualizing the collateral ligaments and for pathologic gapping of the joint surfaces. Intra-articular soft tissue interposition and cement loose bodies can be removed.

Cement Extraction

During revision arthroplasty, extraction of intramedullary cement can be challenging and increase the risk of periprosthetic fracture. Using an arthroscope placed in the humeral or ulnar canal allows direct visualization of the cement and safer, more controlled extraction (Figure 23-4).

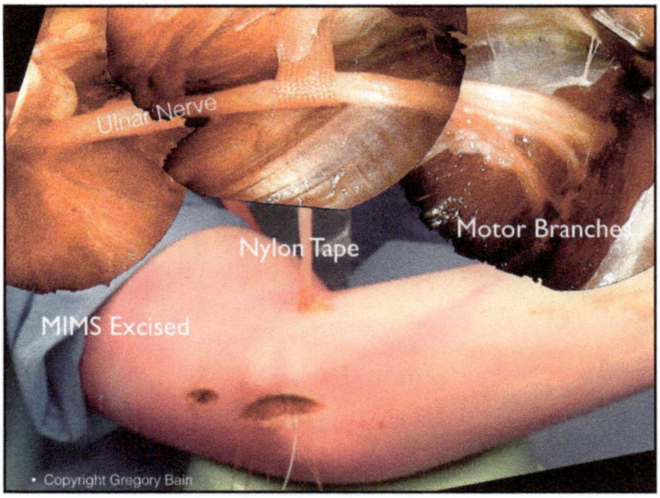

Figure 23-5. Endoscopic ulnar nerve transposition. Below is the elbow with the main working portal over the medial epicondyle. A proximal portal was used to retract the ulnar nerve at the time of resection of the medial intermuscular septum. An anterior portal has a nylon tape to retract the nerve. The compose photo shows the ulnar nerve held transposed by the nylon tape and the multiple motor branches dissected free.

Evaluation of Wear After Hemiarthroplasty

There is a growing interest in distal humeral hemiarthroplasty for trauma. The main concern with this technique is wear of the native ulna and radial head, which is difficult to quantify radiographically. Arthroscopy would provide the most reliable method of evaluating the painful hemiarthroplasty.

Endoscopy of the Elbow

Olecranon Bursoscopy

This is discussed in detail in Chapter 6. The authors developed and now routinely use the extra-bursal endoscopic procedure specifically for the treatment of sterile olecranon bursitis, which is resistant to conservative management.[10] The threshold to surgical intervention may decrease with this less-invasive technique.

A 2- to 3-cm incision distal to the bursa is made to allow introduction of the hooded scope. The subcutaneous tissues are elevated off the bursa and olecranon. Then, via a separate proximal portal, a pituitary rongeur is used to resect the bursa (Figure 23-5). Rheumatoid nodules can be resected in the same manner. Cautery is used to control bleeding to prevent any fluid accumulation in the bursal space postoperatively.

Olecranon spurs can be resected with a burr endoscopically. The fluoroscopy assists in identifying the spur and ensuring it is completely resected.

Previously, the authors have used pressure bandages and drains to prevent the recurrence of the dead space. However, the authors now have the elbow placed in a sling at 90 degrees of flexion because this will close off the dead space.

Endoscopic Ulnar Nerve Release and Transposition

The authors now routinely perform dry endoscopy as their preferred technique for cubital tunnel decompression. They recently described the technique for endoscopic ulnar nerve transposition, which they perform when indicated.[11]

Under general anesthesia, the patient is placed in the lateral decubitus position, and a 3-cm longitudinal incision is made between the medial epicondyle and olecranon (Figure 23-6). Blunt

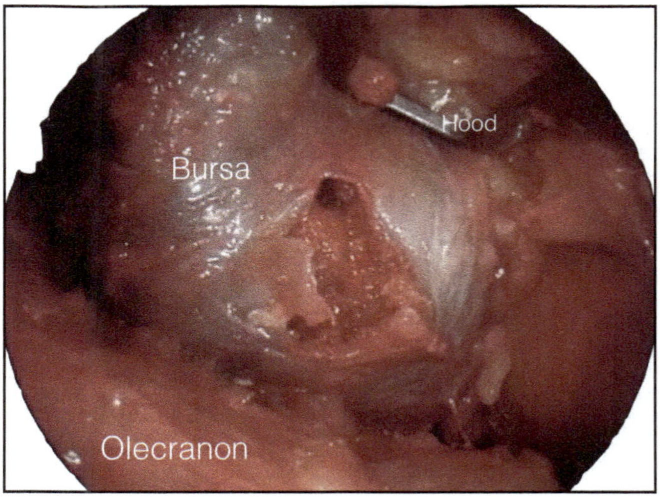

Figure 23-6. Endoscopic olecranon bursa resection. Note that the hood suspends the soft tissues and skin. Therefore, the skin over the olecranon is maintained, and healing is not a problem.

dissection is performed to the level of the cubital retinaculum. The subcutaneous plane at the level of the deep fascia is elevated anterior to the medial epicondyle. The ulnar nerve release is then released endoscopically. The medial intermuscular septum is identified and excised. Care is taken to ensure that any adjacent vessels are protected or cauterized. The ulnar nerve is then mobilized and transferred anterior to the medial epicondyle on a nylon tape.

The nerve should be checked for kinking along its course, following which the subcutaneous fat is then sutured to the soft tissue over the medial epicondyle. The elbow is placed into a sling in flexion for 1 week to ensure that the soft tissues heal and to stabilize the nerve in its new bed.

The authors have also completed releases of the proximal median nerve endoscopically in which an initial open exposure is made to identify the nerve and then the remainder of the release as an endoscopic procedure is performed. Damert et al[12] reported on the endoscopic release of the anterior interosseous nerve. This reduces the morbidity of the procedure while preserving its safety.

Endoscopic Suturing

To be able to perform endoscopic suturing opens an entirely new spectrum of surgery. It invites endoscopic repair of many structures. The authors have used barbed sutures, inserted endoscopically, to repair the deep fascia. The barbed sutures are ideal for endoscopy because they do not require knot tying.

References

1. Angelo RL. Advances in elbow arthroscopy. *Orthopedics.* 1993;16(9):1037-1046.
2. del Piñal F, García-Bernal FJ, Pisani D, Regalado J, Ayala H, Studer A. Dry arthroscopy of the wrist: surgical technique. *J Hand Surg Am.* 2007;32(1):119-123.
3. Hoffmann R, Siemionow M. The endoscopic management of cubital tunnel syndrome. *J Hand Surg Br.* 2006;31(1):23-29.
4. Bain GI, Bajhau A. Endoscopic release of the ulnar nerve at the elbow using the Agee device: a cadaveric study. *Arthroscopy.* 2005;21(6):691-695.
5. New Zealand Orthopaedic Association. *The New Zealand Joint Registry Fourteen Year Report: January 1999 to9 December 2012.* Wellington, New Zealand: New Zealand Orthopaedic Association; 2013. http://www.nzoa.org.nz/system/files/NJR%2014%20Year%20Report.pdf. Accessed August 11, 2015.
6. Australian Orthopaedic Association. National Joint Replacement Registry. *AOA website.* 2014. https://aoanjrr.dmac.adelaide.edu.au/annual-reports-2014. Accessed August 11, 2015.

7. Gay DM, Lyman S, Do H, Hotchkiss RN, Marx RG, Daluiski A. Indications and reoperation rates for total elbow arthroplasty: an analysis of trends in New York State. *J Bone Joint Surg Am.* 2012;94(2)110-117.
8. Dodson CC, Craig EV, Cordasco FA, et al. Propionibacterium acnes infection after shoulder arthroplasty: a diagnostic challenge. *J Shoulder Elbow Surg.* 2010;19(2):303-307.
9. Lutz MF, Berthelot P, Fresard A, et al. Arthroplastic and osteosynthetic infections due to Propionibacterium acnes: a retrospective study of 52 cases, 1995-2002. *Eur J Clin Microbiol Infect Dis.* 2005;24(11):739-744.
10. Tu CG, McGuire DT, Morse LP, Bain GI. Olecranon extrabursal endoscopic bursectomy. *Tech Hand Up Extrem Surg.* 2013;17(3):173-175.
11. Morse LP, McGuire DT, Bain GI. Endoscopic ulnar nerve release and transposition. *Tech Hand Up Extrem Surg.* 2014;18(1):10-14.
12. Damert HG, Hoffmann R, Kraus A, Stowell RL, Lubahn J. Minimally invasive endoscopic decompression for anterior interosseous nerve syndrome: technical notes. *J Hand Surg Am.* 2013;38(10):2016-2024.

The figures and the videos used in this chapter remain the property of Gregory Bain.

Please see videos on the accompanying website at

www.routledge.com/9781630910013

SECTION III

THE ELBOW
Complications

24

Avoiding Complications in Elbow Arthroscopy

Patrick M. O'Brien, MD; E. Rhett Hobgood, MD; and Larry D. Field, MD

Introduction

Elbow arthroscopy is a useful technique in the management of a variety of pathologic conditions. It has demonstrated utility in the treatment of loose bodies, plicae, osteoarthritis, rheumatoid arthritis, osteochondritis dissecans, contracture, fractures, and some causes of elbow instability. However, it is a technically demanding procedure due to the remarkable congruity of the articular surfaces and the close proximity of neurovascular structures. Because of these factors, complications can often occur.

Complications include superficial infection, persistent drainage from portal sites, heterotopic ossification, postoperative contracture, compartment syndrome, septic arthritis, and, most commonly, nerve injury. Some authors have shown the rate of complications after elbow arthroscopy to be much higher (approximately 10%) than that reported after knee or shoulder arthroscopy (1% and 2%, respectively).[1] Although permanent neurologic injuries are uncommon, when they do occur, they can be devastating.

Avoiding complications requires a thorough knowledge of intra- and extra-articular anatomy of the elbow combined with a systematic operative technique. The aim of this chapter is to help surgeons avoid complications by reviewing anatomic considerations, proper positioning, and use of instruments. Specific complications and associated risk factors are also discussed. Finally, the authors present their preferred method of treatment and situations that deserve special consideration.

Anatomic Considerations

Neurovascular injury is the primary concern during elbow arthroscopy. Understanding several important anatomic considerations can help decrease the likelihood of injuring these vital structures. These considerations influence the authors' surgical technique in the following ways: mark anatomic landmarks prior to initiating the procedure; position the elbow in 90 degrees of flexion; understand the effect of joint distention on the relationship between the joint capsule, bone, and

Savoie FH III, Field LD, Steinmann SP, eds. *The Elbow and Wrist: AANA Advanced Arthroscopic Surgical Techniques* (pp 239-249).

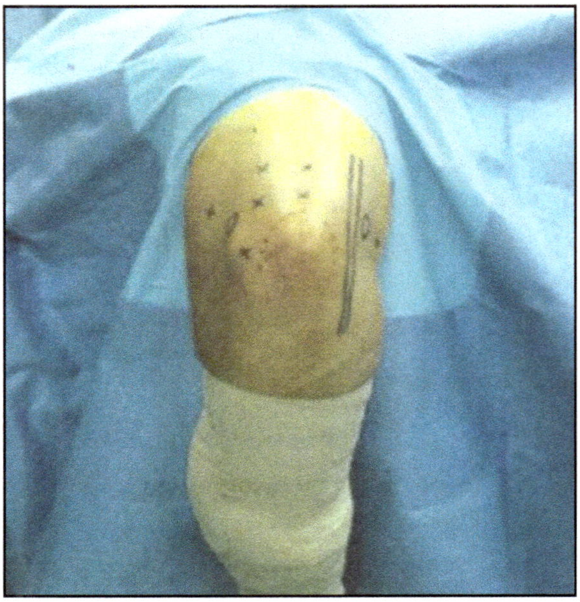

Figure 24-1. Anatomic landmarks are outlined on the skin.

neurovascular structures; incise only the skin to protect the cutaneous nerves; and use proximal portals in the anterior compartment.

The bony landmarks of the elbow, ulnar nerve, and portal sites are marked on the skin prior to joint distention (Figure 24-1). This is important because anatomic landmarks may become obscured secondary to swelling once the procedure is initiated. The important bony landmarks to outline include the medial and lateral epicondyles, radial head, and olecranon. It is especially important to mark the position of the ulnar nerve because subluxation and anterior dislocation can occur in approximately 16% of the population. This can place it at risk during the placement of the anteromedial portal.

Positioning the elbow in 90 degrees of flexion is recommended. In this position, the neural structures are farther away from the bone and capsule than in the extended position. In a cadaveric study, Miller et al[2] demonstrated that the capsule-to-nerve and the bone-to-nerve distances increased for the radial and median nerves in flexed elbows when compared to matched extended elbows. However, they found that the distance between the ulnar nerve and the capsule did not vary with elbow flexion and extension but remained essentially on the capsule in most specimens. Most importantly, elbow extension eliminates the protective effect of insufflation.[2]

Joint insufflation with 20 mL of sterile saline should always be performed prior to portal placement. Insufflation increases the distance between the bone and the radial and median nerves.[2] However, the bone-to-ulnar nerve distance does not change significantly with insufflation. Joint distention does not increase the distance between the joint capsule and adjacent neurovascular structures (Figures 24-2).[3] Therefore, it does not protect these structures from work performed against the joint capsule. An additional benefit is that joint distention makes capsule penetration easier and more reliable. Distention of the joint with more than 25 mL of saline risks capsular rupture. This may result in poor visualization and fluid extravasation during the procedure. In addition, exercise caution when insufflating degenerative or posttraumatic elbows because they may not have the capacity to hold more than 10 mL of fluid.

Cutaneous nerves should be protected during portal placement (Figure 24-3). When establishing portals, the authors advise only incising the skin to protect the subcutaneous nerves. Blunt dissection through the subcutaneous tissues is then performed prior to cannula insertion. Stab incisions should always be avoided.

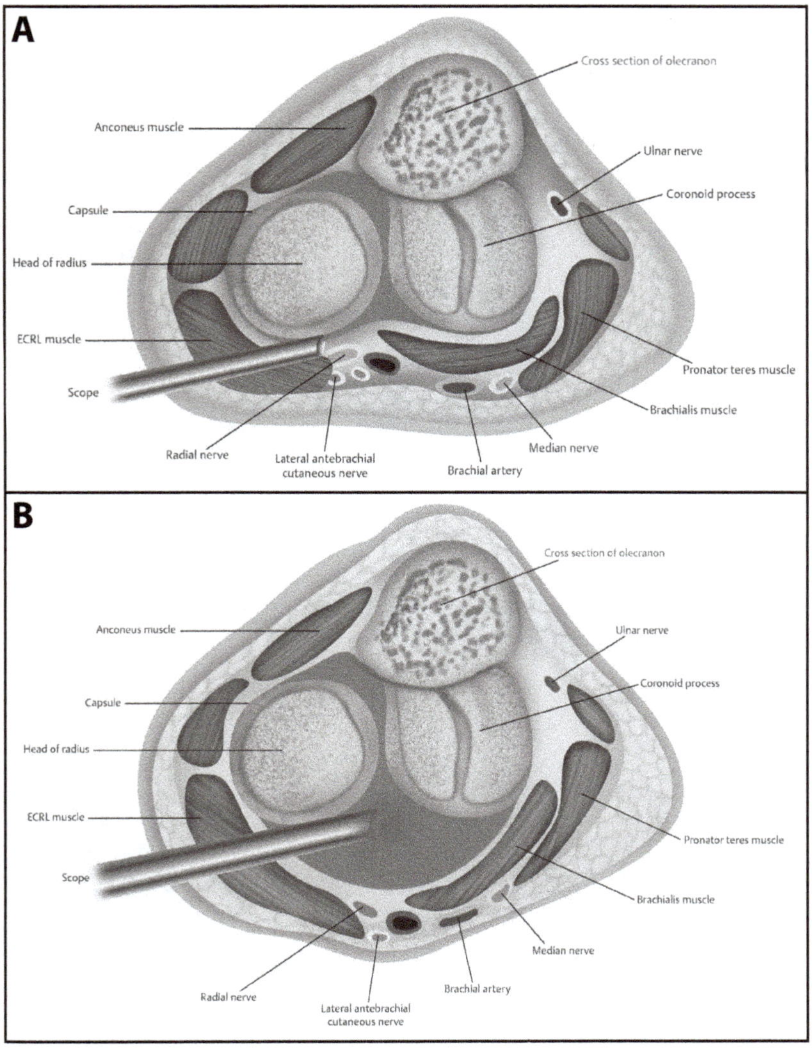

Figure 24-2. (A) Cross-section of a noninsufflated elbow. (B) Cross-section of an insufflated elbow. ECRL, extensor carpi radialis longus.

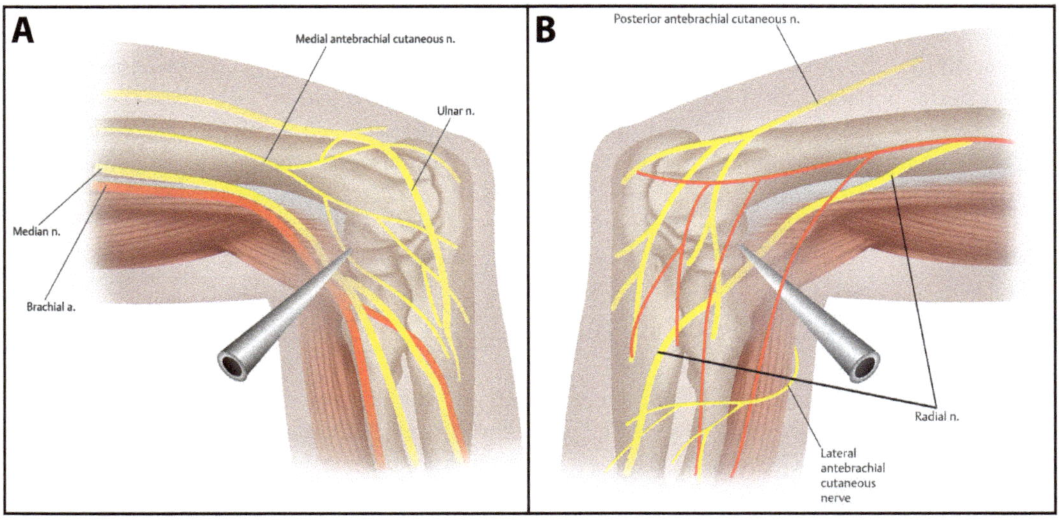

Figure 24-3. (A) Diagram of the medial elbow cutaneous nerves. (B) Diagram of the lateral elbow cutaneous nerves.

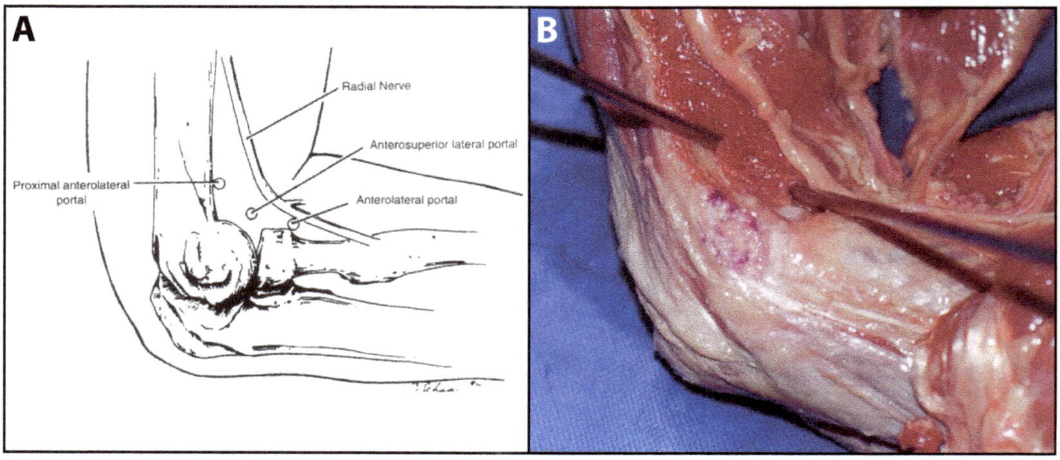

Figure 24-4. (A) Diagram depicting the proximal anterolateral and standard anterolateral portals in relation to the radial nerve. (B) Anatomic dissection of the lateral side of the elbow demonstrating the proximity of the radial nerve to the proximal anterolateral (left) and standard anterolateral (right) portals.

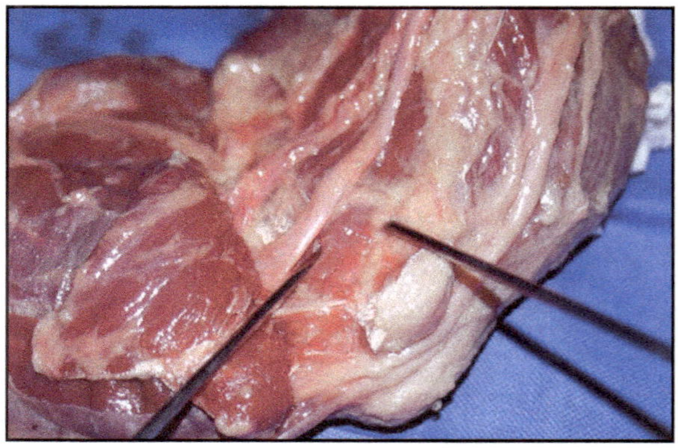

Figure 24-5. Anatomic dissection of the medial side of the elbow demonstrating the proximity of the median nerve to the proximal anteromedial (right) and standard anteromedial (left) portals.

When performing arthroscopy in the anterior compartment, use proximal portals because they are safer than distal portals. Field et al[4] showed that a proximal anterolateral portal is located farther away from the radial nerve than the standard anterolateral portal (Figure 24-4). In addition, they found that the more proximal portal provided equivalent visualization. The proximal anteromedial portal popularized by Poehling et al[5] has also been shown to be safer than the standard anteromedial portal. As Figure 24-5 demonstrates, the median nerve is significantly farther from a more proximally placed anteromedial portal than a standard anteromedial portal. In addition, the more proximal position allows the arthroscope to be directed distally, resulting in the arthroscope being almost parallel to the median nerve in the coronal plane.[3]

Positioning and Equipment

Proper patient positioning and equipment are integral components of a successful arthroscopy. The position of the elbow and the specific types of trocars and cannulas are reviewed in this section. The authors also discuss the use of small osteotomes and retractors to aid in visualization while protecting neurovascular structures.

Placing the elbow in 90 degrees of flexion helps ensure that neural structures are farther away from the bone and capsule than in the extended position. Patients may be positioned in 1 of 4 ways

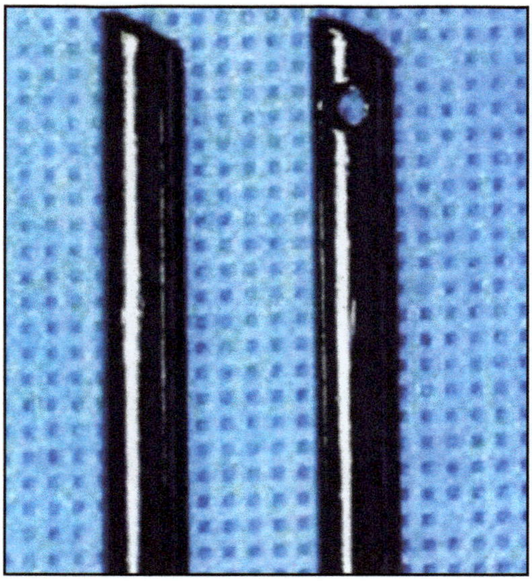

Figure 24-6. Side-vented inflow cannulas (right) should be avoided because the side vents may lie outside of the elbow joint, resulting in fluid extravasation into the surrounding soft tissues. Fluid flow should occur from the end of the cannula (left).

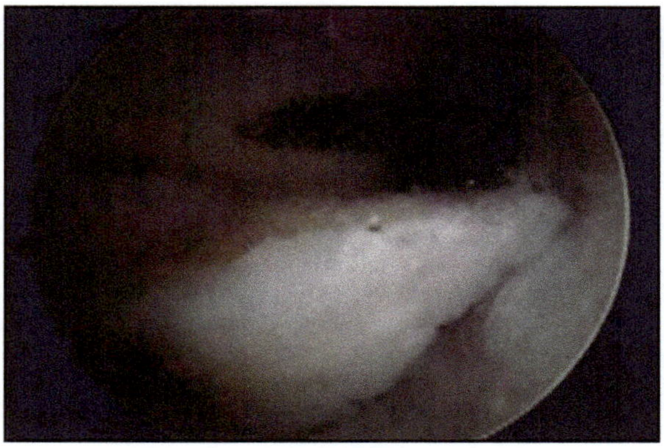

Figure 24-7. Small handheld osteotomes are useful for removing bony spurs and prominences.

to accomplish this, including supine, supine-suspended, prone, and lateral decubitus. Each position has specific advantages and disadvantages, which are described in more detail elsewhere in this book.

The surgeon should be familiar with the type of cannulas and trocars used because there are important differences. Side-vented inflow cannulas should be avoided because the distance between the skin and the joint capsule is often very small (Figure 24-6). This can result in the cannula being intra-articular while the side vents remain extra-articular.[6] This can result in fluid extravasation into the surrounding soft tissues. In addition, trocars should be conical and blunt tipped to decrease the possibility of neurovascular and articular injury during cannula placement.

Small osteotomes are a valuable tool for removing bony spurs and prominences (Figure 24-7). They are easily introduced through a cannula and can be used to remove spurs in a more controlled manner compared to a burr. The loose fragments are then removed with an arthroscopic grasper. This technique is especially useful when bony spurs are adhered to the adjacent capsule where an arthroscopic burr with suction would increase the potential for neurovascular injury.

Retractors should also be used to decrease the likelihood of nerve injury. As shown in Figure 24-8, retractors improve visualization and physically protect specific structures during at-risk procedures. Capsular release and radial head excision are examples of procedures in which retractors can be used to protect neurovascular structures. A summary of the equipment needed to perform elbow arthroscopy is provided in Table 24-1.

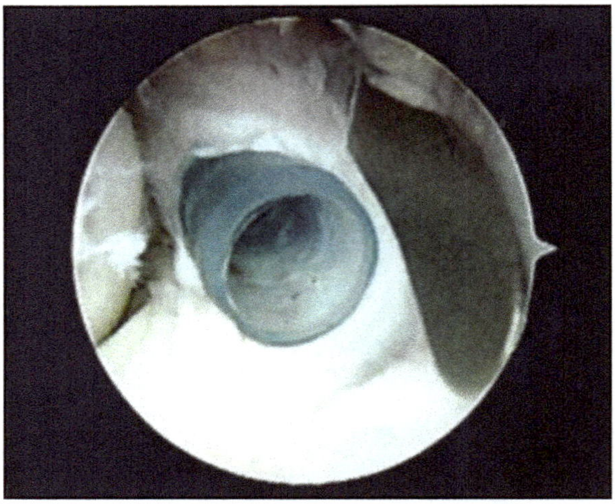

Figure 24-8. Arthroscopic view from the proximal anterolateral portal showing a retractor used to improve visualization and protect neurovascular structures.

Table 24-1. Equipment

- Unsterile tourniquet
- Prone/lateral position arm holder
- 60-cc syringe with 20 to 30 cc normal saline/18-gauge 1.5-inch needle
- Stockinette, 4-inch Coban wrap, standard drapes
- #11 blade, hemostat
- Small and large metal cannulas with blunt trocars
- Single-use clear plastic screw-in cannula with lure lock flow port
- Switching sticks, Wissinger rod
- Gravity inflow setup (tubing)
- Epinephrine 2-mg/5-L bag of fluid
- Standard 4.0-mm arthroscope
- 4.0-mm, full-radius shaver blade, 4.5-mm burr blade
- Small and large handheld graspers
- Small narrow straight osteotomes, freer/elevator

Finally, as with any arthroscopic technique, it is imperative that the surgeon maintains visualization of instruments and the articular surfaces at all times. The risk of inadvertent injury is increased exponentially when the tips of burrs, shavers, or other instruments cannot be visualized.

Potential Complications

The complications associated with elbow arthroscopy include superficial infection, persistent drainage from portal sites, heterotopic ossification, postoperative contracture, compartment syndrome, septic arthritis, and nerve injuries.[7] This section reviews the incidence and treatment of each complication and any risk factors identified in the literature. These are summarized in Table 24-2. This knowledge may assist the treating surgeon in avoiding the complication.

Table 24-2. Common Complications Following Elbow Arthroscopy and Their Incidences

Complication	Incidence, %
Superficial infection	2[8,9]
Persistent drainage	3 to 5[8,9]
Heterotopic ossification	0.9[8]
Postoperative contracture	3[9]
Septic arthritis	0.6 to 0.8[8,9]
Neurologic injury	0 to 14[7]

Superficial Infection

Superficial infection is an uncommon complication when performing elbow arthroscopy. Two of the largest series found an incidence of 2% in 334 and 473 cases of elbow arthroscopy, respectively.[8,9] All infections resolved with a course of oral antibiotics, and no particular risk factors were identified in either study. Attention to sterile technique and use of perioperative antibiotics may help reduce the incidence of this complication.

Persistent Drainage

Drainage from portal sites has been noted in 3% to 5% of elbow arthroscopies.[8,9] The lateral portal sites appear to be most susceptible because the subcutaneous tissues are thin and are often unable to provide a barrier between the joint and the skin. The authors recommend suture closure of portal sites, particularly lateral ones, to help prevent this complication.

Heterotopic Ossification

This is a rare complication occurring in 0.9% of patients in one of the largest series of patients evaluated.[8] One case report involved a young throwing athlete undergoing arthroscopic debridement for posterior impingement. It has also been reported in patients who underwent ulnohumeral arthroplasty for degenerative arthritis.[10] Treatment involved a combination of physical therapy and open excision of the heterotopic bone. The use of perioperative nonsteroidal anti-inflammatory drugs (eg, indomethacin) and single-dose radiation therapy have also been described. No particular risk factors have been identified, although Hughes and Hildebrand noted an occurrence in an individual with prior heterotopic bone formation following total hip arthroplasty.[11] This complication should be considered in patients who are unable to recover full range of motion after elbow arthroscopy.

Postoperative Contracture

Contracture occurred in 3% of elbows undergoing arthroscopy in the largest series in the literature.[9] Motion loss occurred in the flexion-extension plane and was less than 20 degrees in all patients. Most cases were associated with conditions that predispose the elbow to stiffness (eg, inflammatory arthritis and osteochondritis dissecans). The explanation for loss of motion after arthroscopy is uncertain; however, immediate postoperative motion with the assistance of an occupational therapist may help prevent this complication.

Septic Arthritis

This serious complication has been reported in 0.6% to 0.8% of elbow arthroscopies.[8,9] Nelson et al[12] found an increased incidence of deep infections in elbows receiving an intra-articular steroid injection during the procedure. Patients require irrigation and debridement combined with a prolonged course of intravenous antibiotics. Routine administration of preoperative intravenous prophylactic antibiotics, as well as avoiding corticosteroid injections, may help prevent this potentially devastating complication.

Neurologic Injury

Neurologic complications after elbow arthroscopy range from 0% to 14%.[7] Injuries to the radial, median, ulnar, posterior interosseous, and anterior interosseous nerves have been reported. Several case reports detail permanent neurologic injury; however, the majority of injuries are transient. Risk factors associated with the development of a transient nerve palsy include rheumatoid arthritis, contracture, and performance of a capsular release.[9] Nerve injury may be secondary to portal placement, local anesthetic, prolonged tourniquet compression, indwelling catheters, compression due to swelling, and direct injury from instruments.

The posterior interosseous nerve (PIN) is at risk for injury near the inferior aspect of the anterolateral capsule. This complication was reported in 2 case series in which an anterior capsular release was performed.[13,14] Both authors recommend stopping the debridement once the fibers of the brachioradialis or brachialis are visualized. Thus, caution must be exercised when working near the anterolateral capsule just distal to the radiocapitellar joint. Retractors can be used to protect the anterolateral capsule in this area.

Anterior interosseous nerve (AIN) injury is a rare complication. One case report involved a rheumatoid patient who underwent extensive arthroscopic synovectomy with removal of multiple loose bodies.[15] Subsequent surgical exploration revealed diffuse scarring involving the anterior capsule with complete transection of the anterior interosseous branch of the median nerve. Other authors have noted that patients with rheumatoid arthritis have a thin anterior capsule and atrophic brachialis muscle.[15] The authors of this chapter recommend that surgeons maintain extreme caution when performing arthroscopic synovectomy or capsular release in rheumatoid patients because anterior structures, including the median nerve and AIN, are at increased risk for injury.

Ulnar nerve injury can occur for a variety of reasons. Anteromedial portal placement too far posterior risks direct injury to the nerve, and posterior portals should never be placed medial to the midline of the arm.[16] Also, intra-articular work performed near the posteromedial gutter risks injury due to the close proximity of the nerve to the capsule. Stretch-induced ulnar neuropathy is a documented complication after arthroscopic capsular release where flexion is greatly increased. A decreased flexion-extension arc has been identified as a risk factor for neuropathy in one retrospective review of 191 consecutive arthroscopies.[17] Therefore, the current authors recommend routine decompression of the ulnar nerve in patients undergoing capsular release when less than 95 degrees of elbow flexion is present preoperatively. Blonna and O'Driscoll[18] found a significant decrease in the incidence of ulnar neuropathy (11% vs 3%, respectively) when a patient received a prophylactic nerve decompression, with a limited (7- to 8-cm) decompression providing the optimal results with the fewest complications.

Complete transection of nerves is an exceedingly rare complication; however, transection of the median and radial nerves has been reported. Haapaniemi et al[19] described this devastating complication after arthroscopic release of a posttraumatic elbow contracture. They noted that elbow trauma may change anatomy, making correct portal placement difficult. In addition, the capsule has reduced compliance and capacity, leading to markedly reduced fluid distension. This consequently reduces the working distance between the articular surface and the neurovascular structures. An ulnar nerve transection has also been reported following arthroscopic release of

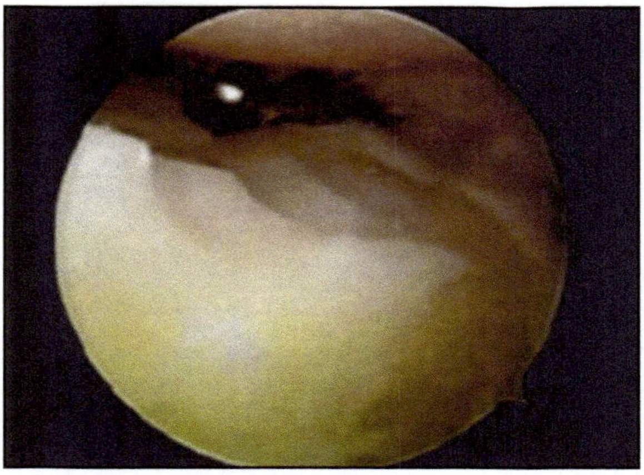

Figure 24-9. Arthroscopic view from the proximal anteromedial portal demonstrating radial head resection.

an elbow contracture in a patient previously treated with an open contracture release, subcutaneous ulnar nerve transposition, and postoperative radiation.[20] All of these factors result in altered anatomy and diminished tissue compliance, increasing the potential for nerve injury.

Special Considerations

There are several situations that require unique technical consideration. These are synovectomy in rheumatoid patients, radial head resection, capsular release, and posttraumatic contractures. These should be considered at-risk procedures, and almost all cases of severe nerve injury have been associated with them. Each situation presents unique challenges and specific recommendations to prevent complications.

Synovectomy in Rheumatoid Patients

Rheumatoid arthritis is a significant risk factor for the development of nerve injury. Patients with rheumatoid arthritis have a thin and filmy anterior capsule. The brachialis muscle, which normally provides a stout barrier to injury of anterior structures, is typically thin and atrophic. Surgeons need to bear in mind the diminished thickness of the anterior capsule and overlying brachialis when performing synovectomy in rheumatoid patients. Injury to the median nerve and brachial artery have been reported with this procedure.[15]

Radial Head Resection

The PIN is at risk for injury because this procedure places instruments adjacent to the inferior capsule (Figure 24-9). In addition, prior trauma may cause the PIN to adhere or scar down to the capsule, increasing the risk.

Capsular Release

Prevention of neurologic injury during arthroscopic anterior capsular release is aided by several measures. The release must be performed on the anterior aspect of the distal humerus and stopped once the muscular layer of the brachialis or brachioradialis is identified (Figure 24-10). In addition, care must be taken not to direct the shaver blade toward the anterolateral capsule just distal to the radiocapitellar joint where the PIN is located. Some experienced elbow arthroscopists consider trauma that produces excessive scarring in the vicinity of the PIN a contraindication to arthroscopic capsular release.

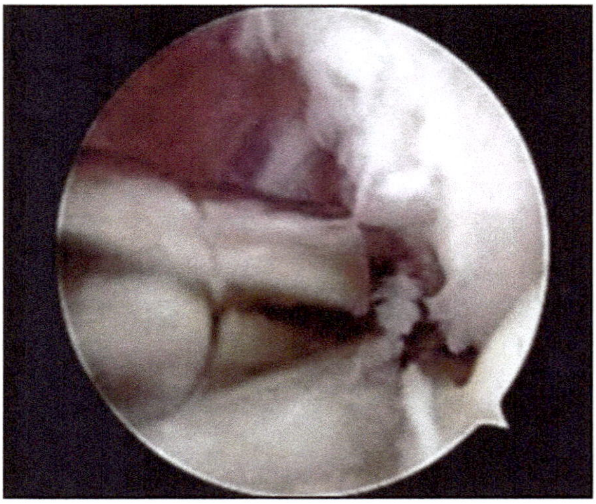

Figure 24-10. Arthroscopic view from the anteromedial portal demonstrating fibers of the brachialis seen during anterior capsular release.

Posttraumatic Contractures

Trauma may change the anatomy, making correct placement of portals difficult. The joint capsule has a reduced compliance and capacity, leading to reduced fluid distension and, consequently, a reduced working distance between the articular surface and neurovascular structures. In addition, a decreased flexion-extension arc preoperatively has been identified as a risk factor for the development of delayed-onset ulnar neuritis postoperatively due to restoration of elbow flexion.[17] Prophylactic ulnar nerve decompression has been shown to decrease this incidence (11% vs 3%) in elbows with less than 95 degrees of elbow flexion preoperatively.[18] However, if delayed-onset ulnar neuritis develops postoperatively, subsequent ulnar nerve decompression and/or transposition may be necessary.

Conclusion

Elbow arthroscopy is a valuable tool that can be used for a variety of pathologic conditions. However, it is a technically challenging procedure due to the anatomic constraints of the joint and the close proximity of neurovascular structures. Avoiding complications requires a thorough understanding of elbow anatomy and a methodical surgical technique.

Top Technical Pearls for the Procedure

1. Define landmarks and palpate the ulnar nerve.
2. Distend the joint prior to portal placement and incise the skin only to protect the cutaneous nerves.
3. Keep the elbow flexed 90 degrees when possible and use proximal anterior portals.
4. Avoid the inferior aspect of the anterolateral capsule (PIN) and posteromedial gutter (ulnar nerve) when possible.
5. Abandon the procedure if visualization/orientation is compromised because prevention of nerve injury in elbow arthroscopy is everything!

References

1. O'Driscoll SW, Savoie FH III. Arthroscopy of the elbow. In: Morrey BF, ed. *Master Techniques in Orthopaedic Surgery: The Elbow*. Philadelphia, PA: Lippincott Williams & Wilkins; 2002:27-45.
2. Miller CD, Jobe CM, Wright MH. Neuroanatomy in elbow arthroscopy. *J Shoulder Elbow Surg*. 1995;4(3):168-174.
3. Abboud JA, Ricchetti ET, Tjoumakaris F, Ramsey ML. Elbow arthroscopy: basic setup and portal placement. *J Am Acad Orthop Surg*. 2006;14(5):312-318.
4. Field LD, Altchek DW, Warren RF, O'Brien SJ, Skyhar MJ, Wickiewicz TL. Arthroscopic anatomy of the lateral elbow: a comparison of three portals. *Arthroscopy*. 1994;10(6):602-607.
5. Poehling GG, Whipple TL, Sisco L, Goldman B. Elbow arthroscopy: a new technique. *Arthroscopy*. 1989;5(3):222-224.
6. Ramsey ML, Naranja RJ. Diagnostic arthroscopy of the elbow. In: Baker CL Jr, Plancher KD, eds. *Operative Treatment of Elbow Injuries*. New York, NY: Springer-Verlag; 2002:163-169.
7. Morrey BF. Complications of elbow arthroscopy. *Instr Course Lect*. 2000;49: 255-258.
8. Thomas R, Savoie FH III, Field LD. Complications of elbow arthroscopy (SS-67). *Arthroscopy*. 2007;23(6):e34.
9. Kelly EW, Morrey BF, O'Driscoll SW. Complications of elbow arthroscopy. *J Bone Joint Surg Am*. 2001;83(1):25-34.
10. Sodha S, Nagda SH, Sennett BJ. Heterotopic ossification in a throwing athlete after elbow arthroscopy. *Arthroscopy*. 2006;22(7):802.e1-802.e3.
11. Hughes SC, Hildebrand KA. Heterotopic ossification—a complication of elbow arthroscopy: a case report. *J Shoulder Elbow Surg*. 2010;19(1):e1-e5.
12. Nelson GN, Wu T, Galatz LM, Yamaguchi K, Keener JD. Elbow arthroscopy: early complications and associated risk factors. *J Shoulder Elbow Surg*. 2014;23(2):273-278.
13. Jones GS, Savoie FH III. Arthroscopic capsular release of flexion contractures (arthrofibrosis) of the elbow. *Arthroscopy*. 1993;9(3):277-283.
14. Park JY, Cho CH, Choi JH, Lee ST, Kang CH. Radial nerve palsy after arthroscopic anterior capsular release for degenerative elbow contracture. *Arthroscopy*. 2007;23(12):1360.e1-1360.e3.
15. Ruch DS, Poehling GG. Anterior interosseus nerve injury following elbow arthroscopy. *Arthroscopy*. 1997;13(6):756-758.
16. Dumonski ML, Arciero RA, Mazzocca AD. Ulnar nerve palsy after elbow arthroscopy. *Arthroscopy*. 2006;22(5):577.e1-577.e3.
17. Huffman GR, O'Driscoll SW. Delayed-onset ulnar neuropathy after arthroscopic elbow contracture release (SS-63). *Arthroscopy*. 2006;22(6):e32.
18. Blonna D, O'Driscoll SW. Delayed-onset ulnar neuritis after release of elbow contracture: preventive strategies derived from a study of 563 cases. *Arthroscopy*. 2014;30(8):947-956.
19. Haapaniemi T, Berggren M, Adolfsson L. Complete transection of the median and radial nerves during arthroscopic release of post-traumatic elbow contracture. *Arthroscopy*. 1999;15(7):784-787.
20. Gay DM, Raphael BS, Weiland AJ. Revision arthroscopic contracture release in the elbow resulting in an ulnar nerve transection: a case report. *J Bone Joint Surg Am*. 2010;92(5):1246-1249.

25

Early Arthroscopic Management of Heterotopic Ossification of the Elbow

Felix H. Savoie III, MD; Michael J. O'Brien, MD; and Matthew Wert, MD

Introduction

The formation of heterotopic ossification (HO) about the elbow commonly follows elbow trauma, closed head injuries, or major burns.[1] Although it can form anywhere in the body, the most commonly involved joints are the hip and elbow.[2] Although the exact etiology is unknown, possible predisposing factors include increased prostaglandin activity, tissue hypoxia, alterations in the sympathetic nervous system, and immobilization.[3,4] This lack of full understanding of the etiology limits preventative measures. Many different preventive and treatment measures have been proposed, including early motion, cryocompression, indomethacin, disphosphonates, and radiation therapy.[5-10] However, none other than radiation therapy has provided consistent success in preventing the formation of HO about the elbow. Once formation begins, traditional management has been to allow the process to mature before excision because it has been reported that early open excision has a high rate of recurrence.[11] Recently, some surgeons have questioned the need for delay, with reports of early open excision of HO with satisfactory results.[12-16] Wert and Savoie[17] reported on the first all-arthroscopic excision with release of early HO with similar excellent results. This chapter presents the arthroscopic technique for excision of HO about the elbow.

Indications

- Discovery of heterotopic bone about the elbow with a progressive loss of motion. The best time for surgical intervention is within the first 6 weeks.

Contraindication

- The primary contraindication is a lack of advanced skills in elbow arthroscopy.

Savoie FH III, Field LD, Steinmann SP, eds. *The Elbow and Wrist: AANA Advanced Arthroscopic Surgical Techniques* (pp 251-256).

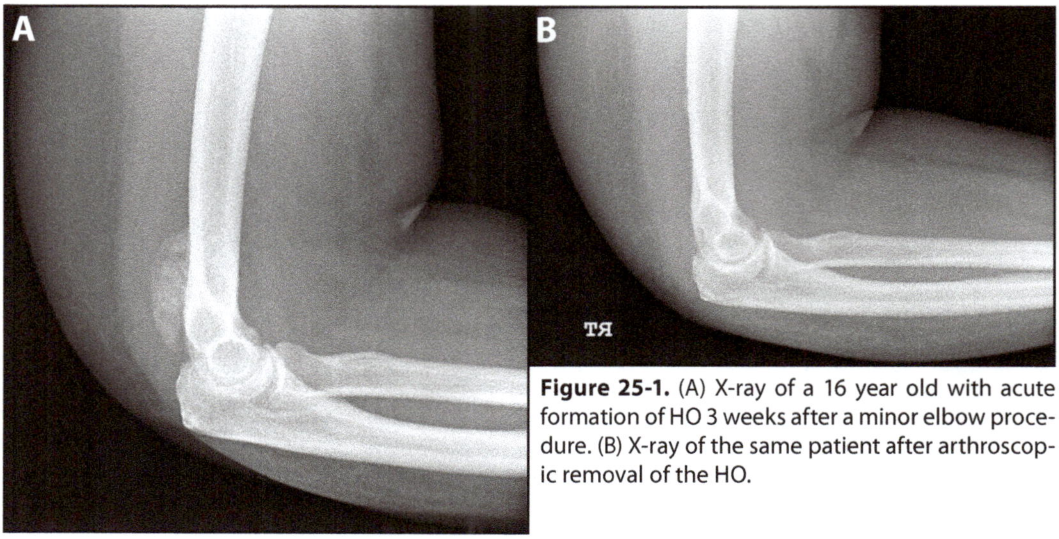

Figure 25-1. (A) X-ray of a 16 year old with acute formation of HO 3 weeks after a minor elbow procedure. (B) X-ray of the same patient after arthroscopic removal of the HO.

Pertinent Physical Findings

Patients with early HO formation present with the following:

- Decreasing elbow range of motion
- Inspection may reveal some localized swelling
- Although there is often no specific area of tenderness to palpation, a generalized, swollen, boggy feel is often noted when palpating the capsule.
- Examination shows decreasing motion, initially with soft and then hard endpoints.

Pertinent Imaging

- X-rays
  - Early x-rays may be completely normal.
  - Once the motion loss occurs, repeat imaging may show wispy bone forming in the soft tissues.
  - Subsequent imaging will reveal more bone formation becoming visible as the HO activity increases (Figure 25-1).
- Magnetic resonance imaging (MRI)
  - Scanning will show the extent of the HO formation because the bone areas visible on early imaging will show only a part of the pathology (Figure 25-2).

Equipment

- Video arthroscopy equipment
- Interchangeable cannula system

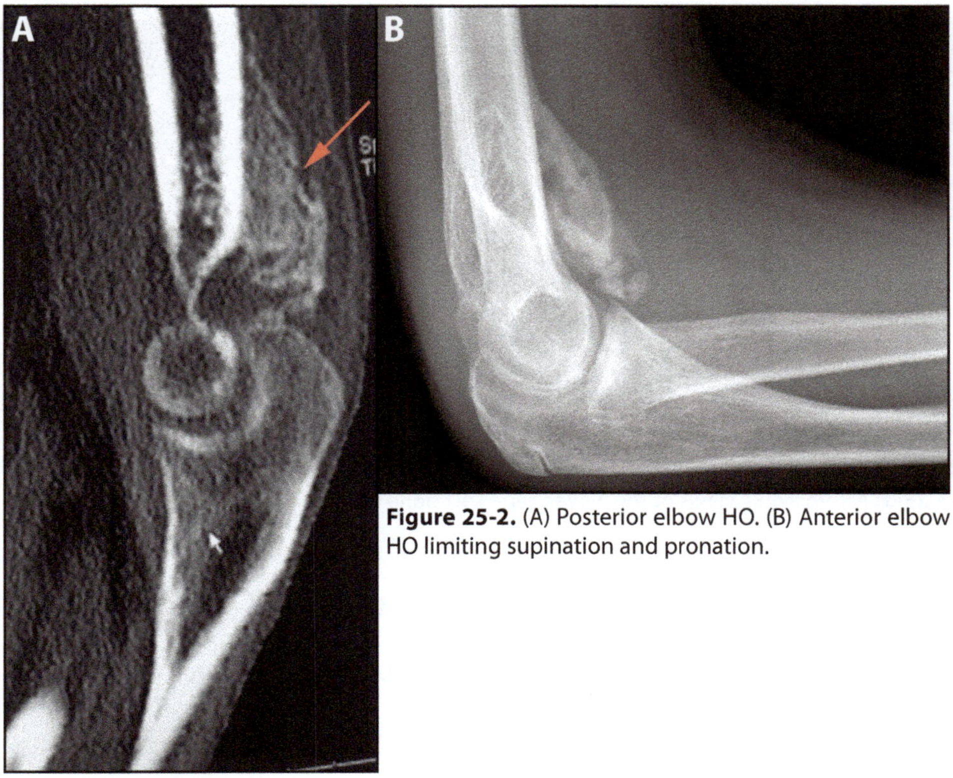

Figure 25-2. (A) Posterior elbow HO. (B) Anterior elbow HO limiting supination and pronation.

- 3.5- and 4.5-mm full-radius shavers
- 4.0-mm motorized burr
- Switching sticks and small blunt freer dissectors to act as arthroscopic retractors
- Side effect cautery system
- Fluoroscopy unit
- Tourniquet
- Arm holder

It is recommended that a standard 4.0-mm arthroscope with an interchangeable cannula system be used. This allows the viewing and operating portals to be changed without removing and reinserting cannulas. A standard 3.5- and 4.5-mm full-radius soft tissue resector, a 4.0-mm burr, side effect cautery, switching sticks, arthroscopic retractors, and a miniature fluoroscopy unit are essential for this surgery.

Positioning and Portals

The patient may be positioned in the prone, supine, or lateral decubitus position. The advantages and disadvantages of each are been discussed in Chapter 1. The authors' preferred position is prone with a small bump placed on a regular arm board under the upper arm to keep it parallel to the floor.[1]

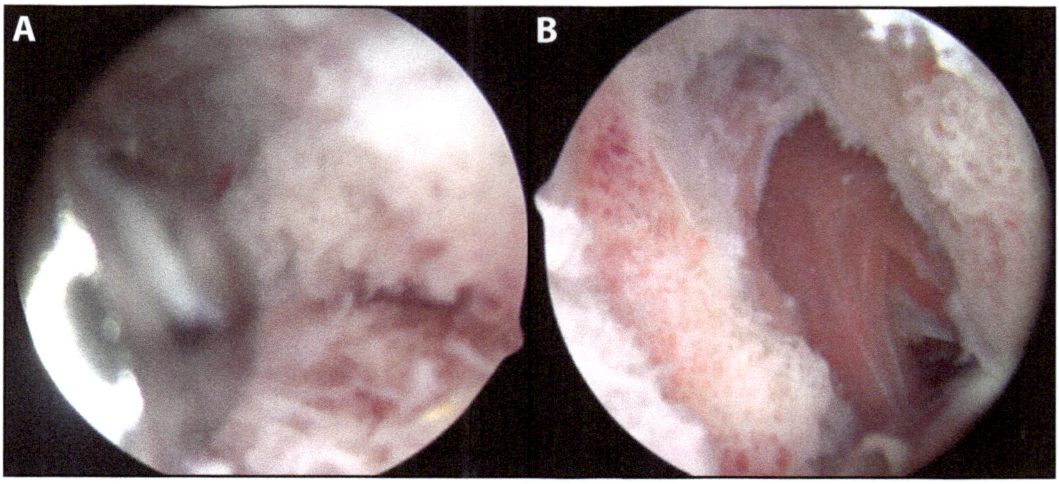

Figure 25-3. Arthroscopic views of the woven type soft bone noted in early HO cases.

Step-by-Step Description of the Procedure

1. Review preoperative imaging to ascertain the exact locations of the HO and its proximity to the neurovascular structures.
2. Place the patient in the prone position with free movement of the elbow.
3. Insufflate the joint via the posterior or soft spot portal.
4. After carefully locating the ulnar nerve, establish a proximal anteromedial portal to visualize the anterior joint capsule.
5. Establish a proximal anterolateral portal via an outside-in technique.
6. The HO anteriorly is usually located anterior to the capsule and posterior to the brachialis, so it may not be readily visualized. The first step is to define the proximal extent by releasing the capsule off the humerus with an electrocautery and then resect the capsule until the HO comes into view. It is soft, woven-type bone adjacent to the humerus (Figure 25-3).
7. Continue visualizing from the proximal anteromedial portal and establish a straight lateral portal with a switching stick so that it can be used to retract the brachialis away from the HO and protect the neurovascular bundle.
8. Using the shaver in the proximal anterolateral portal and visualizing from the proximal anteromedial portal, resect the HO from top to bottom, always staying posterior to the switching stick and brachialis.
9. Switch the arthroscope to the proximal anterolateral portal and the shaver to the proximal anteromedial portal, and remove any remaining HO.
10. Using fluoroscopy confirms complete excision of anterior HO; check for restoration of motion.
11. Posterior excision follows a similar pattern:
    - Establish posterior central and lateral portals.
    - Elevate the triceps off the HO using a switching stick.
    - A superior posterior lateral portal can be established to place a switching stick or retractor to hold the triceps away from the HO and to protect the ulnar nerve medially.
    - The HO posteriorly is usually resected from distal to proximal with the shaver in the posterior central portal and the arthroscope in the posterior lateral portal.

Postoperative Protocol

A Hemovac drain is placed in the anterior and posterior compartments overnight. Continuous passive motion and cryocompression are also used for the first week. Each patient receives radiation therapy within a 24-hour window before or after surgery; the exact amount is determined by the radiation oncologist but is usually around 700 rads. Physical therapy is started within 48 hours of surgery with an emphasis on motion and compression.

Potential Complications

The most fearsome complication is neurovascular injury. It is essential to mark out each of the nerves and know their locations throughout the procedure. This should be considered advanced arthroscopy due to the distortion of normal anatomy by the injury and the subsequent HO formation. Portal drainage due to failure to close the lateral portals occurs in about 10% of cases. Recurrence of the HO is also a potential complication.

Top Technical Pearls for the Procedure

1. Define the extent of the HO on preoperative imaging and evaluate the proximity to associated neurovascular structures.
2. Mark out all the neurovascular structures prior to beginning the procedure.
3. Use retractors to keep the soft tissues off the HO during resection.
4. Excise the HO in a set pattern. Anteriorly, the authors favor proximal to distal and lateral to medial, whereas posteriorly, they favor distal to proximal.
5. Evaluate the excision under fluoroscopy before completing the procedure.

References

1. Viola RW, Hastings H II. Treatment of ectopic ossification about the elbow. *Clin Orthop Relat Res.* 2000;(370):65-86.
2. Hardy AG, Dickson JW. Pathological ossification in traumatic paraplegia. *J Bone Joint Surg Br.* 1963;45:76-87.
3. Baird EO, Kang QK. Prophylaxis of heterotopic ossification - an updated review. *J Orthop Surg Res.* 2009;4:12.
4. Dodds SD, Hanel DP. Heterotopic ossification of the elbow. In: Trumble TE, Budoff JE, eds. *Wrist and Elbow Arthroscopy and Reconstruction.* Rosemont, IL: American Society for Surgery of the Hand; 2006:425-438.
5. Crawford CM, Barghese G, Mani MM, Neff Jr. Heterotopic ossification: are range of motion exercises contraindicated? *J Burn Care Rehabil.* 1986;7(4):323-327.
6. Peterson SL, Mani MM, Crawrord CM, Neff JR, Hiebert JM. Postburn heterotopic ossifcation: insights for management decision making. *J Trauma.* 1989;29(3):365-369.
7. Evans EB. Heterotopic bone formation in thermal burns. *Clin Orthop Relat Res.* 1991;(263):94-101.
8. Nollen AJ. Effects of ethylhydroxydiphosphonate (EHDP) on heterotopic ossification. *Acta Orthop Scand.* 1986;57(4):358-361.

9. Hurvitz EA, Mandac BR, Davidoff G, Johnson JH, Nelson VS. Risk factors for heterotopic ossification in children and adolescents with severe traumatic brain injury. *Arch Phys Med Rehabil.* 1992;73(5):459-462.
10. Stein DA, Patel R, Egol KA, Kaplan FT, Tejwani NC, Koval KJ. Prevention of heterotopic ossification at the elbow following trauma using radiation therapy. *Bull Hosp Jt Dis.* 2003;61(3-4):151-154.
11. Garland DE. A clinical perspective on common forms of acquired heterotopic ossification. *Clin Orthop Relat Res.* 1991;(263):13-29.
12. Viola RW, Hanel DP. Early "simple" release of posttraumatic elbow contracture associated with heterotopic ossification. *J Hand Surg.* 1999;24(2):370-380.
13. McAuliffe JA, Wolfson AH. Early excision of heterotopic ossification about the elbow followed by radiation therapy. *J Bone Joint Surg Am.* 1997;79(5):749-755.
14. Tsionos I, Leclercq C, Rochet JM. Heterotopic ossification of the elbow in patients with burns. Results after early excision. *J Bone Joint Surg Br.* 2004;86(3):396-403.
15. Moritomo H, Tada K, Yoshida T. Early, wide excision of heterotopic ossification in the medial elbow. *J Shoulder Elbow Surg.* 2001;10(2):164-168.
16. Peters WJ. Heterotopic ossification: can early surgery be performed, with a positive bone scan? *J Burn Care Rehabil.* 1990;11(4):318-321.
17. Wert M, Savoie FH III. Early arthroscopic management strategies for patients developing moderate to severe heterotopic ossification of the elbow. *Arthroscopy.* 2013;29(6):e21.

SECTION IV

THE WRIST

Basics

26

Wrist Arthroscopy
Setup, Anatomy, and Portals

Jeffrey B. Witty, MD; Larry D. Field, MD; and Brandon P. Donnelly, MD

Introduction

Wrist arthroscopy was first described by Chen in 1979.[1] In the early stages of development, it provided only partial evaluation of the articular surfaces and was not used therapeutically.[2] It was not until 1986, when Whipple et al[3] advocated distraction techniques and precise portal placement, that the exposure necessary to perform an extensive evaluation of the wrist joint became an option. Even then, diagnosis was the primary function, and therapeutic indications had yet to be developed. Since then, innovations in wrist arthroscopy have expanded treatment indications and promoted widespread acceptance.

Diagnostic and operative forms of arthroscopy have advanced the understanding of wrist anatomy and function, and arthroscopic techniques have facilitated the repair of previously unrecognized pathology. Continued advances in instrumentation and technology will improve the ability to perform challenging and innovative procedures as the principles of open surgical procedures become adapted to arthroscopy.[4]

Wrist arthroscopy allows close visual examination of the carpal articular surfaces and wrist ligaments, which is often inadequate with open procedures and which can be performed in a less invasive manner than traditional arthrotomy.[5] The extremely close evaluation of details provides many benefits and increases appreciation of the subtle differences between normal and pathologic anatomy.[6] This fact alone underscores the importance of a thorough understanding of arthroscopic anatomy. This chapter reviews the pertinent anatomy, setup, currently described portals, and the techniques used to establish them.

Anatomy

The wrist is made of the 8 carpal bones, each with multiple articular surfaces and the intrinsic and extrinsic ligaments, and a triangular fibrocartilage complex (TFCC) that is surrounded by tendons and neurovascular structures (Figure 26-1).[7,8] A thorough understanding of the relationship between the surface anatomy of the wrist and these underlying structures is essential to perform accurate arthroscopic portal placement and adequate arthroscopy. Understanding these

Savoie FH III, Field LD, Steinmann SP, eds. *The Elbow and Wrist: AANA Advanced Arthroscopic Surgical Techniques* (pp 259-274).

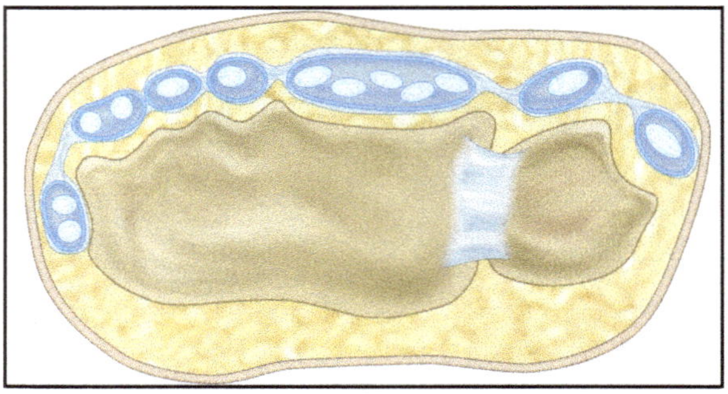

Figure 26-1. Cross-sectional anatomy of the dorsal compartments. (Modified from Geissler WB, Freeland AE, Weiss AP, Chow JC. Techniques of wrist arthroscopy. *Instr Course Lect.* 2000;49:225-237.)

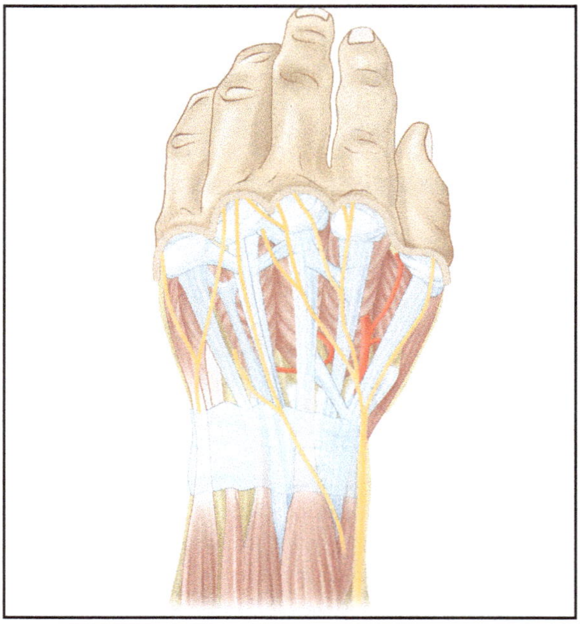

Figure 26-2. Dorsal wrist anatomy.

relationships helps to prevent injury to the cutaneous nerves, tendons, and vascular structures and can minimize the risk to the articular surfaces in the wrist. It also facilitates the use of instruments during procedures, enabling the completion of increasingly complicated arthroscopic wrist procedures.

To accurately place portals, the surface anatomy can be mapped and labeled before making the first incision. Bony landmarks that should be familiar to the surgeon include Lister's tubercle, the radius and ulna with their styloids, the radiocarpal joint level, the radial border of the third ray, and the central portion of the fourth ray. The capitate sulcus (ie, soft spot) should also be palpated.

The extensor retinaculum is an obliquely oriented structure that spans the dorsal distal radius and ulna. It overlies the 12 extensor tendons, which are partitioned into 6 compartments to prevent bowstringing.[4] The extensor pollicis longus (EPL) is the only tendon in the third compartment, and it is easily palpated, especially after application of traction. This structure passes just ulnar to Lister's tubercle and should be appropriately marked. The area bordered by the EPL and extensor pollicis brevis together and the extensor carpi radialis longus (ECRL) define the margins of the anatomic snuffbox. The extensor digitorum communis (EDC) is just ulnar to the EPL. The extensor carpi ulnaris (ECU) and the ECRL and extensor carpi radialis brevis (ECRB) tendons are easily palpated and should be marked. The intersection of these tendons and the bony structures allows accurate identification and precise placement of the arthroscopy portals (Figure 26-2).

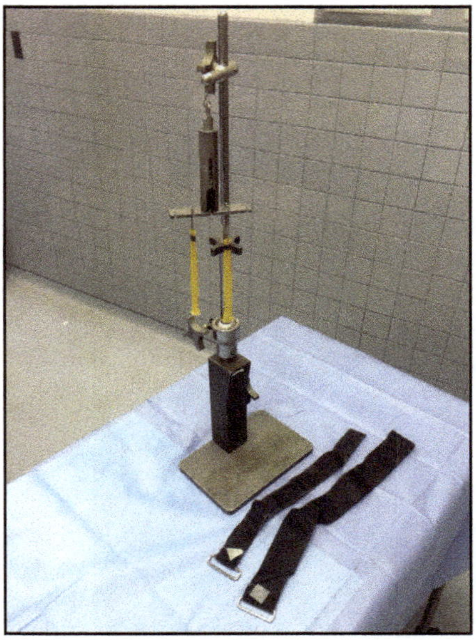

Figure 26-3. Traction tower.

Arthroscopic Technique

Setup

A significant improvement in wrist arthroscopy came with the innovation of wrist distraction. This key element enhanced the surgeon's ability to perform arthroscopic procedures in the confined wrist joint. Distraction is essential to improve visualization and provide adequate space for maneuverability during wrist arthroscopy because distention of the joint alone does not provide adequate room for instrumentation.[2] Several options exist to provide the necessary distraction. A dedicated sterile or nonsterile traction tower is a popular choice. Alternatives include the use of horizontal traction with a pulley and weight system and a nonsterile traction boom device (Figures 26-3 and 26-4). Use of a radiolucent triangle with the fingers curled around the apex and the weight draped over the opposite side onto the floor has recently been described.[9]

The authors prefer a sterile traction tower with nylon finger traps (Figure 26-5). It provides convenient application of wrist distraction in flexion, extension, and radial and ulnar deviation. This system allows adjustability to the distraction force and the position of the wrist and permits easy conversion to open procedures if necessary. The traction tower system maintains the wrist in a stable position for portal preservation during the exchange of instruments.[2]

The arm is placed in an abducted position and the upper arm is secured to the traction tower. A nonsterile tourniquet is applied, and the arm and hand are prepared and draped with the forearm in a vertical position (Figure 26-6A). The authors use sterile soft nylon finger traps to secure the index and long finger to the tower for most procedures. Soft traps increase the surface area and distribute the force better than wire devices. For patients with poor or fragile skin, additional fingers in the traps can decrease the force to the skin.[2] To improve visualization for ulnar-sided pathology, the authors frequently use the index and ring fingers (Figure 26-6B). Most procedures require 5 to 10 lb of traction.

Equipment

Proper equipment is essential to perform a quality wrist arthroscopy. A number of companies have small joint arthroscopes and instrumentation; the specific sizes for each depend on the

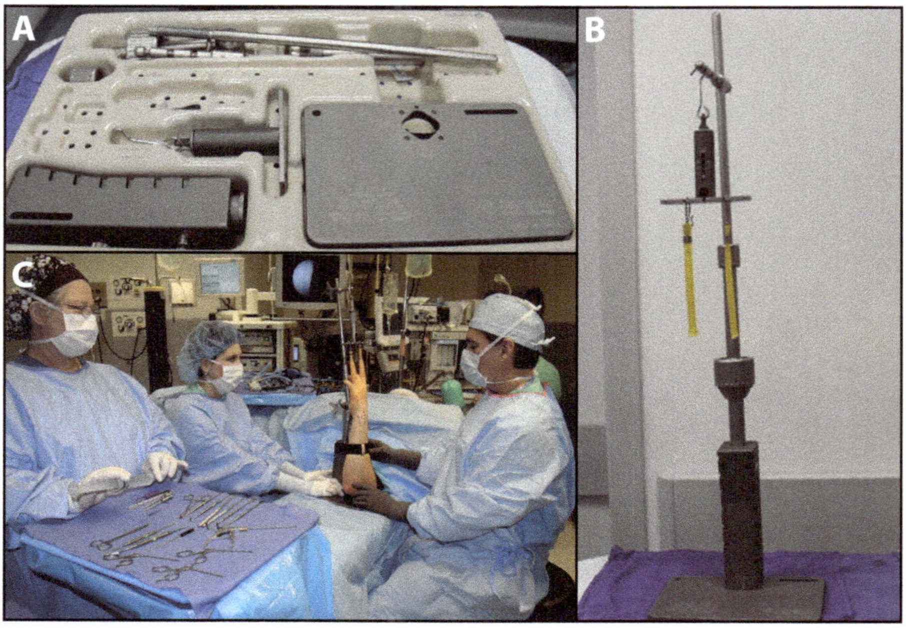

Figure 26-4. (A, B) Sterile traction tower. (C) Operative setup with sterile traction tower.

Figure 26-5. Nylon finger traps for use with the traction tower.

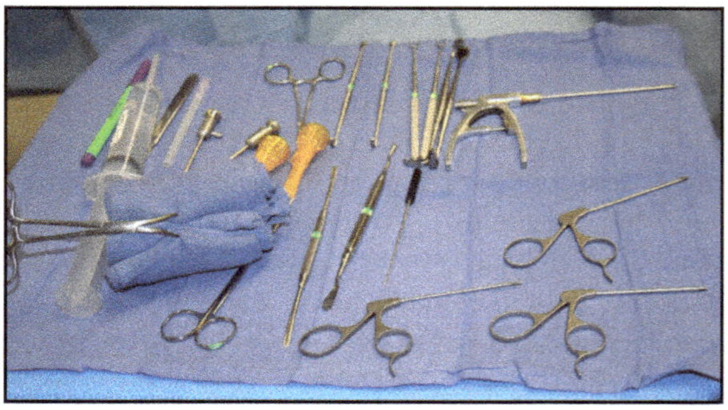

Figure 26-6. Draping and tower placement with the index and ring fingers secured in nylon finger traps.

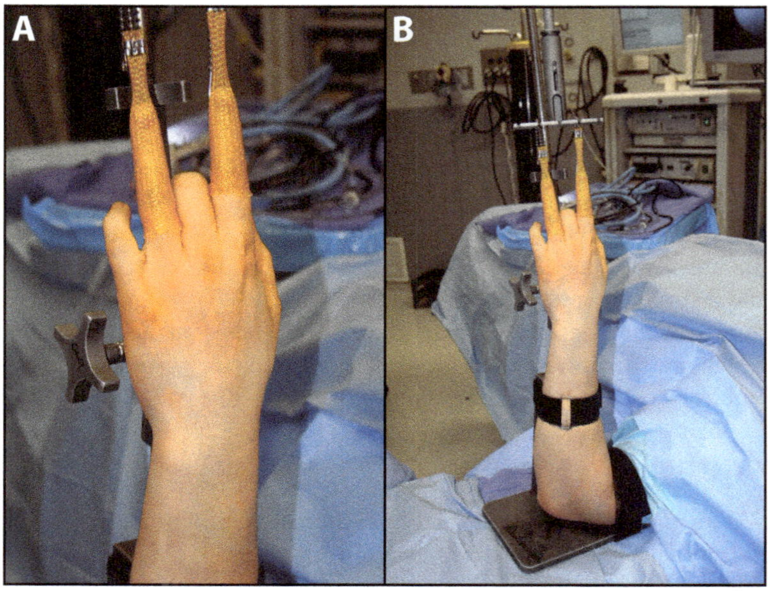

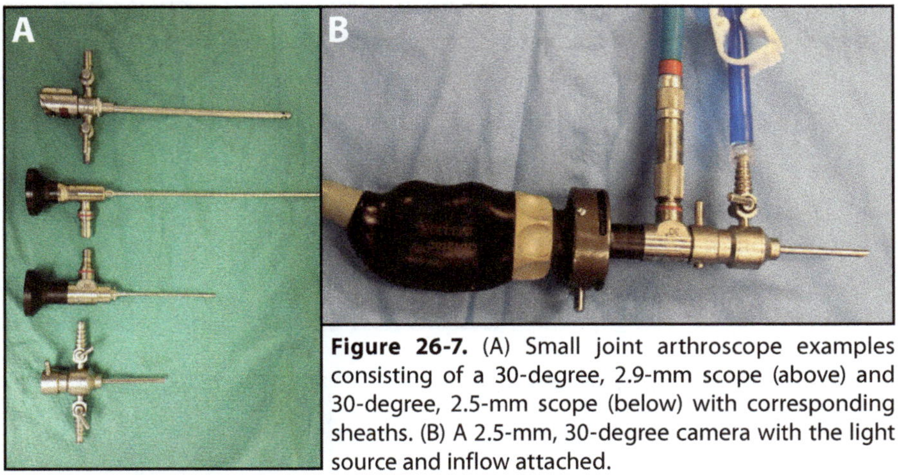

Figure 26-7. (A) Small joint arthroscope examples consisting of a 30-degree, 2.9-mm scope (above) and 30-degree, 2.5-mm scope (below) with corresponding sheaths. (B) A 2.5-mm, 30-degree camera with the light source and inflow attached.

individual company. The typical sizes range between 1.9 and 3.0 mm. A video arthroscope and monitor with a printer and video that allows digital storage is necessary to document the intra-articular findings. In addition to adequate visualization, a major improvement came with the innovation of instruments specifically designed for use in small joints. Larger instrumentation used for knee and shoulder arthroscopy is not adequate for procedures in the wrist. A 2.0- to 3.0-mm diameter arthroscope is essential to allow adequate mobilization without the risk of injury to the surrounding structures and articular surfaces (Figures 26-7A and 26-7B). In addition to the standard 30-degree arthroscope, a 70-degree arthroscope is occasionally useful. Seventy-degree scopes may not be available in sizes smaller than 2.5 mm

Other small joint arthroscopy equipment is available and necessary for mastery of wrist arthroscopy. Equipment includes a small joint shaver (2.7 or 2.9 mm) with multiple tips, a wrist probe (1.7 or 2.0 mm), and many of the smaller versions of large joint arthroscopic instruments.[5,7] As arthroscopy has advanced, more specialized equipment for specific procedures has become available, including TFCC repair kits, retrograde retrievers, ablation shrinkage devices, and fracture fixation devices. Spinal needles and passing sutures are helpful tools that have been adapted from other arthroscopic repair techniques.

Clear physiologic crystalloid solution, such as lactated ringer's solution, is preferable because it can be rapidly absorbed into the tissues and can prevent overdistension. Irrigants can be introduced through the sheath of the arthroscope or by separate inflow and outflow portals. Gravity inflow has proved adequate in the authors' practice. Pinch chambers can introduce small boluses or irrigants to clear the visual field.[2] Fluid pumps that can precisely control the pressure in the joint are available. However, pressurized injection increases the risk of fluid extravasation into the subcutaneous tissue and is usually unnecessary.

Equipment

- Traction options
  - Nonsterile or sterile traction tower (see Figures 26-3 and 26-4)
  - Radiolucent triangle with free-hanging weight[9]
  - Nylon finger traps (see Figure 26-5)
- Video
  - 30- and 70-degree arthroscopes (size ranges from approximately 2.0 to 3.0 mm; see Figure 26-7)

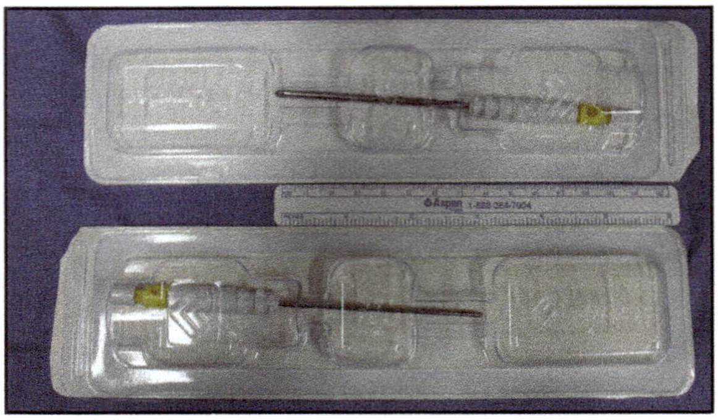

Figure 26-8. Picture showing 2.9- and 2.0-mm full-radius shavers for small joint arthroscopy.

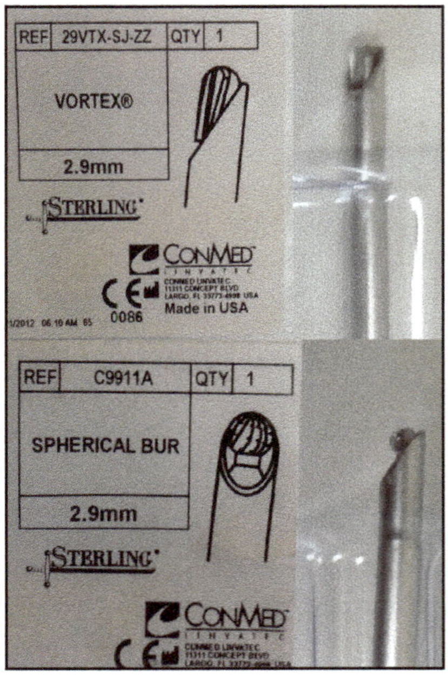

Figure 26-9. Examples of 2.9-mm small joint burr options.

- Fluid management
  - Normal saline or lactated ringer's solution
  - Pump
  - Tubing with pinch chambers
- Instrumentation
  - Small joint shavers (size range approximately 2.0 to 3.0 mm; Figure 26-8)
  - Small joint burrs (size range approximately 2.0 to 3.0 mm; Figure 26-9)
  - Probe (Figure 26-10)
  - Standard, straight, and curved mosquito tip graspers (2.0 and 2.75 mm; Figures 26-11 and 26-12)
  - Blunt tip and scoop tip forceps of various angles (2.0 and 2.75 mm; Figure 26-13)
  - Curettes (2.7 5 mm; Figure 26-14)
  - Dissectors (2.7 5 mm; see Figure 26-14)
  - 18-gauge spinal needles
  - Small joint electrode for cutting and hemostasis (approximately 2.9 mm)

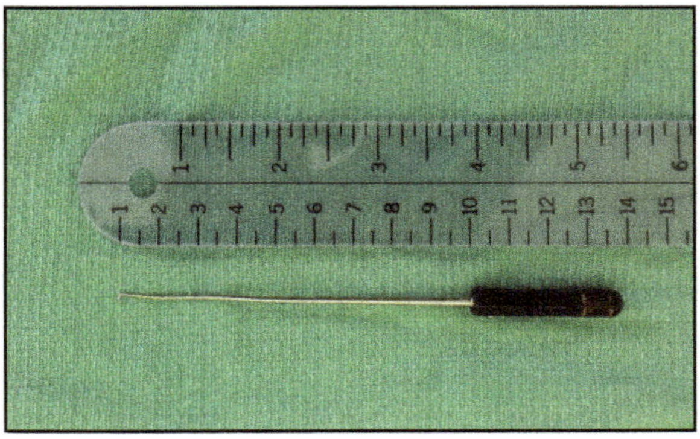

Figure 26-10. Small joint probe.

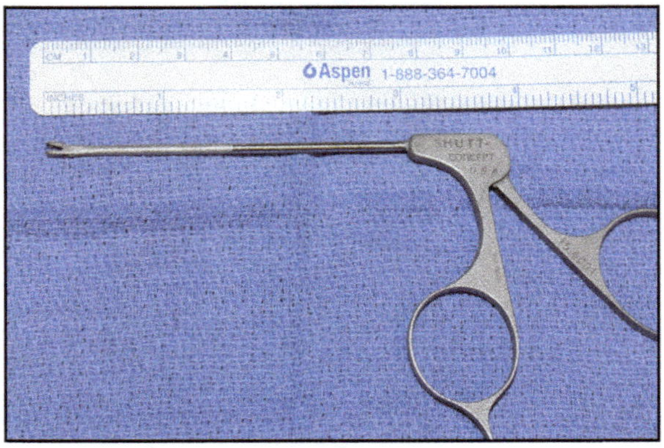

Figure 26-11. Straight tip grasper.

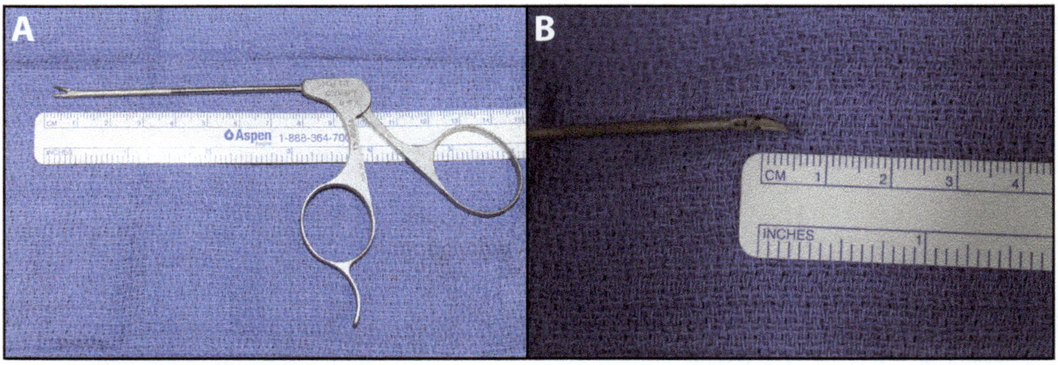

Figure 26-12. Mosquito tip grasper.

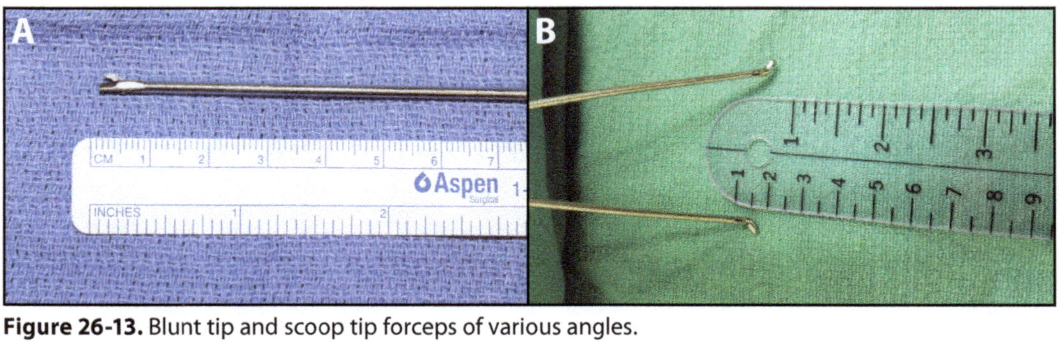

Figure 26-13. Blunt tip and scoop tip forceps of various angles.

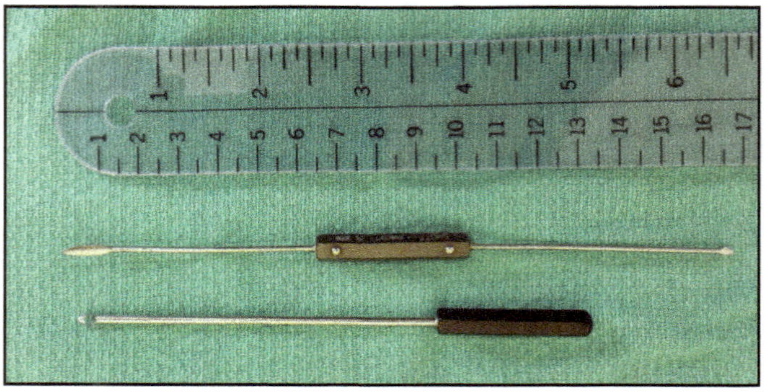

Figure 26-14. Curette and dissector (2.75 mm).

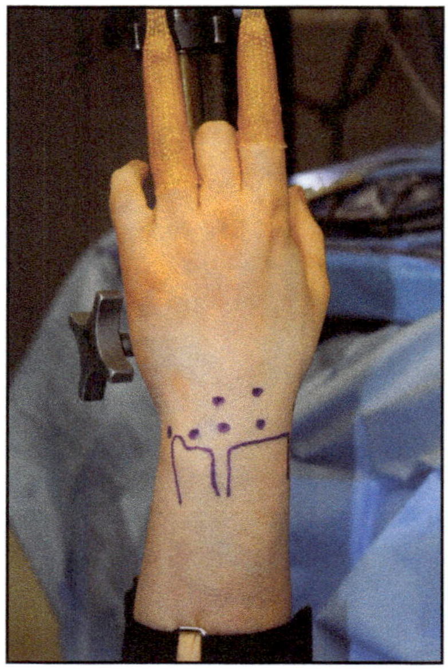

Figure 26-15. Portal sites are marked after the application of traction.

Positioning and Portals

Wrist arthroscopy portals include radiocarpal, midcarpal, distal radioulnar, and volar portals. Traditionally, arthroscopic viewing portals are described by their relation to the 6 extensor compartments of the wrist. They include 6 radiocarpal, 4 midcarpal, and 2 distal radioulnar portals. Two additional volar portals are also used.

Precise portal placement is essential for performing a complete wrist arthroscopy and for minimizing iatrogenic injury to the wrist joint and surrounding structures. Placing the portals in an incorrect manner can result in damage to neurovascular structures and the articular cartilage. All portals and surface landmarks should be marked on the skin. Marking portals after the application of traction helps to prevent distortion and improperly placed portal sites (Figure 26-15). Typically, only the skin is incised, and a blunt instrument is then used to spread to the wrist capsule (Figure 26-16).

Radiocarpal Portals

These portals are named according to the interspace between extensor compartments. The 3-4 portal divides the third and fourth extensor compartments. The 6-R and 6-U portals are named by their relationship to the ECU, with the 6-R on the radial aspect and the 6-U on the

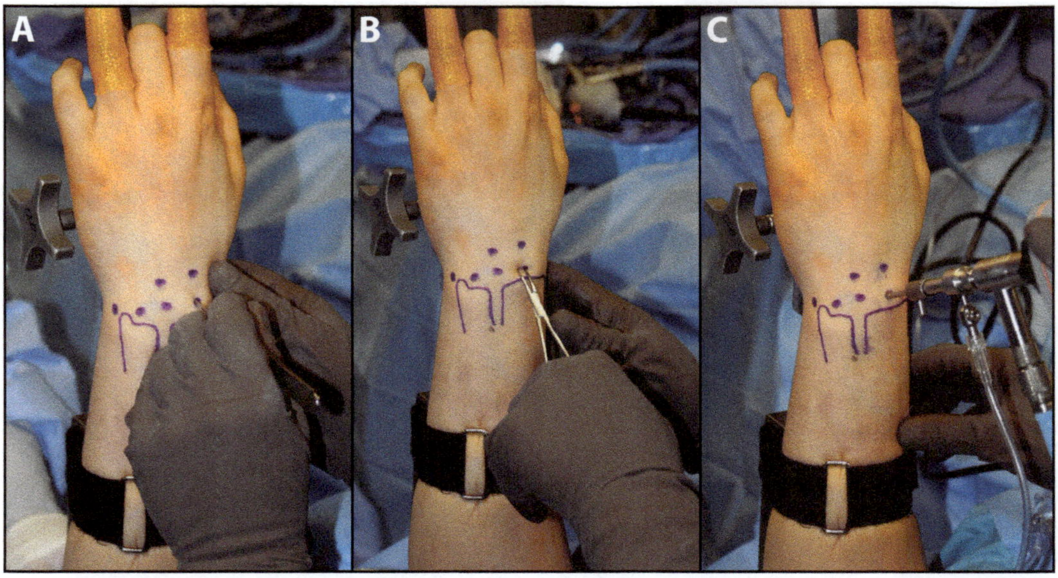

Figure 26-16. Portal placement technique. (A) Only the skin is cut with the scalpel blade. (B) A blunt instrument such as a hemostat is used to spread and open the joint capsule. (C) Insertion of arthroscope.

ulnar aspect. A volar 6-U portal has also been described. Palpation between these compartments demonstrates soft spots of the wrist, which provide the least traumatic entry points into the joint. The carpal articulations appear smooth when viewing through the radiocarpal portals, as opposed to the midcarpal portals, which have a more irregular articulation.[5] The radiocarpal portal locations are illustrated in Figure 26-17.

3-4 Portal

The 3-4 portal is usually the first portal established and is the primary viewing portal. It is bordered on the radial side by the EPL and ECRB, on the ulnar side by the EDC, on the proximal side by the distal radius, and on the distal side by the scapholunate ligament. The 3-4 portal is established 1 cm distal to Lister's tubercle and is located by palpating the distal edge of the radius between the ulnar border of the ECRB and the radial margin of the EDC in line with the radial border of the long finger. This is the soft spot between the third and fourth compartments.[7] A spinal needle is then inserted parallel to the radial articular surface by angling about 10 degrees proximally to match the palmar tilt.

This portal is the workhorse of standard wrist arthroscopy and provides a broad view of most of the radiocarpal joint on the volar side. The portal is relatively safe, with the sensory branch of the radial nerve (SBRN) a mean distance of 16 mm and a mean distance from the radial artery of 26.3 mm.[10]

4-5 Portal

The 4-5 portal is bordered on the radial side by the EDC, on the ulnar side by the extensor digiti quinti (EDQ), proximally by the attachment of the radius and the TFCC, and distally by the lunatein line with the ring metacarpal. It is established 1 cm ulnarly and slightly more proximal to the 3-4 portal because of the inclination of the radius.[7] It can be found by palpating the soft spot directly ulnarly to the EDC. A spinal needle should then be placed just proximal to the lunate. Entry through this portal places instruments directly adjacent to the midportion of the TFCC.[11] The 4-5 portal is typically the main working portal for instrumentation on the ulnar side of the wrist. It may also be used as a viewing portal for ulnar sided structures. This portal has minimal neurovascular risk unless there is an aberrant branch of the SBRN.[10]

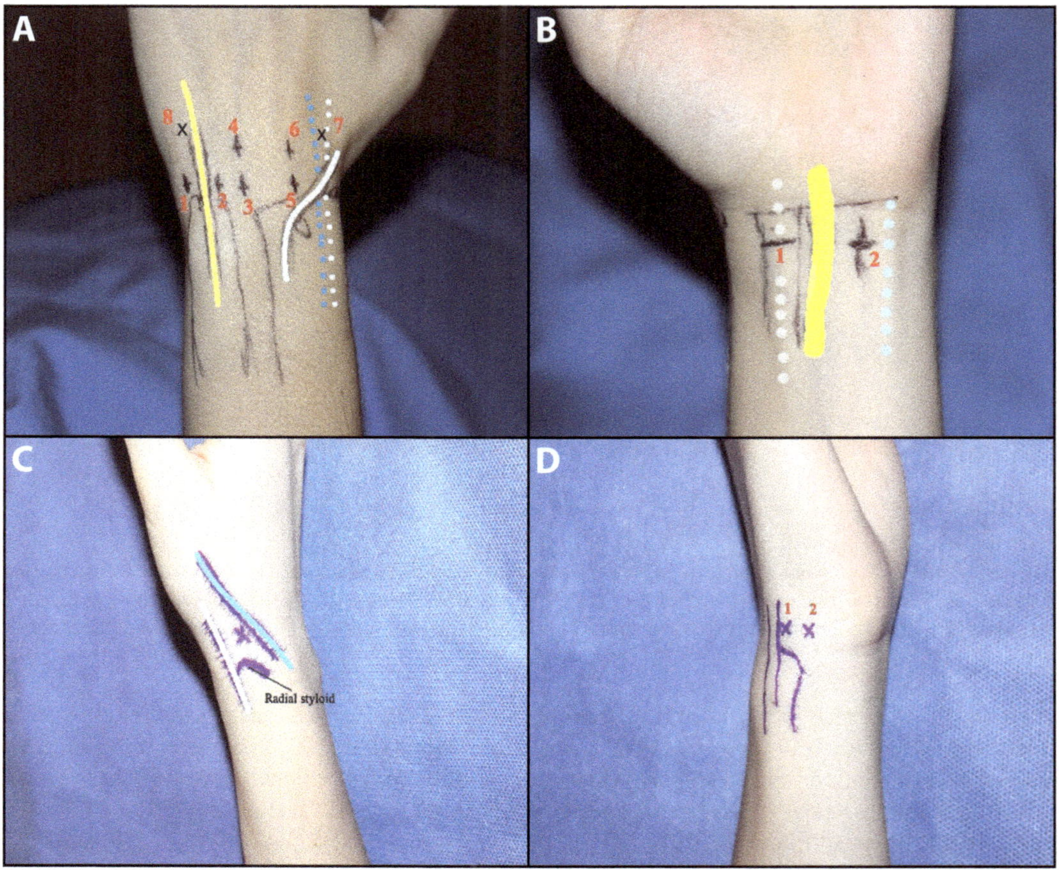

Figure 26-17. Wrist anatomy and portal locations. (A) Dorsal portals consisting of the (1) 6-U portal, (2) 6-R portal, (3) 4-5 portal, (4) ulnar midcarpal portal, (5) 3-4 portal, (6) radial midcarpal, (7) scaphoid-trapezoid-trapezium portal, and (8) triquetrohamate portal. The EPL (white line), ECRB, and ECRL (blue and white dotted lines, respectively), and the ECU (yellow line) are shown. (B) Volar portals consisting of the (1) volar radial portal and the (2) volar ulnar portal. Also shown are the median nerve (yellow line), FCR (dotted white line), and flexor carpi ulnaris (dotted blue line). (C) Radial-sided view with the 1-2 portal marked just radial to the EPL tendon (blue line). The first dorsal compartment is marked by the white line. (D) Ulnar-sided view with the (1) dorsal 6-U and (2) volar 6-U portals labeled.

6-R Portal

Frequently used as an alternative to the 4-5 portal, the 6-R portal is bordered radially by the EDQ, ulnarly by the ECU, proximally by the TFCC, and distally by the lunotriquetral joint. It enters the wrist joint just distal to the ulnar attachment of the TFCC. This portal is found by using the proximal border of the triquetrum rather than the distal ulna as a surface landmark to avoid damaging the TFCC. It is established under arthroscopic guidance by introducing a needle just radial to the ECU. The 6-R has a mean distance of 8.2 mm from the dorsal sensory branch of the ulnar nerve (DBUN).[10]

6-U Portal

The 6-U portal is established volar to the ECU tendon, but because of its proximity to the DBUN, it is not routinely used. The skin incision may be placed as far volar as the dorsal border of the ECU tendon. The portal enters the wrist joint through the prestyloid recess between the

ECU tendon and the ulnar styloid. The portal is distal to the TFCC and dorsal ulnar to the ulnotriquetral ligament. The 6-U portal is typically used for the inflow or outflow cannula. It may be used as an accessory portal for viewing ulnar-sided structures or for instrumentation during TFCC repairs. The mean distance of the portal to the DBUN is 4.5 mm, but the nerve has multiple branches in some patients.[10]

1-2 Portal

The 1-2 portal is not used frequently due to its proximity to neurovascular structures.[12] It is established between the first and second extensor compartments 1 to 2 mm distal to the radial styloid. This portal is placed by finding the soft spot between the first extensor compartment containing the abductor pollicis longus and extensor pollicis brevis and the second compartment with the ECRL and ECRB tendons along the far ulnar part of the anatomic snuffbox. It is located just proximal to the waist of the scaphoid. The radial artery is located at the volar and radial aspect of the anatomic snuffbox. This necessitates placement of this portal as far dorsal as possible to avoid injury to the artery.[11]

The 1-2 portal provides access to the radial styloid, scaphoid, and articular surface of the distal radius, but it allows a limited view of the lunate.[4] There is significant risk with the placement of this portal. Two branches of the SBRN are a mean distance of 3 mm radial and 5 mm ulnar to the portal, and this radial artery is a mean distance of 3 mm radial to the portal.[10]

Midcarpal Portals

Midcarpal evaluation should be done as a routine part of wrist arthroscopy. The 4 midcarpal portals include the midcarpal radial, midcarpal ulnar, triquetrohamate, and triscaphe portals. The most commonly used are the radial and ulnar midcarpal portals. The less common ones are the triscaphe and triquetrohamate portals. The limited room in the midcarpal space requires extra care when entering the joint. Once established, these portals should be maintained to minimize the difficulty in re-establishing them due to fluid extravasation.[7] Normally, there is no communication between the radiocarpal and midcarpal spaces.

Evaluation of wrist instability with midcarpal arthroscopy is better than with radiocarpal arthroscopy alone. Studies show that instability of the scapholunate or lunotriquetral ligament diagnosed with radiocarpal arthroscopy was always seen on midcarpal arthroscopy, but instability seen by midcarpal arthroscopy was not always noticed when performing radiocarpal arthroscopy alone. However, grading of the instability was equal to or greater than that done by midcarpal examination.[13]

Visualization of the scaphoid-trapezoid-trapezium (STT) joint, the midcarpal extrinsic ligaments, the capitohamate joint, and the articular surfaces of the midcarpal bones is improved with midcarpal arthroscopy. Midcarpal arthroscopy can be mastered quickly and adds little time to wrist arthroscopy. It has a low morbidity rate and should be used routinely for a thorough evaluation of the wrist.[13] The midcarpal portal locations are illustrated in Figure 26-17A.

Midcarpal Radial Portal

The radial midcarpal portal is the most commonly used midcarpal portal. It is bordered radially by the ECRB, ulnarly by the EDC, proximally by the scapholunate ligament, and distally by the capitate. It should be established in line with the radial border of the third metacarpal 1 cm distal to the 3-4 portal. A soft spot may be palpated on the radial side of the proximal capitate between the base of the third metacarpal and the dorsal margin of the distal radius. The arthroscope enters between the capitate and scaphoid. This allows evaluation of the midcarpal space and the scapholunate, lunotriquetral, and STT articulations. This portal is relatively safe, with branches of the SBRN found radially at a mean distance of 15.8 mm.[10]

Figure 26-18. Box concept using dorsal and volar portals as the viewing and working portals to encircle the wrist. (Modified from Bain GI, Munt J, Turner PC. New advances in wrist arthroscopy. *Arthroscopy.* 2008;24(3):355-367.)

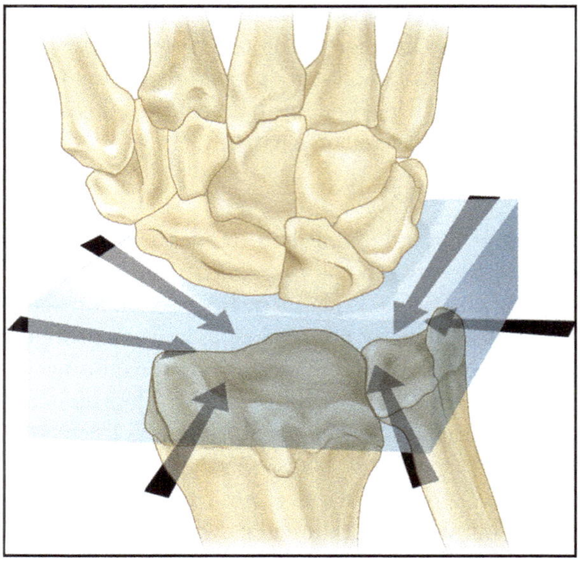

Midcarpal Ulnar Portal

The midcarpal ulnar portal is bordered radially by the EDC, ulnarly by the EDQ, proximally by the lunotriquetral joint, and distally by the capitate hamate joint. It is in line with the center of the fourth metacarpal. As with the radial midcarpal portal, it is placed approximately 1 cm distal to the 4-5 portal and at approximately the same level as the radial midcarpal portal. This portal enters through capitate-hamate-triquetral-lunate interval. It is used primarily for instrumentation within the midcarpal joint. There is minimal risk when making this portal because the SBRN branches are usually remote to this portal.[10]

Triquetrohamate Portal

The triquetrohamate portal is established on the ulnar side of the wrist, distal to the triquetrum and ulnar to the midcarpal ulnar portal. It enters the triquetrohamate joint just ulnar to the ECU tendon. It provides excellent access for an inflow or outflow cannula and can be used for instrumentation in the triquetrohamate joint.

Triscaphe Portal

The triscaphe portal (STT) is on the radial side of the midcarpal space. It is established ulnar to the EPL or radial to the abductor pollicis longus in line with the radial margin of the second metacarpal at the level of the distal pole of the scaphoid. The STT-R portal provides an additional view and access to the STT joint.[14] Staying ulnar to the EPL helps to avoid the radial artery. The ulnar aspect of the ECRL tendon can be used to check the location of this portal because the EPL is quite mobile at the level of the STT joint. Care must be taken to prevent displacing the tendon radially while establishing the STT portal to protect the radial artery. The STT joint can be entered directly through this portal, and it is used primarily for instrumentation in this joint.[11] Care should be taken to avoid the small terminal branches of the SBRN.

Volar Portals

Volar portals have become increasingly popular to complete the view of diagnostic wrist arthroscopy and to provide access for procedures that are not feasible from the dorsal entry sites. Bain et al[4] suggested "The Box Concept" for wrist arthroscopy (Figure 26-18). By using both dorsal and volar portals, the surgeon is able to achieve circumferential visualization and access for instrumentation.[4,15] The viewing and working portals can then be adjusted for the specific diagnostic or therapeutic procedure. The volar portals allow improved treatment for dorsal pathology, such as dorsal rim fractures of the distal radius, dorsal rheumatoid synovial proliferation, and volar segment tears of the scapholunate and lunotriquetral interosseous ligaments.[15] The volar portal locations are illustrated in Figure 26-17B and the volar 6-U portal is in Figure 26-17D.

Volar Radial Portal

To place the volar radial portal, a mini-open technique is used over the flexor carpi radialis on the radial side of the volar proximal wrist crease. An anatomic study found that there was a safe zone that included the width of the flexor carpi radialis and at least 3 mm in all directions at this level from the palmar cutaneous branch of the median nerve (ulnarly) and the radial artery (radially).[16] Because of this safe zone, a 2-cm transverse incision can be made over the flexor carpi radialis tendon. The transverse incision provides superior cosmesis while maintaining minimal risk for the volar structures. The tendon sheath is divided, the radial artery is retracted radially, and the flexor carpi radialis and median nerve are retracted ulnarly. The radiocarpal joint is identified with a spinal needle and the portal is opened with a blunt instrument. This portal is used to assess the dorsal aspect of the scapholunate interosseous ligament and the dorsal radiocarpal ligament.[16]

Volar Ulnar Portal

Placement of the volar ulnar portal uses a mini-open technique. A 2-cm longitudinal incision is centered over the proximal wrist crease along the ulnar edge of the common flexors. The interval between the flexor carpi ulnaris and common flexor tendons is then used. The common flexors are retracted radially, and the flexor carpi ulnaris and the ulnar nerve are retracted ulnarly. The joint space is identified with a spinal needle and the capsule is again opened bluntly. Because there is no true safe zone for the volar ulnar portal, it requires a careful dissection and spread technique.[17] This portal provides access for reduction of a distal radius fracture and a view of the dorsal articular surfaces and dorsal ligaments.

Volar 6-U Portal

According to Moskal et al,[18] this portal is established approximately 5 mm volar to the dorsal 6-U portal. This portal can be established while viewing through a 3-4 portal and can be used for treating lunotriquetral instability by suture plication of the disk-carpal ligaments. A spinal needle is used to pass suture via this portal.[18]

Distal Radioulnar Portals

The DRUJ is difficult to examine, and arthroscopy is not frequently used in these cases. The proximal and distal DRUJ portals are named according to their location proximal or distal to the ulnar head. The DRUJ portals are bordered radially by the EDC and ulnarly by the ECU. The joint is entered from the base of the DRUJ, bordered by the radius and ulna. The proximal portal is placed in this line just proximal to the DRUJ. The forearm is supinated to relax the dorsal capsule, and the arthroscope is then introduced between the radius and ulna underneath the TFCC and proximal to the articular surface. The radioulnar articular surfaces can then be seen. Pronation and supination increase the available surface area during examination.

The distal portal is not always accessible. Use of this portal allows the surgeon to examine the distal articular surface of the ulna and the undersurface of the TFCC. The DRUJ portal uses a mini-open approach. It is located just proximal to the TFCC, and care must be taken to stay below the TFCC to prevent injury to this structure. There is some risk to the posterior interosseous nerve.[8] There is minimal risk to sensory nerves, with the closest being 17.5 mm distally.[10]

Table 26-1. Wrist Arthroscopy Portals

Radiocarpal	3-4	4-5	6-R	6-U	1-2
Midcarpal	Radial	Ulnar	Triquetrohamate	Triscaphe (STT)	
Volar	Radial	Ulnar	6-U		
Distal Radioulnar	Dorsal (proximal, distal)	Volar			

The DRUJ can be accessed via dorsally and volarly based portals. The dorsal DRUJ portal is created by supinating the forearm and introducing the trocar underneath the TFCC in the space between the radius and ulna. The volar DRUJ portal is created in a similar manner as the volar ulnar portal.

A complete list of portals and their locations are summarized in Table 26-1.

Potential Complications

Because of the absence of major neurovascular structures, most wrist arthroscopy uses the dorsum of the wrist. Only the deep branch of the radial artery and the superficial dorsal sensory branches of the radial, ulnar, and lateral antebrachial cutaneous nerves are located on the dorsal side of the wrist.[8] Injury to these structures can cause numbness and, at worst, a painful neuroma and complex regional pain syndrome. Certain portals have an increased risk of iatrogenic neurovascular injury. The greatest risk to the radial artery and dorsal radial and ulnar sensory nerve branches occur with the 1-2, 6-R, and 6-U portals. The midcarpal, 3-4, 4-5, and DRUJ portals are relatively safe.

Risk exists even in safe portals because aberrant sensory nerve branches can be dangerously close.[10] This usually necessitates incisions that are longitudinal and are made by cutting only the skin and bluntly spreading through the subcutaneous tissue. When piercing the capsule, only a blunt trocar should be used. This technique helps protect structures between the dermis and capsule from injury.[10]

Complications arising from wrist arthroscopy can be procedure specific or generally related to wrist arthroscopy, such as traction, arm positioning, and portal site creation. Complication rates have been cited as low as 2%, of which many resolve with observation alone.[4,5] Most of these general complications can be prevented with simple precautions, such as using appropriately sized instrumentation, blunt trocars, taking care to avoid the EPL and EDQ (the tendons most at risk during arthroscopy), using nylon finger traps, and the appropriate amount of traction.[4,19]

Excessive fluid extravasation is possible and may occur in acutely injured patients or if the inflow cannula is inadvertently placed extra-articularly. Halting the inflow and elevating the extremity may help this situation. If significant enough, the arthroscopic portion of the case may need to be stopped. The risk of compartment syndrome is very low, and extravasated fluid is rapidly absorbed and does not increase compartment pressures long enough to compromise circulation.[20]

Postoperative infection is uncommon. Oral antibiotics are typically sufficient for any superficial infection. If a deep infection occurs, irrigation, arthroscopic or open debridement, and intravenous antibiotics are usually required.[21]

Top Technical Pearls for the Procedure

1. Use only soft finger traps, and minimize traction and procedure time if skin quality is poor.
2. To protect neurovascular structures, incise only the dermis by pulling the skin against a scalpel, and bluntly spread tissues before cannula placement. Place the 1-2 portal in the most dorsal portion of the snuff box to protect the radial artery.
3. To protect the articular surfaces, know the precise portal location and anatomy, localize the joint space with a spinal needle before establishing a portal, insert with the angle of radial inclination and volar tilt, and use only blunt instruments and cannulas.
4. Use adequate outflow, and use gravity inflow if possible to prevent fluid extravasation.
5. Carefully pad and protect bony prominences and vulnerable superficial nerves when positioning the patient for arthroscopic wrist surgery.

References

1. Chen YC. Arthroscopy of the wrist and finger joints. *Orthop Clin North Am.* 1979;10(3):723-733.
2. Whipple TL, Cooney WP III, Osterman AL, Viegas SF. Wrist arthroscopy. *Instr Course Lect.* 1995;44:139-145.
3. Whipple TL, Marotta JJ, Powerl JH III. Techniques of wrist arthroscopy. *Arthroscopy.* 1986;2(4):244-252.
4. Bain GI, Munt J, Turner PC. New advances in wrist arthroscopy. *Arthroscopy.* 2008;24(3):355-367.
5. Haisman JM, Matthew B, Scott W. Wrist arthroscopy: standard portals and arthroscopic anatomy. *J Am Soc Surg Hand.* 2005;5:175-181.
6. Berger RA. Arthroscopic anatomy of the wrist and distal radioulnar joint. *Hand Clin.* 1999;15(3):393-413.
7. Geissler WB, Freeland AE, Weiss AP, Chow JC. Techniques of wrist arthroscopy. *Instr Course Lect.* 2000;49:225-237.
8. Gupta R, Bozentka DJ, Osterman AL. Wrist arthroscopy: principles and clinical applications. *J Am Acad Orthop Surg.* 2001;9(3):200-209.
9. Wolf JM, Dukas A, Pensak M. Advances in wrist arthroscopy. *J Am Acad Orthop Surg.* 2012;20(11):725-734.
10. Abrams RA, Petersen M, Botte MJ. Arthroscopic portals of the wrist: an anatomic study. *J Hand Surg Am.* 1994;19(6):940-944.
11. Bettinger PC, Cooney WP III, Berger RA. Arthroscopic anatomy of the wrist. *Orthop Clin North Am.* 1995;26(4):707-719.
12. Sraj S. A simple wrist arthroscopy tower: the wrist triangle. *Am J Orthop (Belle Mead NJ).* 2013;42(12):573-574.
13. Hofmeister EP, Dao KD, Glowacki KA, Shin AY. The role of midcarpal arthroscopy in the diagnosis of disorders of the wrist. *J Hand Surg Am.* 2001;26(3):407-414.
14. Carro LP, Golano P, Fariñas O, Cerezal L, Hidalgo C. The radial portal for scaphotrapeziotrapezoid arthroscopy. *Arthroscopy.* 2003;19(5):547-553.
15. Abe Y, Doi K, Hattori Y, Ikeda K, Dhawan V. A benefit of the volar approach for wrist arthroscopy. *Arthroscopy.* 2003;19(4):440-445.
16. Slutsky DJ. Wrist arthroscopy through a volar radial portal. *Arthroscopy.* 2002;18(6):624-630.
17. Slutsky DJ, Nagle DJ. Wrist arthroscopy: current concepts. *J Hand Surg Am.* 2008;33(7):1228-1244.

18. Moskal MJ, Savoie FH III, Field LD. Arthroscopic capsulodesis of the lunotriquetral joint. *Clin Sports Med*. 2001;20(1):141-153.
19. Beredjiklian PK, Bozentka DJ, Leung YL, Monaghan BA. Complications of wrist arthroscopy. *J Hand Surg Am*. 2004;29(3):406-411.
20. Whipple TL. Precaution for arthroscopy of the wrist. *Arthroscopy*. 1990;6(1):3-4.
21. Botte MJ, Cooney WP, Linscheid RL. Arthroscopy of the wrist: anatomy and technique. *J Hand Surg Am*. 1989;14(2 pt 1):313-316.

27

Diagnostic Wrist Arthroscopy

Jeffrey B. Witty, MD; Larry D. Field, MD; and Brandon P. Donnelly, MD

Introduction

During the past 30 years, wrist arthroscopy has evolved into a valuable tool that has become one of the most reliable and productive means of diagnosing, qualifying, and treating wrist pathology. As the arthroscopic surgeon's technical ability has improved, wrist arthroscopy has increasingly become a more routine and safely performed procedure. The number of indications has continued to grow and comprises a variety of pathology. These include triangular fibrocartilage complex (TFCC) injuries, osteochondral lesions, staging, planning and treatment for wrist arthritis, assessment of carpal instability, fracture care, synovitis, ganglion excision, and contracture release.[1,2]

The arthroscopic approach allows excellent access to the intrinsic and extrinsic ligaments of the wrist and the articular surfaces of the carpal bones, which is not possible without extensive arthrotomy. Access to remote areas of the wrist joint is possible while minimizing morbidity.[2,3] Despite the minimally invasive nature of the procedure, a thorough knowledge of wrist anatomy is essential to minimize complications and allow for the safe identification and treatment of wrist pathology. This chapter reviews the preoperative evaluation and imaging and the essential components of diagnostic wrist arthroscopy. Diagnostic arthroscopy of the wrist involves evaluation of the radiocarpal, midcarpal, and distal radioulnar joints. Potential complications are also briefly discussed.

Indications

Indications for wrist arthroscopy are typically procedure specific, but there are instances when a diagnosis is suggested by history and examination but not corroborated on imaging studies. In these cases, diagnostic arthroscopy may provide more information that may influence treatment, including the following[4]:

- Diagnosis and grading of dynamic instability patterns
- Peripheral TFCC tears

Savoie FH III, Field LD, Steinmann SP, eds. *The Elbow and Wrist: AANA Advanced Arthroscopic Surgical Techniques* (pp 275-284).

- Lunotriquetral interosseous ligament tears
- More precise grading of arthrosis within the carpus, which may help determine if a motion-sparing procedure or fusion is indicated.

Pertinent Physical Findings

Each diagnosis will present with its particular findings on clinical examination. Please see the specific chapter for more details. The following list is not meant to be inclusive but to serve a general overview when evaluating the painful wrist.[5-7]

- Inspection of the wrist for areas of swelling, erythema, warmth, nodules, skin lesions, and deformity (eg, dorsal swelling over the extensor tendons as seen with tenosynovitis)
- Areas of tenderness localized to a specific anatomic structure (eg, anatomic snuffbox for scaphoid fractures or scapholunate interosseous ligament pathology, pisotriquetral pain for arthrosis, and tenderness over the hook of the hamate as seen with fracture)
- Range of motion with attention to any symptomatic snapping or clicking, which may indicate carpal instability
- Grind test for thumb carpometacarpal arthritis
- Watson scaphoid shift test (injury to the scapholunate ligament)
- Ballottement test (injury to the lunotriquetral ligament injury)
- Ulnar axial load test (ulnocarpal abutment and TFCC tears)
- Catch-up clunk test (midcarpal instability)
- Distal radioulnar joint compression (DRUJ; instability or arthritis to the DRUJ)
- Vascular status with capillary refill or Allen's test
- Neurologic exam (eg, Tinel's sign, Durkan's test for carpal tunnel syndrome)

Pertinent Imaging

As is the case with the physical examination, each diagnosis has its own specific x-ray, computed tomography, and magnetic resonance imaging findings. The following list outlines some of the common findings found when imaging the painful wrist.[7,8]

- X-rays
  - Posteroanterior, oblique, lateral, clenched fist, carpal tunnel view, and pronated ulnar deviated view
  - Evaluation for fracture, alignment, congruence of joint space, arthritis change, and mineralization
  - Lateral view is best for carpal alignment, scapholunate angle
  - Clenched fist for possible scapholunate dissociation
  - Carpal tunnel view allows visualization of hook of hamate
  - Pronated ulnar deviated image allows view of unobstructed extended scaphoid
- Computed tomography
  - Best for osseous and articular morphology
  - Evaluation of bony healing after fracture (scaphoid)
  - Difficult-to-visualize areas (hook of hamate)

- Magnetic resonance imaging
  - Evaluation of soft tissue and vascularity
  - Avascular necrosis of carpal bones
  - Occult ganglions
  - Tumors
  - Tendinitis
  - Joint effusions
  - Bony edema and microfractures
  - TFCC (90% sensitivity)
  - Scapholunate ligament tear (accuracy 90%, sensitivity 70% to 89%, specificity 94% to 100%)
  - Lunotriquetral ligament tear (accuracy 50%, sensitivity 50% to 82%, specificity 94% to 100%)
  - Extrinsic ligament injury
  - Partial tears (25% to 67% sensitivity and specificity)
  - Full-thickness tears (accuracy up to 100% with magnetic resonance arthrography)

Equipment

Regional or general anesthesia may be used. The patient is positioned supine with the operative extremity on an arm table. A tourniquet is placed proximally on the upper arm. A small joint 30-degree arthroscope (2.3, 2.5, 2.7, or 3.0 mm), small joint arthroscopic instruments, and gravity flow or pump (typically 30 to 60 mm Hg) are used for the procedure. Seventy-degree arthroscopes are also available. Radiofrequency probes can be used to shrink or debride synovium but should be used with outflow to avoid thermal injury. The operating table is angled so that the surgeon is positioned above the arm table and near the patient's head, and the assistant is positioned directly across the arm table within the patient's axilla.[9]

After preparing and draping, the arm is exsanguinated before inflation of the tourniquet and placed in position on a traction tower. The authors prefer a sterile traction tower with nylon finger traps to provide convenient application of wrist distraction in flexion, extension, and radial and ulnar deviation. The authors use soft nylon finger traps to secure the index and long fingers to the tower in a sterile fashion for most procedures. However, for ulnar-sided pathology, the authors frequently use the index and ring fingers. Five to 15 lb of traction are adequate for most procedures.

- Traction options
  - Nonsterile or sterile traction tower
  - Radiolucent triangle with free-hanging weight
  - Nylon finger traps
- Video
  - Arthroscopes (size range approximately 2.0 to 3.0 mm in size) 30 and 70 degrees
- Fluid management
  - Normal saline or lactated ringer's solution
  - Pump
  - Tubing with pinch chambers

- Instrumentation
  - Small joint shavers (size range approximately 2.0 to 3.0 mm)
  - Small joint burrs (size range approximately 2.0 to 3.0 mm)
  - Probe
  - Standard straight and curved mosquito tip graspers (2.0 and 2.75 mm)
  - Blunt tip and scoop tip forceps of various angles (2.0 and 2.75 mm)
  - Curettes (2.75 mm)
  - Dissectors (2.75 mm)
  - 18-gauge spinal needles
  - Small joint electrode for cutting and hemostasis (approximately 2.9 mm)

Positioning and Portals

Patients undergoing diagnostic wrist arthroscopy are positioned supine, with all bony prominences carefully padded and with the operative extremity at 90 degrees of abduction and neutral rotation. This orients the forearm vertically and allows for its placement in the wrist arthroscopy traction tower.

Step-by-Step Description of the Procedure

Radiocarpal Evaluation

Diagnostic wrist arthroscopy begins with the 3-4 portal and is the primary viewing portal. Palpation and spinal needle localization of this portal are essential before the skin incision is made. Through the 3-4 portal, a needle is inserted and the joint is distended with 5 to 7 mL of saline. Only the skin is incised with a #15 or #11 blade, and a small hemostat is used to spread the soft tissues. Next, the blunt trocar should be inserted at approximately a 20-degree proximal angle to match the distal radius articular slope. This angle can avoid damaging the dorsal articular surface.[3,10,11] Only blunt trocars are used in establishing portals. The inflow and outflow are interchangeable and can be maintained through the arthroscopic cannula or a separate 6-U portal established under direct arthroscopic visualization. The authors prefer the inflow through the arthroscope to push debris away instead of pulling it toward the camera. After a 3-4 portal is established, a diagnostic radiocarpal arthroscopy is performed.

The radial styloid and radial capsule are examined first. The scaphoid superiorly and the distal radial articular surface inferiorly can be evaluated for signs of arthritic change or articular injury (Figure 27-1). The proximal border of the radial facet is examined, as are the volar extrinsic ligaments, radioscaphocapitate ligament, and long radiolunate ligament (Figure 27-2). The volar radial extrinsic ligaments are helpful to confirm orientation and location within the radiocarpal joint. The long radiolunate ligament lies ulnar to the radioscaphocapitate ligament and is usually 2 to 3 times its width.[11,12] The ligaments should be taut on probing because of the traction applied to the wrist. Ulnar to these is the radioscapholunate ligament, also called the ligament of Testut, which is a vascularized tuft of tissue with no significant structural integrity. The tuft marks the scapholunate interval and sagittal ridge.[12-14] Blood vessels are frequently seen along this ligament, and there is a natural redundancy to this ligament that should not be mistaken for a tear. Ganglia often arise from the membranous portion of the scapholunate interosseous ligament and can be seen best from the 6-R portal.

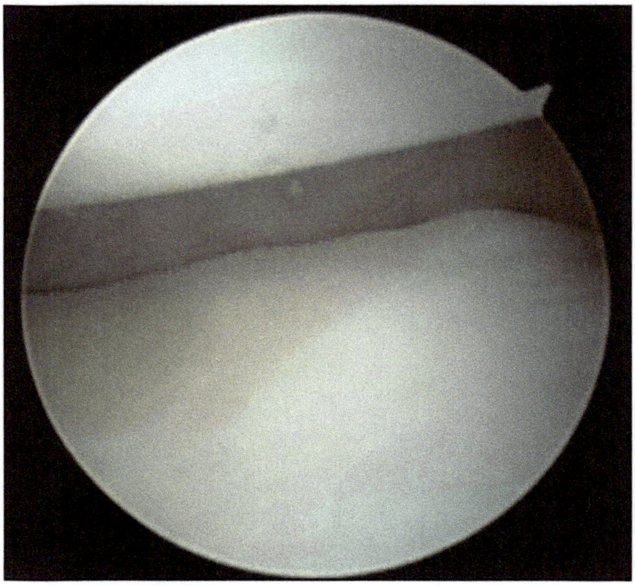

Figure 27-1. The radiocarpal joint is viewed from the 3-4 portal, showing the scaphoid superiorly and distal radius inferiorly.

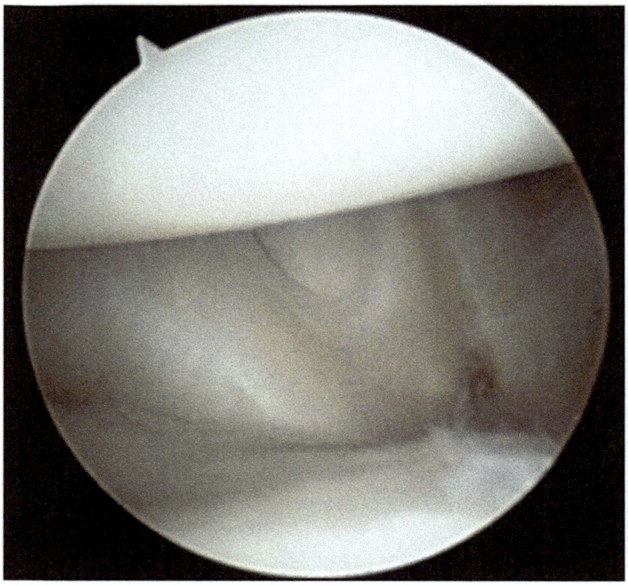

Figure 27-2. Volar extrinsic ligaments are viewed from the 3-4 portal, showing the radioscaphocapitate ligament and the long radiolunate ligament.

Following the scaphoid ulnarly, the slightly concave scapholunate interosseous ligament can be examined for tears or scapholunate diastasis (Figure 27-3). An intact ligament may not be immediately obvious because it mimics the appearance of cartilage. Complete injury to this ligament, however, allows the arthroscope to pass between the scaphoid and the lunate (ie, drive-through sign).[3]

The proximal surface of the lunate and the distal surface of the radius can be evaluated next. The 2 fossae of the distal radius, the scaphoid and the lunate fossae, are separated by a sagittal ridge. Fraying or fissuring of this area, suggestive of chondromalacia, should be documented, and signs of ulnar impaction on the lunate and triquetrum can also be seen. Normally, in the neutral wrist position, one-half of the lunate articulates with the lunate facet and one-half articulates with the TFCC.[12]

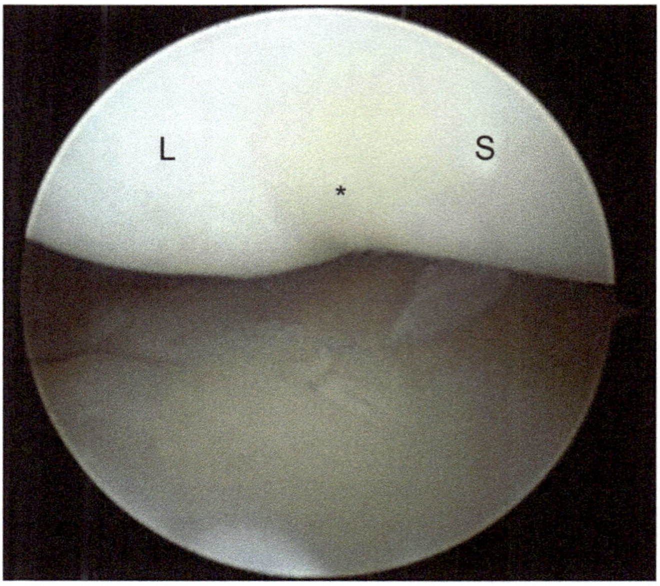

Figure 27-3. The convexity of the scapholunate interosseous ligament (asterisk), scaphoid (S), and lunate (L) can be seen.

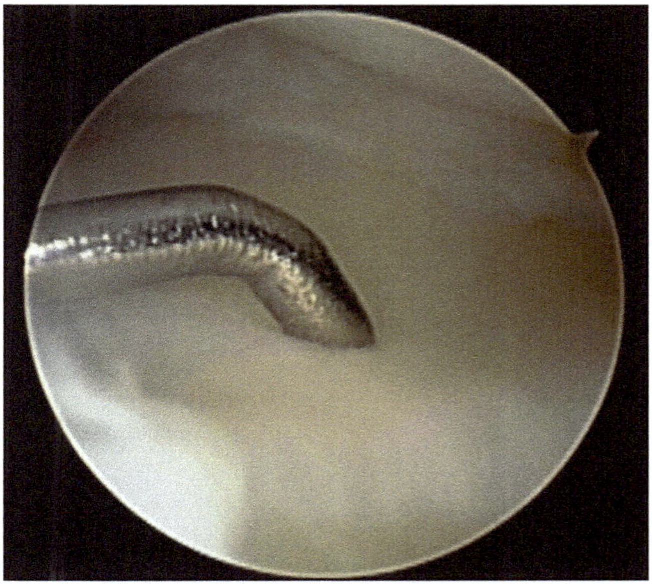

Figure 27-4. For the trampoline test, a probe is used to test the tension of the triangular fibrocartilage.

The radial and central portions of the TFCC are evaluated, as are the volar and dorsal radio-ulnar ligaments. Next, the peripheral attachment of the TFCC and the ulnar prestyloid recess should be examined. The TFCC is wedge shaped in the coronal plane, with a thickened periphery and a thin radial attachment.[14] A probe can be used to evaluate the tension of the TFCC by ballottement (ie, trampoline test; Figure 27-4).[13,15] The TFCC, also known as the *articular disk*, should be taut, and lack of tension raises suspicion of a peripheral TFCC tear. The peripheral 15% to 20% of the TFCC is vascularized and, therefore, has healing potential if torn.[3] The prestyloid ulnar recess is a normal anatomic finding that is approximately 3 to 4 mm wide, and it should not be mistaken for a peripheral tear, which can be distinguished due to signs of synovitis.[12] The arthroscope can be inserted through the 4-5 or 6-R portal to evaluate the integrity of the lunotriquetral ligament. It is evaluated by identifying a sulcus or concavity in the otherwise convex articular surface of the lunate and triquetrum.[15] The ulnolunate and ulnotriquetral ligaments may

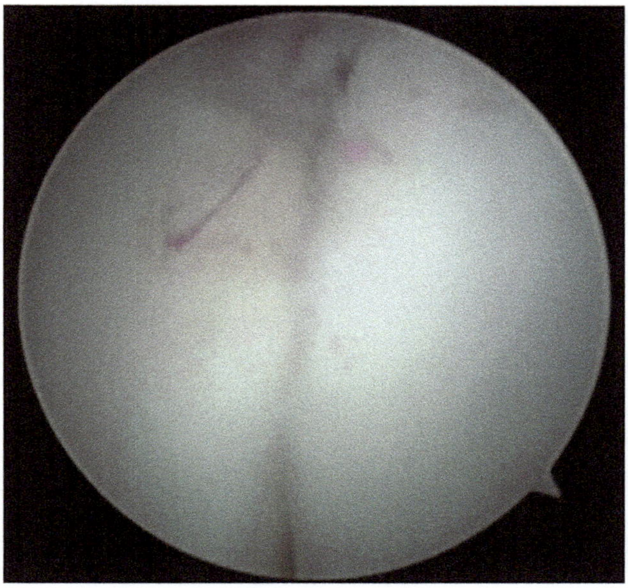

Figure 27-5. The congruent scapholunate joint is viewed from the radial midcarpal portal.

be more easily evaluated by placing the arthroscope in the 4-5 or 6-R portal. These ligaments are identified as capsular thickenings in the volar aspect of the ulnar capsule. One can also evaluate the pisotriquetral joint by advancing the scope into the prestyloid recess.

Midcarpal Evaluation

After a complete examination of the radiocarpal joint has been performed, the arthroscope can be used to evaluate the midcarpal space. The radial midcarpal portal, located approximately 1 cm distal to the 3-4 radiocarpal portal, is typically used to establish a diagnostic arthroscopy portal. The midcarpal joint can be distended with 3 to 5 mL of fluid through the midcarpal radial portal. This allows easier access into the joint with a blunt trocar and minimizes the risk of damaging the articular cartilage.[12] Normally, there is no communication between the radiocarpal and midcarpal spaces.[16]

Care must be taken when entering the radial midcarpal space because it is less than one-half of the depth of the radiocarpal space and does not have the volar tilt of the radiocarpal joint.[3] The ulnar midcarpal portal is created for instrumentation and visualization of the ulnar portion of the midcarpal joint. The arthroscopic evaluation in this area begins with visualization of the convexity of the capitate (superiorly) and the scapholunate joint (inferiorly). This distinct relationship confirms that the arthroscope is in the midcarpal space. The scapholunate joint should be perfectly congruous (Figure 27-5). The scapholunate ligament is not present on the distal edge of the scapholunate joint, and the joint is best viewed from this perspective. Intraoperatively, the stability of the joint may be assessed by performing Watson's scaphoid shift test. The Geissler classification can be used to grade carpal instability.[8,16,17]

The distal surfaces of the lunate and the triquetrum are then evaluated, as is the concave proximal surface of the hamate (Figure 27-6). The lunotriquetral joint is also well visualized from this view, and a ballottement test can be performed to assess stability. Within the distal row, the capitate and capitohamate articulation can be examined from this portal. Farther ulnarly, the triquetrohamate joint is evaluated for degenerative changes. The triquetrohamate joint is a saddle-shaped joint that is normally quite tight and difficult to view across unless pathologic laxity exists.[16]

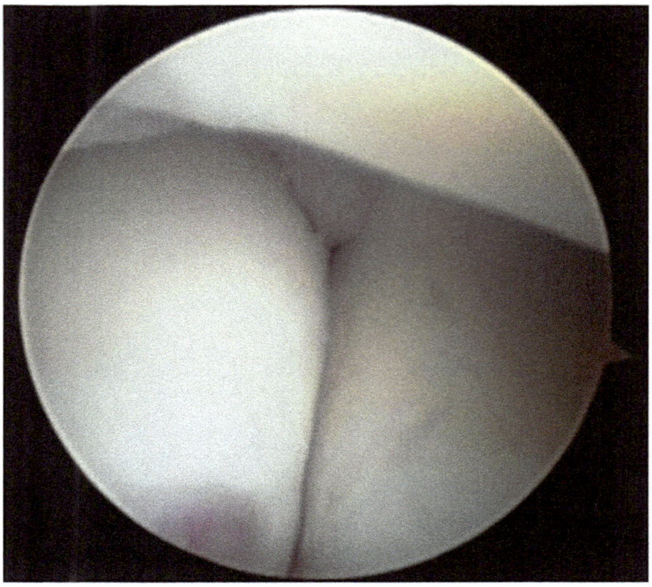

Figure 27-6. The congruent lunotriquetral joint is viewed from the radial midcarpal portal.

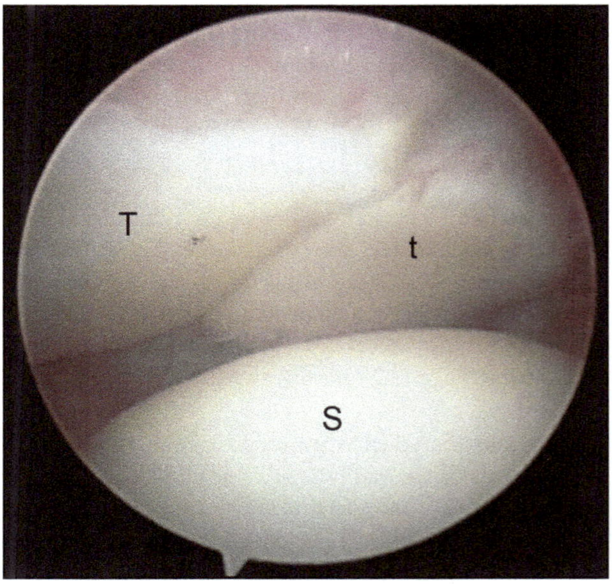

Figure 27-7. The scaphotrapeziotrapezoid joint, including the scaphoid (S), trapezoid (T), and trapezium (t), is viewed from the radial midcarpal portal.

The scaphotrapeziotrapezoid (STT) joint can be seen by passing the arthroscope radially, and early osteoarthritic changes, which are common in this area, should be identified.[18] In the STT joint, the trapezoid is in the foreground, and the trapezium is in the background (Figure 27-7). Bubbles frequently collect here and may impair visualization of the joint. These bubbles may be evacuated with a 21-gauge needle, and debridement can be performed with a small motorized shaver through an accessory STT portal.[16]

Distal Radioulnar Joint Evaluation

On completion of the diagnostic midcarpal arthroscopy, a proximal DRUJ portal can be established, and the ulnar surface of the radius, the radial surface of the ulna, the distal surface of the ulnar head, and the proximal surface of the TFCC can be evaluated. DRUJ arthroscopy is performed with the forearm in supination and suspended in the wrist traction device but with no traction applied. A blunt trocar is angled slightly distal and placed in the joint. If required, outflow can be created by placing an 18-gauge needle into the distal portion of the joint. Through pronation and supination of the wrist, the articular margin of the ulna can be passed in front of the arthroscope lens. This approach is useful for lysis of adhesions, debridement, exostectomy, or capsulotomy of the DRUJ.[3,19]

Postoperative Protocol

The postoperative protocol will depend on the specific procedure being performed.

Potential Complications

Complications after wrist arthroscopy have been reported to range between 4.7% and 5.2%. These include nerve injuries, inclusion cysts, ganglion cysts, tendon sheath fistula formation, sympathetic dystrophy, tendon lacerations/rupture, wrist stiffness, infection, arterial injury, and hematoma. Specific nerve injuries include transection of the transverse radioulnar branch of the dorsal sensory branch of the ulnar nerve when establishing the 6-R portal. Other nerve injuries include transient neuropraxia of the ulnar and sensory branch of the radial nerve. Burn injuries using electrocautery devices have also been reported. The risk of certain complications will depend on the nature of the procedure, including portals used and instrumentation.[4,9]

Top Technical Pearls for the Procedure

1. After the initial skin incision, use a small blunt hemostat to enter the joint capsule and spread the tissues.
2. Angle the trocar to coincide with the radial tilt to avoid damage to the articular surface.
3. Have an assistant maintain fluid flow through the joint with a finger pressure pump.
4. Place the inflow on the camera to push debris away from the scope.
5. Take care when establishing midcarpal portals to minimize the risk of iatrogenic articular cartilage injury.

References

1. Sennwald G. Diagnostic arthroscopy: indications and interpretations of findings. *J Hand Surg Br.* 2001;26(3):241-246.
2. Ringler MD. MRI of wrist ligaments. *J Hand Surg Am.* 2013;38(10):2034-2046.
3. Geissler WB. *Wrist Arthroscopy.* New York, NY: Springer; 2005:1-13.
4. Trumble TE, Budoff JE, Cornwall R. *Hand, Elbow and Shoulder: Core Knowledge in Orthopaedics.* Philadelphia, PA: Mosby Elsevier; 2006.
5. Brown DE, Lichtman DN. The evaluation of chronic wrist pain. *Orthop Clin North Am.* 1984;15(2):183-192.
6. Watson HK, Ashmead D IV, Makhlouf MV. Examination of the scaphoid. *J Hand Surg Am.* 1988;13(5):657-660.

7. Nagle DJ. Evaluation of chronic wrist pain. *J Am Acad Orthop Surg.* 2000;8(1):45-55.
8. Wolf JM, Dukas A, Pensak M. Advances in wrist arthroscopy. *J Am Acad Orthop Surg.* 2012;20(11):725-734.
9. Ahsan ZS, Yao J. Complications of wrist arthroscopy. *Arthroscopy.* 2012;28(6):855-859.
10. Geissler WB, Freeland AE, Weiss AP, et al. Techniques in wrist arthroscopy. Instructional course lecture. *J Bone Joint Surg Am.* 1999;81:1184-1197.
11. Bettinger PC, Cooney WP III, Berger RA. Arthroscopic anatomy of the wrist. *OrthopClin North Am.* 1995;26:707-719.
12. North ER, Thomas S. An anatomic guide for arthroscopic visualization of the wrist capsular ligaments. *J Hand Surg Am.* 1988;13(6):815-822.
13. Roth JH, Poehling GG, Whipple TL. Arthroscopic surgery of the wrist. *Instr Course Lect.* 1988;37:183-194.
14. Berger RA. Arthroscopic anatomy of the wrist and distal radioulnar joint. *Hand Clin.* 1999;15(3):393-413.
15. Hofmeister EP, Dao KD, Glowacki KA, Shin AY. The role of midcarpal arthroscopy in the diagnosis of disorders of the wrist. *J Hand Surg Am.* 2001;26(3):407-414.
16. Viegas SF. Midcarpal arthroscopy: anatomy and portals. *Hand Clin.* 1994;10(4):557-587.
17. Viegas SF. Advances in skeletal anatomy of the wrist. *Hand Clin.* 2001;17(1):1-11.
18. Whipple TL, Cooney WP III, Osterman AL, Viegas SF. Wrist arthroscopy. *Instr Course Lect.* 1995;44:139-145.
19. Wagner J, Ipaktchi K, Livermore M, Banegas R. Current indications for and the technique of wrist arthroscopy. *Orthopedics.* 2014;37(4):251-256.

Please see videos on the accompanying website at

www.routledge.com/9781630910013

28

Wrist Arthroscopy
Triangular Fibrocartilage Debridement and Arthroscopically Assisted Ulnar Shortening

Daniel J. Nagle, MD, FACS, FAAOS and Alex Soneru, MD

Introduction

The triangular fibrocartilage is the primary stabilizer of the distal radioulnar joint (DRUJ). It attaches radially on the distal lip of the sigmoid notch. Ulnarly, the triangular fibrocartilage inserts at the base of the ulnar styloid via a continuation of the dorsal and palmar radioulnar ligaments and the fibers of the ligamentum subcruentum (Figure 28-1).[1]

A patient with an ulnar abutment syndrome (Figure 28-2) typically presents with a central tear of the triangular fibrocartilage complex (TFCC). Chondromalacia can be seen at the ulnar aspect of the lunate and the distal radial surface of the ulnar head. Ulnocarpal synovitis is usually present.

Tears of the triangular fibrocartilage are typically the result of a fall on the outstretched upper extremity. The ulna is driven distally and compresses the TFCC between itself and the lunate, producing a central/radial tear of the articular disk. This same mechanism can result in lunatotriquetral tears and peripheral TFCC tears, neither of which are discussed here.

Forceful ulnar deviation, such as noted in racquet sports and golf, can lead to TFCC tears. The combination of ulnar axial load and torque noted during these sports can be sufficient to tear the triangular fibrocartilage. Gymnastics, with its significant axial loading of the wrists, can also lead to a TFCC tear.

At least 50% of intra-articular distal radius fractures are associated with tears of the triangular fibrocartilage. However, many of these remain asymptomatic and require no treatment.

An ulnar abutment syndrome can develop as a result of distal radial fracture fragment settling. The radial collapse leads to a relative lengthening of the ulna. Palmer et al[2] demonstrated an increase in the ulnocarpal load with increasing ulnar variance.

Repetitive axial loading of the wrist in a patient with an ulnar zero or ulnar plus variance can lead to an attritional tear of the triangular fibrocartilage and ulnar abutment syndrome.

The failure of nonoperative treatment (splinting, rest, nonsteroidal anti-inflammatory drugs, activity modification, and therapy) leads the surgeon and patient to choose surgical treatment.

Savoie FH III, Field LD, Steinmann SP, eds. *The Elbow and Wrist: AANA Advanced Arthroscopic Surgical Techniques* (pp 285-293).

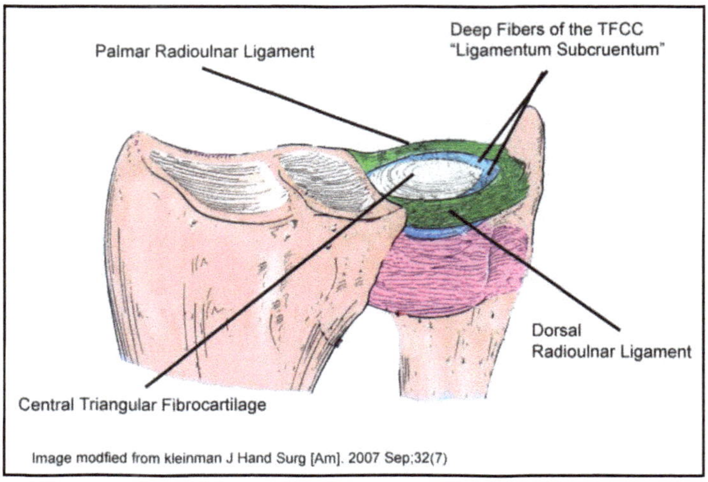

Figure 28-1. Triangular fibrocartilage anatomy. (Modified from Kleinman WB. Stability of the distal radioulna joint: biomechanics, pathophysiology, physical diagnosis, and restoration of function what we have learned in 25 years. *J Hand Surg Am.* 2007;32(7):1086-1106.)

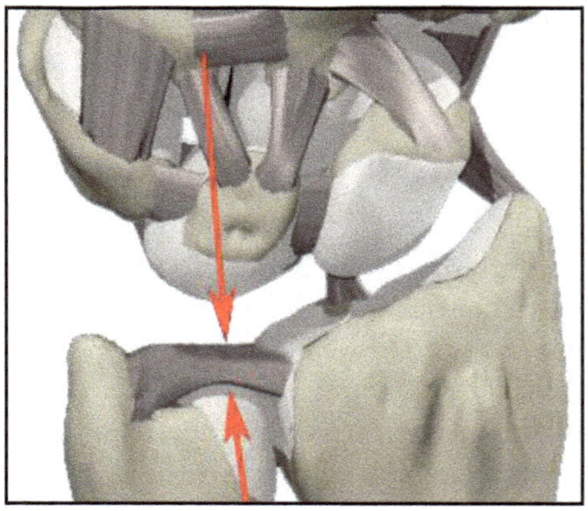

Figure 28-2. Ulnar abutment. The TFCC is compressed between the proximal ulnar lunate and the distal ulnar head. The arrows represent the compression of the TFCC between the lunate and distal ulna.

Pertinent Physical Findings

Ulnocarpal palpation can give some insight into the condition of the TFCC. The synovitis associated with a TFCC tear can render simple palpation of the ulnocarpal joint uncomfortable.

The ulnocarpal compression test (Figure 28-3) is particularly helpful in assessing patients with a suspected ulnar abutment syndrome. In this test, the patient sits in front of the examiner with the wrist in supination. The wrist is simultaneously ulnarly deviated and axially loaded while the forearm is supinated and pronated. A patient with an ulnar abutment syndrome will note pain at the ulnocarpal joint with or without popping and grinding during this maneuver.

A variation of the ulnocarpal compression test is the Lester press test (Figure 28-4).[3] The patient sits in a chair with sturdy arms and lifts his or her self off of the chair seat. Pain at the ulnocarpal joint is considered pathognomonic for a TFCC tear.

Pertinent Imaging

The radiographic evaluation of a patient with an ulnar abutment should include a standard wrist series and a Palmer 90 x 90 view (Figure 28-5).

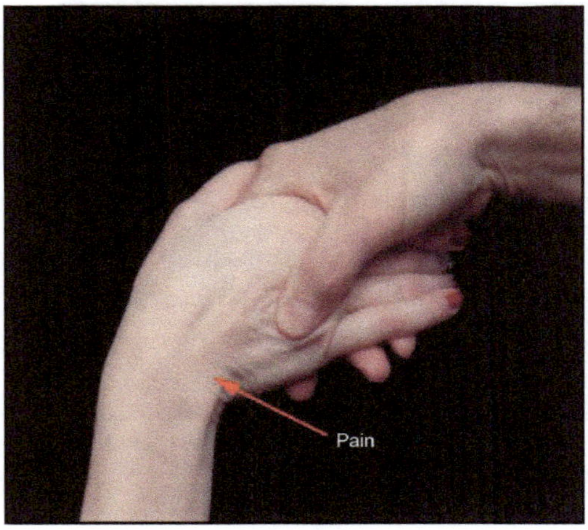

Figure 28-3. Ulnocarpal compression test.

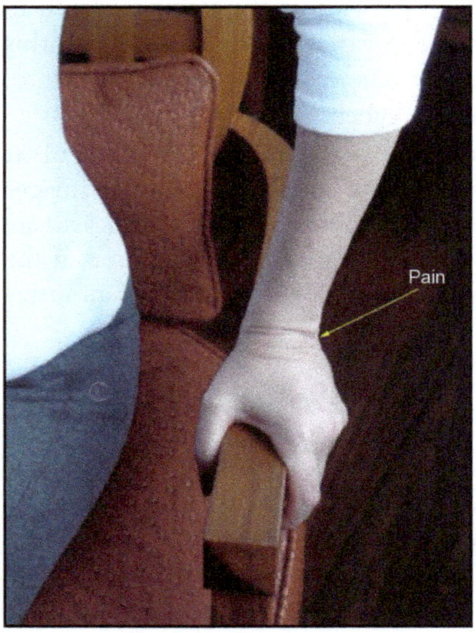

Figure 28-4. The Lester press test.

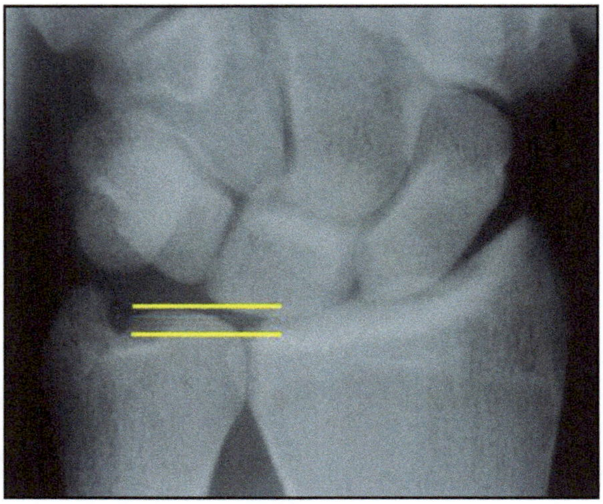

Figure 28-5. Ulnar plus variance noted on 90 x 90 view.

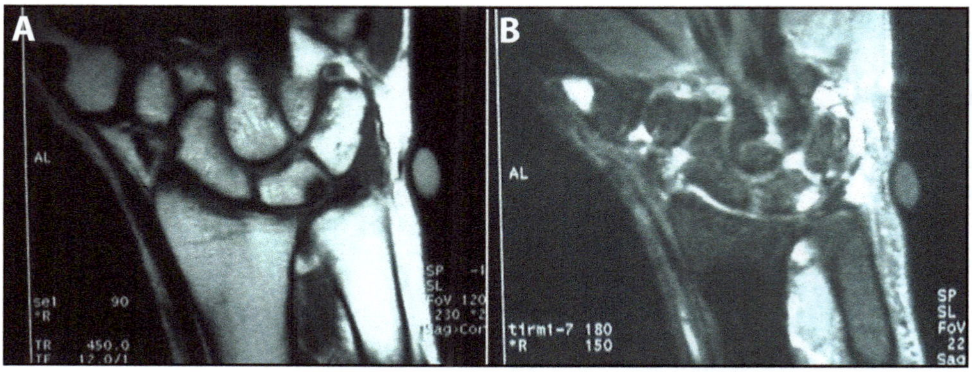

Figure 28-6. MRI of a wrist with an ulnar abutment demonstrating the change in signal at the ulnar proximal lunate on (A) T1- and (B) T2-weighted images.

The Palmer 90 x 90 view places the forearm in neutral rotation while the elbow is flexed to 90 degrees and the shoulder is abducted to 90 degrees.[4] The ulnar variance is calculated from this view. An ulnar abutment can be suspected in a patient with an ulnar zero or ulnar minus variance. The ulnar aspect of the lunate should be carefully examined for subchondral cysts.

Magnetic resonance imaging (MRI) should be considered when evaluating the patient for ulnar abutment. The MRI will demonstrate increased signal in the lunate on the T2-weighted images (Figure 28-6). This corresponds to a cyst or intraosseous edema. The triangular fibrocartilage can also be evaluated on the MRIs. Whether an MR arthrogram is needed is a function of the MR resolution. The accuracy of lower-resolution MR is increased with the addition of an intra-articular gadolinium injection.

Preoperative Planning

Preoperative evaluation should include wrist x-rays composed of a wrist series and a 90 x 90 view described by Palmer.[4] An MRI with or without an arthrogram can also be helpful.

The patient must be informed that an arthroscopically assisted ulnar shortening may not be possible should there be laxity of the ulnocarpal ligaments, a peripheral TFCC tear, or lunotriquetral laxity. The amount of shortening should be calculated preoperatively. It is generally thought that an arthroscopically assisted ulnar shortening is indicated if the ulnar plus variance is less than 4 mm.

Equipment

- Standard wrist arthroscopy equipment
- 1.9-mm wrist arthroscope
- Outflow system
- Wrist distraction tower
- Nerve hook (probe)
- Holmium:YAG laser with 70-degree side-firing laser fiber
- Radiofrequency generator and angled small joint probes
- Small joint motorized shaver with small joint shavers and burrs

Positioning and Portals

The patient is placed in the supine position. A pneumatic tourniquet it is placed on the proximal arm. The patient's involved extremity is prepped and draped in the usual fashion. The wrist is distracted using a commercially available wrist traction device.

Step-by-Step Description of the Procedure

Triangular Fibrocartilage Complex Debridement: Mechanical

The standard 3-4 and 4-5 and/or 6-R wrist arthroscopy portals are used for TFCC debridement. These portals should be wide enough to permit the easy passage of instruments. Prior to debriding the TFCC, a thorough and systematic examination of the radiocarpal, ulnocarpal, and midcarpal joints should be performed because associated intrinsic ligament injury, extrinsic ligament injury, articular pathology, and synovial pathology could impact the treatment plan. Ulnocarpal synovectomy should be performed to assure clear visualization of that joint. Initial debridement of the radial, palmar, and dorsal aspects of the TFCC tear is accomplished with a scope in the 3-4 portal while the instruments enter through the 4-5 portal. Small joint punches (straight and angled), graspers, mini-banana blades, and mini-hook knives are used to debride the TFCC. The suction punch is particularly useful. Care should be taken to not injure the overhanging lunate and triquetrum.

Once the radial and palmar aspects of the TFCC have been debrided, the arthroscope is moved to the 4-5 portal. The debridement of the ulnar aspect of the triangular fibrocartilage is accomplished by passing the instruments through the 3-4 portal. Three points must be kept in mind during debridement of the ulnar aspect of the TFCC. First, avoid injuring the ulnar attachment of the triangular fibrocartilage at the base of the ulnar styloid. Second, avoid injuring the dorsal or palmar radioulnar ligaments. If the ulnar attachment of the TFCC is transected or if the dorsal and palmar radioulnar ligaments are injured, DRUJ instability will result. Third, avoid scuffing the articular surfaces while passing the cutting/grasping instruments from the 3-4 portal across the radiocarpal joint into the ulnocarpal joint.

The dorsal aspect of the TFCC tear can usually be debrided using the 3-4 and 4-5 portals. Occasionally, however, the instruments need to be passed through the 6-U portal while the scope is placed in the 3-4 portal. Injury to the dorsal sensory branch of the ulnar nerve is avoided when using the 6-U portal by using a longitudinal portal incision and blunt dissection to reach the ulnocarpal joint capsule.

Once the TFCC has been debrided with the punches and knives, the rough edges of the debrided TFCC are smoothed using the motorized full-radius cutters. The 2.0-mm cutters are small but relatively ineffective. The 2.9-mm cutters are effective but must be controlled to avoid collateral damage to the adjacent articular surfaces.

The end point of the TFCC debridement is reached when the ulnar head is visible through the TFCC and a stable TFCC perimeter is created. Typically, a central defect measuring at least 1 cm in diameter is created (Figure 28-7).

Triangular Fibrocartilage Complex Debridement: Laser and Radiofrequency Technique

Mechanical debridement of the triangular fibrocartilage has been successful, although it can be challenging, particularly in regard to the debridement of the ulnar and dorsal aspects of the triangular fibrocartilage tear. There are 2 potential problems with mechanical TFCC debridement.

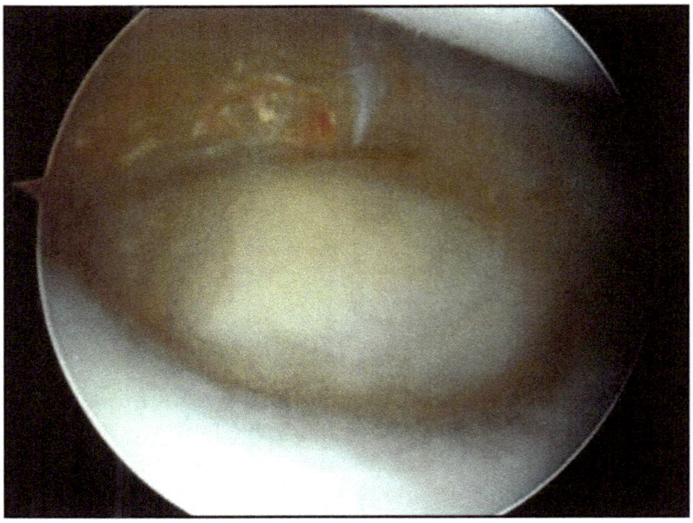

Figure 28-7. The TFCC has been debrided back to a stable edge. The ulnar head is visible.

First, the passage of the instruments across the radiocarpal joint places those joints at risk of scuffing. Second, the close proximity of the scope to the operative site (TFCC) can distort the operator's perception of the ulnocarpal joint.

The technique of laser-assisted triangular fibrocartilage debridement is similar to that of mechanical debridement of the triangular fibrocartilage, except the arthroscope can be left in the 3-4 portal while the laser probe is kept in the 4-5 portal. The laser is set to 1.4 to 1.6 J at a frequency of 15 pulses per second. With the help of a side-firing, 70-degree laser tip, the triangular fibrocartilage can be rapidly and precisely debrided. The 70-degree laser tip permits ablation of not only the radial and palmar portions of the TFCC tear, but also the ulnar and dorsal components. There is no need to bring the laser probe in through the 3-4 portal.

Radiofrequency devices have become increasing popular for TFCC debridement because of the small probe size and relatively low cost. The technique is similar to that used for laser-assisted TFCC debridement. Mono- and bipolar radiofrequency devices are currently in use. The instrument settings to be used vary with the device. Monopolar probes have a theoretical disadvantage in that the energy imparted to the TFCC flows through the adjacent tissue in the direction of the grounding pad. This could lead to tissue damage beyond the TFCC. The flow of irrigation fluid must be sufficient to cool the joint when using the radiofrequency devices and lasers.

Arthroscopic Ulnar Shortening

Arthroscopic ulnar shortening is accomplished by placing the scope in the 3-4 portal and introducing the instruments through the 4-5 portal. Occasionally, the 6-U portal can be used, as can the DRUJ portal. Although the Holmium:YAG laser is useful for ulnar shortening, the barrel abrader can also be used alone or in combination with the laser. If the Holmium:YAG laser is used, it is introduced through the 4-5 portal, and the cartilage and subchondral bone of the ulnar seat of the distal ulna are rapidly vaporized. The laser becomes less efficient once the trabeculae of the distal ulna are visible. At that point, the 2.9-mm barrel abrader is brought in to finish the shortening (Figure 28-8). It is important to avoid injury to the sigmoid notch, and frequent fluoroscopic monitoring of the amount of bone resected is mandatory. Care must be taken to fully supinate and pronate the wrist to adequately debride the ulnar head. All instruments are removed at the end of the procedure, and the wrist is ulnarly deviated, axially loaded, and supinated and pronated to be sure no clicking or popping is noted. If any clicking or popping is noted to be emanating from the area of the surgery, further ulnar resection may be required. The goal of the surgery is to create

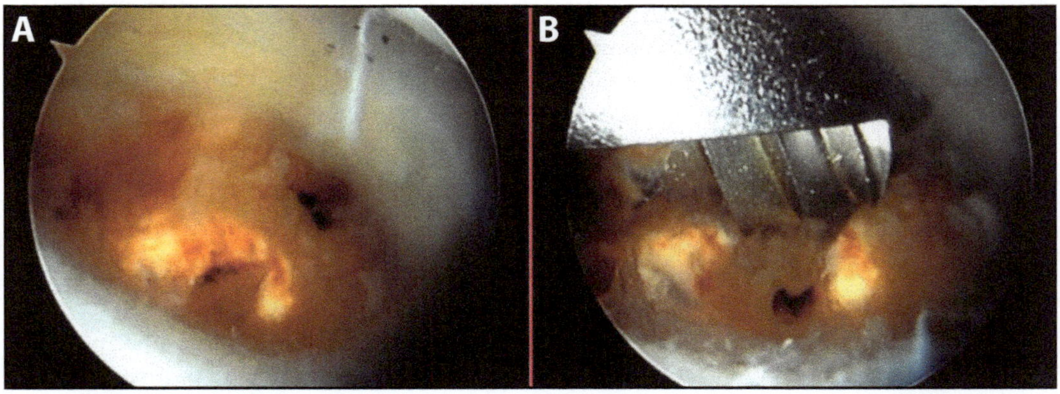

Figure 28-8. (A) The hyaline cartilage of the ulnar seat has been debrided with the laser. (B) The subchondral bone is being debrided using the barrel abrader.

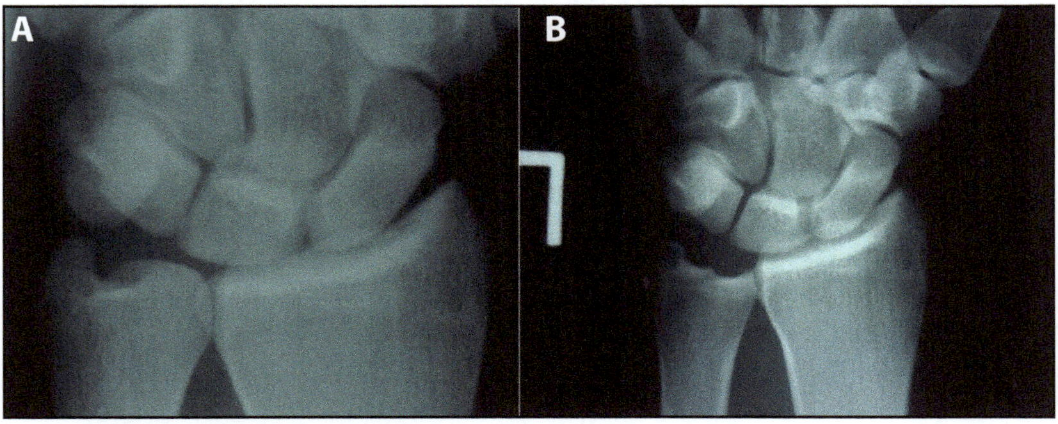

Figure 28-9. (A) Preoperative x-ray. (B) Postoperative x-ray.

an ulnar minus variance of 2 mm. Any irregularities of the remaining distal ulna should be minimized. Small irregularities, however, tend to flatten out with time (Figure 28-9).

Postoperative Protocol

The postoperative care of these patients includes the application of a volar splint followed by early range of motion. Early range of motion is critical as it leads to suppler scar and a better range of motion. The sutures (wounds are closed using subcuticular sutures of 4-0 Prolene [Ethicon]) are removed at 2 weeks. Strengthening exercises can be started at 6 weeks if needed. Premature resumption of heavy lifting or repetitive activities will lead to ulnocarpal synovitis. The patient is instructed to avoid heavy lifting for 3 months. Typically, patients are able to return to unrestricted activities in 12 weeks, although they may experience some discomfort for 6 to 12 months.

Conclusion

The results of arthroscopic debridement of traumatic triangular fibrocartilage tears have been good.[5,6] However, Minami et al[5] noted that degenerative tears (Palmer type 2) have a less favorable prognosis due to the associated ulnar wrist pathology in these patients. The authors' results[7] and those reported by Osterman,[8] Wnorowski et al,[9] and Tomaino and Weiser[10] suggest that arthroscopically assisted ulnar shortening in the properly selected patient population provides excellent and good results in more than 80% of patients. Vandenberghe et al[11] found, as did the authors,[12] no significant difference in the outcomes of arthroscopically assisted ulnar shortening and formal ulnar shortening osteotomy for the treatment of ulnar abutment syndrome.

Top Technical Pearls for the Procedure

1. Arthroscopically assisted ulnar shortening should not be combined with other procedures that require postoperative wrist immobilization because early mobilization is critical after an ulnar shortening.
2. The 4-5 and 6-R portals should be placed just distal to the distal surface of the TFCC because distal placement of the portals can lead to scuffing of the lunate and triquetrum. The surgeon should be mindful of the presence of the dorsal branch of the ulnar nerve. This nerve is at risk during the creation of all ulnar portals.
3. Injury to the underlying tendons and nerves can be avoided by creating portals using a #15 blade held gently against the skin, which is moved beneath the blade. Small transverse incisions in Langer's lines closed with a subcuticular Prolene produce a superior cosmetic result. Once the skin is cut, blunt dissection with a Hartman hemostat should be used to dissect through the subcutaneous tissue and penetrate the wrist joint capsule. The curve of the Hartman hemostat follows the palmar tilt of the distal radius.
4. The 1.9-mm arthroscope is perfectly suited to wrist arthroscopy. Its small size lessens the likelihood of scuffing the wrist joint articular surfaces.
5. Debridement of the TFCC tear must be performed carefully to avoid injury to the peripheral attachments of the TFCC and the dorsal and palmar radioulnar ligaments. Overaggressive debridement can lead to DRUJ instability.
6. A systematic approach to the excision of ulnar head is critical. The assistant must take the wrist from full supination to full pronation while the surgeon maintains the arthroscope in the 3-4 portal and the instruments in the ulnar portals. The ulnar head is debrided because it is presented to the surgeon by the assistant during the rotation of the DRUJ.
7. Rehabilitation is essential to the ultimate success of the procedure. The wrist should not be loaded for at least 4 to 6 weeks.

References

1. Kleinman WB. Stability of the distal radioulna joint: biomechanics, pathophysiology, physical diagnosis, and restoration of function what we have learned in 25 years. *J Hand Surg Am.* 2007;32(7):1086-1106.
2. Palmer AK, Glisson RR, Werner FW. Relationship between ulnar variance and triangular fibrocartilage complex thickness. *J Hand Surg Am.* 1984;9(5):681-682.
3. Lester B, Halbrecht J, Levy IM, Gaudinez R. "Press test" for office diagnosis of triangular fibrocartilage complex tears of the wrist. *Ann Plast Surg.* 1995;35(1):41-45.
4. Palmer AK, Glisson RR, Werner FW. Ulnar variance determination. *J Hand Surg Am.* 1982;7(4):376-379.
5. Minami A, Ishikawa J, Suenaga N, Kasashima T. Clinical results of treatment of triangular fibrocartilage complex tears by arthroscopic debridement. *J Hand Surg Am.* 1996;21(3):406-411.

6. Westkaemper JG, Mitsionis G, Giannakopoulos PN, Sotereanos DG. Wrist arthroscopy for the treatment of ligament and triangular fibrocartilage complex injuries. *Arthroscopy.* 1998;14(5):479-483.
7. Nagle DJ, Bernstein MA. Laser-assisted arthroscopic ulnar shortening. *Arthroscopy.* 2002;18(9):1046-1051.
8. Osterman AL. Arthroscopic debridement of triangular fibrocartilage complex tears. *Arthroscopy.* 1990;6(2):120-124.
9. Wnorowski DC, Palmer AK, Werner FW, Fortino MD. Anatomic and biomechanical analysis of the arthroscopic wafer procedure. *Arthroscopy.* 1992;8(2):204-212.
10. Tomaino MM, Weiser RW. Combined arthroscopic TFCC debridement and wafer resection of the distal ulna in wrists with triangular fibrocartilage complex tears and positive ulnar variance. *J Hand Surg Am.* 2001;26(6):1047-1052.
11. Vandenberghe L, Degreff I, Didden K, Moermans A, Koorneef P, DeSmet L. Ulnar shortening or arthroscopic wafer resection for ulnar impaction syndrome. *Acta Orthop Belg.* 2012;78(3):323-326.
12. Bernstein MA, Nagle DJ, Martinez A, Stogin JM Jr, Wiedrich TA. A comparison of combined arthroscopic triangular fibrocartilage complex debridement and arthroscopic wafer distal ulna resection versus arthroscopic triangular fibrocartilage complex debridement and ulnar shortening osteotomy for ulnocarpal abutment syndrome. *Arthroscopy.* 2004;20(4):392-401.

29

Arthroscopic Excision of Dorsal Wrist Ganglions

A. Lee Osterman, MD and Ashkon Razavi, MD

Introduction

Ganglions (also known as *ganglion cysts*), the most frequently encountered soft tissue tumor of the hand and wrist, are cystic masses associated with synovial joints or tendon sheaths that contain mucinous fluid. Its nomenclature is derived from the Greek word *ganglion*, meaning knot of tissue. Descriptions of ganglions have been found dating back to the day of Hippocrates, who contended that the masses contained mucoid flesh.[1]

Ganglions tend to present in young adults in the second to fourth decades of life and are 2 to 4 times more likely in women than men.[2-4] They may appear suddenly over the course of weeks or days or more insidiously. Symptoms associated with ganglions are largely dependent on their proximity to surrounding structures, or they may be asymptomatic. Commonly, patients present with a 1- to 2-cm fluctuant mass on the dorsum wrist over the dorsal scapholunate (SL) ligament and complain of a dull ache, which is likely the result of compression of the terminal branches of the posterior interosseous nerve. Patients may also complain of pain with active range of motion and often of the cosmesis of the mass.

The clinical work-up for a suspected ganglion begins with a comprehensive history. Aside from the traditional questions regarding duration, chronicity, and exacerbating factors, every attempt should be made to tease out details of prior injuries. A thorough physical examination should be conducted, including provocative maneuvers that attempt to detect ligamentous injuries of the carpus, particularly involving the SL ligamentous complex. Plain x-rays are commonly unremarkable. Magnetic resonance imaging (MRI) can be clinically valuable, however, to confirm the diagnosis and elucidate the relationship of the ganglion to the surrounding neurovascular structures. In addition, MRI can be useful to clarify if a ganglion arises from the SL ligament and to visualize an associated stalk. Ultrasound imaging[5] is another useful tool to define the diagnosis of a ganglion compared to other types of similar wrist masses, such as lipoma and carpometacarpal boss.

There are numerous theories regarding the etiology and pathoanatomy of these masses. Cross-sectional studies suggest that they arise from a mucoid degeneration process, whereas other investigators, using arthrographic MRI and ultrasound modalities, demonstrated that a unidirectional

Savoie FH III, Field LD, Steinmann SP, eds. *The Elbow and Wrist: AANA Advanced Arthroscopic Surgical Techniques* (pp 295-303).

valve mechanism between the wrist joint and the ganglion is responsible.[6,7] Trauma that leads to acute or chronic ligamentous injury, most notably at the junction between the dorsal fibers of the SL ligament and the dorsal wrist capsule, has also been proposed as a potential cause.[6,8] It is reasonable to conclude that a combination of these mechanisms are at play and result in a final common pathway.

An estimated 25,000 resections are performed yearly to remove ganglions, making it one of the most frequently performed procedures in hand surgery. The theoretical advantages of arthroscopic resection include faster recovery, less capsular scarring and stiffness, and the ability to diagnose concomitant pathology. The primary indication for surgical resection is a painful mass on the dorsum wrist that limits activities of daily living. Occasionally, concerns regarding the cosmesis of the deformity may justify resection. However, patients should be reminded, particularly if a traditional open technique is contemplated, of the old adage that they would be trading a bump for a scar. This may be why arthroscopic resection has gained in popularity and acceptance.

Indications

- Dorsal wrist ganglia
- Volar wrist ganglia

Controversial Indications

- Recurrent wrist ganglia
- Occult wrist ganglia
- Intraosseous carpal ganglia

Indications and contraindications for arthroscopic dorsal wrist ganglion resection are evolving. The authors' indications include primary and recurrent dorsal ganglia. It is assumed that the majority of dorsal wrist ganglia originate from the SL interval. Given the capsular limitation in the wrist, however, this interval is only partially visualized from the radiocarpal joint. One study[9] observed that cysts communicated with the midcarpal joint in 75% of cases. Although the majority of cysts may be resected successfully through an isolated radiocarpal portal, some cysts may need supplemental debridement from the midcarpal joint.

Regarding recurrent cysts, one group of investigators[10] suggested that recurrent cysts following previous open surgical excision should be considered a contraindication for arthroscopic resection. Appropriate concerns are the risk of extensor tendon injury due to their potential displacement by the scar from the previous surgery. Thus, most previous studies have used recurrence as an exclusion criterion. In the authors' experience, successful results can be achieved arthroscopically in patients with a recurrent ganglion. In the authors' series[3] in which 15% of patients had recurrent ganglia, results were comparable to outcomes of primary cyst resections.

Pertinent Physical Findings and Imaging

- Palpable soft mass on dorsum of wrist in area of the SL joint
- Normal wrist x-rays
- Positive ultrasound

The clinical work-up for a suspected ganglion begins with a comprehensive history. The first question to answer when a patient presents with a mass is whether it is a cyst or a tumor. Occurrence, progression, size, shape, texture, the presence or absence of pain, and association with traumatic or repetitive activities should be addressed. Cysts can decrease in size, whereas tumors usually do not become smaller. On physical examination, transillumination can be helpful in differentiating a cyst from a tumor. This is performed by holding a penlight up against the lesion. A cystic lesion will allow the light to transmit through its fluid medium.

Although the appearance and feel of the mass are fairly classic, a thorough physical examination should be conducted, including provocative maneuvers that attempt to detect ligamentous injuries of the carpus, particularly involving the SL ligamentous complex.

Plain x-rays are commonly unremarkable. An MRI can be clinically valuable, however, to confirm the diagnosis and to elucidate the relationship of the ganglion to surrounding neurovascular structures. In addition, an MRI can be useful to clarify if a ganglion arises from the SL ligament and to visualize an associated stalk. Ultrasound imaging[5] is another useful tool to define the diagnosis of a ganglion compared to other types of similar wrist masses, such as lipoma and carpometacarpal boss.

Controversy of Intra-Articular Associations

The dorsal ganglion may be an overt sign of intra-articular pathology. Povlsen and Peckett[11] found intra-articular abnormalities in 75% of patients with painful ganglia. They concluded that, similar to popliteal cysts in the knee, the dorsal ganglion was a marker of joint abnormality. Osterman and Raphael[2] found abnormalities in 42% predominated by findings at the SL ligament (24%), triangular fibrocartilage (8%), lunotriquetral ligament (3%), and significant chondromalacia. Despite only the ganglion being treated, wrist pain resolved in all cases. Edwards and Johansen[12] elaborated on this notion by showing that the majority of ganglia are associated with type II and III SL and type III lunotriquetral laxity. Langner[13] found a high incidence of triangular fibrocartilage injuries. Although it is reasonable to propose that increased intercarpal pathology may contribute to ganglion formation, the actual significance is unclear given that the natural incidence of these ligamentous laxities in the general population is not known.

Equipment

- 2.7- and 2.9-mm arthroscope
- Wrist traction tower
- 2.9- and 3.5-mm shaver
- Small suction punch
- Radiofrequency probe (optional)

Positioning and Step-by-Step Description of the Procedure

The patient is positioned in the supine position, and regional or general anesthesia is administered. A tourniquet should be placed on every patient as a precaution and inflated in the event that intra-articular bleeding obscures visualization. Although the patient's arm is suspended in a traction, finger traps should be placed around all 4 fingers and suspended from a traction tower. The tower should be adjusted to position the wrist in neutral to mild flexion, and 10 to 15 lb of traction is applied. Several surface anatomical landmarks are identified, including Lister's tubercle, the course of the extensor carpi ulnaris tendon, the ulnar styloid, and the perimeter of the ganglion itself. The location of the 6-R portal is then established by identifying the soft spot

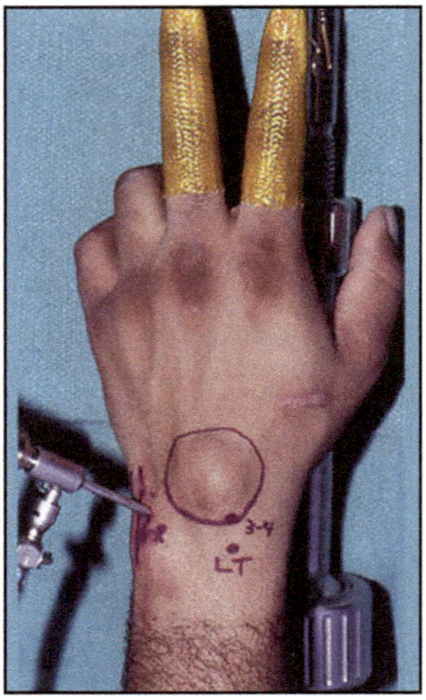
Figure 29-1. Ganglion marked with entry portal 6-R.

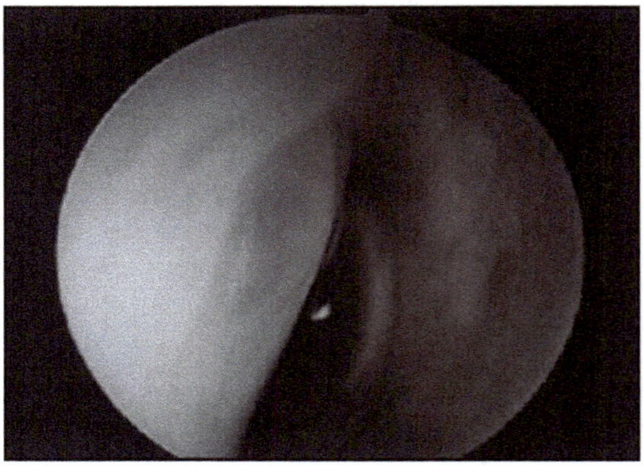
Figure 29-2. Sessile intraligamentous stalk at the juncture of the membranous and fibrous juncture of the SL ligament seen 40% of time.

just lateral to the extensor carpi ulnaris and distal to the end of the ulna (Figure 29-1). Care should be taken to ensure entry does not damage the triangular fibrocartilage. The more radial 3-4 or 4-5 portals are avoided at this time to prevent inadvertently decompressing the cyst. An 18-gauge needle, attached to a syringe filled with 10 cc of normal saline, is inserted into the portal, and the joint is insufflated. This injection often further inflates the ganglion. It can also identify if there are abnormal flow connections to the distal radioulnar joint or the midcarpal joints. A #11 blade is then used to make a stab incision, taking care to advance the blade no deeper than the dermal layer of the skin to minimize risk of iatrogenic injury to subcutaneous veins, extensor tendons, and more importantly, the dorsal cutaneous nerves. A small straight or curved hemostat is then used to dilate the incision by spreading in a proximal-distal direction and advanced into the joint with the correct entry point identified by a return of the injected saline. The trocar for a standard 2.7-mm arthroscope is then inserted at the same trajectory.

The 2.7-mm arthroscopic camera is directed across the radiocarpal joint to the membranous portion of the SL ligament. Once there, the scope is directed dorsally up the ligament toward the dorsal capsule. The ganglion stalk usually arises at the juncture of the membranous and dorsal fibrous portion of the SL ligament (Figure 29-2). Often, the ganglion is transilluminated. The stalk of the ganglion may be enhanced by applying gentle outside pressure to the ganglion. Yao and Trindade[14] suggested the use of methylene blue to help identify the stalk and confirm its excision.

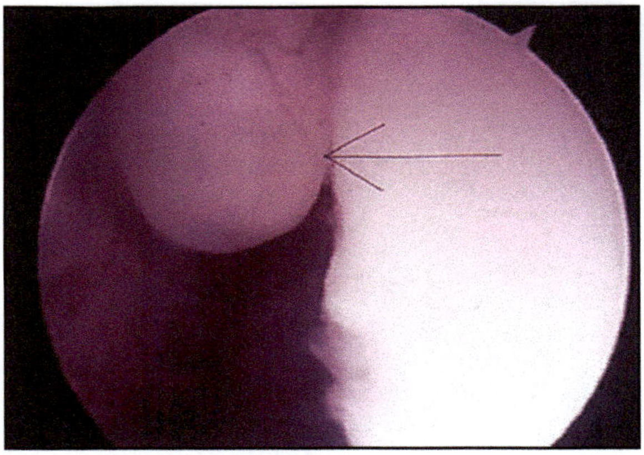

Figure 29-3. Pedunculated stalk seen 35% of time. Arrow is pointing at the peduculated ganglion stalk.

Three patterns of ganglion stalk have been seen.[2] In 40% of them, there was a sessile cyst seen directly arising from the SL ligament. In 35%, a pedunculated stalk (Figure 29-3) was noted, and in 25%, no defined stalk was present, but there was a large amount of redundant capsule with or without synovitis in this area instead of an actual cystic stalk.

The authors recommend a method that attempts to avoid decompressing the cyst with the shaver prior to actual excision to observe the possibility of an undisturbed cystic stalk and its path elsewhere outside the radiocarpal joint. The working portal is created adjacent to the immediate area of the cyst, rather than directly over the 3-4 portal. Consequently, this modified working portal is usually just distal and sometimes slightly radial to the actual 3-4 portal. A 2.9-mm, full-radius shaver is introduced through this modified portal, with every attempt not to decompress the cyst with simple introduction of the shaver. If the cyst is decompressed too soon, the surgeon cannot confirm by palpation whether the cyst was adequately resected or simply decompressed.

Although the procedure implies that the cyst is removed by the arthroscopy, in actuality, the arthroscopic resection disrupts the joint origin of the cyst and the communication between the cyst and the joint, leaving a deflated sac behind that cannot reinflate. Eventually, the empty sac is resorbed.

The focus of the resection begins at the site of ganglion stalk or the redundant capsular material. The presence or absence of a defined stalk has shown no effect on the outcomes of the resection.

When a landmark of a stalk is found, the surgeon may begin capsulotomy. If no stalk is identified, the debridement begins adjacent to the dorsal SL ligament and distal capsular reflection. Commonly, the cyst travels within the capsular reflection as it communicates with the SL joint. Upon initial debridement of the capsular reflection, viscous cystic fluid may occasionally be visualized escaping into the joint.

Debridement continues until approximately 1 cm of capsule has been removed (Figure 29-4). This should be done carefully because it is easy to inadvertently cut into an extensor tendon dorsal to the capsule or into the adjacent dorsal fibrous component of the SL ligament.

A common mistake is to make the capsulotomy too small, which is easy to do under magnification. Using the 2.9-mm shaver as a reference is helpful in gauging the size of the capsulotomy. Another common mistake is to create an incomplete capsulotomy, which fails to communicate with the extra-articular space. The authors no longer advise direct visualization of the extensor tendons to verify that complete capsulotomy has been performed, but rather rely upon the arthroscopic visualization of the capsular resection and the palpable disappearance of the ganglion. The arthroscope itself is then inserted, and a step-wise evaluation of the proximal carpal row, intrinsic and extrinsic ligaments, and triangular fibrocartilage complex is undertaken to evaluate for coexisting pathology. A needle with air and fluid is placed in the midcarpal to check for any abnormal communications between the mid- and radiocarpal joints (ie, bubbles appearing across the SL ligament).

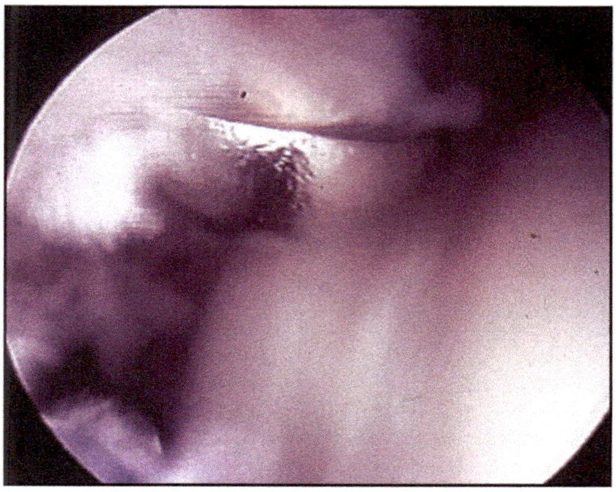

Figure 29-4. Redundant capsule being resected.

Once the capsulotomy and cyst excision have been completed from the radiocarpal joint and any coexistent pathology has been addressed, the camera is removed, and the dorsal wrist is palpated to determine the efficacy of the debridement. If a portion of the cyst remains, this implies some degree of communication between the cyst and the midcarpal joint that has not yet been addressed. To remedy this, the arthroscopic camera is introduced through an ulnar midcarpal portal, and a similar capsulotomy is performed adjacent to the SL interval through the radial midcarpal portal. During debridement from the midcarpal joint, a fenestration is often created between the midcarpal and radiocarpal joint through the capsular reflection. Even if no midcarpal communication is present, the surgeon should always complete the midcarpal portion of the arthroscopic examination to check for pathology, such as hamate impingement on a type II lunate. Upon removing the arthroscopic equipment, the wrist is palpated again to ensure that the cyst has been completely excised.

Removing the extra-articular ganglion sac is not necessary because it often resorbs over time once detached from its origin at the joint. If the cyst is particularly large, resorption may take some time, and patients may complain about the residual prominence on the dorsum of the hand. Removal of such a large sac is done by enlarging the 3-4 portal and manually pulling out the sac with a hemostat.

Some surgeons close each arthroscopic portal with one simple nonabsorbable suture, but other surgeons leave them open with no cosmetic detriment. Because open arthroscopic portals rarely form sinus tracts,[8] the authors prefer to close their wounds. A sterile wrist dressing and a splint supporting the wrist and metacarpal phalangeal joints to protect any inadvertent injury to the extensor tendons are used in all cases.

Postoperative Protocol

Immediately, postoperative digital motion is encouraged in the bandage, and sutures are removed in 7 to 10 days. Supervised therapy is seldom required. If there is residual fullness over the ganglion or its portal, the use of elastomer as a pressure scar modulator may be helpful. Activity is resumed as tolerated and the patient is advised against forceful loading of the wrist for 6 weeks. Reduced recovery times, less postoperative pain, and quicker return to work and athletics have been reported after arthroscopic ganglion resection.[3,7,12,15-19]

Potential Complications

- Ganglion recurrence
- Extensor tendon injury
- SL injury
- Portal fistula

The overall complication rate of wrist arthroscopy is estimated to be 2%, although some speculate that this figure is an underestimate.[20,21] Reported complications include superficial infections, fistula cysts,[8,22] iatrogenic injury to the cutaneous nerves (the terminal branches of the superficial branch of the radial nerve and particularly the transverse radioulnar branch of the dorsal sensory branch of the ulnar nerve), complex region pain syndrome/reflex sympathetic dystrophy, extensor tendon injuries,[23] and chondral damage. The dorsal sensory branch of the ulnar nerve is particularly vulnerable because of its anatomical variability near the 6-R portal.[20,24] Risk of nerve injury can be minimized by strict adherence to the technique previously described when establishing portals (ie, incision of only the dermal layer of the skin followed by longitudinal dilatation by a blunt hemostat). Iatrogenic injury to the articular cartilage can be minimized by precise placement of portals and avoiding forceful introduction and use of instruments.

Results

Open excision of a dorsal wrist ganglion is not always a simple procedure. Faithful and Seeto[25] reported on 59 open ganglionectomies followed for more than 5 years. This group had a recurrence rate of 14%. Of the patients, 28% had residual pain or functional limitations and 8% were frankly unhappy with the procedure.

Clinical outcomes following arthroscopic ganglion resection have been investigated and compared to those of the open technique by several authors.[2,3,7,9,10,12,15,16,18,19,26-29] The authors' prospective study[2] included 38 patients with palpable ganglions with an average size of 9 mm and all of whom had failed aspiration. The average age was 26 years, with 28 women and 10 men. At follow-up averaging 39 months, no patient was lost and the satisfaction rate was 100%. There were no recurrences. Two patients had residual discomfort. All patients reported full wrist functionality.

Rizzo et al[18] found improved postoperative motion and grip strength, no cases of SL instability, and recurrences in 2 (4.9%) of their 41 patients. Shih et al[29] concluded that the arthroscopic technique is a reasonable alternative compared to open excision despite experiencing a recurrence rate of 15.6% in their 32 patients. Kang et al[28] presented a prospective, randomized study comparing arthroscopic resection with more traditional open techniques. This study evaluated patients at 4 to 8 weeks and again at 1 year postoperatively and found no difference in outcomes other than improved cosmesis and faster return of wrist motion. At 12-month follow-up, this study demonstrated that the recurrence rates with arthroscopic resection (3 of 28 patients, 10.7%) were comparable to those of open excision (2 of 23 patients, 8.7%). Aslani et al[15] also compared pre- and postoperative metrics and found statistically significant increases in wrist flexion (mean, 12.7 degrees), wrist extension (mean, 10.5 degrees), and grip strength (6.4 mm Hg). Edwards and Johansen[12] prospectively evaluated grip strength, wrist motion, and Disabilities of the Arm, Shoulder, and Hand scores in 55 patients with dorsal wrist ganglions who underwent arthroscopic resection with a minimum follow-up of 24 months. At 2 years, all patients demonstrated motion to within 5 degrees of preoperative measurements, and there were no recurrences, although 10 patients had recurrent ganglions previously treated with open resection. In addition, preoperative Disabilities of the Arm, Shoulder, and Hand scores improved from 14.2 to 1.7 at 6 weeks and remained stable at 2 years.

Despite a paucity of studies that prospectively compare arthroscopic ganglion resection with traditional open excision, these studies suggest that the less invasive arthroscopic method offers patients substantial increases in function and pain relief. Moreover, the incidence of ganglion recurrence seems to be comparable between the 2 methods. In addition to having the theoretical advantages of resulting in less wrist stiffness and allowing faster surgical recovery, arthroscopic ganglion resection has also become common practice due to its low complication rate.

Top Technical Pearls for the Procedure

1. Mark out the ganglion perimeter.
2. The initial visualization portal is the 6-R portal and the operative portal is the 3-4 portal made through the ganglion.
3. Evaluate the dorsal aspect of the SL ligament prior to making the 3-4 portal.
4. Resect the cyst, any redundant capsule, and the ganglion stalk, including the origin from the SL ligament, and palpate the area to confirm complete excision of the cyst.
5. Always scope the midcarpal joint to complete the arthroscopic evaluation.

References

1. Soren A. Pathogenesis and treatment of ganglion. *Clin Orthop Relat Res.* 1966;48:173-179.
2. Osterman AL, Raphael J. Arthroscopic resection of dorsal ganglion of the wrist. *Hand Clin.* 1995;11(1):7-12.
3. Osterman AL, Jander R. Arthroscopic excision of wrist ganglia. In: Trumble TE, ed. *Wrist and Elbow Reconstruction and Arthroscopy: A Master Skills Publication.* Rosemont, IL: American Society for Surgery of the Hand; 2006:267-275.
4. Singh D, Culp RW. Arthroscopic ganglionectomy. *J Am Soc Surg Hand.* 2002;2(1):33-38.
5. Yamamoto M, Kurimoto S, Okui M, Tatebe M, Shinohara T, Hirata H. Sonography-guided arthroscopy for wrist ganglion. *J Hand Surg Am.* 2012;37(7):1411-1415.
6. Andrén L, Eiken O. Arthrographic studies of wrist ganglions. *J Bone Joint Surg Am.* 1971;53(2):299-302.
7. Nishikawa S, Toh S, Miura H, Arai K, Irie T. Arthroscopic diagnosis and treatment of dorsal wrist ganglion. *J Hand Surg Br.* 2001;26(6):547-549.
8. Naam NH. Synovial fistula as a complication of recurrent dorsal wrist ganglion excision: case report. *J Hand Surg Am.* 2012;37(6):1225-1228.
9. Geissler WB. Arthroscopic excision of dorsal wrist ganglia. *Tech Hand Up Extrem Surg.* 1998;2(3):196-201.
10. Kim JP, Seo JB, Park HG, Park YH. Arthroscopic excision of dorsal wrist ganglion: factors related to recurrence and postoperative residual pain. *Arthroscopy.* 2013;29(6):1019-1024.
11. Povlsen B, Peckett WR. Arthroscopic findings in patients with painful wrist ganglia. *Scan J Plast Reconstr Surg Hand Surg.* 2001;35(3):323-328.
12. Edwards SG, Johansen JA. Prospective outcomes and associations of wrist ganglion cysts resected arthroscopically. *J Hand Surg Am.* 2009;34(3):395-400.
13. Langner I, Krueger PC, Merk HR, Ekkernkamp A, Zach A. Ganglions of the wrist and associated triangular fibrocartilage lesions: a prospective study in arthroscopically-treated patients. *J Hand Surg.* 2012;37(8):1561-1567.
14. Yao J, Trindade MC. Color-aided visualization of dorsal wrist ganglion stalks aids in complete arthroscopic excision. *Arthroscopy.* 2011;27(3):425-429.
15. Aslani H, Najafi A, Zaaferani Z. Prospective outcomes of arthroscopic treatment of dorsal wrist ganglia. *Orthopedics.* 2012;35(3):e365-e370.

16. Chassat R, Nourissat G, Chaumeil G, Dumontier C. Arthroscopic treatment of dorsal ganglion cyst at the wrist. About 54 cases [in French]. *Chir Main.* 2006;25(3-4):146-151.
17. Wiedrich T, Osterman A. Arthroscopic excision of dorsal carpal ganglion cysts. *Oper Tech Plast Reconstr Surg.* 2003;9(4):118-123.
18. Rizzo M, Berger RA, Steinman SP, Bishop AT. Arthroscopic resection in the management of dorsal wrist ganglions: results with a minimum 2-year follow-up period. *J Hand Surg.* 2004;29(1):59-62.
19. Rocchi L, Canal A, Pelaez J, Fanfani F, Catalano F. Results and complications in dorsal and volar wrist ganglia arthroscopic resection. *Hand Surg.* 2006;11(1-2):21-26.
20. Ahsan ZS, Yao J. Complications of wrist arthroscopy. *Arthroscopy.* 2012;28(6):855-859.
21. Gupta R, Bozentka DJ, Osterman AL. Wrist arthroscopy: principles and clinical applications. *J Am Acad Orthop Surg.* 2001;9(3):200-209.
22. Shirley DS, Mullet H, Stanley JK. Extensor tendon sheath fistula formation as a complication of wrist arthroscopy. *Arthroscopy.* 2008;24(11):1311-1312.
23. Cooper AR, Elfar JC. Extensor tendon lacerations from arthroscopic excision of dorsal wrist ganglion: case report. *J Hand Surg Am.* 2013;38(10):1957-1959.
24. Warhold LG, Ruth RM . Complications of wrist arthroscopy and how to prevent them. *Hand Clin.* 1995;11(1):81-89.
25. Faithfull DK, Seeto BG. The simple wrist ganglion--more than a minor surgical procedure? *Hand Surg.* 2000;5(2):139-143.
26. Gallego S, Mathoulin C. Arthroscopic resection of dorsal wrist ganglia: 114 cases with minimum follow-up of 2 years. *Arthroscopy.* 2003;26(12):1675-1682.
27. Head L, Gencarelli JR, Allen M, Boyd KU. Wrist ganglion treatment: systematic review and meta-analysis. *J Hand Surg Am.* 2015;40(3):546.e8-553.e8.
28. Kang L, Akelman E, Weiss AP. Arthroscopic versus open dorsal ganglion excision: a prospective, randomized comparison of rates of recurrence and of residual pain. *J Hand Surg Am.* 2008;33(4):471-475.
29. Shih JT, Hung ST, Lee HM, Tan CM. Dorsal ganglion of the wrist: results of treatment by arthroscopic resection. *Hand Surg.* 2002;7(1):1-5.

Please see videos on the accompanying website at

www.routledge.com/9781630910013

Section V

THE WRIST
Advanced Procedures

30

Lunotriquetral Tears

Mike Moskal, MD

Introduction

Arthroscopic capsulodesis of the lunotriquetral (LT) joint is an all-arthroscopic suture plication procedure combined with arthroscopic reduction and LT joint pinning. The LT ligament complex is composed of the volar, middle, and dorsal portion of the LT ligament[1] and the ulnocarpal ligament. The volar LT ligament is the primary restraint for LT translation, and the dorsal portion resists rotation.[2] The ulnocarpal ligament is composed of the ulnolunate (UL), ulnotriquetral (UT), and ulnocapitate (UC) ligaments. The UL and UT ligaments originate from the volar radioulnar ligament of the triangular fibrocartilage complex (TFCC) and inserts into the lunate, triquetrum, and volar LT ligament; the UC is just volar to the UL and UT ligaments, originates from the palmar fovea, and inserts upon the ulnar volar portion of the capitate.[3]

Isolated LT injuries may be due to a dorsally applied force with wrist flexion, resulting in injury of the LT joint while sparing injury to the volar radiolunotriquetral ligament.[4,5] However, LT injuries are typically associated with wrist hyperextension and radial deviation, such as a fall or lifting injuries. Loading the hypothenar eminence from a fall on an outstretched hand in maximal extension and radial deviation allows for loading in a reverse of the lesser arc pattern of perilunate injury and results in isolated LT injury. Wrist hyperextension or hyperextension–radial deviation results in substantial strain to the UC and UT ligaments and on the foveal and palmar styloid insertions of the TFCC.[6-8] Carpal ligament injuries form a spectrum from elastic elongation to permanent stretch to tear.[9]

After arthroscopic evaluation of the LT complex spectrum of injury, arthroscopic reduction and pinning of the LT joint with concomitant ulnocarpal ligament suture plication is designed to augment the volar LT joint while shortening the ulnocarpal ligament length to act as a checkrein on excessive LT motion while tightening the prestyloid recess tension in the ulnar distal radioulnar joint capsule. Tightening of the ulnocarpal ligaments and TFCC has been the proposed mechanism associated with reduced symptoms associated with ulnar shortening osteotomy.[10-12]

Savoie FH III, Field LD, Steinmann SP, eds. *The Elbow and Wrist: AANA Advanced Arthroscopic Surgical Techniques* (pp 307-313).

Indications

The primary indication for arthroscopic stabilization of LT injuries is failure of nonoperative management and the absence of static volar intercalated segment instability. Clinical scenarios appropriate for arthroscopic treatment may involve the following anatomical pathology:

- Isolated LT instability
- LT instability associated with TFCC traumatic and/or degenerative tears
- LT instability, degenerative TFCC tears in combination with ulnar abutment syndrome

Controversial Indications

- Compromise of the dorsal extrinsic ligaments (dorsal radiotriquetral and scaphotriquetral) with LT instability producing a static volar intercalated segment instability deformity and/or disruption of the ulnocarpal ligament

Pertinent Physical Findings

A more comprehensive physical examination should include the following:

- Inspection
- Range of motion
- Palpation

Although there is no best test, the following are helpful:

- LT shear (involves dorsal translation force to the pisiform/triquetrum while volarly translating the lunate)
- LT ballottement (attempts to volarly and dorsally translate the pisiform/triquetrum while the lunate is stabilized)
- LT compression (comprises a radial-directed compression force upon the triquetrum [from the ulnar wrist] into the lunate)

For each test, appropriate reproducible pain response is assessed. Ballottement and shear translation should be compared to the contralateral wrist; crepitus may accompany an unstable LT joint.

Pertinent Imaging

- X-rays
  - Zero rotation posteroanterior view
  - True lateral views
  - Particular attention should be focused toward ulnar variance, LT interval and the integrity of the subchondral joint surfaces, greater and lesser arc continuity, and LT joint widening, and carpal angles should be recorded. Wrist x-rays with LT ligament tears do not often reveal abnormality; a posteroanterior clenched fist stress view and radial and ulnar deviated posteroanterior view may provide evidence of dynamic instability.
- Magnetic resonance arthrography (MRA)
  - Beneficial for bone, cartilage, and soft tissue evaluation. In general, reliability of magnetic resonance imaging assessment has been called into question for LT ligament injuries;

however, variation in technical assessment and radiologist oversight has a role in imaging assessment.

- Multidetector computed tomography arthrography
  - Has been shown to be more sensitive than MRA, especially for partial LT ligament tears[13]
- Combined multidetector computed tomography arthrography and MRA
  - Can provide enhanced articular and nonarticular structures of the wrist but may be cost prohibitive

Equipment

- Hand table and wrist traction tower system with mesh nylon finger traps
- Sterile tourniquet, marking pen, #11 blade
- Gravity or mechanical infusion pump for fluid management
- Hemostats
- 18-gauge spinal needle
- Small joint (2.5- or 2.7-mm) scope with small hand instrument
- Small joint power instruments, including shaver and thermal probe, if desired
- Sutures (2-0 monofilament polydioxanone)
- Smooth K-wires (1.1 mm)
- Have available a TFCC repair kit and arthroscopic burr in case of TFCC repair and wafer procedure

Positioning and Portals

The patient is placed supine on the operating bed with a hand table attached to the bed so that his or her arm is in the middle of the hand table. Often, shifting the patient to the operative side of the bed enhances arm position. A fluoroscopy unit should be brought in to ensure that adequate imaging is possible. Typically, the arthroscopic video and power system are positioned on the opposite side of the patient to allow a clear view of the monitor by the surgeon and assistant. A Mayo stand is used to place the camera, power instruments, and handheld instruments. The Mayo stand is initially positioned near the video tower and then brought over the patient after definitive draping. Initially, position the arm with 90 degrees abduction, 90 degrees of elbow flexion, and forearm pronation.

Step-by-Step Description of the Procedure

An examination under anesthesia should be performed. Draw bone and soft tissue landmarks, including approximate portal sites, once the wrist is placed into the traction tower and after applying longitudinal traction upon the wrist.

Radiocarpal portals used during arthroscopic capsulodesis are the 3-4, 6-R, and volar 6-U. The volar 6-U portal is located just volar to the 6-U portal at the level of the volar wrist. The volar 6-U portal position is designed to optimize suture passage around the ulnocarpal ligaments. Depending on the individual clinical situation, a 4-5 portal is helpful. During LT reduction and pinning, the radial midcarpal and ulnar midcarpal portals are used.

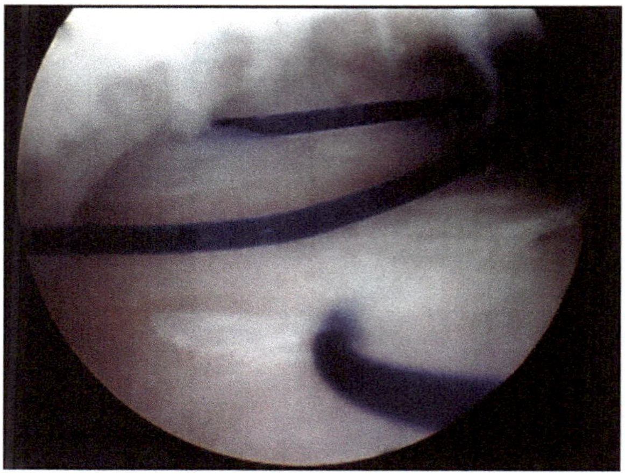

Figure 30-1. Ulnar styloid (right). The 2 ulnocarpal ligament sutures have been passed around the ulnocarpal ligaments, and suture has been passed through the ulnar distal radioulnar joint capsule.

Create the initial 3-4 portal and then create the 6-R portal under direct visualization. For the diagnostic portion, view from the 3-4 and 6-R portals. Included in the diagnostic assessment is special reference to ulnar structures. Midcarpal assessment begins by viewing through the radial midcarpal portal; the ulnar midcarpal portal is the primary working portal. The LT joint is assessed for congruency and laxity of the triquetrum. In the absence of a separate lunate facet, the lunate and triquetrum should be collinear. In the presence of a separate lunate facet, the radial articular edge of triquetrum should be aligned with the most ulnar articular edge of the hamate facet of the lunate. Laxity should be assessed upon triquetral rotation and separation from the lunate; laxity can be referenced in relation to the scapholunate joint. The dorsal portion of the triquetrum articular surface may be distal to the lunate with excessive laxity.

While viewing from the 3-4 portal, debride the LT ligament complex. A cleft or interval is seen between the UL and the UT ligaments; the interval identifies the volar aspect of the LT joint. Should additional pathology be present, such as a peripheral TFCC tear, initial debridement should be performed. Create the volar 6-U portal, which is just dorsal to the ulnocarpal ligaments.

Pass an 18-gauge spinal needle through the volar 6-U portal and briefly stop at the ulnar edge of the UT ligament. The goal is to pass the needle just volar to the ulnocarpal ligaments and approximately 5 mm distal to the joint surface; provisionally check the likely pathway of the spinal needle. As the needle is passed just volar to the ulnocarpal ligaments, the spinal needle re-enters the radiocarpal joint at the radial edge of the UL ligament. Pass a 2-0 polydioxanone suture through the spinal needle. Retrieve the suture sequentially through the 6-R and then the volar 6-U using a grasper or directly through the volar 6-U using a wire loop suture retriever or a grasper. Place a hemostat on the suture ends to complete the first suture plication.

Place tension on the first plication suture by having an assistant pull on the sutures in an ulnar-to-proximal direction. Pass the spinal needle in likewise fashion approximately 5 mm distal and parallel to the first plication suture; place a hemostat on the suture ends of the second plication suture. Tension on the first stitch often facilitates a second needle passage through the UL and UT ligaments. Adequacy of the plication (tension the stitch) and its effect on LT interval stability should be assessed after each suture passage. Occasionally, 3 sutures are used across the ulnocarpal ligaments. Through volar 6-U portal, place a plication suture through the volar distal radioulnar joint capsule at the prestyloid recess and volar peripheral TFCC edge. In Figure 30-1, the 2 ulnocarpal ligament sutures and the volar capsule suture have been passed. The suture is again retrieved out of the volar 6-U portal. The plication sutures will be tied after LT joint reduction and pinning.

Insert the arthroscope into the midcarpal radial portal. While viewing, pass a spinal needle from ulnar to radial across the distal aspect of the LT joint to use as a guide for pin placement into the triquetrum. Through the ulnar midcarpal joint, maintain a congruent LT joint, such as using a blunt trocar. With fluoroscopy readily available, pass the initial K-wire 2 to 3 mm proximal to

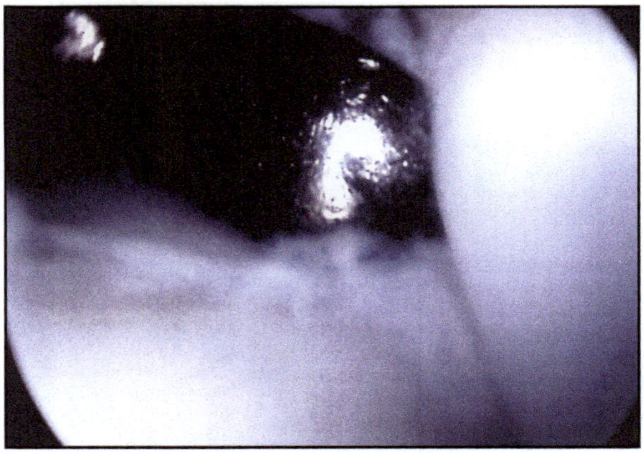

Figure 30-2. The lunate (left) and the triquetrum (right). The unstable LT joint results in a lax joint, with the triquetrum rotated resulting in an incongruous joint.

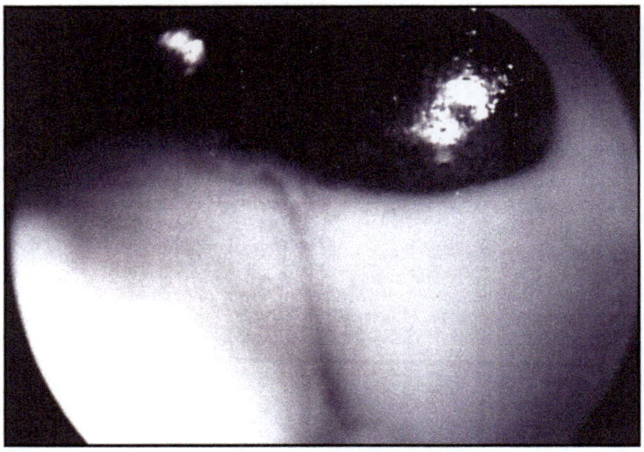

Figure 30-3. The lunate (left) and the triquetrum (right). The LT joint has been reduced and pinned, maintaining a congruous LT joint.

the distal aspect of the triquetrum. The first pin is advanced across the LT interval from ulnar to radial under fluoroscopic guidance and the second pin is placed using the first pin as a guide to placement. In Figure 30-2, the triquetrum (right) is rotated and the articular surface is distal to the lunate (left). In Figure 30-3, the triquetrum and lunate are reduced and are congruent after LT pinning. After satisfactory reduction and LT pinning (Figure 30-4), attention is directed back to the plication sutures.

Insert the arthroscope into the radiocarpal joint; a knot pusher can be used to pass over the sutures to ensure the absence of soft tissue entanglement and to assist in knot tying. Release traction, and with the forearm held in neutral rotation, tie each of the 3 plication suture sets. In Figure 30-5, each of the plication sutures have been tensioned and tied. The K-wires are cut and left in a subcutaneous position or the ends are bent and left outside the skin.

In a case of LT joint and peripheral TFCC tear, repair the TFCC after passing the plication sutures and tie the LT complex plication sutures and TFCC sutures after LT pinning. In case of LT joint and degenerative TFCC tear with or without ulnar impaction syndrome, debride the central avascular portion of the TFCC to a stable rim; perform wafer, if needed; then begin LT capsulodesis as described previously. As in TFCC surgery, dissect sufficiently to reduce chances of ulnar sensory branch injury.

Postoperative Protocol

After surgery, apply a long-arm splint or, alternatively, a Muenster splint, with the forearm in neutral rotation and wrist in neutral flexion and extension. At 1 to 2 weeks, immobilize for

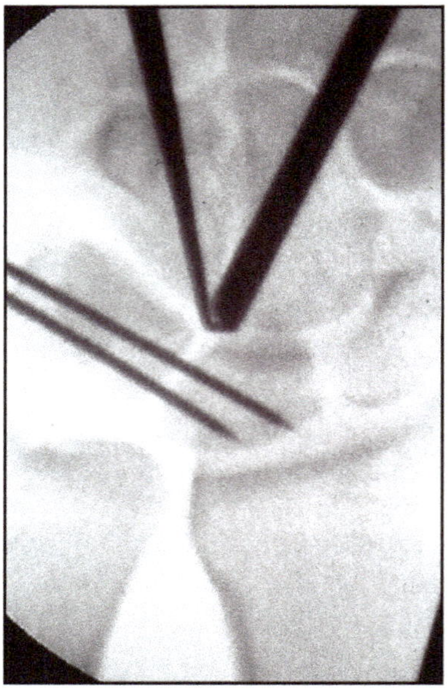

Figure 30-4. Fluoroscopic image demonstrating satisfactory reduction and 2 K-wires across the LT joint.

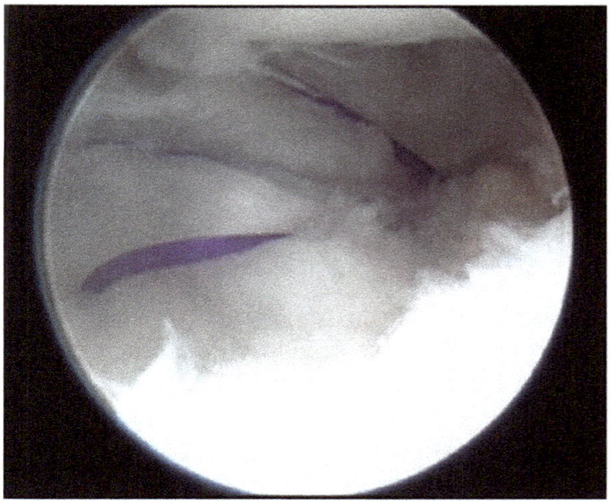

Figure 30-5. Ulnar styloid (right). The 3 placation sutures have been tied.

6 weeks in a Muenster cast or equivalent (forearm and wrist in neutral), and approximately 6 weeks after surgery, remove the K-wires. Encourage finger range of motion. A removable wristlet is offered during the initial phase of wrist rehabilitation; use of the brace should be weaned after about 2 weeks and off completely by the tenth week after surgery. The initial goal of rehabilitation is motion followed by strengthening, which may occur concomitantly with motion efforts. Strengthening is individualized.

Potential Complications

A complete list of complications cannot be offered. Common complications are related to localized irritation due to polydioxanone knots, ulnar sensory nerve irritation, and pin site cellulitis.

Top Technical Pearls for the Procedure

1. Radiological imaging is radiologist and pathology dependent; know which tests to order as well as unique characteristics of imaging available. Recognize that central LT ligament perforations without clinical significance occur and are not uncommon.
2. Patient complaints and physical examination should be consistent with LT compromise and correlate to pathoanatomy.
3. An assistant significantly facilitates the procedures. Set up the fluoroscopy unit so that you can easily manipulate imaging during reduction and pinning.
4. Lightly debride the ulnocarpal ligaments and LT ligament to facilitate scarring response; use the volar 6-U as a working portal as needed. Pass all sutures (plication and, if needed, TFCC) before LT reduction and pinning.
5. Confirm pin placement, then tie sutures with the wrist in neutral.

References

1. Ritt MJ, Bishop AT, Berger RA, Linscheid RL, Berglund LJ, An KN. Lunotriquetral ligament properties: a comparison of three anatomic subregions. *J Hand Surg Am.* 1998;23(3):425-431.
2. Berger RA. The anatomy of the ligaments of the wrist and distal radiolunar joints. *Clin Orthop Relat Res.* 2001;(383):32-40.
3. Moritomo H. Anatomy and clinical relevance of the ulnocarpal ligament. *J Wrist Surg.* 2013;2(2):186-189.
4. Lichtman DM, Noble WH III, Alexander CE. Dynamic triquetrolunate instability: case report. *J Hand Surg Am.* 1984;9(2):185-188.
5. Alexander C, Lichtman D. Triquetrolunate instability. In: Lichtman DM, Alexander AH, eds. *The Wrist and Its Disorders.* 2nd ed. Philadelphia, PA: WB Saunders; 1997:307-316.
6. Reagan DS, Linschied RL, Dobyns JH. Lunotriquetral sprains. *J Hand Surg Am.* 1984;9(4):502-514.
7. Linscheid RL, Dobyns JH. Athletic injuries of the wrist. *Clin Orthop Relat Res.* 1985;(198):141-151.
8. Murray PM, Palmer CG, Shin AY. The mechanism of ulnar-sided perilunate instability of the wrist: a cadaveric study and 6 clinical cases. *J Hand Surg Am.* 2012;37(4):721-728.
9. Pin PG, Nowak M, Logan SE, Young VL, Gilula LA, Weeks PM. Coincident rupture of the scapholunate and lunotriquetral ligaments without perilunate dissociation: pathomechanics and management. *J Hand Surg Am.* 1990;15(1):110-119.
10. Palmer AK. Triangular fibrocartilage disorders: injury patterns and treatment. *Arthroscopy.* 1990;6(2):125-132.
11. Darrow JC Jr, Linscheid RL, Dobyns JH, Mann JM III, Wood MB, Beckenbaugh RD. Distal ulnar recession for disorders of the distal radioulnar joint. *J Hand Surg Am.* 1985;10(4):482-491.
12. Gupta R, Bingenheimer E, Fornalski S, McGarry MH, Osterman AL, Lee TQ. The effect of ulnar shortening on lunate and triquetrum motion–a cadaveric study. *Clin Biomech (Bristol, Avon).* 2005;20(8):839-845.
13. Moser T, Dosch JC, Moussaoui A, Dietemann JL. Wrist ligament tears: evaluation of MRI and Combined MDCT and MR arthrography. *AJR Am J Roentgenol.* 2007;188(5):1278-1286.

Please see videos on the accompanying website at

www.routledge.com/9781630910013

31

Arthroscopic Treatment of Scapholunate Instability and Indications and Techniques for Arthroscopic Management of Scapholunate Injuries

Scott P. Steinmann, MD and Julie E. Adams, MD

Introduction

Optimal treatment of scapholunate (SL) instability remains a subject of discussion. In the acute or subacute situation, treatment aims to restore the normal relationship between the scaphoid and lunate to prevent carpal malalignment. The ultimate goals are relief of symptoms in the short term and preventing progression to arthritis in the form of SL advanced collapse wrist.

Arthroscopy has a role in diagnosis and staging of SL injuries as well as in treatment. Arthroscopic treatment options include assessment and arthroscopically assisted fixation of the scaphoid and lunate with use of smooth pins or a variety of screw constructs, such as in the reduction association of the scaphoid and lunate procedure, adjunctive use of thermal capsulorrhaphy, or arthroscopic debridement alone. In addition, arthroscopy may be used as a diagnostic and staging tool to determine how to proceed next. The definitive procedure may take the form of a ligament reconstruction or other open arthrotomy procedure.

Indications

- Known or suspected SL injuries
- Use of arthroscopy as a diagnostic and staging tool
  - Geissler et al[1] described an arthroscopic staging system, which is useful to document the extent of tears.
- Those with chronic injury and/or known or suspected chondral changes (although arthroscopy is most useful in the setting of acute or subacute injuries without known arthritis)
  - X-rays and magnetic resonance imaging (MRI) underestimate or fail to demonstrate the extent of chondral changes, and presence of arthritis may be apparent upon arthroscopic visualization but may not be demonstrated on imaging studies; thus, arthroscopy can be a tool to determine the most appropriate treatment procedure.

Savoie FH III, Field LD, Steinmann SP, eds. *The Elbow and Wrist: AANA Advanced Arthroscopic Surgical Techniques* (pp 315-321).

Controversial Indications

- Arthritis as seen on plain x-rays. Geissler et al's[1] series documents symptomatic improvement following arthroscopic debridement alone in patients who decline salvage-type procedures; however, the durability and the completeness of pain relief remain uncertain.

Pertinent Physical Findings

Patients with a suspected SL injury may recall a specific mechanism of injury. Although the believed mechanism of injury is a fall on the outstretched wrist, this injury may not be recalled or may commonly be thought to be a wrist sprain. This injury may be neglected by the patient or the examining provider; initial x-rays may be unremarkable.

- Tender to palpation over the dorsal SL interval:
  - This is easy to find because it is located at the 3-4 portal site. One can palpate Lister's tubercle over the distal radius, and then approximately 1 cm distal to that area is a soft spot, which represents the SL interval. Even in acute situations in which patients may have a distal radius fracture or other injury, careful palpation over the SL interval can demonstrate presence or absence of discomfort and suggest presence or absence of injury.
- In addition, the Watson test or SL shift test is helpful to evaluate for injury.
  - The examiner places his thumb on the scaphoid tubercle volarly and moves the wrist from ulnar to radial deviation with an axial load. The examiner assesses for the presence of a clunk and discomfort. It is important to assess the contralateral side and document the presence of discomfort. Many patients will have a clunk but no pain, which is deemed to be a normal finding.[2,3]

Pertinent Imaging

- X-rays
  - Initial imaging studies include posteroanterior (PA), lateral, and oblique x rays of the injured wrist as well as stress dynamic views of the bilateral wrists (PA grip view).
  - Commonly, as in the setting of predynamic and dynamic SL injuries, plain x-rays will be unremarkable. Occasionally, however, widening of the SL interval or a dorsal intercalated segmental instability deformity may be apparent. These findings are suggestive of a complete SL ligament injury with concomitant injury to the secondary stabilizers (static instability) of the carpus or, more commonly, a chronic situation. It is important to get comparison views of the contralateral wrist because some patients will have symmetric widening of the SL interval, which is physiologic rather than pathologic.[4]
  - PA grip views or clenched fist views are helpful to assess the SL interval and apply a dynamic stress to this interval. Nonstress views may be normal; however, stress views may demonstrate incompetence of the SL interval in the setting of dynamic instability.
- Other imaging modalities
  - MR arthrography is helpful to increase the sensitivity and specificity for SL injury; however, it cannot exclude anatomic perforations, which may be a normal finding.[5]
  - It is helpful to look at the axial cuts of the MRI, in which one can look specifically at the dorsal, volar, and membranous portions of the SL interosseous ligament.

- MRI may also demonstrate subtle chondral changes; however, it is often insensitive to early chondral changes, and astute surgeons should be prepared at the time of arthroscopy to find more substantial chondral changes than suggested by MRI, particularly in the chronic setting, and be prepared to alter the planned procedure as necessary.

Equipment

- Wrist arthroscopy traction tower
- Finger traps
- Upper-arm tourniquet (18 to 24 inches)
- 10-mL syringe
- 18- or 19-gauge hypodermic needles
- Small tubing for outflow (optional)
- Joint arthroscope (2.7- to 2.9-mm) and 1.9-mm arthroscope (optional)
- Blunt trocars and cannulas
- Small joint RF ablators or arthroscopic cautery devices
- Arthroscopic shavers (2.0 to 2.5 mm)
- Small probe (2-mm tip)
- K-wires (0.045-, 0.054-, and 0.062-inch; optional)
- Mini or micro suture anchors (optional)
- Mini fluoroscopy unit
- Open ligament reconstruction:
  - K-wires (0.045-, 0.054-, and 0.062-inch)
  - Cannulated drill bits (2.5 to 3.5 mm)
  - Hewson suture passer
  - Bunnell tendon passer
  - Mini or micro suture anchors (optional)
  - Tendon braider or mini right angle
  - 2-0 and 3-0 braided nonabsorbable suture on a taper needle
  - Synovial rongeur
  - Plaster for a thumb spica splint postoperatively

The standard wrist arthroscopy tower is used. The surgeon will find a 2-mm probe helpful, as well as the standard 2.7- to 2.9-mm arthroscope. For small wrists and for the midcarpal joint, it is helpful to have a small arthroscope, such as a 1.9-mm scope. Blunt trocars are used. Standard radiofrequency (RF) ablators or arthroscopic cautery devices are used, as well as shavers, such as a 2.0- or 2.5-mm shaver. A 10-mL syringe and 18- or 19-gauge needle is helpful for starting the procedure. Likewise, outflow can be achieved through an 18- or 19-gauge needle with or without small tubing.

A variety of devices may be used to fixate the SL interval, including smooth pins (typically 0.054-inch size), purpose-made screws, and other constructs. For open procedures for ligament repair (which is rarely possible as an isolated procedure) or for concomitant capsulodesis or reconstruction procedures (more commonly), one may find mini or micro suture anchors useful. For ligament reconstruction with a tendon graft, such as a Brunelli procedure, it is helpful to have cannulated drill bits (2.5 to 3.5 mm) and K-wires.

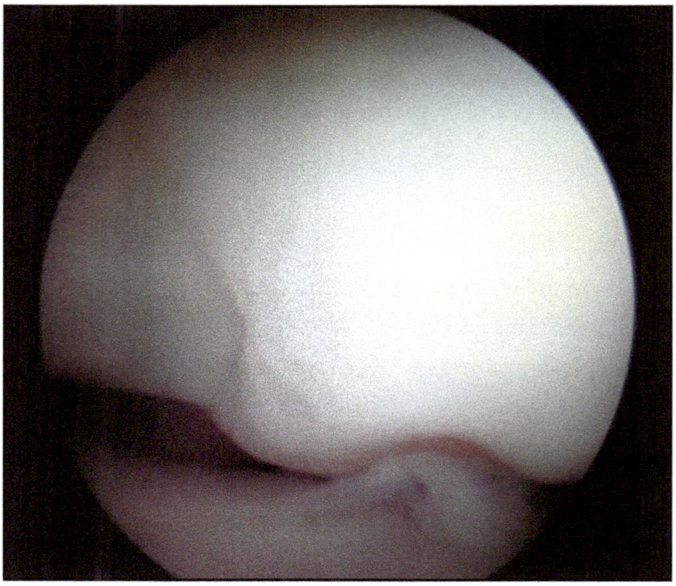

Figure 31-1. Arthroscopic view from the radiocarpal joint. The SL interosseous ligament is visualized as patulous and lax rather than the normal tight tissue. (Reprinted with permission of Julie Adams, MD.)

A mini-fluoroscopy unit is helpful to assess adequacy of SL reduction and to document appropriate hardware positioning.

Positioning and Portals

The patient is positioned supine with the operative arm resting on an arm table. The arm is prepped and draped to a nonsterile upper-arm tourniquet set at 200 to 250 mm Hg. The arm is suspended in a traction tower by the 4 fingers.

Step-by-Step Description of the Procedure

The procedure starts with a diagnostic wrist arthroscopy. The joint is first insufflated via the 3-4 portal by an 18- or 19-gauge needle and a 10-mL syringe filled with saline. Wrist arthroscopy proceeds in the usual fashion with creation of portal sites with incision through the skin only and dissection bluntly down to the capsule. The 3-4 portal is used for initial visualization with the initial working portal at the 6-R portal and outflow via the 6-U site. The cartilage surfaces of the radiocarpal joint, particularly at the scaphoid facet of the distal radius and the scaphoid, are assessed. The SL interosseous ligament interval is assessed with direct visualization through the arthroscope and extent of ligament injury documented with respect to the Geissler classification (Figure 31-1). Visualization through the 6-R portal is performed to assess the LT interval and any changes on the ulnar aspect of the wrist. While visualizing with the arthroscope in the radiocarpal joint, an air fluid arthrogram may be performed by placing a combination of air and fluid via one of the midcarpal portals. The surgeon watches for bulging of the SL ligament and for passage of bubbles into the radiocarpal joint, which may suggest an SL ligament tear. The diagnostic arthroscopy continues with visualization through the midcarpal joint via the radial and ulnar midcarpal portals (Figure 31-2). The findings from visualization via the radiocarpal joint and the midcarpal joint are used to classify the ligament injury with respect to the Geissler classification; grade I represents attenuation or hemorrhage of the ligament visualized from the radiocarpal joint without malalignment, grade II represents a stepoff seen via the midcarpal joint, grade III represents

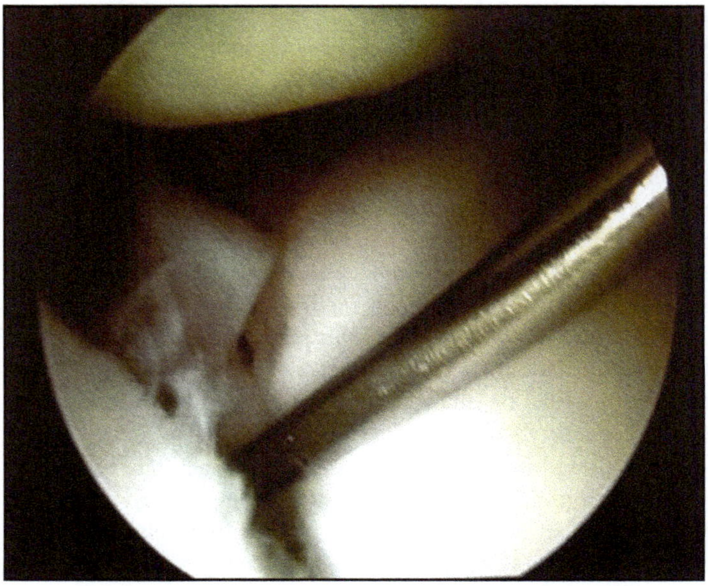

Figure 31-2. Arthroscopic view from the midcarpal joint. The probe can be readily turned in the SL interosseous ligament interval, demonstrating pathological laxity. (Reprinted with permission of Julie Adams, MD.)

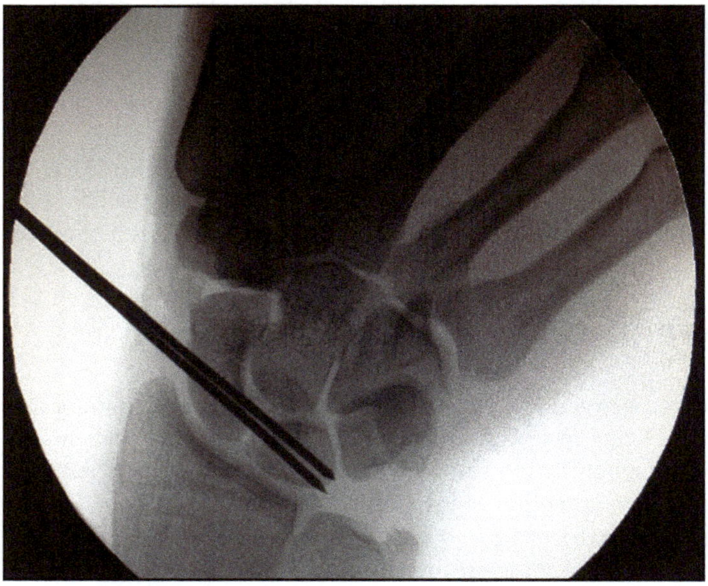

Figure 31-3. The SL interosseous ligament interval has been pinned with 2 smooth K-wires. (Reprinted with permission of Julie Adams, MD.)

incongruity or stepoff visualized via the radiocarpal and midcarpal joints, and grade IV represents gross instability with a so-called *drive-through sign*.[1]

Following completion of the diagnostic portion of the procedure, treatment considerations can be made. In a patient with acute predynamic instability with obvious SL injury on arthroscopy (Geissler I to III injury), the author typically pins the SL interosseous interval with 2 smooth 0.054-inch K-wires (Figure 31-3). Synovitis may be ablated with an RF ablator or coagulator. Thermal capsulorrhaphy may be considered for the dorsal portion of the SL interosseous ligament and the dorsal wrist capsule; spot application of the RF probe in a striped fashion is performed.

In the setting of a complete SL interosseous ligament tear with or without static carpal malalignment, one might consider SL ligament reconstruction as an open procedure. For the author, this is restricted to patients who are less than the age of approximately 50 years and those who have no chondral changes visualized with the arthroscope. In addition, the carpal malalignment must be reducible. Patients with existing carpal malalignment and a static gap are more likely to have recurrence of gap following surgery; nevertheless, pain relief may be substantial and the resulting symptomatic improvement is often an adequate reason to consider the tenodesis procedure.

Following completion of the arthroscopic portion of the procedure, the instruments are withdrawn. A dorsal longitudinal incision is made and dissection proceeds to the wrist capsule. In general, a minimal capsulotomy is performed to visualize the SL interval. A chondrodesis is performed between the scaphoid and the lunate by roughing up these surfaces with a small rongeur. The intended exit hole through the dorsum of the scaphoid is exposed. Attention is then turned to the volar aspect of the distal forearm and carpus. A longitudinal incision or a series of incisions are made over the flexor carpi radialis (FCR) tendon. Dissection proceeds, isolating one-third to one-half of the FCR, which is detached proximately and left attached distally. A K-wire is advanced through the tuberosity of the scaphoid, exiting dorsally in a transverse fashion. A 2.7- to 3.2-mm cannulated drill bit is used to overdrill this area. The smaller drill bits are used in females or small wrists, whereas larger drill bits are used in larger patients.

The harvested portion of the FCR is passed from volar to dorsal. This is facilitated by use of a Hewson passer. The transversely oriented path of the drill hole allows tension upon the FCR graft to cause the scaphoid to extend out of its abnormally flexed posture and help correct the carpal malalignment. K-wires in the scaphoid and lunate may also be used as joysticks to correct the dorsal intercalated segmental instability deformity and reduce the SL gap.

Two 0.054-inch K-wires may be prepositioned for passage through the scaphoid into the lunate via a small radial-sided incision. Care is taken to avoid the radial sensory nerve and radial artery. Following the reduction of the carpal alignment and SL interval, the pins are passed and the neoligament is woven through the dorsal radiotriquetral ligament and sutured into place and then back about itself and through the capsule, performing a concomitant capsulodesis.

There is also a role for debridement alone in patients with SL injuries and early arthritic changes. These patients have simple start arthroscopy with debridement of synovitis with the RF probe and the shaver in the usual wrist arthroscopy fashion. No planning of the SL interval is performed.

Postoperative Protocol

Patients who undergo ligament reconstruction are immobilized in a thumb spica splint or cast with the interphalangeal joint free. Digital motion is initiated immediately. Reliable patients for whom a splint is used may remove the splint for dart thrower's motion. Pins are generally removed at approximately 6 weeks, and gradual wrist motion and rehabilitation is initiated.

For patients who have SL pinning with thermal shrinkage or SL pinning alone, the postoperative protocol is similar, with pins left in place for approximately 6 weeks and gradual wrist rehabilitation beginning following pin removal.

Patients undergoing debridement alone, as in the setting of SL injury and early arthritic changes, are splinted for comfort for a brief period of time, and then mobilization proceeds. No restrictions are placed on the wrist.

Potential Complications

The risks associated with wrist arthroscopy and potential complications include chondral injury, tendon injury, etc. In addition, there is a risk of failure of the procedure to relieve symptoms. Recurrence of the SL gap or progression of carpal malalignment are possible; however, patients may have durable pain relief despite radiographic changes. If ligament reconstruction is performed with drilling of the scaphoid, there is a risk of scaphoid fracture or avascular necrosis of the scaphoid.

Top Technical Pearls for the Procedure

1. Use of arthroscopy as a diagnostic and staging tool is important, and assessment of the SL ligament via the radiocarpal and midcarpal joints is essential to understand the extent of injury, document any chondral changes or concomitant injuries, and determine appropriate treatment options.
2. Preoperative comparison views of the injured wrist and contralateral wrist including dynamic stress views, such as the PA grip view, are essential to rule out normal physiological widening of the SL interval.
3. Patient selection for the procedure is essential for good outcomes. In patients who are older, have limited goals, have poor physiology, or have chondral changes, a salvage procedure, such as a limited wrist arthrodesis or proximal row carpectomy, may be better choices then a reconstructive procedure.
4. Pinning the SL interval can be facilitated by ulnar deviation of the wrist and by making an open incision with dissection down to the scaphoid to avoid injury to the radial sensory nerve and the radial artery.
5. If thermal capsulorrhaphy is to be performed, it is done in a striping fashion rather than a whitewashing fashion, and the wrist is immobilized for several weeks to allow the collagen fibrils to shrink and repair.

References

1. Geissler WB, Freeland AE, Savoie FH, McIntyre LW, Whipple TL. Intracarpal soft-tissue lesions associated with an intra-articular fracture of the distal end of the radius. *J Bone Joint Surg Am.* 1996;78(3):357-365.
2. Watson HK, Ashmead D IV, Makhlouf MV. Examination of the scaphoid. *J Hand Surg Am.* 1988;13(5):657-660.
3. Easterling KJ, Wolfe SW. Scaphoid shift in the uninjured wrist. *J Hand Surg Am.* 1994;19(4):604-606.
4. Vitello W, Gordon DA. Obvious radiographic scapholunate dissociation: x-ray the other wrist. *Am J Orthop (Belle Mead NJ).* 2005;34(7):347-351.
5. Hobby JL, Tom BD, Bearcroft PW, Dixon AK. Magnetic resonance imaging of the wrist: diagnostic performance statistics. *Clin Radiol.* 2001;56(1):50-57.

32

Midcarpal Instability
Arthroscopic Techniques

David J. Slutsky, MD

Introduction

Midcarpal instability (MCI) is a form of nondissociative carpal instability with instability between the proximal and distal carpal rows. It represents several distinct clinical entities that differ in the cause and direction of subluxation but share the common characteristic of abnormal force transmission at the midcarpal joint. Lichtman consolidated the different forms into intrinsic or extrinsic types. The intrinsic types are palmer MCI (PMCI), dorsal MCI (DMCI), and combined.[1] There are no objective methods to quantify the magnitude of the instability. There are no arthroscopic findings that are characteristic of MCI. Extrinsic MCI as described by Taleisnik and Watson[2] is due to a dorsally malunited distal radius fracture. This is typically treated by a distal radius osteotomy to restore the normal palmar tilt and falls outside the scope of this discussion.

Indications

- Midcarpal instability to rule out associated intercarpal ligament pathology and to inspect the midcarpal joint to assess for chondral damage. Milder forms of PMCI can be treated with a thermal capsulorrhaphy.

Controversial Indications

- A variety of open soft tissue procedures have been generally ineffective for severe forms of MCI; hence, arthroscopic treatment should be approached with caution, especially in patients with self-induced palmar midcarpal translation.

Savoie FH III, Field LD, Steinmann SP, eds. *The Elbow and Wrist: AANA Advanced Arthroscopic Surgical Techniques* (pp 323-328).

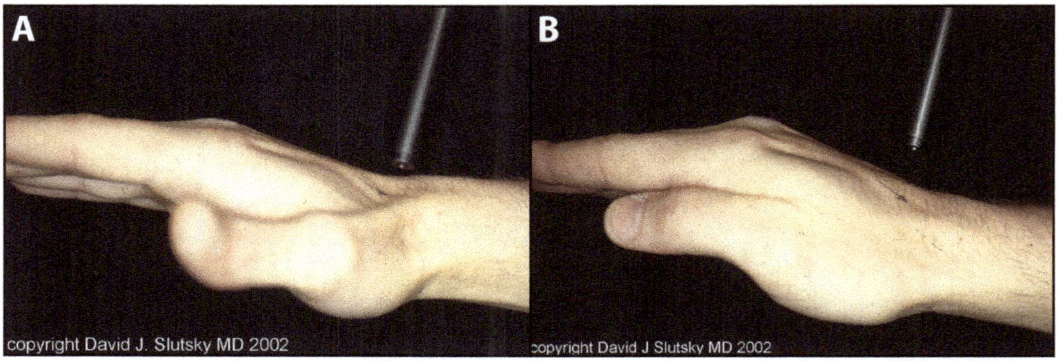

Figure 32-1. Palmer MCI. (A) Note the sag in the midcarpal joint with the wrist in radial deviation. (B) The carpus is reduced in ulnar deviation and the sag disappears.

Pertinent Physical Findings

- PMCI
  - Patients present with a history of clunking of their wrist.
  - Patients complain of posttraumatic chronic pain, weakness, and wrist clicking.
  - Tight grasping, especially in supination, aggravates the symptoms.
  - Patients can often reproduce the clunk on both sides because generalized ligamentous laxity frequently coexists. The patient may have a trivial injury, however, which accentuates this normal laxity, resulting in a painful clunk.
  - On physical examination, close inspection will reveal a sag of the midcarpal joint with the wrist in radial deviation, which is reduced with active or passive ulnar deviation (Figure 32-1).
  - The clunk may be reproduced by performing the midcarpal shift test as described by Lichtman et al.[3] This test is performed by placing the patient's wrist in neutral with the forearm in pronation. A palmar force is then applied to the hand at the level of the distal capitate. The wrist is simultaneously loaded and deviated ulnarly. The test result is positive if a painful catch-up clunk occurs that reproduces the patient's symptoms.
- Dorsal MCI
  - A history of an extension injury may be present.
  - The physical examination also reveals palmar sagging of the ulnar wrist.
  - A dorsal capitate displacement test is performed by applying dorsal pressure to the scaphoid tuberosity while longitudinal traction and flexion are applied to the wrist. There is an associated painful click as the lunate is abruptly shifted dorsally and ulnarly.

Pertinent Imaging

- Static x-rays are typically normal but occasionally reveal a mild volar intercalated segmental instability (VISI) pattern with the wrist in the neutral position.
  - In static radial deviation views, the entire proximal row is flexed, which results in a foreshortened appearance of the scaphoid and a positive ring sign, whereas in static ulnar deviation views following the catch-up clunk, the carpus appears normal (Figure 32-2). However, this also occurs in the normal wrist.

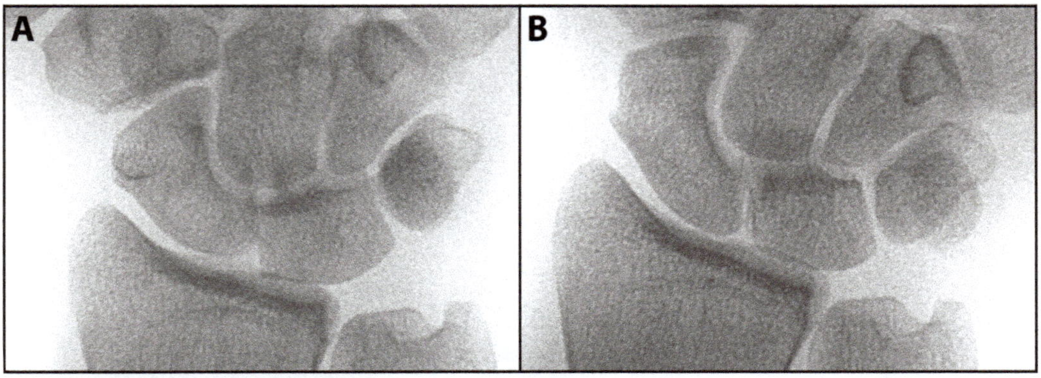

Figure 32-2. (A) In static radial deviation views, the entire proximal row is flexed, which results in a foreshortened appearance of the scaphoid and a positive ring sign. (B) In static ulnar deviation views following the catch-up clunk, the carpus appears normal.

- Arthrograms are normal unless there are associated intracarpal or triangular fibrocartilage complex tears.
- Magnetic resonance imaging findings are nonspecific.
- Dynamic ultrasound can also be used to demonstrate midcarpal dyskinesia, including the characteristic triquetral catch-up clunk.
- Magnetic resonance arthrography and computed tomography arthrography can demonstrate tears of the extrinsic ligaments, but intact yet redundant ligaments are more difficult to identify.
- Dynamic fluoroscopy provides the hallmarks for diagnosis of this condition.
  - With normal wrist kinematics, the proximal carpal row rotates synchronously from flexion to extension as ulnar deviation of the wrist is achieved. With PMCI, the proximal row maintains a volar flexed position until terminal ulnar deviation is reached, at which time it suddenly snaps into extension (MCI video).
  - In dynamic dorsal MCI, x-rays are usually normal. In chronic cases, the x-rays often show a VISI pattern. The capitolunate displacement test shows dorsal subluxation of the proximal carpal row in addition to dorsal subluxation of the capitate from the lunate (Figure 32-3).[4] This led Louis et al[5] to coin the term *capitolunate instability pattern* or *CLIP wrist*.

Equipment

A 2.7-mm, 30-degree angle arthroscope and a fiber-optic light source and camera setup are used. A full-radius resector with suction is used for debridement as necessary, and a 3-mm small joint hook probe is used for palpation. Some type of diathermy unit is used for the thermal shrinkage.

Step-by-Step Description of the Procedure

1. The patient is placed in a supine position on the operating table with the arm suspended vertically in a traction tower with 10 to 15 lb of traction applied to the index and long fingers.
2. After exsanguination, an upper arm tourniquet is inflated to 250 mm Hg. Large bore outflow cannulas are desirable to provide rapid joint irrigation to minimize the risk of chondral damage through heat necrosis.

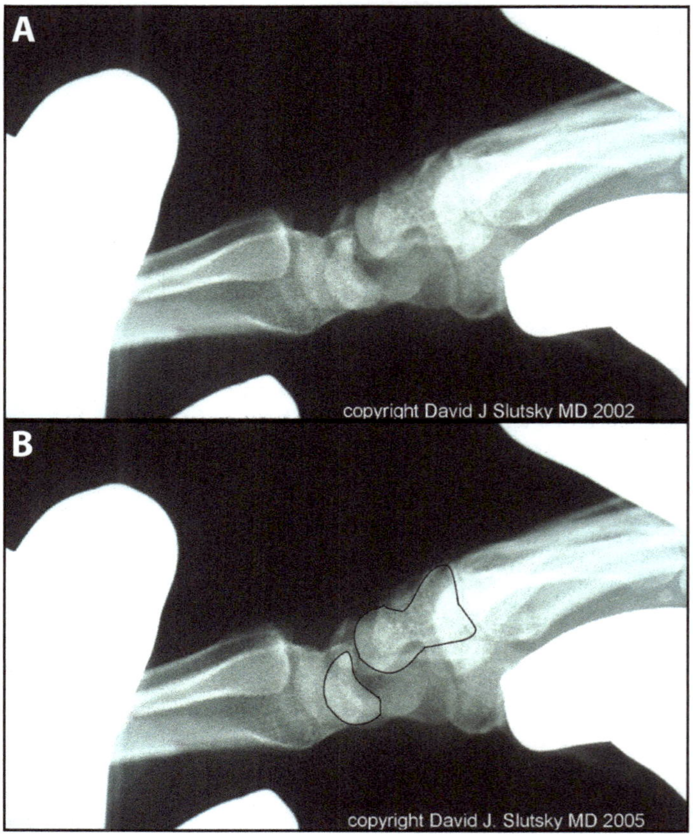

Figure 32-3. Capitolunate displacement test. (A) Lateral x-ray demonstrating dorsal subluxation of the capitate on the lunate. (B) Same view with the lunate and capitate outlined for clarity.

3. The standard dorsal portals, including a 3-4 and 4-5 portal, are used for an arthroscopic survey. A radial and ulnar midcarpal portal are used to assess the arcuate ligament and the scapholunate and lunotriquetral joint laxity.
4. The radiocarpal joint is identified 1 cm distal to Lister's tubercle at the 3-4 portal, and the 2.7-mm arthroscope is introduced. Outflow is established through the 6-R portal. Any associated triangular fibrocartilage tears or lunotriquetral ligament tears are noted and treated by debridement or repair. The ulnar extrinsic ligaments are assessed for laxity. If laxity is noted, a 1.5-mm electrothermal probe (Arthrocare or Oratec) is introduced through the 6-R portal. The ulnolunate and ulnotriquetral ligaments are painted with the probe using a stripe technique, leaving sections of untouched ligament in between.
5. A midcarpal radial portal is then established. The scapholunate and lunotriquetral joints are inspected and probed for laxity. A midcarpal ulnar portal is established and used for introduction of the thermal probe. A thermal probe is applied to the ulnar arm of the arcuate ligament (ulnocapitate, ulnotriquetral, and triquetrocapitate ligaments) as well as the radial arm (radioscaphocapitate, long and short radiolunate ligaments) and accessible parts of the dorsal capsule in the radiocarpal and midcarpal joints (Figure 32-4).
6. A volar radial portal is now established by making a 2-cm longitudinal incision in the proximal wrist crease, exposing the flexor carpi radialis (FCR) tendon sheath. The sheath is divided and the FCR tendon is retracted ulnarly. The radiocarpal joint space is identified with a 22-gauge needle, and the joint is inflated with saline. A blunt trocar and cannula are introduced through the floor of the FCR sheath, which overlies the interligamentous sulcus between the radioscaphocapitate ligament and the long radiolunate ligament. A 2.7-mm, 30-degree arthroscope is inserted through the cannula. The dorsal radiocarpal ligament can

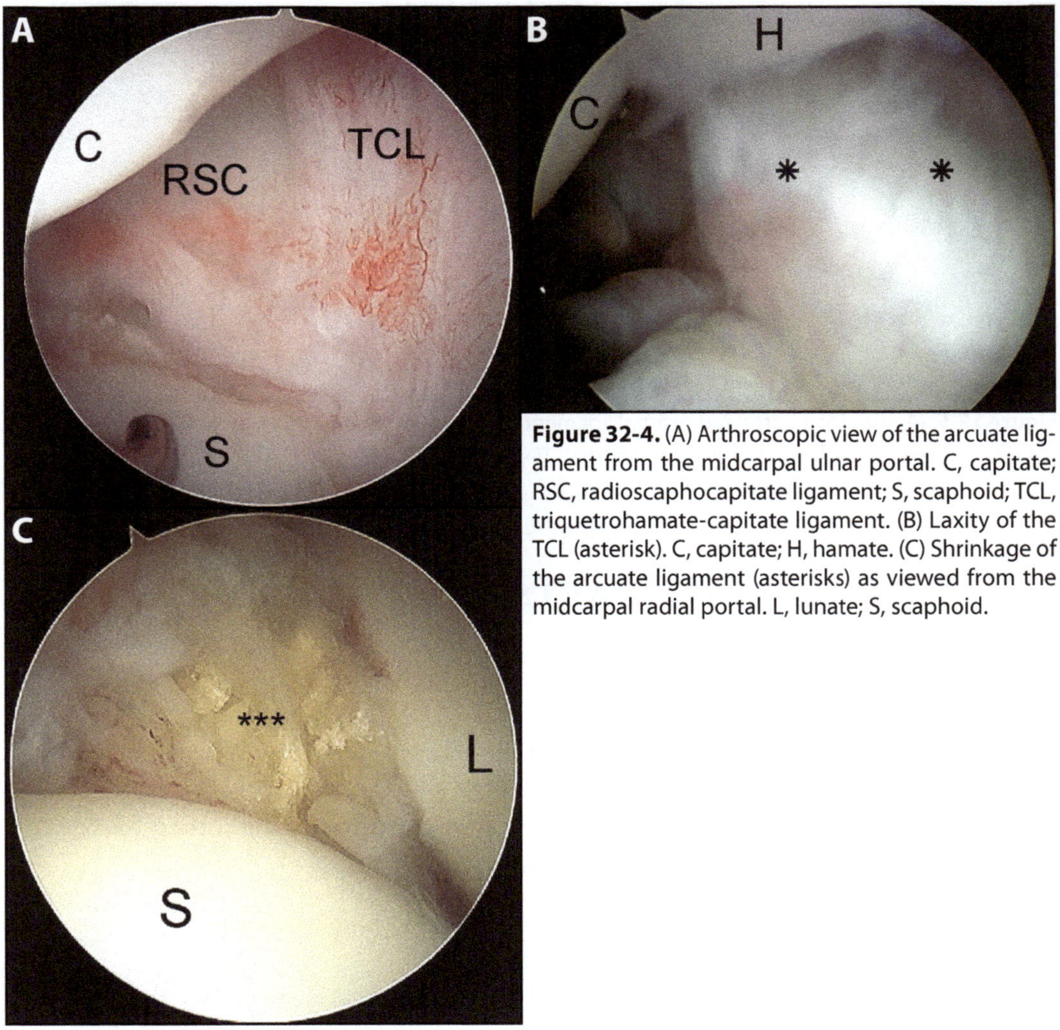

Figure 32-4. (A) Arthroscopic view of the arcuate ligament from the midcarpal ulnar portal. C, capitate; RSC, radioscaphocapitate ligament; S, scaphoid; TCL, triquetrohamate-capitate ligament. (B) Laxity of the TCL (asterisk). C, capitate; H, hamate. (C) Shrinkage of the arcuate ligament (asterisks) as viewed from the midcarpal radial portal. L, lunate; S, scaphoid.

be seen ulnar to the 3-4 portal and lying underneath the lunate. When laxity is present, the electrothermal probe is introduced through the 3-4 and 4-5 portals and is used to shrink the dorsal radiocarpal ligament (Figure 32-5).

Postoperative Protocol

Following an arthroscopic shrinkage, the patient's wrist is immobilized for 6 weeks followed by range of motion exercises and gradual strengthening.

Potential Complications

The main complication is a failure to correct the PMCI. Sensory nerve injury and/or tendon secondary to portal placement can occur in addition to skin and/or tendon necrosis and rupture due to the use of a thermal probe that is too close to these structures.

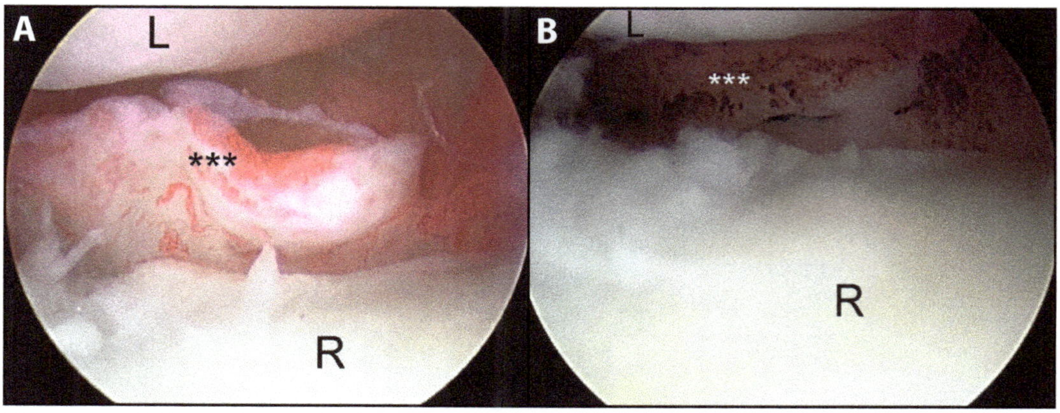

Figure 32-5. (A) View of a dorsal radiocarpal ligament tear (asterisks) from the volar radial portal. L, lunate; R, radius. (B) View of a dorsal radiocarpal ligament tear after shrinkage.

Top Technical Pearls for the Procedure

1. Examine the opposite wrist for MCI.
2. Examine for a painful midcarpal clunk.
3. Dynamic fluoroscopy demonstrates loss of the normal synchronous motion from physiologic dorsal intercalated segmental instability to VISI.
4. Perform arthroscopy to assess and treat any associated intercarpal ligament pathology.
5. Perform capsular shrinkage for milder forms of MCI.

References

1. Lichtman DM, Wroten ES. Understanding midcarpal instability. *J Hand Surg Am.* 2006;31(3):491-498.
2. Taleisnik J, Watson HK. Midcarpal instability caused by malunited fractures of the distal radius. *J Hand Surg Am.* 1984;9(3):350-357.
3. Lichtman DM, Schneider JR, Swafford AR, Mack GR. Ulnar midcarpal instability-clinical and laboratory analysis. *J Hand Surg Am.* 1981;6(5):515-523.
4. White SJ, Louis DS, Braunstein EM, Hankin FM, Greene TL. Capitate-lunate instability: recognition by manipulation under fluoroscopy. *AJR Am J Roentgenol.* 1984;143(2):361-364.
5. Louis DS, Hankin FM, Greene TL. Chronic capitolunate instability. *J Bone Joint Surg Am.* 1987;69(6):950-951.

Please see videos on the accompanying website at

www.routledge.com/9781630910013

33

Arthroscopic Management of Displaced Intra-Articular Distal Radius Fractures

William B. Geissler, MD and Aaron M. Weber, DO

Introduction

The purpose of this chapter is to describe various arthroscopic techniques in the management of displaced intra-articular fractures of the distal radius. With practice, using wrist arthroscopy as an adjunct can minimally increase operative time and improve the intra-articular reduction. Particularly, wrist arthroscopy with volar plate fixation results in anatomic restoration of the joint surface and stable fixation. This combination allows for early range of motion (ROM).

Wrist arthroscopy is a valuable adjunct in the management of complex displaced intra-articular fractures of the distal radius. Displaced articular surface fragments of the distal radius may be viewed under bright light and magnified conditions with the wrist arthroscope as compared to open arthrotomy. Fracture fragments are frequently rotated and can easily be viewed arthroscopically. These same fragments, however, are often difficult to detect under fluoroscopy. Fracture hematoma and loose bodies can be arthroscopically lavaged and may improve the patient's final ROM. Intra-articular soft tissue lesions are often associated with intra-articular fractures of the distal radius and may affect the final prognosis. These are easily detected arthroscopically and can be managed at the same setting as they may have an important impact on the patient's final prognosis and explain why some patients complain of pain postoperatively despite radiographic anatomic fracture reduction. Patients frequently continue to complain of ulnar-sided wrist pain after surgery, which may be attributed to injury to the triangular fibrocartilage complex (TFCC).

A high incidence of associated intra-articular soft tissue injuries have been shown to be associated with fractures of the distal radius. In 2 separate wrist arthrogram studies, Mohanti and Kar[1] and Fontes et al[2] had a high incidence of injury to the TFCC associated with fractures of the distal radius. Mohanti and Kar[1] noted a 45% incidence of tears to the TFCC in 60 patients. Fontes et al[2] revealed a 66% incidence of tears of the TFCC in 58 patients. Arthroscopic studies also demonstrate similar findings. In a series by Geissler et al,[3] 49% of 60 patients with intra-articular distal radius fractures had a tear of the TFCC, of which the majority were peripheral and repairable. Injury to the scapholunate (SL) interosseous ligament was identified in 32% of patients, and tears to the lunotriquetral (LT) interosseous ligament were reported in 15% of patients. Lindau,[4]

Savoie FH III, Field LD, Steinmann SP, eds. *The Elbow and Wrist: AANA Advanced Arthroscopic Surgical Techniques* (pp 329-346).

Table 33-1. Geissler Arthroscopic Classification of Carpal Instability

Grade	Description	Management
I	Attenuation/hemorrhage of interosseous ligament as seen from the radiocarpal joint. No incongruency of carpal alignment in the midcarpal space.	Immobilization
II	Attenuation/hemorrhage of the interosseous ligament as seen from the radiocarpal joint. Incongruency/step-off as seen from the midcarpal space. A slight gap (less than the width of a probe) between the carpal bones may be present.	Arthroscopic reduction and pinning
III	Incongruency/step-off of carpal alignment is seen in both the radiocarpal and midcarpal space. The probe may be passed through gap between the carpal bones.	Arthroscopic/ open reduction and pinning
IV	Incongruency/step-off of carpal alignment is seen in the radiocarpal and midcarpal space. Gross instability with manipulation is noted. A 2.7-mm arthroscope may be passed through the gap between the carpal bones.	Open reduction and repair

in a similar arthroscopic study of 50 patients, noted that tears of the TFCC occurred in 78% of patients. Tears to the SL interosseous ligament were identified in 54% of patients, whereas LT interosseous ligament tears were found in 16% of the patients. Hanker,[5] in his arthroscopic study, reported that TFCC tears were common and present in 55% of patients. Common to these studies was the high incidence of injury to the TFCC associated with displaced intra-articular fractures of the distal radius.

Geissler et al[3] described an arthroscopic classification of interosseous ligament injuries based on his work in arthroscopic management of intra-articular distal radius fractures. He noted that the interosseous ligament stretches, attenuates, and eventually tears from a volar to dorsal direction around increased rotation between the carpal bones. This arthroscopic classification of carpal instability is based on observation of the interosseous ligament from the radiocarpal and midcarpal spaces. It functions to evaluate injuries to the SL and LT interosseous ligaments (Table 33-1).

Wrist arthroscopy takes advantage of its ability to view the articular surface under bright light and magnified conditions. Two millimeters of articular displacement has become a well-known established criterion in congruency of the distal radius over the past several years. Knirk and Jupiter[6] demonstrated that patients whose articular reduction was greater than 2 mm at final follow-up had higher incidences of degenerative changes within their wrists. Bradway et al[7] reported similar findings. Fernandez and Geissler[8] noted that the complication rate was substantially lower when the articular reduction was within 1 mm or less. Trumble et al[9] reported that the factors that most strongly result in successful outcomes included the amount of residual radial shortening and articular incongruence.

Edwards et al[10] described the advantage of viewing the intra-articular reduction by wrist arthroscopy compared to monitoring under fluoroscopy alone. In his series of 15 patients who underwent arthroscopic evaluation of the articular surface following reduction and stabilization under fluoroscopy, he reported 33% of the patients still had articular step-off of 1 mm or more. Frequently, the fracture fragment was rotated. He noted that wrist arthroscopy was particularly useful in judging rotation of the fracture fragments, which is not readily identifiable under fluoroscopy alone.

The literature is sparse regarding the results of arthroscopically assisted fixation of displaced intra-articular fractures of the distal radius. Stewart and Berger[11] presented a comparison study of 12 open and 12 arthroscopically assisted reductions of comminuted AO type C fractures of the distal radius. In the arthroscopic group, the authors reported results of 5 excellent, 6 good, and 1 fair. The open group reported no excellent results. The arthroscopic group had increased ROM compared to the group that underwent open stabilization in similar fracture patterns. Doi et al[12] reported similar results in a comparison study of 38 patients who underwent arthroscopically assisted fixation with open reduction and fixation. They also noted that the arthroscopic group had improved ROM.

Geissler and Freeland[13] reported on 33 patients who underwent arthroscopically assisted reduction of extra-articular distal radius fractures. In their series, 25 patients had anatomic reduction of the articular surface and 8 had a 1-mm step-off. In addition, they analyzed their results based on associated soft tissue injuries. They noted that a Geissler grade II injury of the SL interosseous ligament did not affect the final prognosis. However, in patients for whom a Geissler grade III or IV tear was present with an AO type C fracture, it significantly affected the final result.

Wrist arthroscopy has proven to be a valuable adjunct in the management of intra-articular distal radius fractures. Wrist arthroscopy allows for visualization of the articular reduction under bright light and magnified conditions. When wrist arthroscopy is combined as an adjunct to volar plating, precise reduction of the articular surface, combined with the stability of a volar plate, allows for early ROM. The importance of anatomic restoration of the articular surface has been confirmed by several studies.[6,7,9] In addition, arthroscopic lavage of fracture hematoma and debris may improve the patient's final ROM. Comparison studies by Stewart and Berger[11] and Doi et al[12] have shown improved ROM in patients who underwent arthroscopic reduction compared to open reduction alone.

Indications

- Displaced intra-articular fractures of the distal radius
- Radial styloid fractures
- Dye-punch fractures
- Three- and 4-part fractures with or without metaphyseal comminution
- Distal radius fractures with suspected distal radioulnar instability
- Dorsal comminution with more than 20 degrees of dorsal tilt
- Extensive dorsal comminution volar to the mid-axial line of the distal radius
- Initial radial shortening greater than 4 mm when compared to the ulna
- Significant intra-articular involvement in patients older than 60 years

Controversial Indications

- Open fractures

Pertinent Physical Findings

- Soft tissue swelling
- Pain with ROM
- Obvious deformity
- Assess neurovascular status to assess for traumatic carpal tunnel syndrome

Pertinent Imaging

- Standard posteroanterior, oblique, and lateral wrist x-rays
- Anteroposterior and lateral x-rays of the forearm and elbow
- Computed tomography studies for highly comminuted fractures

Equipment

A radiolucent traction tower is usually preferred in fracture management, allowing simultaneous arthroscopy and fluoroscopy with removing the traction. The patient is positioned supine with the arm on a stable arm table that is also radiolucent. Additional equipment includes multiple 18-gauge spinal needles, K-wires and wire driver, cannulated screw set, and distal radial plates.

Positioning and Portals

- The patient is placed in the supine positioned with the wrist suspended in a wrist arthroscopy traction tower.
- Joint fluid inflow is through the 6-U portal.
- The standard 3-4 and 4-5 or 6-R working portals are used for instrumentation during the procedure.

Step-by-Step Description of the Procedure

Swelling associated with wrist fractures can make it difficult to palpate the extensor tendon landmarks traditionally used for arthroscopy. However, the bony landmarks are usually easily palpated and are useful. These bony landmarks include the base of the metacarpals, the ulnar head, and the dorsal lip of the radius.[14] Small joint instrumentation is essential for arthroscopically assisted reduction of intra-articular distal radius fractures. The small joint scopes measuring 2.7 mm in diameter or smaller may be used. In addition, a small joint shaver ($\leq$3.5 mm) is mandatory to clear fracture hematoma and debris to improve visualization. An oscillating drill is useful when inserting K-wires for visual and stabilization to prevent injury to the dorsal cutaneous nerves that surround the wrist.

A traction tower is essential to arthroscopic management of distal radius fractures. The traction tower allows the surgeon to flex, extend, and radially and ulnarly deviate the wrist to help facilitate reduction of the fracture fragments while maintaining constant traction for visualization. Previous towers that suspended the wrist used a traction bar to extend the forearm and hand, which made simultaneous fluoroscopic evaluation of the reduction difficult. Newer traction towers have been designed to allow the surgeon to simultaneously reduce the intra-articular fracture of the distal radius while monitoring the reduction under fluoroscopy. The traction bar is uniquely placed at the side of the wrist rather than at the center so that it does not block fluoroscopic visualization. The wrist can be manipulated in traction to help reduce the fracture fragments. The tower may also be flexed to allow the surgeon to perform wrist arthroscopy in the vertical or horizontal plane, depending on the surgeon's preference. If a traction tower is not available, the wrist may be suspended with finger traps suspended in a shoulder holder or over the end of a hand table. A small bump may be placed in the volar aspect of the wrist to help maintain slight wrist flexion when weights are being used over the end of the hand table.

The standard 3-4 portal is made between the third and fourth dorsal extensor compartments. The 3-4 portal is made in line with the radial border of the long finger when the extensor tendons cannot be palpated. It is useful to place an 18-gauge needle into the proposed location of the 3-4 portal prior to committing to a skin incision. The arthroscope may be placed within the fracture itself if the portal is placed too proximal or can injure the articular cartilage of the carpus if the portal is placed too distally. Once the precise location of the portal is determined, the portal is made upon the skin against the surgeon's thumb with the tip of a #11 blade. In this manner, injury to the dorsal sensory cutaneous branches is decreased. Blunt dissection is then continued with a hemostat to the level of the joint capsule, and the arthroscope is then introduced with a blunt trocar into the 3-4 portal.

Intra-articular fractures of the distal radius are usually associated with abundant fracture hematoma and debris.[15] Thorough irrigation of the fracture hematoma is required to evaluate the fracture fragments and, particularly, to improve the field of view to judge rotation to the fracture fragments. Inflow may be provided through the wrist arthroscopic cannula or through a 14-gauge needle inserted into the 6-U portal. Because the small cannula in wrist arthroscopy does not allow much space for fluid irrigation into the joint, it is strongly recommended to have a separate inflow through the 6-U portal. Outflow is provided through the arthroscopic cannula with intravenous extension tubing, which drains into a basin on the hand table so the fluid does not go into the surgeon's lap or onto the floor. A separate inflow and outflow limits fluid extravasation into the soft tissues. The 4-5 or 6-R working portal may be made to debris fracture hematoma to improve visualization. The 4-5 working portal is made in line with the mid-axis of the ring metacarpal when the extensor tendons cannot be palpated. The 6-R portal may be made just radial to the extensor carpi radialis tendon. Similar to initially making the 3-4 portal, an 18-gauge needle should be inserted into the proposed location and viewed arthroscopically prior to committing to a skin incision.

Dry Arthroscopy

Extravasation of arthroscopic fluid can be problematic, especially in light of highly comminuted intra-articular fractures. Dry arthroscopy uses an inert gas to insufflate the joint and has the benefit of reducing soft tissue infiltration of arthroscopic fluid. This will reduce the risk of potential compartment syndrome and allow for more open procedures due to better maintenance of soft tissue integrity. In addition, larger portals may be used because there is no worry about bubbling secondary to air infiltration into the joint as occurs when using a wet technique. Using larger portals can facilitate rapid and efficient manipulation of fracture fragments, reducing total surgical time.

Del Piñal,[16] who is a pioneer in dry arthroscopy, addressed many difficulties of dry arthroscopy, primarily focusing on problems in maintaining a clean camera lens and joint during the procedure in the absence of a flushing fluid solution. He recommends leaving airflow on at all times with the scope valve open to allow continuous circulation. This ensures that when suction is used during shaving and burring, the joint space will not collapse and soil the camera lens. Furthermore, when using suction to remove debris from the joint, only open the suction when aspirating from the joint. Leaving the suction on can result in similar collapse of the joint space. If the joint needs to be flushed, a small syringe may be attached to the side valve of the scope. Once suction is turned on through the shaver or burr, the negative pressure will pull fluid from the syringe into the joint, flushing out any debris. When using this technique, one must realize that they will not have a pristine view of the joint. This is not necessary for the task of reducing fracture fragments, and attempting to attain such an arthroscopic view can waste valuable operating room time.

The ideal timing for arthroscopically assisted reduction of intra-articular distal radius fractures is usually between 3 and 10 days.[17] Other attempts at arthroscopic fixation may result in troublesome bleeding, which may obscure visualization. Fractures older than 10 days may be difficult to disimpact and mobilize percutaneously.

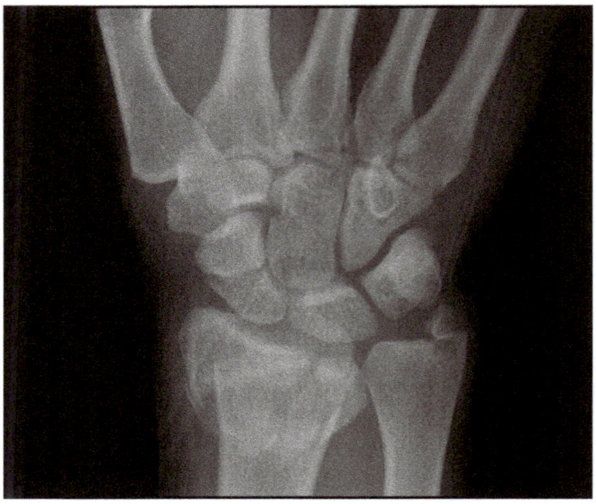

Figure 33-1. Posteroanterior x-ray of a transradial, transscaphoid, perilunate dislocation. This is a greater arc injury involving a fracture of the capitate and greater triquetral instability.

Radial Styloid Fractures

An isolated fracture of the radial styloid is an ideal fracture pattern to manage arthroscopically, particularly if one is just beginning to gain experience in arthroscopic management of wrist fractures. Several techniques are possible. The simplest technique is to advance 2 guide wires under fluoroscopy into the tip of the radial styloid fragment and not across the fracture site. It is important to make a small incision to insert the guide wires through a soft tissue protector or with an oscillating drill to limit injury to the cutaneous nerves. The positions of the guide wires into the radial styloid fragment are evaluated under fluoroscopy. The wrist is then suspended in the traction tower, and standard portals are made. The radiocarpal space is cleared of hematoma and fracture debris to help facilitate visualization and to judge rotation of the radial styloid fragment. The arthroscope is then transferred over to the 6-R or 4-5 portal to view the reduction of the radial styloid fragment by looking across the wrist. It is easier to judge rotation of the fracture fragment by looking across the wrist joint. The previously placed guide wires are then used as joysticks, and the fracture is manipulated under direct observation and anatomically reduced back to the radial shaft. A trocar inserted into the 3-4 portal may be useful to further aid the reduction of the radial styloid fragment and control rotation. The guide wire is then advanced across the fracture site into the radial shaft once the fracture reduction is judged anatomic. The articular reduction and the position of the guide wires are evaluated under fluoroscopy. Initially, K-wires are used alone. Headless screws are now recommended to stabilize the fracture because they provide good stability while decreasing soft tissue irritation and potential pin tract infections compared to K-wires. Headless screws allow potentially earlier ROM as well (Figures 33-1 and 33-2).

An alternative technique is to perform a closed reduction and percutaneous stabilization of the radial styloid fragment under fluoroscopy and advance the guide wires across the fracture site. The wrist is then suspended in the traction tower and the fracture hematoma is debrided. The arthroscope is subsequently placed in the 4-5 or 6-R portal to look across the wrist and evaluate the articular reduction. If the fracture fragment is rotated, the guide wires may be backed out of the shaft, leaving them only in the radial styloid fragment to use as joysticks to re-reduce the fracture and then advanced across the fracture site.

Radial styloid fractures have a high incidence of associated injury to the SL interosseous ligament. The zone of injury may pass through the fracture and continue distally through the SL interosseous ligament. Following reduction of the fracture, the SL interosseous ligament is evaluated from the radial carpal and midcarpal spaces.

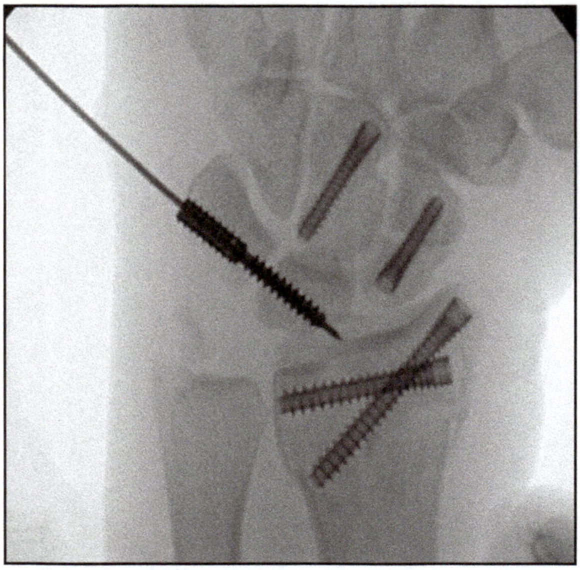

Figure 33-2. Fixation of a distal radius and scaphoid with Geissler grade IV tear to the LT interosseous ligament. The distal radius and scaphoid fractures were fixed arthroscopically. Percutaneous fixation was performed of the capitate fracture. A SLIC screw (Acumed) was percutaneously inserted to stabilize the LT interval. This entire case was treated arthroscopically or percutaneously for this severe wrist injury.

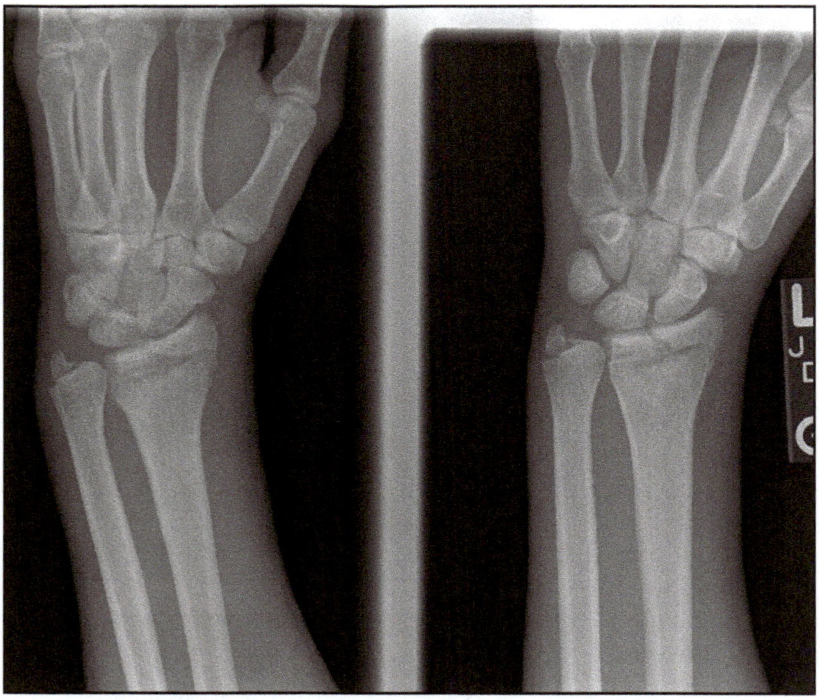

Figure 33-3. Oblique and posteroanterior plain films of a 3-part intra-articular fracture of the distal radius with an associated ulnar styloid base fracture.

Three-Part Fractures Without Metaphyseal Comminution

Displaced 3-part fractures involve radial styloid and lunate facet fracture fragments (Figure 33-3). The radial styloid fragment may almost always be reduced by closed manipulation (Figure 33-4). The radial styloid fragment is reduced and provisionally stabilized to the shaft with K-wires inserted by an oscillating drill. The wrist is then suspended in a traction tower and the fracture debris and hematoma are evacuated (Figures 33-5 to 33-7). The reduced radial styloid fragment may now be used as a landmark to reduce the depressed lunate facet fracture fragment (Figure 33-8). The arthroscope is placed in the 3-4 portal, and an 18-gauge needle is

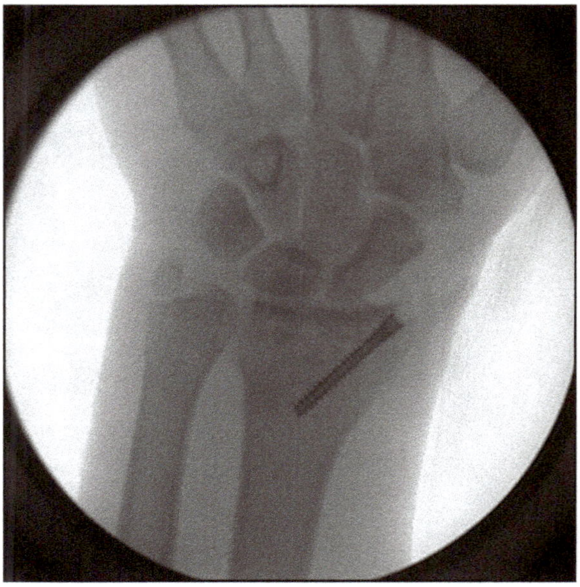

Figure 33-4. The radial styloid is closed reduced, and a headless cannulated screw is inserted to support the fracture fragment.

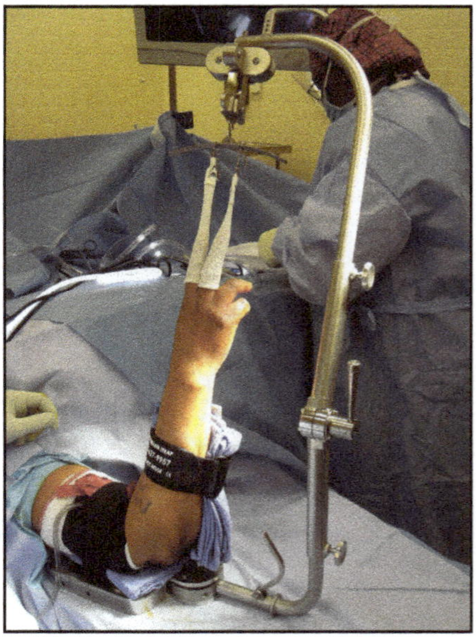

Figure 33-5. A wrist suspended in the traction tower (Acumed).

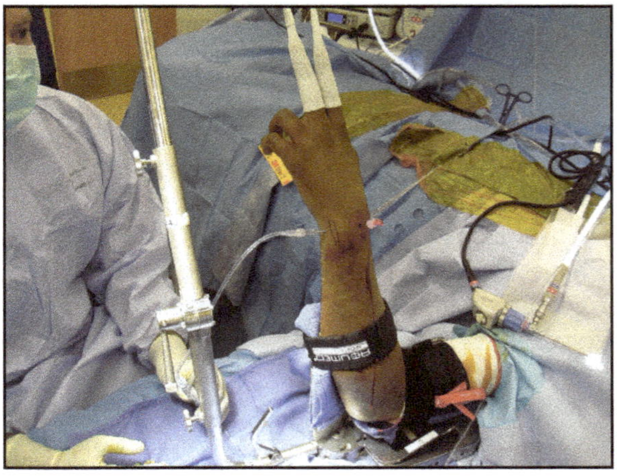

Figure 33-6. Patients with fractures of the distal radius usually present with swollen wrists. It is useful to identify the proposed portal with an 18-gauge needle prior to committing to a skin incision.

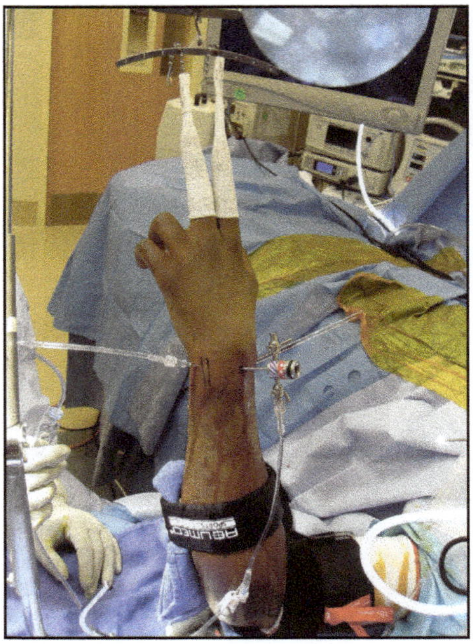

Figure 33-7. It is useful to wash out the fracture hematoma and debris to improve visualization. A separate inflow is provided through a needle through 6-U, and outflow is provided through an extension through the arthroscopic cannula.

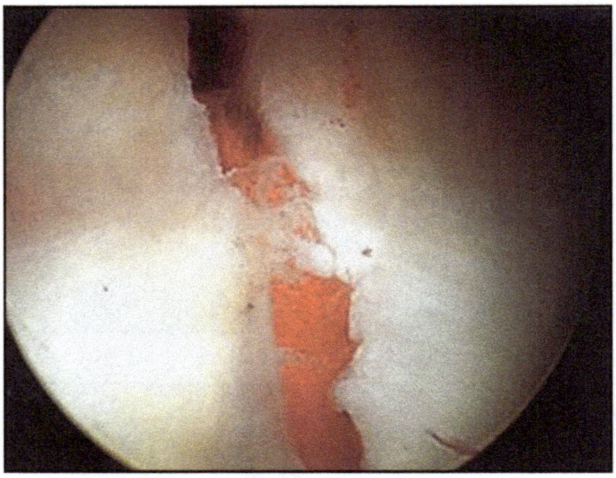

Figure 33-8. The depressed lunate facet fragment is identified with the arthroscope in the 3-4 portal.

placed percutaneously into the radial carpal space over the depressed lunate facet fragment. A large K-wire may then be placed approximately 2 cm proximal to the 18-gauge needle to elevate the depressed lunate facet fragment (Figure 33-9). A bone tenaculum is also helpful to further reduce the fracture gap between the fragments. Guide wires are then placed transversely from the radial styloid just beneath the articular surface into the lunate facet fragment once the fracture fragments are anatomically reduced as viewed arthroscopically (Figures 33-10 to 33-12). If a dorsal dye-punch fragment is present, it is important to aim the transverse wires dorsally to capture and stabilize this dorsal fragment. Following placement of the transverse guide wires, the forearm is pronated and supinated to ensure the guide wires have not violated the distal radial ulnar joint. Headless cannulated screws may then be placed over the guide wires to stabilize the radial styloid fragment and the impacted lunate facet fragment. Generally, one headless screw is used to stabilize the radial styloid fragment (Figures 33-13 and 33-14). One or 2 headless screws placed volar and dorsal to the radial styloid screw may then be used to stabilize the lunate facet fragment. Further stabilization of the lunate facet fragment may be performed by adding bone graft through a small incision placed between the fourth and fifth dorsal compartments to avoid late settling of the fracture fragments. Cancellous allograft bone chips or bone substitutes may be used.

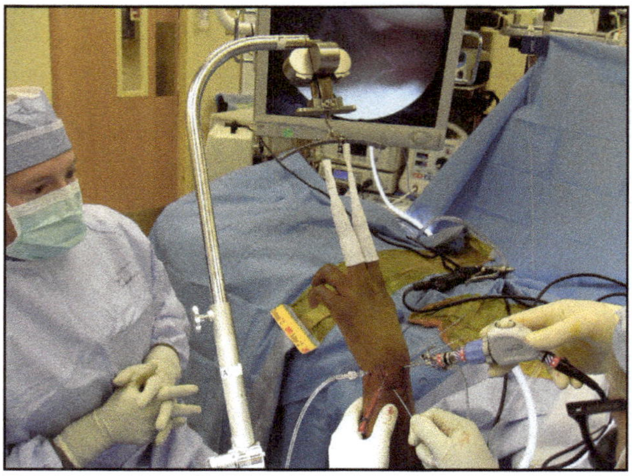

Figure 33-9. With the arthroscope in the 3-4 portal, the depressed fragment is percutaneously elevated with a large K-wire inserted approximately 2 cm proximal to the fracture, and it is elevated as viewed directly arthroscopically.

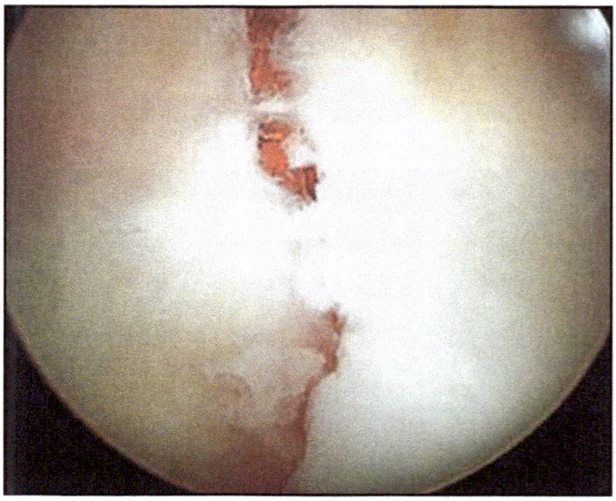

Figure 33-10. Arthroscopic view showing reduction of the impacted lunate facet fragment. Once the fragment is elevated, transverse guide wires are placed through the radial styloid into the impacted lunate facet fragment.

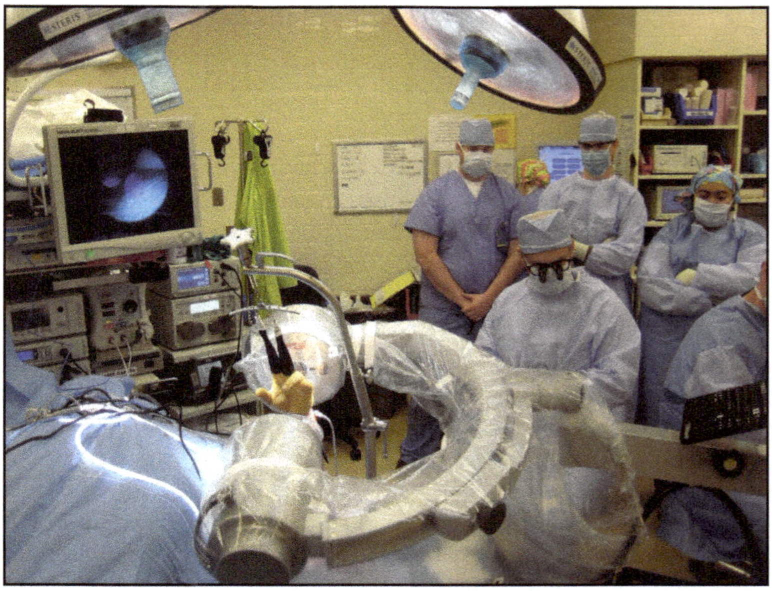

Figure 33-11. The Acumed wrist traction tower is mini C-arm friendly. The Orthoscan C-arm is brought in to confirm the articular reduction to the lunate facet and position of the guide wires.

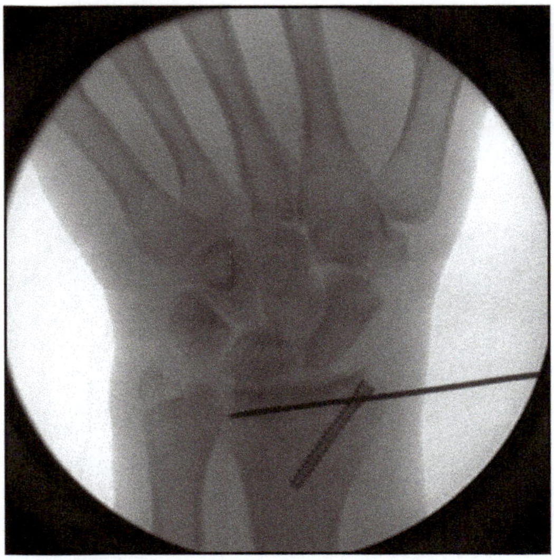

Figure 33-12. Fluoroscopic view confirming anatomic reduction to the articular surface and ideal placement of the guide wires volar and dorsal to the previous hemi-screw inserted into the radial styloid.

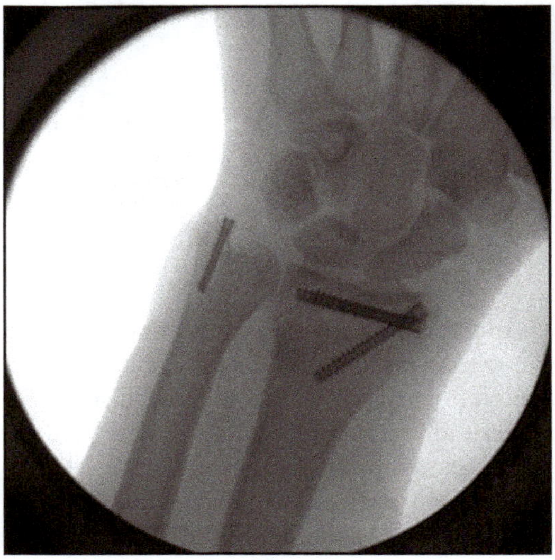

Figure 33-13. Postoperative fluoroscopic view showing anatomic reduction to the articular surface and ideal placement of the headless cannulated screws. The articular disk had lost its tension when palpated, and no peripheral tear was identified. In this instance, a micro Acutrak (Acumed) was placed through the ulnar styloid fragment.

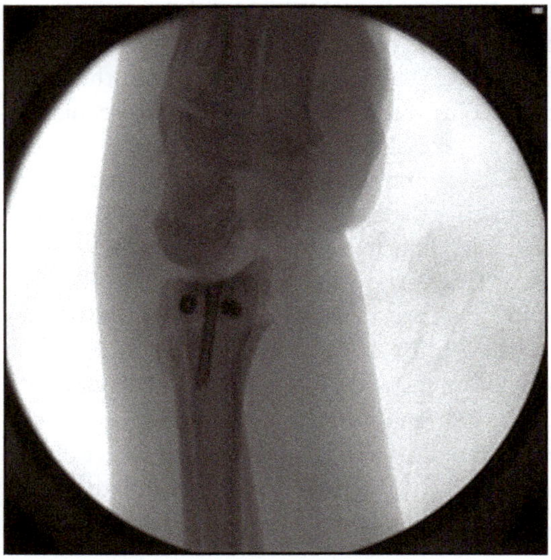

Figure 33-14. Fluoroscopic lateral view confirming anatomic reduction to the articular surface with headless screws placed anterior/posterior to the radial styloid screw.

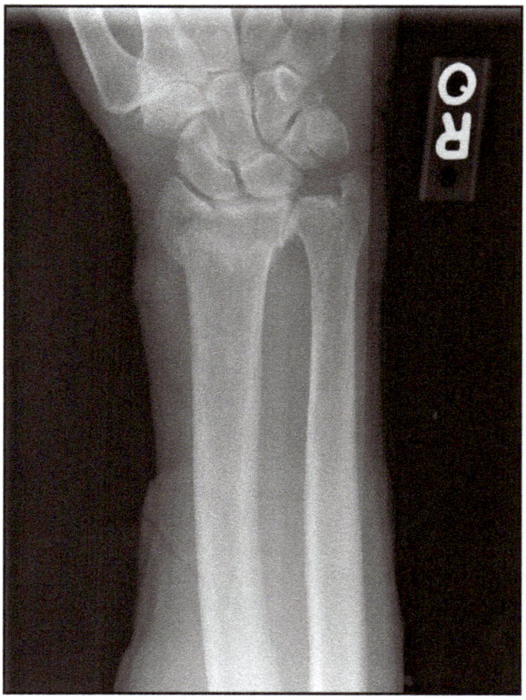

Figure 33-15. Posteroanterior x-ray showing a displaced intra-articular fracture of the distal radius with radial shortening.

Three- and Four-Part Fractures With Metaphyseal Comminution

In this scenario, a standard volar approach is made to the distal radius over the radial side of the flexor carpi radialis tendon. The flexor pollicis longus tendon is identified and retracted to protect the median nerve, and the pronator quadratus is released from the radial border of the distal radius. The brachioradialis may be further released from the radial styloid to facilitate fracture reduction. It is important not to open the joint capsule during the approach and subsequent dissection. The fracture is provisionally reduced and stabilized with a volar plate. The initial screw is placed in the offset hole of the volar plate in order to stabilize the plate to the radial shaft. The fracture fragments are manipulated to attain a reduction that is as anatomic as possible when viewed under fluoroscopy. Provisional stabilization with K-wires to the plate is performed.

The wrist is then suspended in the traction tower and the articular reduction is viewed arthroscopically. If the articular reduction is not anatomic, the pins are removed from the plate, and the reduction is fine-tuned. Once the reduction is judged to be anatomic arthroscopically, the pins are placed back through the plate to provide provisional stabilization to the fracture fragments. It is important to have the wrist solidly flexed in the traction tower to help reduce the distal radius to the plate so there is no gap. A nonlocking distal screw is initially placed in the distal aspect of the plate to further reduce the fracture fragments to the plate. The remaining distal screws are inserted and the reduction is viewed under fluoroscopy and arthroscopy. Particularly, in distal dorsal lip fragments, arthroscopy is useful to judge fragment stability as the distal screws are being inserted. Dorsal lip fragments are best seen with the arthroscope in the 6-R portal or through a volar radial portal between the radial scaphocapitate and long radial lunate ligament.

In 4-part fractures, the lunate facet is divided into volar and dorsal fragments (Figures 33-15 and 33-16). The volar ulnar fragment is reduced to the radial styloid fragment under direct observation through the volar approach and pinned (Figure 33-17). The volar distal radius plate is used to provisionally stabilize the radial styloid and volar ulnar fragments (Figures 33-18 and 33-19).

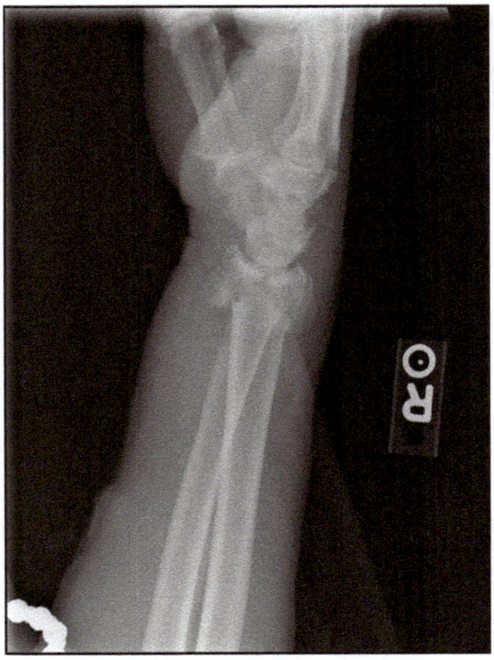

Figure 33-16. The lateral view demonstrates a 4-part fracture of the distal radius with a displaced volar ulnar fragment. This fracture cannot be closed reduced and requires open reduction and stabilization.

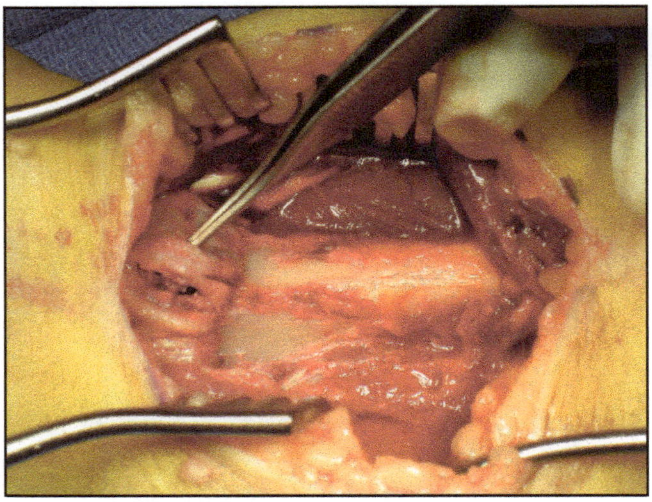

Figure 33-17. Intraoperative view showing reduction of the radial styloid and the volar ulnar fragment back to the radial shaft.

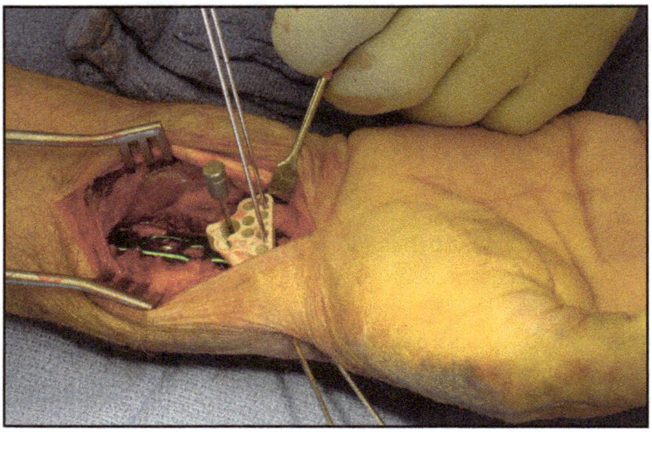

Figure 33-18. The Acumed Acu-Loc is placed through the volar incision. The fracture is provisionally stabilized with K-wires placed through the radial styloid and through the plate to support the articular surface reduction.

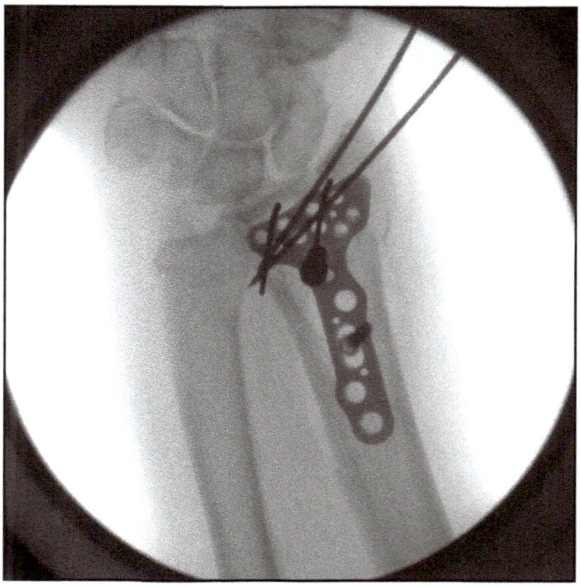

Figure 33-19. Fluoroscopic view demonstrating the provisional articular reduction to the distal radius.

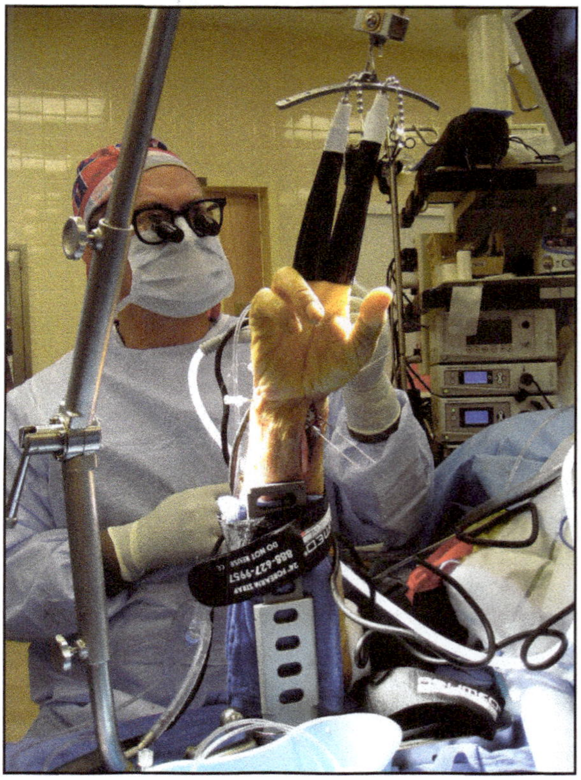

Figure 33-20. The wrist is then suspended in the Acumed wrist traction tower, and articular reduction is evaluated. The tower gives full exposure to the volar aspects of the wrist so the K-wires can be removed and replaced if the articular surface reduction is not satisfactory.

The wrist is then suspended in the traction tower. With the arthroscope in the 6-R portal, the dorsal lunate fragment is then visualized and percutaneously elevated (Figure 33-20). Once the articular surface is anatomic as seen arthroscopically, the provisional fixation is advanced from volar to dorsal to stabilize the dorsal fragment (Figures 33-21 and 33-22). The distal screws are then placed in the volar plate (Figures 33-23 and 33-24).

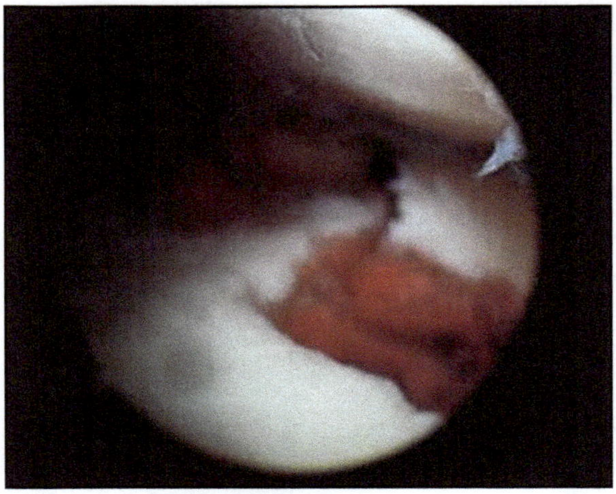

Figure 33-21. Arthroscopic view with the arthroscope in the 6-R portal showing displacement to the dorsal ulnar fragment.

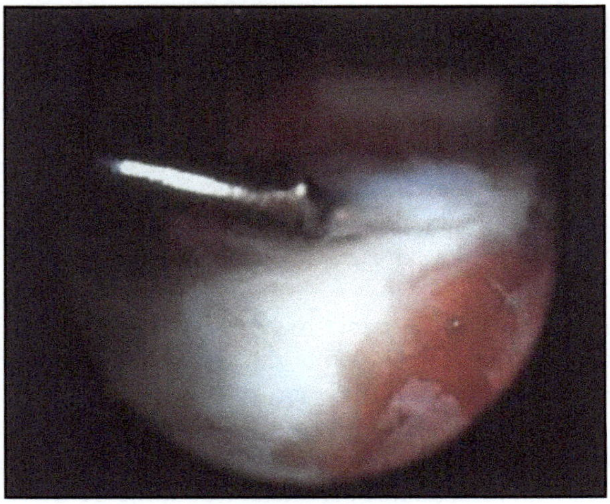

Figure 33-22. Arthroscopic view showing reduction of the dorsal ulnar fragment back to the volar ulnar fragment as viewed arthroscopically with the arthroscope in the 6-R portal.

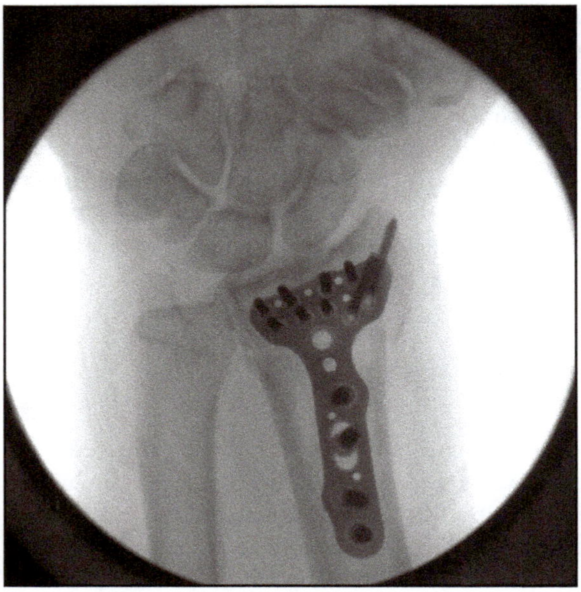

Figure 33-23. Posteroanterior fluoroscopic view showing placement of the Acu-Loc plate (Acumed) and anatomic restoration to the articular surface.

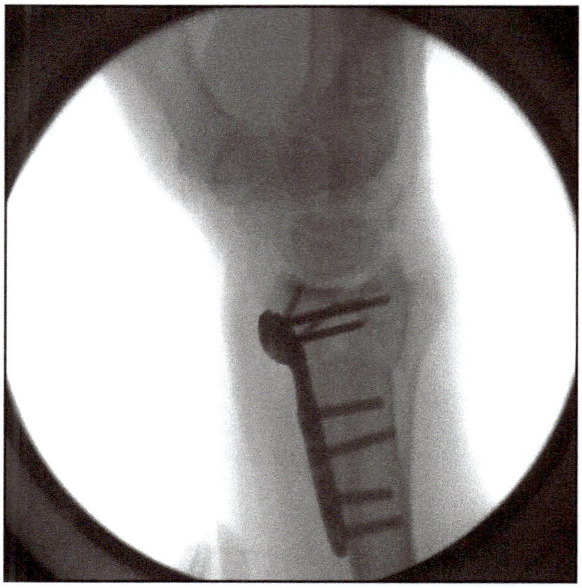

Figure 33-24. Lateral fluoroscopic view confirming anatomic reduction to the articular surface with reduction of the volar and dorsal lunate facet fracture fragments.

Volar plate stabilization using wrist arthroscopy as an adjunct to view the articular reduction is preferred if metaphyseal comminution is present. This allows a stable construct and early ROM and rehabilitation compared to K-wires or headless screws alone. Late settling of the fracture fragments is likely to be seen with volar plate stabilization compared to percutaneous K-wires or cannulated screws.

Recommendations for stabilization of an associated ulnar styloid fragment are controversial. Following anatomic reduction of a distal radius fracture, the tension of the articular disk is palpated with a probe. The arthroscope is placed in the 3-4 portal, the probe is inserted through the 6-R portal, and the tension of the disk is evaluated. The majority of the fibers of the TFCC are still attached to the base of the ulna as opposed to the displaced ulnar styloid fragment when there is good tension noted to the articular disk with palpation. A peripheral tear of the TFCC is suspected if there is loss of tension to the disk. A peripheral tear is often covered with hematoma or synovitis, and it is important to debride the hematoma to obtain direct visualization of the periphery to the articular disk. A peripheral tear is repaired arthroscopically when detected. Stabilization of a large ulnar styloid fragment is considered when there is loss of tension to the articular disk and no peripheral ulnar tear of the articular disk is identified. In this case, the majority of the fibers of the articular disk are attached to the ulnar styloid fragment. The incision is made between the interval of the extensor carpi ulnaris and flexor carpi ulnaris, and blunt dissection is carried down to protect the dorsal sensory branch of the ulnar nerve, which runs along the volar aspect of the incision. The ulnar styloid fragment is anatomically reduced and may be stabilized with a tension band, K-wire, or, preferably, a small headless cannulated screw.

Postoperative Protocol

Postoperatively, the wrist is placed in a volar resting splint to allow for soft tissue rest. The patient is encouraged to keep the extremity elevated and perform finger exercises to reduce swelling and prevent stiffness. At 2 weeks postoperatively, the splint is removed, plain x-rays are obtained, and sutures are removed. If postoperative swelling has resolved sufficiently, the wrist is placed in a custom fabricated splint that is worn at all times except to perform gentle ROM exercises. After 6 weeks postoperatively, the splint is discontinued and exercises focusing on strength and grip are added. At 12 weeks postoperatively, the patient is progressed to activity as tolerated and often may be discharged from care.

Potential Complications

Adding wrist arthroscopy as an adjunct to the operative treatment of distal radius fractures is relatively safe. Traditionally, wrist arthroscopy has enjoyed a relatively low complication rate. Beredjiklian et al[18] reported 11 complications in a series of 211. Of these, 2 major complications occurred, including permanent wrist stiffness after a synovectomy and the formation of a ganglion cyst. Minor complications included neuropraxia form portal placement, portal site infection, and skin burns. Theoretically, arthroscopy in the light of wrist trauma could lead to excess extravasation of fluid into the soft tissues during a prolonged arthroscopic procedure. This could result in postoperative joint stiffness, increased difficulty with tissue dissection during adjunct open procedures, or iatrogenic compartment syndrome. Many of these complications can be avoided by careful portal placement attentiveness to the amount of fluid extravasation during the procedure.

Top Technical Pearls for the Procedure

1. Precise portal placement is mandatory in wrist arthroscopy. Therefore, with a swollen wrist, it is important to know the external landmarks that can usually be palpated to help in portal placement. The 3-4 portal is made in line with the radial border of the long finger. The 4-5 portal is in line with the mid-axis of the ring finger. The 6-R portal is just radial to the extensor carpi ulnaris tendon. It is important to place a needle into a portal location prior to committing to a skin incision.
2. Take the time to wash out fracture hematoma and debris to improve visualization.
3. It is easier to judge rotation of a fracture fragment by looking across the wrist from the fragment. A radial styloid fragment is best visualized with the arthroscope in the 6-R portal, and a depressed lunate facet fragment is best visualized with the arthroscope in the 3-4 portal.
4. Be wary of the cutaneous sensory nerves about the wrist. Insert guide wires through a small incision, through a trocar, or in oscillation mode.
5. Using wrist arthroscopy as an adjunct combining with volar plating in fractures with extensive metaphyseal involvement allows for anatomic restoration of the joint surface and good stability, which allows an early ROM program.

References

1. Mohanti RC, Kar N. Study of triangular fibrocartilage of the wrist joint in Colles' fracture. *Injury.* 1980;11(4):321-324.
2. Fontes D, Lenoble E, de Somer B, Benoit J. Lesions of the ligaments associated with distal fractures of the radius. 58 intraoperative arthrographies [in French]. *Ann Chir Main Memb Super.* 1992;11(2):119-125.
3. Geissler WB, Freeland AE, Savoie FH, et al. Carpal instability associated with intraarticular distal radius fractures. Presented at: Proceedings, American Academy Orthopedic Surgeons Annual Meeting; February 18-23, 1993; San Francisco, CA.

4. Lindau T. Treatment of injuries to the ulnar side of the wrist occurring with distal radial fractures. *Hand Clin*. 2005;21(3):417-425.
5. Hanker GJ. Wrist arthroscopy in distal radius fractures. Presented at: Proceedings, Arthroscopy Association North America Annual Meeting; October 6-10, 1993; Albuquerque, NM.
6. Knirk JL, Jupiter JB. Intra-articular fractures of the distal end of the radius in young adults. *J Bone Joint Surg Am*. 1986;68(5):647-659.
7. Bradway JK, Amadio PC, Cooney WP. Open reduction and internal fixation of displaced comminuted intra-articular fractures of the distal end of the radius. *J Bone Joint Surg Am*. 1989;71(6):839-847.
8. Fernandez DL, Geissler WB. Treatment of displaced articular fractures of the radius. *J Hand Surg*. 1991;16(3):375-384.
9. Trumble TE, Schmitt SR, Vedder NB. Fractures affecting functional outcome of displaced intra-articular distal radius fractures. *J Hand Surg Am*. 1994;19(2):325 340.
10. Edwards CC II, Harasztic CJ, McGillivary GR, Gutow AP. Intra-articular distal radius fractures: arthroscopic assessment of radiographically assisted reduction. *J Hand Surg*. 2001;26(6):1036-1041.
11. Stewart NJ, Berger RA. Comparison study of arthroscopic as open reduction of comminuted distal radius fractures. In: Presented at the 53rd Annual Meeting of the American Society for Surgery of the Hand (Programs and Abstracts); January 11, 1998; Scottsdale, AZ.
12. Doi K, Hatturi T, Otsuka K, Abe T, Tamamoto H. Intra-articular fractures of the distal aspect of the radius: arthroscopically assisted reduction compared with open reduction and internal fixation. *J Bone Joint Surg Am*. 1999;81(8):1093-1110.
13. Geissler WB, Freeland AE. Arthroscopically assisted reduction of intraarticular distal radial fractures. *Clin Orthop Relat Res*. 1996;(327):125-134.
14. Geissler WB, Savoie FH. Arthroscopic techniques of the wrist. *Mediguide to Orthopedics*. 1992;11:1-8.
15. Geissler WB. Arthroscopically assisted reduction of intra-articular fractures of the distal radius. *Hand Clin*. 1995;11(1):19-29.
16. Del Piñal F. Technical tips for (dry) arthroscopic reduction and internal fixation of distal radius fractures. *J Hand Surg Am*. 2011;36(10):1694-1705.
17. Geissler WB. Intra-articular distal radius fractures: the role of arthroscopy? *Hand Clin*. 2005;21(3):407-416.
18. Beredjiklian PK, Bozentka DJ, Leung YL, Monaghan BA. Complications of wrist arthroscopy. *J Hand Surg Am*. 2004;29(3):406-411.

Please see videos on the accompanying website at

www.routledge.com/9781630910013

SECTION VI

WRIST ARTHROSCOPY
Special Techniques

34

Carpal, Metacarpal, and Phalangeal Fractures

Michael P. Gaspar, MD; Brian D. Norton, MD;
Randall W. Culp, MD; and A. Lee Osterman, MD

Introduction

Carpal, metacarpal, and phalangeal fractures are the most common injuries treated by hand surgeons. Historically, 10% of all fractures occur in the metacarpals or phalanges. Of these fractures, 80% are isolated to the tubular bones of the hands.[1-3] In the early twentieth century, most carpal and hand fractures were treated nonoperatively regardless of the amount of displacement. Even today, nondisplaced or minimally displaced fractures are viewed as stable and treated conservatively with closed reduction and cast immobilization. Unstable fractures require surgical fixation to restore alignment, length, and rotation. Fixation methods include percutaneous pinning, external fixation, open reduction and internal fixation, and arthroscopically assisted reduction and internal fixation. Arthroscopically assisted fixation has gained increased popularity with the advances in technology and increases in surgeons' arthroscopic skill sets.

Background

Indications for arthroscopic surgery of the wrist and finger joints have rapidly evolved since Chen first reported his findings in 1979.[4] Current indications include the diagnosis and treatment of numerous wrist disorders, including fractures, soft tissue pathology, and arthritis. However, arthroscopy of smaller joints, including the metacarpophalangeal (MCP) and interphalangeal joints, has lagged in comparison to wrist arthroscopy.[5] In 1995, Ryu and Fagan[6] described treating the ulnar collateral ligament Stener lesion in 8 thumbs with success. In 1999, Rozmaryn and Wei[7] reported the technical aspects of MCP arthroscopy with general references to the potential use of this technique in treating juxta- and intra-articular fractures. In the same year, Slade and Gutow[8] published a review article on arthroscopy of the MCP joint. They offered detailed technical explanations and emphasized that small joint arthroscopy requires specialized instruments and a thorough knowledge of the anatomy within these specialized joints. In 2006, Badia[9] reported encouraging results in treating bony gamekeeper's thumb with arthroscopically assisted reduction and internal fixation (AARIF).

Savoie FH III, Field LD, Steinmann SP, eds. *The Elbow and Wrist: AANA Advanced Arthroscopic Surgical Techniques* (pp 349-359).

Anatomy

Due to the relatively small working space in the MCP and interphalangeal (IP) joints, knowledge of normal wrist and hand anatomy, precise portal placement, and appropriately selected instrumentation are critical to success when performing small joint arthroscopy of the hand and fingers. Fracture fixation of small joints presents unique challenges that test the skills necessary to successfully restore articular congruity in AARIF.

Anatomically, the MCP joint is composed of several critical structures. These include the osseous metacarpal head, the proximal phalangeal base, and soft tissue restraints, including the Stout volar plate, collateral ligaments, and relatively thin and flimsy dorsal capsule. The thumb carpometacarpal (CMC) joint is described in detail by Bettinger et al.[10] The authors describe the 16 ligaments surrounding the CMC joint. Strong extensor tendons run dorsal to the dorsal capsule and are held in check to the capsular fibers and the sagittal bands. On either side of the joint are the insertions of the intrinsic muscles on the extensor mechanism. The digital neurovascular bundles rest volar to the joint, along with the flexor tendons. The terminal branches of the dorsal sensory nerves are less predictably centered over the dorsum of the joint.

Indications

- Juxta- or intra-articular fractures of CMC and MCP joints.
- Simple 2-part fracture with displacement greater than 1 mm involving the metacarpal head or base of the proximal phalanx[11]
- Avulsion fracture with a rotated fragment from the collateral ligament insertion
- Treatment of dye punch articular fractures of the proximal phalangeal base
- Salter-Harris type III physeal fractures

Conservative Management

- Poor soft tissue coverage
- Open fractures
- Active cellulitis[11]
- Fractures with 3 or more fragments
- Comminution, or associated diaphyseal extension that cannot be easily reduced percutaneously
- Patients with frail or thin-appearing skin, as is often associated with chronic diseases and/or steroid use

Pertinent Physical Findings

- Inability to fully flex and extend the digit
- Tenderness and swelling about the affected joint
- A suspicious laceration or cut in the region of the injured joint should heighten the awareness for an open articular fracture.
- Rotational malalignment of the digit is often associated with a displaced articular fragment and indicates an unstable fracture pattern.

Particular attention should be paid to patients with frail or thin-appearing skin, which is often associated with chronic diseases and chronic steroid use. If small joint arthroscopy is performed on these patients, inadvertent damage to the skin can occur from the traction applied across the joint during the arthroscopic procedure.

Pertinent Imaging

- Plain radiographs provide most of the information necessary to diagnose lesions of the MCP joints.
- Special views, including oblique and Brewerton views to evaluate the metacarpal head, may be useful in addition to traditional posteroanterior and lateral x-rays in the evaluation of articular displacement.
- Computed tomographic scans can also help to define step-offs of intra-articular fractures.
- Bone scans can be useful to rule out a questionable fracture of the metacarpal head.

Equipment

- Wrist traction tower with appropriate sized finger traps
- Sterile Coban for positioning fingers and securing finger traps
- High-pressure Inflow system: The small radius of the inflow cannulas requires higher pressures to ensure adequate irrigation.[8] A gravity system using a pinch pump and small joint or a standard arthroscopy pump set to maintain the pressure between 50 and 80 mm Hg may be used.
- Mini C-arm fluoroscope
- Small hand wire driver
- Mini curette(s)
- Mini-fragment screws
- Power drill (for final implant placement)
- Specialized small joint instruments are necessary for arthroscopy of small joints
- 1.9-mm, 30- degree arthroscope is used in conjunction with a 2.2-mm cannula
- Instruments and shavers between the sizes of 2.0 and 2.5 mm in diameter
- Small grasper(s)/biter(s)
- Small radiofrequency ablation probe
- 18-gauge needle
- #11 or #15 blade scalpel

Positioning and Portals

- The patient is placed supine on the operating room table and a tourniquet is placed on the upper arm and preset to 250 mm Hg.
- The affected arm is positioned on a radiolucent arm table, and the surgeon is positioned at the cephalic side of the arm.

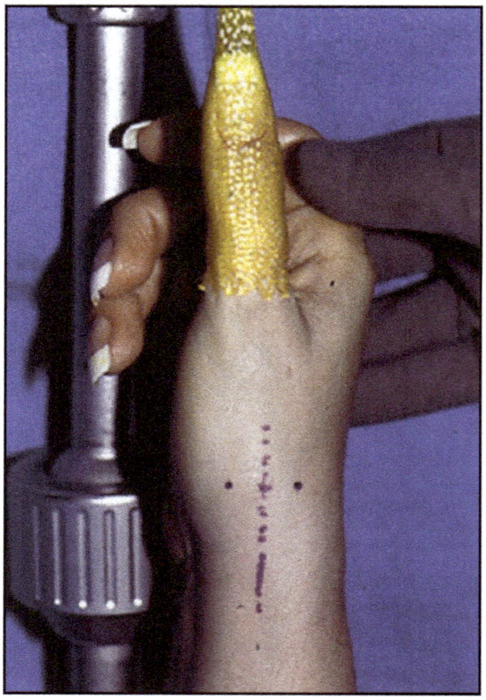

Figure 34-1. Standard small joint arthroscopy set up with Chinese finger traps suspending the thumb.

- Using finger traps, 5 lb of longitudinal traction is typically applied to the thumb or affected digit, with the possibility of increasing traction to as much as 10 or 12 lb (Figure 34-1).
- Place the operative finger in the line of axis of traction, with the other 2 surrounding digits providing rotational control.[10]
- Coban is used to wrap the wrist in place against the wrist tower and provides additional stabilization for the thumb or digits if the finger trap is loose fitting (Figure 34-2).
- The mini C-arm fluoroscopy machine is positioned parallel to the table, out of the way of the operating surgeon (Figure 34-3).

Step-by-Step Description of the Procedure

The authors present a broad overview of AARIF of small joint fractures and offer additional insight into specific small joint fracture pattern. General or regional anesthesia is appropriate for AARIF as long as adequate sedation is achieved to allow painless elevation of the tourniquet for the necessary time.

Thumb Carpometacarpal Base and Trapezial Fractures

Intra-articular fractures of the thumb metacarpal base include the more common Bennett's fracture and a less common Rolando variant (Figure 34-4). Fractures of the trapezium are rare (less than 5% of all small bone fractures) and may occur when forced radial deviation of the thumb results in avulsion due to capsular strain (see Figure 34-1).

Step 1

After elevation of the tourniquet, the joint of interest is localized with an 18-gauge needle. The skin is incised with a #11 or #15 blade. Special care is taken to remain superficial to avoid injury to

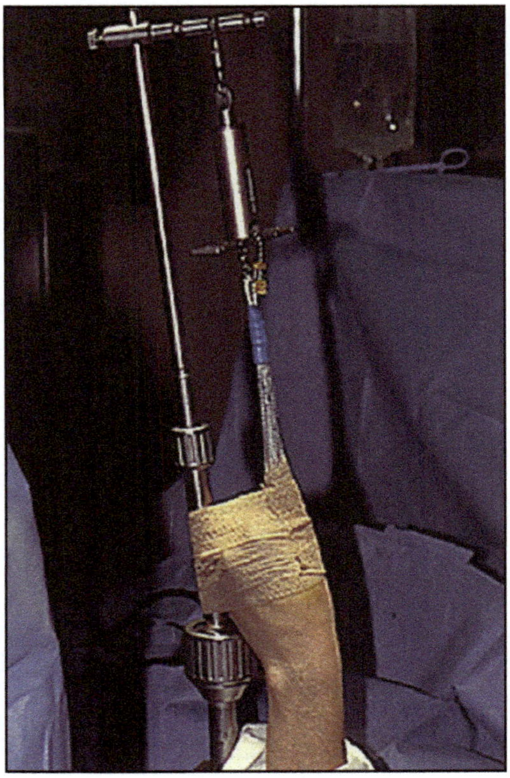

Figure 34-2. Coban was used to set and maintain the hand in the proper position.

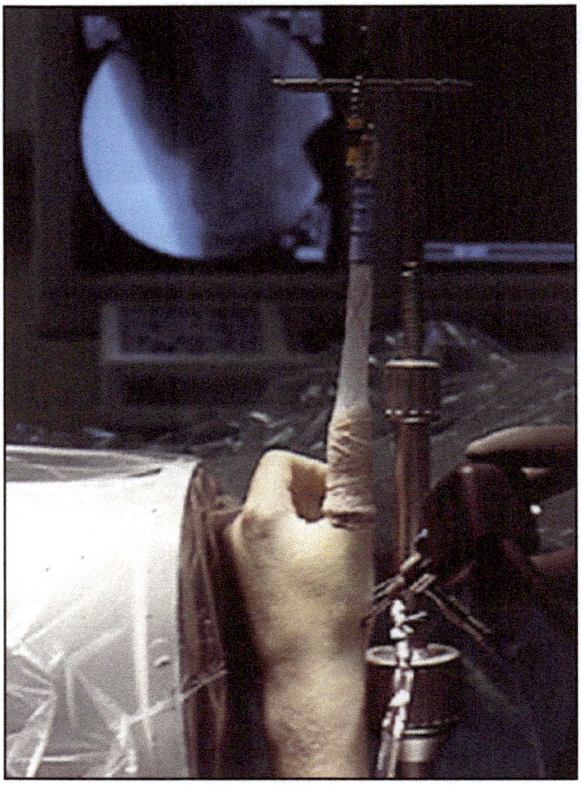

Figure 34-3. The typical set up for a shell, with the C-arm appropriately positioned adjacent to the traction tower but away from the surgeon, providing unobstructed access to the joint of interest.

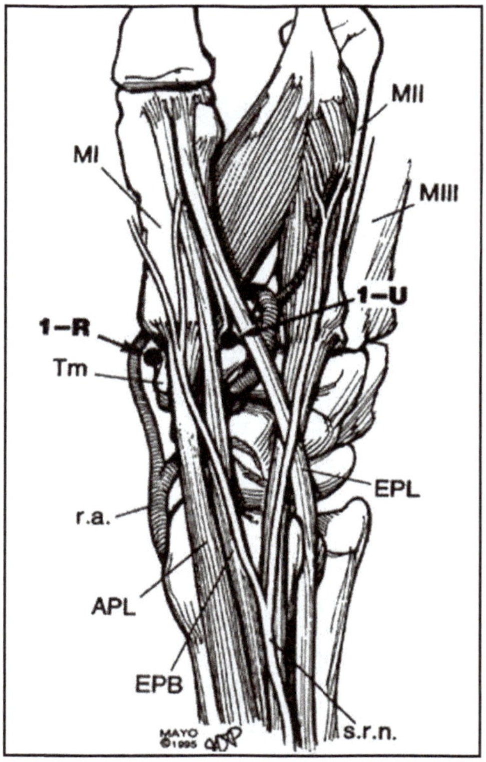

Figure 34-4. Incision for the 1-R (radial) portal is placed just volar to the abductor pollicis longus (APL) tendon, where the incision for the 1-U (ulnar) portal is made just ulnar to the extensor pollicis brevis (EPB) tendon.

branches of dorsal sensory nerves. The authors prefer to bluntly insert the trocar and arthroscopic camera with one smooth stroke, thereby achieving a "suction seal" with the portal. Alternatively, a small, curved clamp can be inserted into the joint capsule before inserting the arthroscope. With either method, care should be taken so that the trocar is introduced into the joint in an atraumatic fashion.

Step 2

For fractures at the thumb CMC base, the base of the first metacarpal is identified and palpated. The incision for the 1-R (radial) portal is placed just volar to the abductor pollicis longus tendon, and the incision for the 1-U (ulnar) portal is made just ulnar to the extensor pollicis brevis tendon (see Figures 34-1 and 34-5). For trapezial fractures, the portals may be placed slightly more proximal to allow for evaluation of the scaphotrapeziotrapezoid joint. Before the skin incision is made, the CMC joint is distended by injecting 2 mL of normal saline. A 1.9-mm arthroscope is atraumatically introduced into the joint at the 1-R portal. The 1-U working portal is then established under direct visualization using a similar technique. Viewing and working portals are interchanged to ensure complete visualization of the critical ligamentous structures, including the dorsal radial, posterior oblique, ulnar collateral, and anterior oblique ligaments.

Step 3

After the thumb CMC joint has been entered, it is often necessary to debride synovitis and fracture hematoma debris with an arthroscopic shaver (Figure 34-6). A systematic approach is used to visualize critical structures such as the anterior oblique ligament and fracture fragments.

After debridement and evacuation of hematoma, the fracture fragments are manipulated into position with a probe or K-wire (Figure 34-7). A 0.035- or 0.045-inch K-wire is useful for this purpose and can be used as a joystick to reduce and pin the fragments. The authors introduce the K-wire and advance it just proximal to the fracture site while holding the fracture fragment reduced with a probe before advancing the K-wire or across the fracture site.

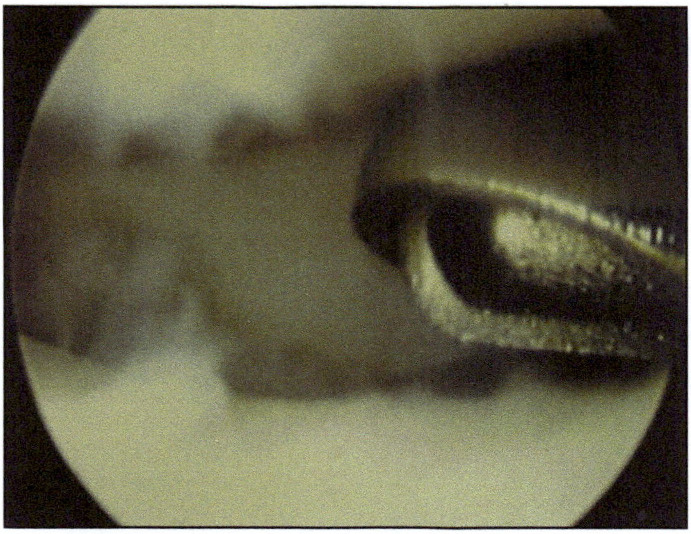

Figure 34-5. A specialized shaver used for debriding synovitis within the small joint to improve fracture visualization.

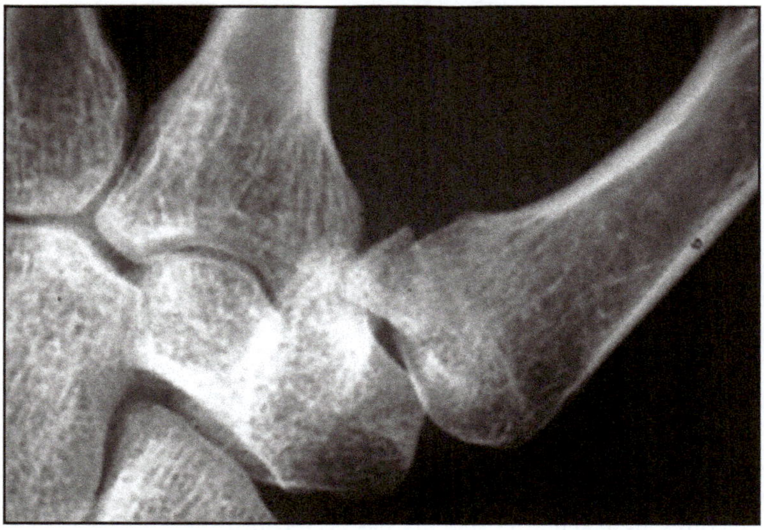

Figure 34-6. The radiograph demonstrates the characteristic appearance of a Bennett fracture, the most common fracture pattern at the base of the thumb metacarpal. This fracture is intra-articular, begins at the ulnar base of the thumb metacarpal, and is rotated in supination by the pull of the abductor pollicis longus (APL).

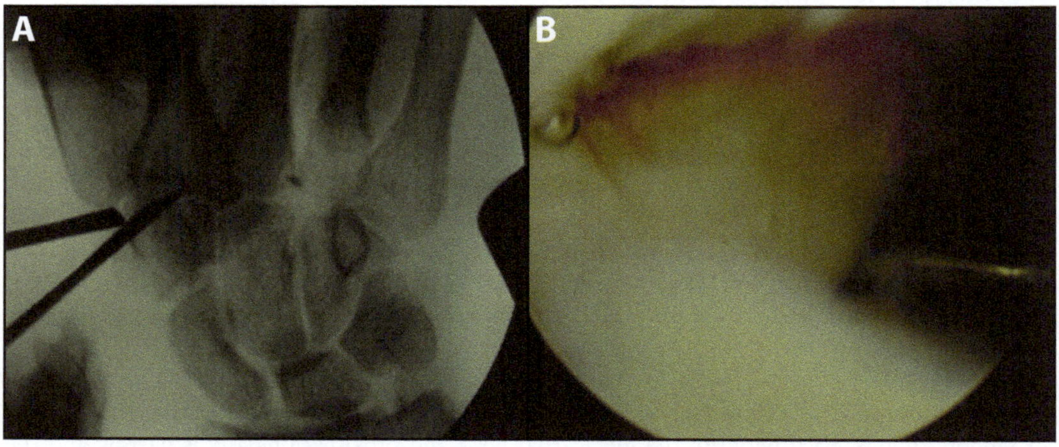

Figure 34-7. (A) The fluoroscopic image shows a probe holding the volar fracture fragment in good position. (B) The arthroscopic view verifies the anatomic reduction of an intra-articular Bennett fracture. The probe was holding the reduction before K-wire fixation.

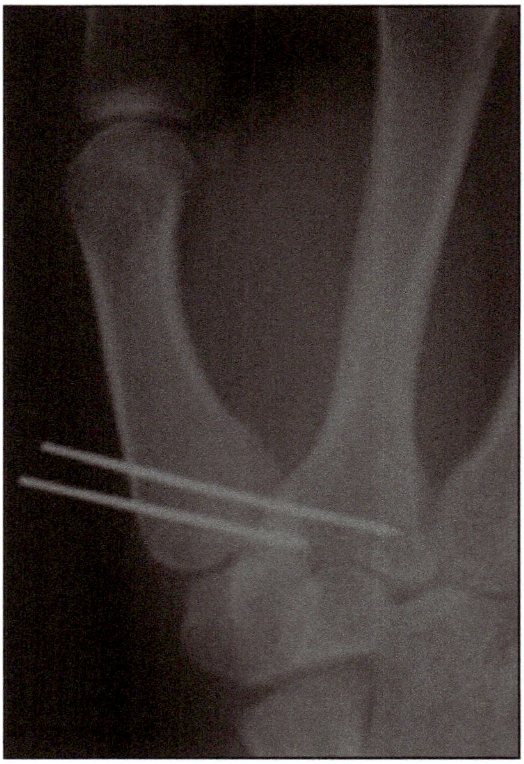

Figure 34-8. The postoperative radiograph demonstrates percutaneous fixation of a Bennett fracture in an excellent position.

Step 4

After the fracture has been adequately reduced, the guide wire is inserted perpendicular to the fracture plane. A second guide wire is then inserted to maintain rotational control and either provide definitive fixation or stability during placement of the cannulated screw (Figure 34-8). If the surgeon elects to use cannulated screws, proper screw length is measured and the appropriate screws inserted over the guide wire with the reduction is visualized as a screw is inserted. C-arm fluoroscopy is useful during fixation and final reduction. After fixation is obtained, the arthroscope may be used to verify anatomic reduction and to ensure proper position of the K-wire or screw. Final fluoroscopic pictures are taken after stability has been confirmed and the joint is taken through a final range of motion (Figure 34-9). Skin incisions are closed with 4-0 nylon.

Thumb and Digital Metacarpophalangeal Fractures

Small joints of the hand offer minimal joint spaces and considerable iatrogenic injury may be caused if care is not taken. In acutely injured hands, excessive swelling may obscure superficial landmarks. In these cases, the surgeon should not hesitate to use C-arm fluoroscopy to assist in localizing the joint.

When treating thumb radial collateral ligament avulsion fractures, the patient is positioned and the thumb is suspended as previously described. The principles of thumb MCP and digital MCP AARIF are quite similar to those for CMC arthroscopy.

Step 1

The portals for MCP arthroscopy are simple because they lie on either side of the visible extensor tendon. The interval between the metacarpal head and proximal phalanx is narrow and the joint space is localized with an 18-gauge needle before a skin incision is made. The arthroscope is introduced at the same angle. A thorough inspection of the joint is performed, along with

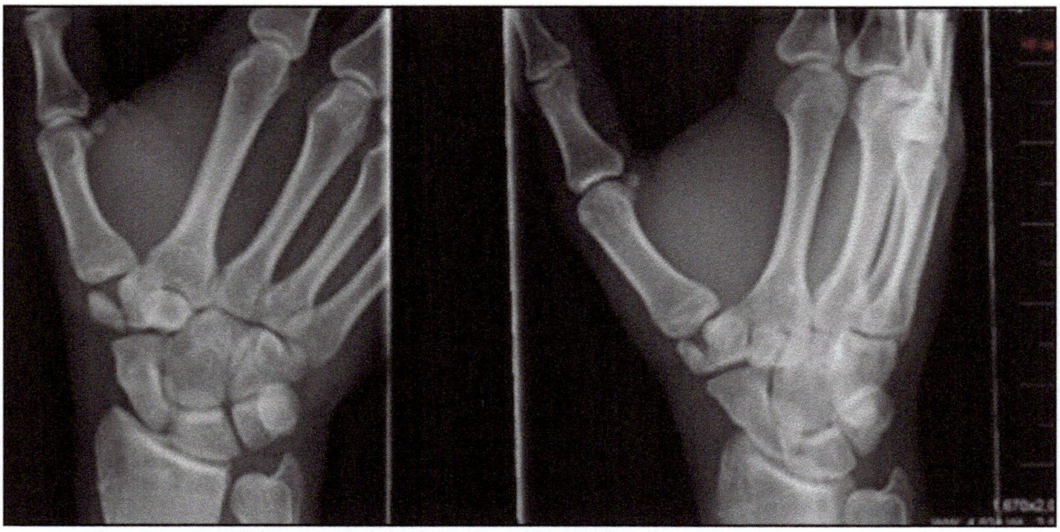

Figure 34-9. The radiograph demonstrating a displaced fracture of trapezium.

synovectomy and debridement of the fracture hematoma. Fracture reduction is achieved with use of a probe, and a K-wire is introduced to maintain anatomic reduction of the fracture.

Step 2

Portal incisions are once again made with a #11 or #15 blade knife. The camera is introduced as previously described. As before, debridement may be necessary to adequately view the joint. Systematic evaluation of the joint, beginning with assessment of one collateral ligament, followed by the volar plate and finally the contralateral collateral ligament, should be performed as described by Badia.[5] This is followed by evaluation of the dorsal capsule, extensor mechanism, and articular surface of the proximal phalanx and metacarpal head.

Step 3

After performing any necessary debridement and visualization of important structures, reduction and pinning should be performed as described previously. Intra-articular fractures with impaction, known as *die punch fractures*, require a more delicate approach to fixation. Care must be taken not to disengage the fragment, thereby destabilizing it and creating a loose body in the joint. A percutaneous K-wire can be used to fine-tune the reduction, while the probe is used to reduce the fragment. Definitive fixation is achieved with a subcutaneous buttress pin. Additional pins may be required to hold the fixation.

Step 4

After fixation, the arthroscope can be utilized to directly evaluate joint congruity. Final radiographs should then be taken to confirm anatomic reduction with no intra-articular step-off or deformity in order to minimize the likelihood of future posttraumatic arthritis. Skin incisions are closed with 4-0 nylon.

Postoperative Protocol

The usual postoperative protocol involves a short-arm thumb spica splint for MCP or CMC arthroscopy and a dorsal MCP block splint in flexion for digital MCP arthroscopy. Splinting in the safe position allows the collateral ligaments to heal in their most taut position to prevent loss of motion. The IP joints are left free. Sutures are removed 7 to 10 days postoperatively and K-wires are removed at approximately 4 weeks. AARIF of small joints offers the benefit of minimal capsular, collateral ligament, and tendon scarring. Consequently, there is faster recovery of the full digital range of motion.[9] Formal occupational therapy is initiated if necessary, but most patients are able to follow a home exercise program.

Potential Complications

Complications are rarely encountered but may include pin tract infection, K-wire migration, neurovascular injury, and digital stiffness. Careful preoperative patient selection, with particular attention to skin quality and presence of infection is critical for prevention of infection. Use of cannulated screws, when appropriate, avoids the potential for wire migration, while also mitigating the potential for infection due to exposed hardware. Careful surgical dissection is necessary to avoid neurovascular injury, particularly to dorsal sensory nerves. Finally, proper postoperative management including appropriate splint placement and proper therapy regimen are crucial in minimizing the risk of postoperative stiffness.

Top Technical Pearls for the Procedure

1. When inserting the trocar into the joint, use a steady, smooth stroke to create a "suction seal" effect. Use of a curved hemostat to open the capsule is often unnecessary if the joint is entered smoothly.
2. When attempting to capture a disengaged fragment, introduce a K-wire to the fracture site while holding it steadily in place with a probe. After the fracture is anatomically reduced, advance the K-wire through the fragment for definitive fixation.
3. If screw fixation is chosen, an additional K-wire is necessary to maintain reduction and rotational control while engaging the fracture fragment with the screw.
4. For large fracture fragments, use a fracture reduction clamp to assist with rotational control before attempting to pin the fracture fragment with a K-wire.
5. For die-punch fractures, use a probe in the joint to reduce a fracture while simultaneously manipulating the impacted fragment with a percutaneous K-wire.

References

1. Green DP, Rowland SA, Hotchkiss RN. Fractures and dislocation in the hand. In: Wolfe SW, Pederson WC, Hotchkiss RN, Kozin SH. *Green's Operative Hand Surgery.* New York, NY: Churchill Livingstone; 1991:709-771.
2. Kelsey JL, Pastides H, Kreiger N. *Upper Extremity Disorders: A Survey of Their Frequency and Cost in the United States.* St. Louis, MO: CV Mosby; 1980.
3. Emmett JE, Breck LW. A review and analysis of 11,000 fractures seen in a private practice of orthopaedic surgery, 1937-1956. *J Bone Joint Surg Am.* 1958;40(5):1169-1175.
4. Chen YC. Arthroscopy of the wrist and finger joints. *Orthop Clin North Am.* 1979;10(3):723-733.

5. Badia A. Arthroscopy of the trapeziometacarpal and metacarpophalangeal joints. *J Hand Surg Am.* 2007;32(5):707-724.
6. Ryu J, Fagan R. Arthroscopic treatment of acute complete thumb metacarpophalangeal ulnar collateral ligament tears. *J Hand Surg Am.* 1995;20(6):1037-1042.
7. Rozmaryn LM, Wei N. Metacarpophalangeal arthroscopy. *Arthroscopy.* 1999;15(3):333-337.
8. Slade JF III, Gutow AP. Arthroscopy of the metacarpophalangeal joint. *Hand Clin.* 1999;15(3):501-527.
9. Badia A. Arthroscopic reduction and internal fixation of bony gamekeeper's thumb. *Orthopedics.* 2006;29(8):675-678.
10. Bettinger PC, Linscheid RL, Berger RA, Cooney WP 3rd, An KN. An anatomic study of the stabilizing ligaments of the trapezium and trapeziometacarpal joint. *J Hand Surg Am.* 1999;24(4):786-798.
11. Barbieri RA. Arthroscopic treatment of metacarpophalangeal joint fractures in the hand. In: Capo J, Tan V, eds. *Atlas of Minimally Invasive Hand and Wrist Surgery.* New York, NY: Informa Healthcare; 2008:235-238.

Please see videos on the accompanying website at
www.routledge.com/9781630910013

35

Arthroscopic Treatment of Wrist Arthritis

Stephanie C. Petterson, MPT, PhD; Michael L. Mangonon, DO; and Kevin D. Plancher, MD, MS

Introduction

Wrist arthritis, a common condition encountered by hand surgeons, can be idiopathic (eg, rheumatoid arthritis [RA] or osteoarthritis) or posttraumatic in nature. The wrist is almost always affected by RA. Patients commonly present with active synovitis along the dorsum of the wrist and, in advanced stages of disease, present with loss of mobility due to fibrous or bony ankylosis. The progression of degenerative arthritis in the wrist typically occurs first in the radial styloid and distal scaphoid articulation followed by the scaphocapitate joint, and then midcarpal joints, including the scaphoid, capitate, and lunate.[1,2] In the wrist with scaphoid nonunion advanced collapse, the first signs of arthritis are first visualized in the radial styloid area and then progress to the scaphocapitate and capitolunate joints.[1,3]

The clinical manifestation of wrist arthritis includes loss of wrist function, decreased grip and pinch strength, and limited hand function caused by significant pain with loss of range of motion (ROM) and weakness. Arthroscopy of the wrist is not only a therapeutic modality but also an excellent diagnostic tool for bony and soft tissue pathology. The arthroscope allows for examination of the joint articular surfaces, diagnosis of degenerative triangular fibrocartilage lesions, and the ability to perform synovial biopsy. It can also be used as a therapeutic modality to remove loose bodies and debride the wrist of early-stage arthritis.

Arthroscopy has advantages over the traditional, open treatments including less invasive techniques and faster healing and recovery times.[4-6] Arthroscopic synovectomy has been well described.[7] The goal of arthroscopic synovectomy is to excise the inflamed synovium to remove and eliminate the effusion and inflammatory substrate. The outcomes of arthroscopic synovectomy are dependent on preoperative function and etiology of arthritis[8-10]; however, the procedure may be effective in delaying more complex procedures, such as arthrodesis or total wrist arthroplasty.[11] Early results demonstrate decreased pain, decreased swelling, and improved joint function.

Chondral defects are also a common source of occult pain in the wrist. Abrasion chondroplasty takes advantage of this phenomenon to fill articular defects. The goals of abrasion chondroplasty are to reduce mechanical symptoms and minimize intra-articular debris by smoothing out the chondral lesions.[12-14]

Savoie FH III, Field LD, Steinmann SP, eds. *The Elbow and Wrist: AANA Advanced Arthroscopic Surgical Techniques* (pp 361-372).

Aggressive arthroscopic debridement including arthroscopic radial styloidectomy and partial resection of the scaphoid has also been described for the treatment of radial styloid wrist arthritis. The arthroscopic technique ensures preservation of the volar ligaments, to maintain radial stability of the wrist, and enhances precision in resecting the appropriate amount of styloid.[7] Similar benefits are also found with arthroscopic proximal hamate resection indicated for patients with proximal hamate arthritis.

Indications

- Failed conservative management, including the following:
  - Removable thermoplastic splints customized to maintain the wrist in the functional position of neutral or slight dorsiflexion
  - Nonsteroidal anti-inflammatory drugs
  - Antirheumatic medications for patients with RA
  - Steroid injections
- Arthroscopic synovectomy[8-10,15]
  - RA: Synovectomy for RA is indicated in the early stages of disease development when complete synovectomy is more feasible. This procedure has been shown to slow and halt the progression of the disease.[10,16]
  - Juvenile RA
  - Outerbridge grade I to III chondral lesions: The Outerbridge classification system, originally developed for patients with chondromalacia patellae, can be used to classify disease progression.[14]
  - Systemic lupus erythematosus
  - Postinfectious arthritis
  - Posttraumatic joint contractures
  - Septic arthritis after failed systemic antibiotics and lavage
- Arthroscopic abrasion chondroplasty
  - Focal grade IV chondral lesions: Lesions smaller than 5 mm have been reported to yield the best outcomes.[17]
  - Radiocarpal arthrosis
  - Proximal pole of the hamate arthrosis: Proximal hamate arthritis is influenced by lunate morphology. The presence of an additional distal medial articular facet for the hamate, a type II lunate, leads to a greater incidence of proximal hamate arthritis (44%) compared to a type I lunate, where there is one distal articular facet for the hamate (2%).[7,18-24] It is the second medial facet during contact loading of the proximal pole of the hamate that increases the risk of developing arthritis. Patients with a type II lunate defect exhibit excellent outcomes following abrasion chondroplasty.
- Arthroscopic radial styloidectomy
  - Radial styloid arthritis
  - Radioscaphoid arthritis as a result of scapholunate advanced collapse, scaphoid nonunion advanced collapse, Kienböck's disease, impingement after scaphotrapeziotrapezoidal fusion, proximal row carpectomy, or 4-corner fusion (Figure 35-1). Patients with preserved wrist ROM and good grip strength but have a positive Watson test and painful wrist radial deviation are considered ideal candidates.[25]

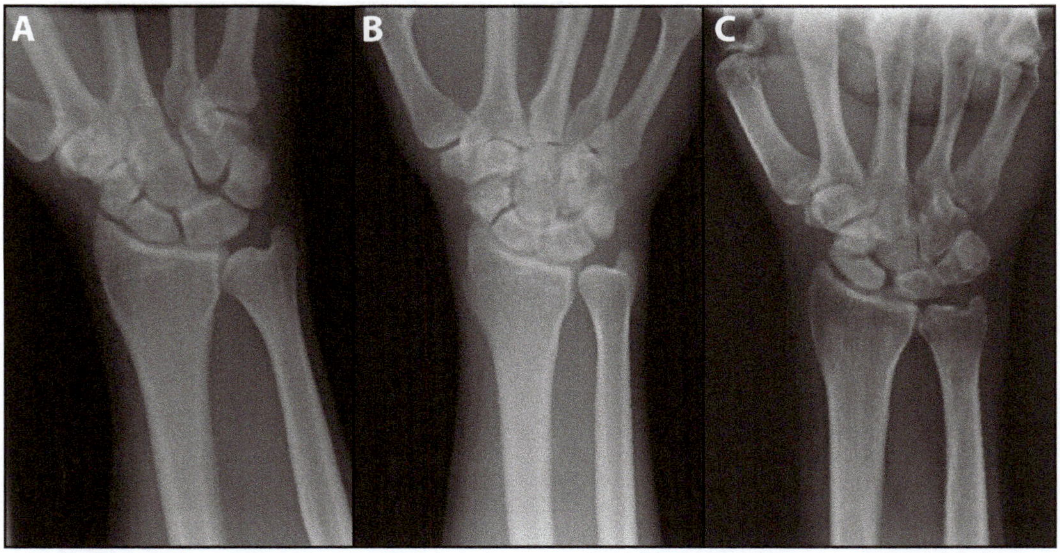

Figure 35-1. Radiocarpal arthritis secondary to a scaphoid nonunion fracture (scaphoid nonunion advanced collapse wrist). Note the penciling of the radial styloid, which is pathognomonic of this condition.

- Arthroscopic proximal hamate resection
- Proximal pole of the hamate arthrosis, particularly in the presence of a type II lunate[22,26]: Arthroscopic resection of the proximal hamate can aid in unloading the additional facet in a type II lunate, leading to good symptomatic relief with Outerbridge grade IV lesions.[7]

Contraindications

- RA not medically controlled
- Active infectious processes in areas outside of the wrist
- Radial styloidectomy is contraindicated in patients with long-standing rheumatoid disease and disruption of the radioscaphocapitate (RSC) ligament as a result of a distal radius fracture or radiocarpal dislocation due to increased risk of ulnar translocation.[27,28]
- Abrasion chondroplasty is contraindicated in cases of widespread articular cartilage damage.

Pertinent Physical Findings

- Pain at extreme wrist ROM in the early stages of disease, progressing throughout the full available ROM in advanced stages of disease
- Loss of wrist extension ROM limits the tenodesis effect (eg, passive flexion of the digits with passive wrist extension and passive extension of the digits with passive wrist flexion).
- Decreased grip and pinch strength
- Crepitus with motion
- Physical deformity in RA: Classically, the wrist is observed in a position of radial deviation with resultant ulnar head prominence in patients with early stage RA. In more advanced stages, inspection may reveal supination and ulnar translation of the carpus and volar subluxation of the radiocarpal joint.

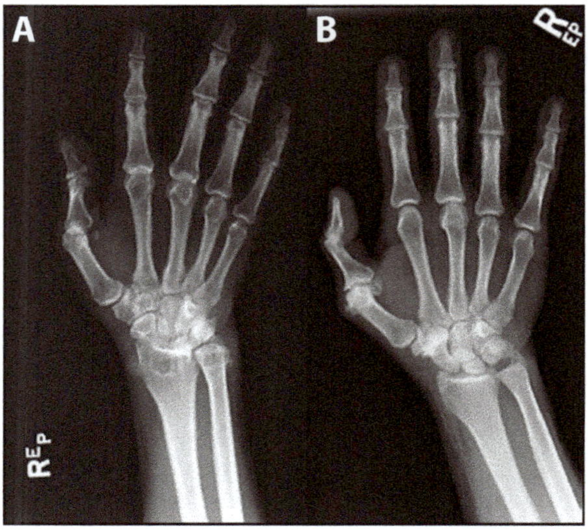

Figure 35-2. Wrist x-rays demonstrating wrist arthritis. (A) Scapholunate advanced collapse wrist stage III/IV with styloscaphoid arthritis, radiocarpal arthritis, and joint space narrowing of the capitolunate junction. (B) Scaphotrapeziotrapezoidal arthritis with joint space narrowing and sclerotic changes.

- Patients with RA may also exhibit enlargement of the wrist and metacarpophalangeal joints as well as subluxation of the radiocarpal and inferior radioulnar joints.

Pertinent Imaging

- Plain x-rays (eg, zero posteroanterior view, zero lateral view, oblique view, ulnar and radial deviation, and grip views; Figure 35-2)
- Magnetic resonance imaging is an important diagnostic modality. The Outerbridge classification of cartilage defects was initially developed for articular cartilage pathologies of the knee and has been adapted with great success for wrist defects.[13,29] Strong indicators of an evolving arthritic disease process include signs of synovitis, enhancement with bone erosion-like changes, and bone marrow edema.[30,31] Magnetic resonance imaging is also a sensitive method for excluding the diagnosis of early avascular necrosis and for evaluating the extent to which fibrocartilaginous repair tissue has formed postoperatively. These cartilages lesions are confirmed during the diagnostic arthroscopy.

Equipment

The availability, setup, and testing of equipment prior to the actual surgery is crucial to performing successful wrist arthroscopic procedures. Continuous traction for wrist arthroscopy is important. Several sterile wrist traction towers are available that can be placed on the hand table and provide vertical traction with the ability to adjust the wrist angle in flexion, extension, radial deviation, and ulnar deviation. Some towers also allow for horizontal traction and have less view obstruction when used in conjunction with a fluoroscopy unit.

A 2.5-mm, 30-degree arthroscope is used for viewing. A short bridge arthroscope with a lever arm of 100 mm allows for better control. For synovial debridement, a motorized shaver system with a 3.5-mm small joint shaver with a synovial resector blade is essential. For tissue shrinkage, if desired by the surgeon, a thermal ablation system is needed. Specially designed awls (2.5/3.5 mm) are used in abrasion chondroplasty, and a 2.9-mm burr is used for bony resections. A 22-gauge needle attached to arterial line tubing is effective for use as a drainage port at the 6-U portal. A

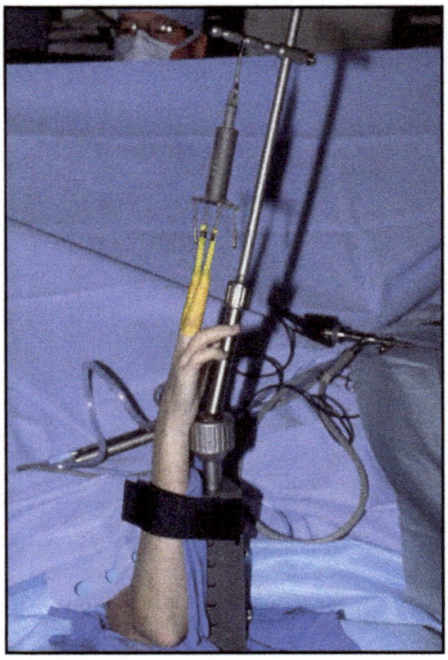

Figure 35-3. Wrist arthroscopy setup. The index and long fingers are placed in finger traps. Ten to 15 lb of traction is applied to allow for better access and mobility inside the wrist joint.

small straight Jacobsen clamp with blunt tip is best used to enter the radiocarpal joint and spread open the tract without damaging the articular surfaces. A 3-mm hook probe is useful in examining and palpating the bony and soft tissue structures without doing harm to the articular surfaces.

Positioning and Portals

General or regional anesthesia can be used for arthroscopic wrist procedures. The patient is positioned supine on the operating table with the shoulder along the table's edge and abducted 70 to 90 degrees. The elbow is placed on the hand table and flexed 90 degrees. The wrist is placed in traction setup with 10 to 15 lb of traction to assist in opening the joint (Figure 35-3). The index and long fingers are placed in finger traps from an articulating arm attached to the operating table, allowing for the forearm to be suspended vertically. In patients with RA or older patients with delicate skin, several fingers may be used to suspend the forearm to allow for an even force distribution. A tourniquet is placed above the elbow and inflated to 250 mm Hg. A sling with 7 to 10 lb of weight is placed over the tourniquet to provide downward counter traction and distraction of the wrist joint. The wrist is placed into 5 to 10 degrees of wrist flexion to open the dorsal side and mimic the palmar tilt of the radius. Ulnar or radial deviation can be provided by adjusting the wrist traction to open up the side of interest for better viewing and use of instrumentation. Extreme caution should be taken to avoid tractioning the brachial plexus. Portals used for each of the described arthroscopic interventions are detailed in Table 35-1. Prior to the start of the procedure, a complete examination of the wrist is performed, and all landmarks are palpated and drawn on the dorsum of the hand and wrist to delineate portal placement (Figure 35-4).

Step-by-Step Description of the Procedure

Arthroscopic Synovectomy

Arthroscopic synovectomy uses the 3-4, 4-5, 6-R, and 6-U portals. A 22-gauge needle is used to establish the 3-4 portal in the soft spot, 1 cm distal to Lister's tubercle. The needle is angled 5 to

Table 35-1. Arthroscopic Wrist Portals: Technique and Function

PORTAL	TECHNIQUE	FUNCTION
Dorsal		
1-2	Inserted in the extreme dorsum of the snuffbox just radial to the EPL tendon to avoid the radial artery	Provides access to the radial styloid, scaphoid, lunate, and articular surface of the distal radius
3-4	The portal is 1 cm distal to Lister's tubercle between the tendons of the third and fourth compartments.	Primary working portal, gives a wide range of movement and view
4-5	Between the common extensor fourth compartment and EDQ in the fifth compartment	Alternative to the 6-R portal
6-R	Located distal to the ulnar head and radial to the ECU tendon. Established under direct vision of the arthroscope by use of a needle. Avoids damage to the TFCC	Primary working portal
6-U	Established under direct visualization similar to the 6-R portal. Blunt dissection is always used to avoid the dorsal branches of the ulnar nerve.	6-U and 6-R portals allow visualization back toward the radial side and access to the ulnar-sided structures
MCR	Created 1 cm distal to the 3-4 portal	Allows instrument access to the ulnar midcarpal joint
MCU	Created 1 cm distal to the 4-5 portal	Allows instrument access to the radial midcarpal joint

6-R, 6-radial; 6-U, 6-ulnar; ECU, extensor carpi ulnaris; EDQ, extensor digiti quinti proprius; EPL, extensor pollicis longus; MCR, midcarpal radial; MCU, midcarpal ulnar; TFCC, triangular fibrocartilage complex.

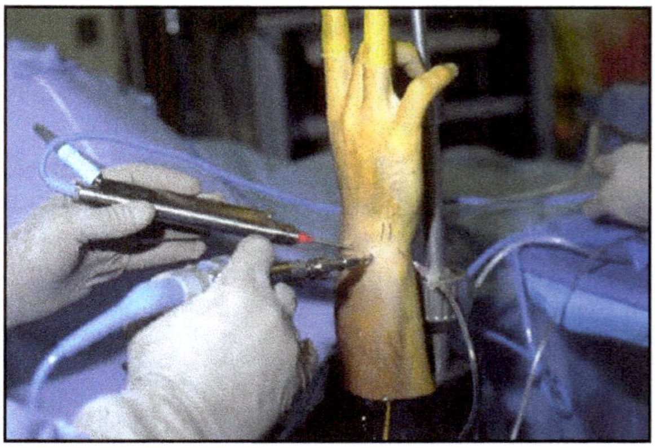

Figure 35-4. Wrist arthroscopy setup with instrumentation. Note arthroscope and instruments can be interchanged between portals to obtain the proper vantage point.

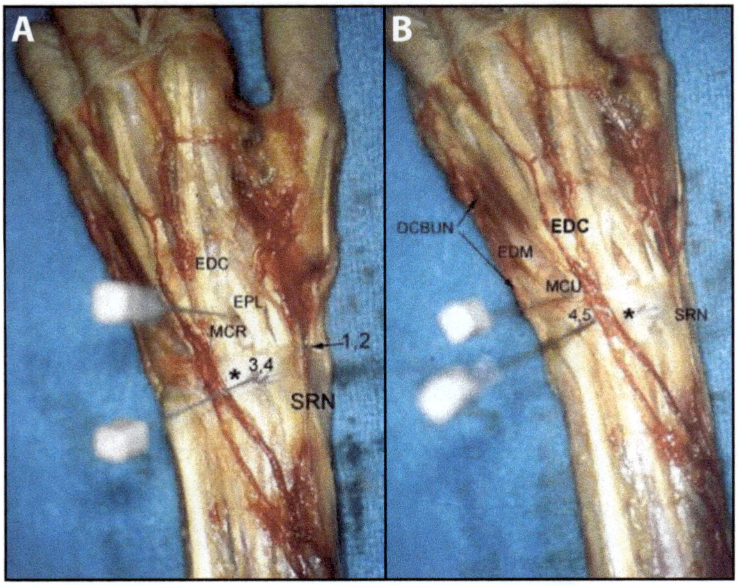

Figure 35-5. Dorsal portal anatomy. (A) Cadaver dissection of the dorsal aspect of a left wrist demonstrating the relative positions of the dorsoradial portals. (B) Relative positions of the dorsoulnar portals. *, Lister's tubercle; DCBUN, dorsal cutaneous branch of the ulnar nerve; EDC, extensor digitorum communis; EDM, extensor digiti minimi; EPL, extensor pollicis longus; MCR, midcarpal radial portal; MCU, midcarpal ulnar portal; SRN, superficial radial nerve.

10 degrees in the volar direction, parallel to the joint surface, to decrease the risk of articular cartilage damage. Five to 10 cc of saline are then injected into the radiocarpal joint to open the joint and help stretch the capsule (Figure 35-5). If no resistance is felt upon injection, successful entry into the radiocarpal joint is confirmed. A #15 blade is used to create a longitudinal incision over the 3-4 portal through the dermis only to avoid injury to the nerves and superficial veins. A small blunt straight clamp is used to dissect longitudinally down to the wrist capsule. The radiocarpal joint is entered in the same direction as the previously placed needle and the capsule is longitudinally spread open. A blunt trocar is inserted along the same path and enters the joint. A rush of irrigation out the skin represents confirmation of placement within the radiocarpal joint through the trocar upon insertion. The 2.5-mm scope is inserted and examination of the radiocarpal joint is performed. Passive infusion of irrigation (eg, lactated ringer's solution) is accomplished with gravity infusion (ie, no pump required) through the scope or with a pump at a low (eg, ≤ 30 mm Hg) pressure.

Subsequent portals, including the 4-5 or 6-R portal used for a radiocarpal portal, are established using an outside-in technique in which the needle is introduced in the joint. They are identified using transillumination and introduction of the needle radial to the extensor carpi ulnaris (ECU) tendon or ulnar to the common extensor tendons and distal to the triangular fibrocartilage complex (TFCC). The radial and ulnar midcarpal portals are used to access the midcarpal joints. An outflow port is placed under visualization at the 6-U portal using a 22-gauge needle attached to arterial line tubing that will provide continuous drainage throughout the procedure. Caution must be taken when creating the skin incision for the 6-U portal to avoid laceration or a painful neuroma of the dorsal sensory branch of the ulnar nerve. The second working portal, created at the 4-5 interval, is the working portal used for shaving. The probe is placed in the 4-5 portal with the arthroscope placed in the 3-4 portal. A complete examination is performed, including inspection of the radial styloid recess, radioscapholunate ligament, ulnar prestyloid recess, and dorsoulnar region beneath the ECU sub-sheath. A 3.5-mm small joint shaver is then used to debride all inflamed synovial tissue (Figure 35-6). Classically, the tissue is hypertrophic with inflamed wispy fraying and injected erythematous tissue. The distal radioulnar joint can be inspected through a central defect in the horizontal portion of the TFCC, and the synovectomy can be performed through an additional 6-R portal. If this defect is not present, a separate distal radioulnar portal immediately proximal to the TFCC can be used for shaving while viewing through the radiocarpal joint.

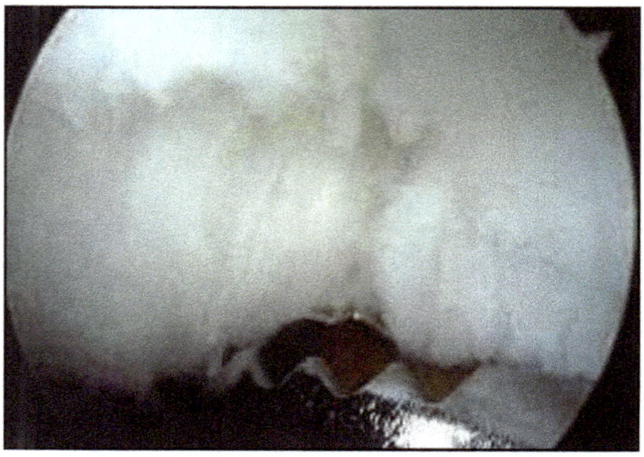

Figure 35-6. The rotator shaver is used to perform the synovectomy and remove all fibrillated cartilage.

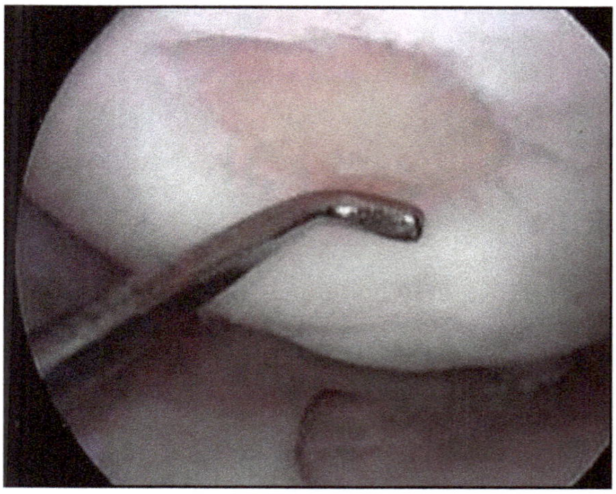

Figure 35-7. The chondral lesion is debrided and ready for chondroplasty.

Arthroscopic Abrasion Chondroplasty

Radiocarpal arthritis is treated with abrasion chondroplasty as described by Steadman et al[32] for the knee. Portals are created at the 3-4, 4-5, and 6-R intervals, with outflow from the 6-U interval for abrasion chondroplasty as previously described. Examination of the entire visual field is performed with focus on the chondral surfaces. Articular cartilage lesions are graded by the Outerbridge classification system. Any loose bodies are removed during the diagnostic arthroscopy. Focal areas of chondral damage with exposed subchondral bone are treated with microfracture awls (2.5 and 3.5 mm). Multiple perforations, or microfractures, are made in the subchondral bone plate and are spaced as close together as possible (approximately 1 to 2 mm apart). This allows for an adequate bony bridge between perforations but not so close as to break into one another (Figures 35-7 and 35-8). A shaver with a closed cage may be used on the articular cartilage to remove loose debris. The released marrow elements (eg, mesenchymal stem cells, growth factors, and other healing proteins) will form a surgically induced super-clot that will provide an enriched environment for new tissue formation. This new tissue is fibrocartilage, not hyaline cartilage. Resolution of symptoms occurs with this technique.

Arthroscopic Radial Styloidectomy

As this procedure does not address the underlying cause, it is often a palliative procedure rather than a long-term solution. The radial styloid is the insertion point for the radial collateral and

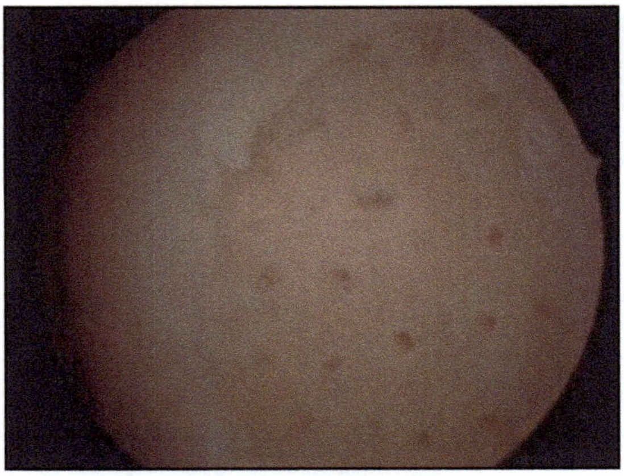

Figure 35-8. Microfractures created in the subchondral bone 1 to 2 mm apart using specially designed awls.

radioscaphocapitate ligaments approximately 4 and 10 mm from the tip of the styloid process, respectively. The amount of bone resection should therefore be minimal (less than 4 mm) to decrease the risk of radial instability, ulnar translocation, and progressive weakening of the volar radiocarpal ligaments, specifically the radioscaphoid ligament.[33,34]

Radial styloidectomy can be performed arthroscopically when indicated to alleviate symptoms associated with wrist arthritis. Arthroscopy aids in visualization to ensure complete resection of the arthritic portion of the styloid without sacrificing the ligamentous support of the wrist. Visualization is performed through the 3-4 portal, and the 1-2 portal is used as the working portal. The 1-2 portal is created in the palmar and proximal portion of the anatomic snuffbox, and a volar radial portal may also be used through the floor of the flexor carpi radialis tendon sheath at the level of the proximal palmar crease if needed. A 22-gauge needle is used to confirm the location of the joint space. To minimize damage to the scaphoid, the cannula and blunt trochar and then the 3-mm hooked probe are inserted with the wrist in ulnar deviation. A 2.9-mm burr is inserted into the 1-2 portal to access the radial styloid. The diameter of the burr is a good benchmark to gauge the amount of styloid to be removed, ideally less than 4 mm. A 22-gauge needle can be introduced into the bone to mark the end point of the styloid resection and is verified by fluoroscopy. The origins of the RSC and long radiolunate ligaments on the distal radius mark the ulnar extent of the resection. Care must be taken when using the osteotome to avoid compromise of the radial joint capsule and radial artery in the anatomical snuffbox. Final confirmation can be performed using continuous fluoroscopy to visualize any remaining impingement between the scaphoid and radial styloid during radial deviation of the wrist with the traction released (Figure 35-9).

Arthroscopic Proximal Hamate Resection

Portals are created at the midcarpal radial (MCR) and midcarpal ulnar (MCU) intervals in addition to the 3-4 and 4-5 working portals. The scope is initially placed in the MCR portal, which allows the MCU portal to be placed under visualization. A complete arthroscopic examination with careful attention to the lunate articular surface and the TFCC is performed prior to proceeding with any intervention. The distal chondral surface of the ulnar head can be inspected if there is a perforation in the TFCC. The 4-5 portal is best used to inspect the lunotriquetral interosseous ligament. A midcarpal synovectomy is performed as needed to inspect the proximal pole of the hamate, best visualized through the MCU portal, and instability of the lunotriquetral interval is also assessed with the scope in the MCR portal and a probe in the MCU portal.

A 3.5-mm full-radius resector is used to expose the subchondral bone of the proximal hamate. Then, a 2.9-mm burr is inserted through the MCU portal and approximately 2 to 4 mm of the proximal pole of the hamate is resected. This allows complete unloading of the hamatolunate articulation without affecting the loading characteristics of the triquetrohamate articulation. The

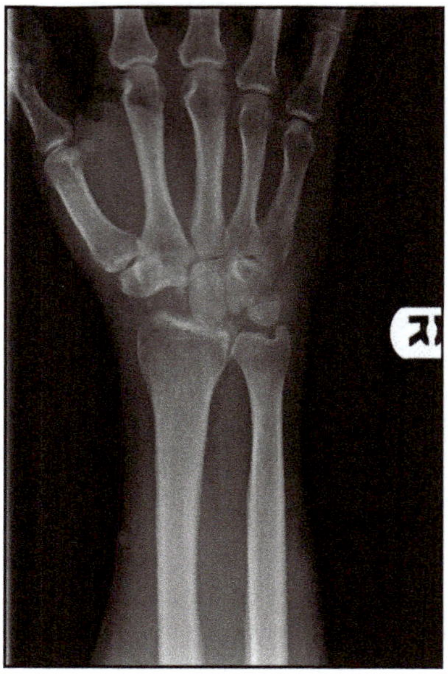

Figure 35-9. Radial styloidectomy performed in conjunction with a proximal row carpectomy. Approximately 4 mm were removed off the radial styloid decompressing the articular surface of the scaphoid and the radius.

MCR and MCU portals will typically be used interchangeably to obtain complete proximal pole resection. Specifically, the scope should be placed in the MCU portal during the volar resection of the proximal hamate. The burr can be used to assess the extent of bone resection, and the depth of resection can also be visualized fluoroscopically.

Postoperative Protocol

Upon completion of any arthroscopic procedure, the wrist is re-examined and the instrumentation is removed under visualization. The portals are closed using absorbable or nonabsorbable sutures. If warranted, the 22-gauge needle outflow port may be left in place after instrumentation removal and upon closure of the portals for placement of any injection that can be given. The wounds and wrist are then dressed, and a short-arm volar splint is placed with the thumb and fingers free for 7 to 10 days when a simple arthroscopy is performed. Digital motion is encouraged to avoid stiffness and edema and maintain tendon gliding. Wrist motion is initiated during postoperative week 1 with a certified hand therapist, and a protective custom-molded volar splint is used. Therapy is advanced and the splint is weaned over the following 6 weeks, at which time the patient is cleared for return to activities of daily living.

Potential Complications

Portal placement must also be precise to avoid vital neurovascular structures. Similarly, when using the thermal ablator, thermal damage to the subchondral bone and adjacent normal articular cartilage must be avoided. During arthroscopic synovectomy, care must be taken to avoid injury to the dorsal sensory branch of the ulnar nerve when creating the 6-R or 6-U portals and avoid potential complications of reflex sympathetic dystrophy.[35] The radial artery in the anatomical snuffbox is at risk with placement of the 1-2 portal and, therefore, should be placed near the extensor carpi radialis longus tendon dorsally. The most significant complication of radial styloidectomy is ulnar translocation due to excessive resection of the radial styloid and RSC and long radiolunate ligaments resulting in destabilization of the capitate. The capitate will no longer rest on the lunate, leading to radial instability. The 1-2 portal poses risk to the superficial radial nerve and radial artery; therefore, caution must be taken when establishing this portal to avoid these structures. Finally, the durability of the fibrocartilage repair tissue that forms following the creation of microfractures is unknown with abrasion chondroplasty.

Conclusion

Wrist arthritis, irrespective of its etiology, limits hand and wrist function. Wrist arthroscopy has led to improvements in surgical techniques to intervene earlier in the disease process through less invasive means. Literature that demonstrates the effectiveness of each of the described techniques, including arthroscopic synovectomy, abrasion chondroplasty, radial styloidectomy, and resection of the proximal hamate, is scarce, and there is a need for prospective, randomized studies. Symptomatic relief in patients afflicted with wrist arthritis has been found.

Top Technical Pearls for the Procedure

1. Adequate irrigation is needed during thermal ablation to avoid heat buildup.
2. A minimum of 15 lb of traction should be used to extract the joint and aid in visualization of an already compromised joint.
3. Limit subcutaneous dissection during portal creation to avoid extravasation of irrigation into the subcutaneous tissue.
4. The arthroscope should be placed with a blunt trocar to avoid iatrogenic chondral damage. Abrasion chondroplasty or microfracture should be performed using commercially available picks, with a minimum of 1 to 2 mm between perforations to avoid defects.
5. Debridement and resection of the radial styloid should not be below the level of the radial scaphocapitate ligament to avoid compromise to wrist stability.

References

1. Watson HK, Ballet FL. The SLAC wrist: scapholunate advanced collapse pattern of degenerative arthritis. *J Hand Surg Am.* 1984;9(3):358-365.
2. Cooney WP III. *The Wrist: Diagnosis and Operative Treatment.* 2nd ed. Philadelphia, PA: Wolters Kluwer/Lippincott Williams & Wilkins Health; 2010.
3. Shah CM, Stern PJ. Scapholunate advanced collapse (SLAC) and scaphoid nonunion advanced collapse (SNAC) wrist arthritis. *Curr Rev Musculoskelet Med.* 2013;6(1):9-17.
4. Ekman EF, Poehling GG. Principles of arthroscopy and wrist arthroscopy equipment. *Hand Clin.* 1994;10(4):557-566.
5. Gupta R, Bozentka DJ, Osterman AL. Wrist arthroscopy: principles and clinical applications. *J Am Acad Orthop Surg.* 2001;9(3):200-209.
6. Wolf JM, Dukas A, Pensak M. Advances in wrist arthroscopy. *J Am Acad Orthop Surg.* 2012;20(11):725-734.
7. Yao J, Osterman AL. Arthroscopic techniques for wrist arthritis (radial styloidectomy and proximal pole hamate excisions). *Hand Clin.* 2005;21(4):519-526.
8. Adolfsson L. Arthroscopic synovectomy in wrist arthritis. *Hand Clin.* 2005;21(4):527-530.
9. Chung CY, Yen CH, Yip ML, Koo SC, Lao WN. Arthroscopic synovectomy for rheumatoid wrists and elbows. *J Orthop Surg (Hong Kong).* 2012;20(2):219-223.

10. Adolfsson L. Arthroscopic synovectomy of the wrist. *Hand Clin.* 2011;27(3):395-399.
11. Feldkamp G. Possibilities of wrist arthroscopy. Even for patients with arthritis? [in German]. *Z Rheumatol.* 2008;67(6):478-484.
12. Kuo AC, Rodrigo JJ, Reddi AH, Curtiss S, Grotkopp E, Chiu M. Microfracture and bone morphogenetic protein 7 (BMP-7) synergistically stimulate articular cartilage repair. *Osteoarthritis Cartilage.* 2006;14(11):1126-1135.
13. Amrami KK, Askari KS, Pagnano MW, Sundaram M. Radiologic case study. Abrasion chondroplasty mimicking avascular necrosis. *Orthopedics.* 2002;25(10):1107-1018.
14. Outerbridge RE. The etiology of chondromalacia patellae. *J Bone Joint Surg Br.* 1961;43:752-757.
15. Park MJ, Ahn JH, Kang JS. Arthroscopic synovectomy of the wrist in rheumatoid arthritis. *J Bone Joint Surg Br.* 2003;85(7):1011-1015.
16. Chepeha DB, Taylor RJ, Chepeha JC, et al. Functional assessment using Constant's Shoulder Scale after modified radical and selective neck dissection. *Head Neck.* 2002;24(5):432-436.
17. Whipple TL. Chronic wrist pain. *Instr Course Lect.* 1995;44:129-137.
18. Nakamura K, Patterson RM, Moritomo H, Viegas SF. Type I versus type II lunates: ligament anatomy and presence of arthrosis. *J Hand Surg Am.* 2001;26(3):428-436.
19. Nardin RA, Rutkove SB, Raynor EM. Diagnostic accuracy of electrodiagnostic testing in the evaluation of weakness. *Muscle Nerve.* 2002;26(2):201-205.
20. Malik AM, Schweitzer ME, Culp RW, Osterman LA, Manton G. MR imaging of the type II lunate bone: frequency, extent, and associated findings. *AJR. Am J Roentgenol.* 1999;173(2):335-338.
21. Dautel G, Merle M. Chondral lesions of the midcarpal joint. *Arthroscopy.* 1997;13(1):97-102.
22. Viegas SF, Wagner K, Patterson R, Peterson P. Medial (hamate) facet of the lunate. *J Hand Surg Am.* 1990;15(4):564-571.
23. Viegas SF. The lunatohamate articulation of the midcarpal joint. *Arthroscopy.* 1990;6(1):5-10.
24. Harley BJ, Werner FW, Boles SD, Palmer AK. Arthroscopic resection of arthrosis of the proximal hamate: a clinical and biomechanical study. *J Hand Surg Am.* 2004;29(4):661-667.
25. Culp RW. *Operative Wrist Arthroscopy.* 5th ed. Philadelphia, PA: Churchill Livingstone; 2005.
26. Viegas SF, Patterson RM, Hokanson JA, Davis J. Wrist anatomy: incidence, distribution, and correlation of anatomic variations, tears, and arthrosis. *J Hand Surg Am.* 1993;18(3):463-475.
27. Dumontier C, Meyer zu Reckendorf G, Sautet A, Lenoble E, Saffar P, Allieu Y. Radiocarpal dislocations: classification and proposal for treatment. A review of twenty-seven cases. *J Bone Joint Surg Am.* 2001;83(2):212-218.
28. Jebson PJ, Adams BD, Meletiou SD. Ulnar translocation instability of the carpus after a dorsal radiocarpal dislocation: a case report. *Am J Orthop (Belle Mead NJ).* 2000;29(6):462-464.
29. Haims AH, Moore AE, Schweitzer ME, et al. MRI in the diagnosis of cartilage injury in the wrist. *AJR. Am J Roentgenol.* 2004;182(5):1267-1270.
30. Edwards PK, Ackland T, Ebert JR. Clinical rehabilitation guidelines for matrix-induced autologous chondrocyte implantation on the tibiofemoral joint. *J Orthop Sports Phys Ther.* 2014;44(2):102-119.
31. Kosta PE, Voulgari PV, Zikou AK, Drosos AA, Argyropoulou MI. The usefulness of magnetic resonance imaging of the hand and wrist in very early rheumatoid arthritis. *Arthritis Res Ther.* 2011;13(3):R84.
32. Steadman JR, Rodkey WG, Rodrigo JJ. Microfracture: surgical technique and rehabilitation to treat chondral defects. *Clin Orthop Relat Res.* 2001;(391 suppl):S362-S369.
33. Siegel DB, Gelberman RH. Radial styloidectomy: an anatomical study with special reference to radiocarpal intracapsular ligamentous morphology. *J Hand Surg Am.* 1991;16(1):40-44.
34. Nakamura T, Cooney WP III, Lui WH, et al. Radial styloidectomy: a biomechanical study on stability of the wrist joint. *J Hand Surg Am.* 2001;26(1):85-93.
35. Lourie GM, King J, Kleinman WB. The transverse radioulnar branch from the dorsal sensory ulnar nerve: its clinical and anatomical significance further defined. *J Hand Surg Am.* 1994;19(2):241-245.

Please see videos on the accompanying website at

www.routledge.com/9781630910013

36

Arthroscopic Proximal Row Carpectomy

Randall W. Culp, MD; Michael P. Gaspar, MD;
Eric S. Wroten, MD; and Jennifer A. Hertz, MD

Introduction

Proximal row carpectomy (PRC) is a motion-sparing salvage procedure that consists of excising the scaphoid, lunate, and capitate, thus converting a complex link joint into a simple hinge.[1] Although the procedure has historically been criticized for loss of motion and strength, progressive radiocapitate arthritis, and unpredictability of outcome, recent studies have shown good survivorship of the procedure at 20-year follow up.[2] The advantages of PRC include preservation of a functional arc of motion, satisfactory strength, pain relief, and high patient satisfaction.

Wrist motion has been shown to be equal or slightly less than preoperative motion. Grip strength has been reported to range between 64% and 100% of the contralateral normal wrist.[3-11] In addition, patients may be converted to a wrist arthrodesis or arthroplasty if painful osteoarthritis develops. The disadvantages of PRC include loss of carpal height, an incongruous joint, and possible progression of radiocapitate arthrosis. Imbriglia et al[11] showed that the radius of curvature of the capitate is approximately two-thirds of the lunate fossa of the distal radius. Using cineradiography, they demonstrated that the motion of the capitate on the distal radius is translational with a moving center of rotation. Thomas et al[12] reported that 12 of 27 patients in his long-term follow-up study developed radiographic evidence of cartilage space narrowing without clinical consequence.

Literature regarding arthroscopic PRC (APRC) is sparse.[13] There are no long-term studies, although short-term results are promising. Of 16 patients treated with APRC in a 24-month follow-up, Weiss et al[14] reported clinical results showing maintenance of 80% flexion/extension, 78% radial/ulnar deviation, and 81% grip strength of the contralateral side. No patient needed revision surgery and no radiocarpal subluxation was evident despite early mobilization.

Savoie FH III, Field LD, Steinmann SP, eds. *The Elbow and Wrist: AANA Advanced Arthroscopic Surgical Techniques* (pp 373-379).

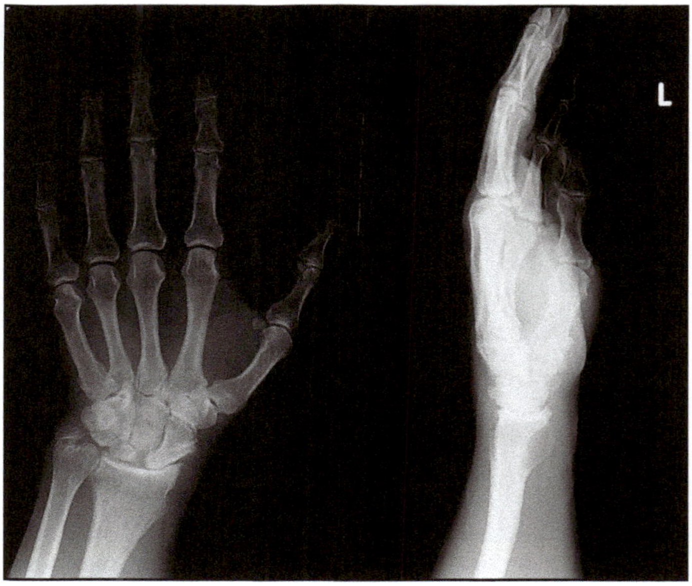

Figure 36-1. Preoperative x-rays showing posttraumatic arthritis with dorsal intercalated segment instability.

Indications

- Symptomatic arthritic disease secondary to scapholunate dissociation[15]
- Symptomatic arthritic disease secondary to scaphoid nonunion[16]
- Symptomatic arthritic disease secondary to Kienböck's disease (Figure 36-1)

Controversial Indications

- Failed carpal implants
- Cerebral palsy
- Spasticity
- Acute and chronic fractures and dislocations[17]
- Replantation: The authors do not recommend APRC in this subset of patients. Due to the high failure rate of open PRC in patients with inflammatory arthropathy (eg, rheumatoid arthritis), Culp et al[3] and Ferlic et al[18] do not recommend its use in these patients.

Pertinent Physical Findings

- Decreased range of motion (ROM)
- Pain and crepitus with ROM
- Dorsal radial swelling

Pertinent Imaging

- Plain radiographs provide the information necessary; no additional imaging is recommended

Equipment

- Wrist traction tower with appropriate sized finger traps
- High-pressure inflow system: A gravity system using a pinch pump and small joint or a standard arthroscopy pump set to maintain the pressure between 50 and 80 mm Hg may be used
- Mini C-arm fluoroscope
- Radiolucent hand table
- Arm tourniquet
- Small sharp osteotomes
- Mini curette(s)
- Hook probe
- Pituitary rongeurs
- 2.7-mm arthroscope
- 4.0-mm burr
- 2.9-mm shaver or small radiofrequency ablation probe
- 18-gauge needle
- #11 or #15 blade scalpel

Positioning and Portals

- The patient is placed supine on the operating room table and a tourniquet is placed on the upper arm and preset to 250 mm Hg.
- The affected arm is positioned on a radiolucent arm table and the surgeon is positioned at the cephalic side of the arm.
- The wrist is suspended in a traction tower with 10 to 15 lbs of longitudinal traction applied.
- A mini C-arm fluoroscopy machine is positioned parallel to the table, out of the way of the operating surgeon.

Step-by-Step Description of the Procedure

After distraction is obtained, landmarks are outlined on the dorsum of the wrist and the portals are made. The tourniquet is inflated without additional exsanguination. Routinely, the 3-4 portal is the initial viewing portal. After the 2.7-mm arthroscope is placed into the joint, outflow is established through the 6-R portal identified by triangulation and direct visualization upon entering the joint at the prestyloid recess. A mechanical pump is used to maintain a constant intra-articular pressure and flow rate. Initially, a routine evaluation of the joint is performed (Figure 36-2). Particular attention is given to the lunate fossa of the distal radius. The radial volar extrinsic ligaments, particularly the radioscaphocapitate ligament, are identified and preserved during the procedure. The arthroscope is then directed ulnarly and the triangular fibrocartilage complex and extrinsic ulnar ligaments are identified.

Next, the midcarpal joint must be well visualized to ensure an adequate proximal capitate cartilaginous surface. If the status of the capitate head is questionable, one of the following alternative procedures is performed: 4-corner fusion,[19] capitolunate arthrodesis, PRC with interposition arthroplasty, open PRC with biologic resurfacing of the capitate,[20] or wrist arthrodesis.

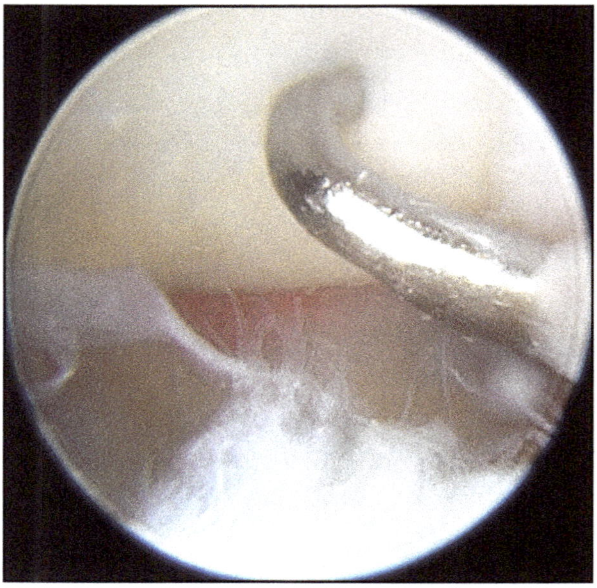

Figure 36-2. Arthroscopic visualization showing loss of cartilage and chondromalacia.

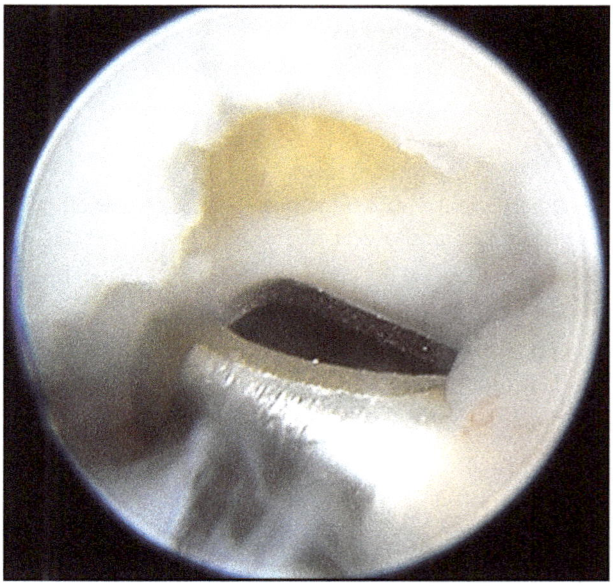

Figure 36-3. Use of a 4-0 burr to remove the lunate.

Assessment of the midcarpal articular surfaces is accomplished through the radial midcarpal portal, which is approximately 1 cm distal to the 3-4 portal.

After the cartilage status of the proximal pole of the capitate and the lunate fossa is deemed appropriate, the first step in performing the PRC is to remove the scapholunate and lunatotriquetral ligaments with a shaver or radiofrequency device. This is performed through the 4-5 and/or 6-R portal. Next, the core of the lunate is removed with a burr; a 4.0-mm burr can be used (Figure 36-3). Care is taken to avoid damaging the lunate fossa and proximal capitate by leaving an eggshell rim of lunate, which is morcellized with a pituitary rongeur under direct vision and/or with image intensification.

Next, using the 3-4 or 4-5 portal as a working portal, the scaphoid and triquetrum are fragmented with an osteotome and burr under image intensification and are removed piecemeal with a pituitary rongeur. Coring out and fragmenting the carpal bones allows for easy removal and

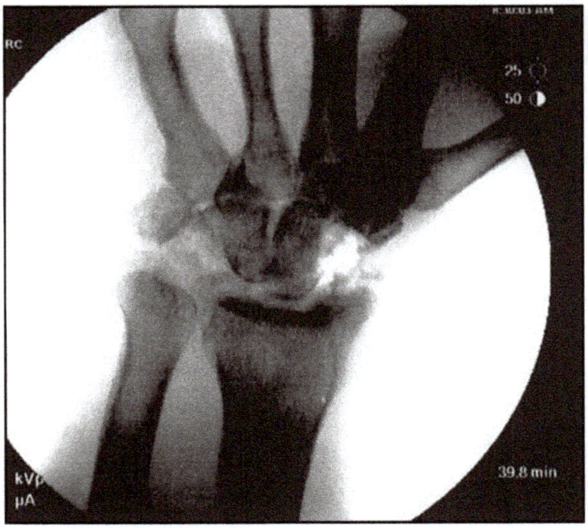

Figure 36-4. Fluoroscopic anteroposterior image of the wrist after the APRC.

protection of the articular cartilage. Great care is taken to avoid damaging the articular cartilage and the volar extrinsic ligaments, especially the radioscaphocapitate, which is responsible for maintaining the stability of the capitate in the lunate fossa.

After the entire proximal row is removed, the wrist is examined under radiographic image intensification (Figure 36-4). Care is taken to ensure that there is no impingement of the trapezium against the radial styloid. Some authors advocate a modest styloidectomy.[21] Although the authors of this chapter rarely perform this procedure, if necessary, it can be done arthroscopically with the aid of image intensification.

Posterior interosseous neurectomy may be performed through a separate 1.5-cm longitudinal incision just ulnar to Lister's tubercle. The fourth compartment is partly opened on the radial side. One centimeter of the nerve is resected with bipolar electrocautery. The retinaculum is then repaired with absorbable suture. All wounds are closed with 4-0 nylon monofilament suture.

Postoperative Protocol

Patients are initially placed in a short-arm plaster splint. Sutures from the portals are removed at 7 to 10 days. Patients are then converted to a short-arm thermoplastic splint for comfort and are allowed to begin wrist ROM and wean out of the splint as tolerated.

Potential Complications

There are several potential complications associated with APRC. Iatrogenic damage to articular cartilage must be avoided by careful instrument placement. Care must be taken to avoid disrupting the volar extrinsic carpal ligaments, particularly the radioscaphocapitate ligament, during excision of the proximal carpal row. To avoid ligamentous injury, a thin shell of cortical bone may be left attached to the volar radiocarpal ligaments. In addition, the potential exists to irritate the nerves (particularly the dorsal ulnar sensory branch) and damage the median and ulnar nerves (particularly the ulnar nerve) while using the osteotomes.

Because the dorsal capsuloligamentous structures have been minimally disrupted during the procedure, there is a theoretical complication that dorsal instability may occur secondary to less dorsal scar formation. Some would argue that not disrupting the dorsal soft tissues provides improved stability and allows for early mobilization.[13] Although this complication has not occurred in the authors' patients, should dorsal capsular laxity become evident, concurrent or subsequent electrothermal capsulorrhaphy may be considered.

Top Technical Pearls for the Procedure

1. Leave thin eggshell sections of bones to avoid damage to the cartilage of the proximal capitate and the lunate fossa.
2. Similarly, care must be taken to avoid iatrogenic ligament injury, particularly to the radioscaphocapitate ligament.
3. Liberal use of fluoroscopy may be warranted to judge preservation of cortical shells.
4. Do not remove the pisiform bone.
5. Avoid damage to extensor tendons and median and ulnar nerves.

References

1. Stamm TT. Excision of the proximal row of carpus. *Proc R Soc Med.* 1944;38:74-75.
2. Wall LB, Didonna ML, Kiefhaber TR, Stern PJ. Proximal row carpectomy: minimum 20-year follow up. *J Hand Surg Am.* 2013;38(8):1498-1504.
3. Culp RW, McGuigan FX, Turner MA, Lichtman DM, Osterman AL, McCarroll HR. Proximal row carpectomy: a multi- center study. *J Hand Surg Am.* 1993;18(1):19-25.
4. Tomaino MM, Delsignore J, Burton RI. Long-term results following proximal row carpectomy. *J Hand Surg Am.* 1994;19(4):694-703.
5. Jebson PJ, Hayes EP, Engber WD. Proximal row carpectomy: a minimum 10-year follow-up study. *J Hand Surg Am.* 2003;28(4):561-569.
6. DiDonna ML, Kiefhaber TR, Stern PJ. Proximal row carpectomy: study with a minimum of ten years of follow-up. *J Bone Joint Surg Am.* 2004;86(11):2359-2365.
7. Begley BW, Engber WD. Proximal row carpectomy in advanced Kienböck's disease. *J Hand Surg Am.* 1994;19(6):1016-1018.
8. Nevaiser RJ. On resection of the proximal carpal row. *Clin Orthop Relat Res.* 1986;(202):12-15.
9. Nevaiser RJ. Proximal row carpectomy for posttraumatic disorders of the carpus. *J Hand Surg Am.* 1983;8(3):301-305.
10. Clendenin MB, Green DP. Arthrodesis of the wrist-complications and their management. *J Hand Surg Am.* 1981;6(3):253-257.
11. Imbriglia JE, Broudy AS, Hagberg WC, McKernan D. Proximal row carpectomy: clinical evaluation. *J Hand Surg Am.* 1990;15(3):462-530.
12. Thomas AA, Rodriguez E, Segalman K. Keinböck's disease in an elderly patient treated with proximal row carpectomy. *J Hand Surg Am.* 2004;29(4):685-688.
13. Culp RW, Osterman AL, Talsania JS. Arthroscopic proximal row carpectomy. *Tech Hand Up Extrem Surg.* 1997;1(2):116-119.
14. Weiss ND, Molina RA, Gwin S. Arthroscopic proximal row carpectomy. *J Hand Surg Am.* 2011;36(4):577-582.
15. Wyrick JD, Stern PJ, Kiefhaber TR. Motion-preserving procedures in the treatment of scapholunate advance collapse wrist: proximal row carpectomy versus four-corner arthrodesis. *J Hand Surg Am.* 1995;20(6):965-970.
16. Culp RW, Williams CS. Proximal row carpectomy for the treatment of scaphoid nonunion. *Hand Clin.* 2001;17(4):663-669.

17. van Kooten EO, Coster E, Segers MJ, Ritt MJ. Early proximal row carpectomy after severe carpal trauma. *Injury*. 2005;36(10):1226-1232.
18. Ferlic DC, Clayton ML, Mills MF. Proximal row carpectomy: review of rheumatoid and nonrheumatoid wrists. *J Hand Surg Am*. 1991;16(3):420-424.
19. Cohen MS, Kozin SH. Degenerative arthritis of the wrist: proximal row carpectomy versus scaphoid excision and four-corner arthrodesis. *J Hand Surg Am*. 2001;26(1):94-104.
20. Dang J, Nydick J, Polikandroitis JA, Stone J. Proximal row carpectomy with capitate osteochondral autograft transplantation. *Tech Hand Up Extrem Surg*. 2012;16(2):67-71.
21. Gelberman RH. Proximal row carpectomy. In: *Master Techniques in Orthopaedic Surgery: The Wrist*. New York, NY: Raven Press; 1994:331-343.

Please see videos on the accompanying website at

www.routledge.com/9781630910013

37

Arthroscopic Treatment of Trapeziometacarpal Degenerative Joint Disease

Julie E. Adams, MD

Introduction

Trapeziometacarpal joint osteoarthritis is common.[1,2] Surgical options include open or arthroscopic removal of the arthritic trapeziometacarpal joint surface by removing all or part of the trapezium. In addition, arthroscopic shrinkage of the ligaments or debridement alone without removal of the distal trapezium have been described as treatment. Interposition of material may be included as part of the procedure, although recent series suggest good outcomes without interposition of any material.[3-5]

Indications

- Trapeziometacarpal arthritic symptoms recalcitrant to nonoperative means, such as splinting, injections, and therapy protocols.

Historically, most surgeons have considered arthroscopic shrinkage, debridement, and/or distal partial trapeziectomy in the setting of Eaton stage I, II, or III osteoarthritis. However, recent series suggest that Eaton stage IV arthritis may also be amenable to removal of the distal portion of the trapezium or debridement alone.[3,6,7] In the author's opinion, scaphotrapeziotrapezoidal (STT) arthritis is commonly asymptomatic and may be an incidental finding that does not necessarily preclude the use of this procedure. Careful examination of the patient should help clarify the pain-generating joints.

Pertinent Physical Findings

- Patients will often have a shoulder sign in which the trapezium metacarpal joint is subluxated with the metacarpus shifted dorsoradially relative to the trapezium.

Savoie FH III, Field LD, Steinmann SP, eds. *The Elbow and Wrist: AANA Advanced Arthroscopic Surgical Techniques* (pp 381-386).

- Hyperextension of the metacarpophalangeal (MCP) joint may be present as a compensatory finding.
- Patients will commonly have pain with pinch, grip, and grasp and have decreased grip and pinch strength.
- A positive trapeziometacarpal grind test, in which pain is elicited with axial loading of the first metacarpal on the trapezium, is typical.
- Patients may also have pain with ballottement of the first metacarpal across the trapezium. Palpable or audible crepitance may be present.

Pertinent Imaging

Imaging studies of the wrist and hand focused at the first trapeziometacarpal joint are essential prior to the procedure and include the following:

- A pronated anteroposterior or Roberts view of the thumb, which is obtained by hyperpronation of the forearm and which allows one to visualize the 4 articulations of the trapezium. The Roberts view represents a true anteroposterior view of the thumb.
- The Betts view represents a true lateral view of the trapeziometacarpal joint. The palm is placed flat on the x-ray cassette with the hand pronated between 15 and 35 degrees, and the x-ray beam is distracted at an angle 15 degrees distally.
- Trapeziometacarpal joint stress views maybe useful to document joint subluxation.

Equipment

Standard wrist arthroscopy equipment is used, including a traction tower and finger traps. The thumb is suspended by a single finger trap. The standard wrist arthroscopy 2.3- to 2.9-mm arthroscope and equipment are used; however, for small hands, a 1.9-mm arthroscope may be useful. A small joint shaver, such as 2.0 to 3.5 mm, and burrs of the same size are useful, as are coagulators or radiofrequency ablators.

Positioning and Portals

The patient is positioned supine with the arm on an arm table. The thumb is suspended from a traction tower via a single finger trap.

Step-by-Step Description of the Procedure

The 2 portals used are the 1-R and 1-U portals. The 1-R portal is between the abductor pollicis longus and the flexor carpi radialis tendon. The 1-U portal is just ulnar to the extensor pollicis brevis tendon (Figure 37-1). Portals are created in the usual fashion following insufflation of the joint. It is helpful to have a mini fluoroscopy unit to ensure that the trapeziometacarpal joint is entered and not the STT joint. Portals are made with the skin incision oriented longitudinally and blunt dissection down to the capsule to avoid injury to underlying structures, such as the superficial radial nerve or the radial artery. When the portals are created, it is helpful to

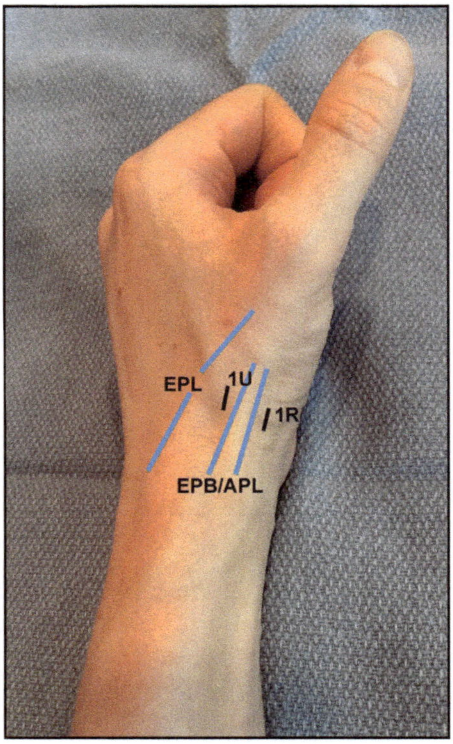

Figure 37-1. The location of the 1-R and 1-U portals are shown. APL, abductor pollicis longus; EPL, extensor pollicis longus. (Reprinted with permission of Julie Adams, MD.)

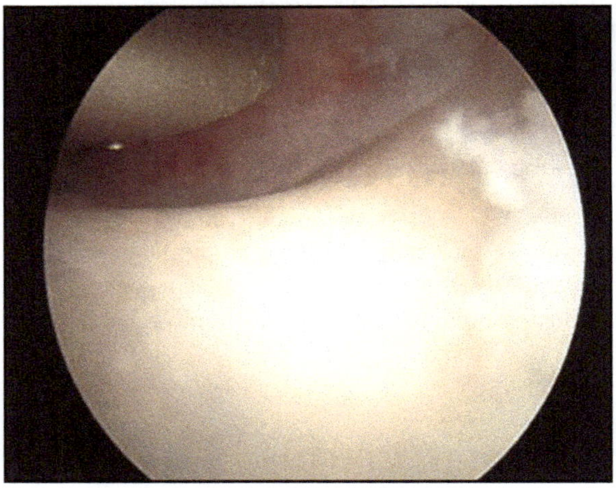

Figure 37-2. The typical biconcave saddle shape trapezium is visualized; in this patient, the distal trapezium is eburnated bone with full-thickness cartilage loss. (Reprinted with permission of Julie Adams, MD.)

use the blunt trocar to sweep across the joint to remove any synovitis and create a visualization space. Following appropriate portal placement and visualization, the working portal is used with a shaver and ablator or coagulator to remove any synovitis to improve visualization. The typical saddle-shaped trapeziometacarpal joint is visualized (Figure 37-2) and the presence and extent of arthritis are documented. Loose bodies may be extracted as they are visualized with a hemostat or small joint grasper.

If debridement alone is performed, it is done with the shaver and the coagulator. Ligaments may be shrunk to address any laxity. In most cases, the surgeon will wish to remove part of the distal trapezium, which may be done with a 2.0- to 3.5-mm burr. Essentially, the distal 2 to 4 mm of the distal trapezium is removed. Care is taken to remove the osteophytes ulnar edge of the second

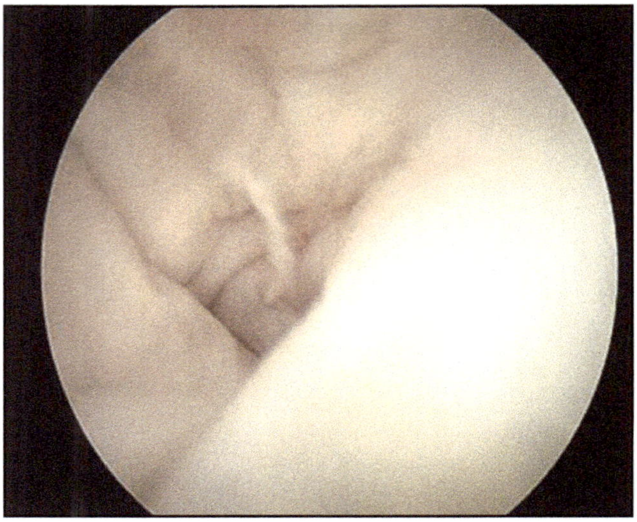

Figure 37-3. Following distal trapeziectomy, the interposition material may be placed into the joint and placement confirmed by arthroscopic visualization. (Reprinted with permission of Julie Adams, MD.)

metacarpal. Fluoroscopy is used to assess adequacy of resection along with the direct visualization through the arthroscope. Historically, interposition of a variety of materials has been proposed. This may include autograft tissue, such as palmaris longus, synthetic materials, or allograft tissue.[8-16] More recently, open and arthroscopic series have suggested that interposition may not be necessary.[3-5,17-20] If a substance is interposed, it is introduced via one of the portals, and a hemostat may be used to spread out the material and pull it through the joint. The arthroscope may be used to visually confirm interposition into the joint (Figure 37-3). The need to address MCP hyperextension remains a subject of discussion. There is some evidence that patients with compensatory MCP hyperextension may not require treatment of this deformity.[3]

Postoperative Protocol

Postoperatively, the patient is placed into a thumb spica splint with the interphalangeal joint free. Immobilization time is 4 to 6 weeks in a removable splint or a cast, similar to open procedures. The patient then initiates a supervised therapy program focusing on thumb rehabilitation and muscular re-education.

Potential Complications

Complications documented in the literature include transection of tendons during arthroscopy or weakening of the tendons presenting as a late rupture, thermal burns, or injury to superficial radial nerve or the radial artery. In addition, thumb subsidence, extrusion of interposed material, and recurrent or residual symptoms may be problematic.[3]

Top Technical Pearls for the Procedure

1. Use of a mini fluoroscopy unit is helpful to ensure that the trapeziometacarpal joint is entered rather than the STT joint.
2. It is important to remove the osteophytes at the ulnar aspect of the joint near the second metacarpal base. Failure to do so can lead to residual symptoms.
3. If interposition material is used, it is pulled into the joint by a hemostat via the 2 portals. Traction can then be let down from the finger trap and the thumb is held as the splint is applied.
4. Preoperative examination to exclude symptomatic STT arthritis is important in patients who have Eaton stage IV disease and who are considered for this procedure.
5. Although proposed advantages of the procedure include its minimally invasive nature and smaller incisions than open procedures, the superiority of this procedure over traditional open procedures has not been established. Nevertheless, published outcome studies in the literature suggest a high rate of symptomatic improvement.

References

1. Martou G, Veltri K, Thoma A. Surgical treatment of osteoarthritis of the carpometacarpal joint of the thumb: a systematic review. *Plast Reconstr Surg.* 2004;114(20:421-432.
2. Pellegrini VD Jr. Osteoarthritis at the base of the thumb. *Orthop Clin North Am.* 1992;23(1):83-102.
3. Noland SS, Saber S, Endress R, Hentz VR. The scaphotrapezial joint after partial trapeziectomy for trapeziometacarpal joint arthritis: long-term follow-up. *J Hand Surg Am.* 2012;37(6):1125-1129.
4. Tropet Y, Gallinet D, Lepage D, Gasse N, Obert L. Treatment of trapeziometacarpal osteoarthritis by partial trapeziectomy and costal cartilage autograft. A review of 100 cases. *Chir Main.* 2012;31(3):145-151.
5. Adams JE. Does arthroscopic débridement with or without interposition material address carpometacarpal arthritis? *Clin Orthop Relat Res.* 2014;472(4):1166-1172.
6. Adams JE, Merten SM, Steinmann SP. Arthroscopic-assisted treatment of coronoid fractures. *Arthroscopy.* 2007;23(10):1060-1065.
7. Adams JE, Steinmann SP, Culp RW. Bone-preserving arthroscopic options for treatment of thumb basilar joint arthritis. *Hand Clin.* 2011;27(3):355-359.
8. Abzug JM, Osterman AL. Arthroscopic hemiresection for stage II-III trapeziometacarpal osteoarthritis. *Hand Clin.* 2011;27(3):347-354.
9. Berger RA. A technique for arthroscopic evaluation of the first carpometacarpal joint. *J Hand Surg.* 1997;22(6):1077-1080.
10. Hofmeister EP, Leak RS, Culp RW, Osterman AL. Arthroscopic hemitrapeziectomy for first carpometacarpal arthritis: results at 7-year follow-up. *Hand (N Y).* 2009;4(1):24-28.
11. Landström JT. Radial portal tendon harvest and interposition in arthroscopic treatment of thumb basilar joint osteoarthritis. *J Hand Surg Am.* 2008;33(3):442-445.
12. Menon J. Partial trapeziectomy and interpositional arthroplasty for trapeziometacarpal osteoarthritis of the thumb. *J Hand Surg Br.* 1995;20(5):700-706.
13. Menon J. Arthroscopic management of trapeziometacarpal joint arthritis of the thumb. *Arthroscopy.* 1996;12(5):581-587.

14. Pegoli L, Parolo C, Ogawa T, Toh S, Pajardi G. Arthroscopic evaluation and treatment by tendon interpositional arthroplasty of first carpometacarpal joint arthritis. *Hand Surg.* 2007;12(1):35-39.
15. Chu PJ, Lee HM, Chung LJ, Shih JT. Electrothermal treatment of thumb basal joint instability. *Arthroscopy.* 2009;25(3):290-295.
16. Diaconu M, Mathoulin C, Facca S, Liverneaux P. Arthroscopic interposition arthroplasty of the trapeziometacarpal joint. *Chir Main.* 2011;30(4):282-287.
17. Edwards SG, Ramsey PN. Prospective outcomes of stage III thumb carpometacarpal arthritis treated with arthroscopic hemitrapeziectomy and thermal capsular modification without interposition. *J Hand Surg Am.* 2010;35(4):566-571.
18. Furia JP. Arthroscopic debridement and synovectomy for treating basal joint arthritis. *Arthroscopy.* 2010;26(1):34-40.
19. Jones NF, Maser BM. Treatment of arthritis of the trapeziometacarpal joint with trapeziectomy and hematoma arthroplasty. *Hand Clin.* 2001;17(2):237-243.
20. Kuhns CA, Emerson ET, Meals RA. Hematoma and distraction arthroplasty for thumb basal joint osteoarthritis: a prospective, single-surgeon study including outcomes measures. *J Hand Surg Am.* 2003;28(3):381-389.

38

Arthroscopy of the Metacarpophalangeal and Proximal Interphalangeal Joints for Degenerative Joint Disease

Alejandro Badia, MD, FACS and Juan Manuel Ríos Ruh, MD

Introduction

Small joint arthroscopy has been present, albeit infrequently used, since the early 1970s. As in larger joints, it has allowed the possibility of using the scope to resolve similar pathology in a small joint environment. Use of arthroscopy in the smaller joints remains a little-explored technique among few members of the hand surgery community and remains virtually unheard of among general orthopedic surgeons, even though it has been available for almost 40 years. The explanation of this may lie in the combination of limited scientific literature regarding the technique and its outcomes and poor delineation of the indications and its obvious benefits.

In 1979, Chen[1] first outlined the concept of small joint arthroscopy and presented a broad treatise on arthroscopy of the wrist and finger joints. He described cadaver arthroscopic anatomy and clinical cases involving the wrist, metacarpophalangeal (MCP) joint, and proximal interphalangeal (PIP) joints of the hand. The thumb trapeziometacarpal joint was not addressed. Chang described the use of a #24 Watanabe Arthroscope, the precursor of today's small joint and microarthroscope. The first clinical report of MCP joint arthroscopy was published in 1985, when Vaupel and Andrews[2] published a case report of diagnostic and operative arthroscopy of the thumb MCP joint in a professional golfer with 1 year of pain, swelling, and stiffness in his nondominant thumb. The technique was briefly described and the clinical indication and results were outlined. Arthroscopy of the PIP joint was outlined in 2002 when Thomsen et al[3] described the clinical indications and arthroscopic portals in a brief report.

The fact that open management of a small joint injury may end up destabilizing the joint makes arthroscopy a compelling technique when it comes to dealing with such clinical issues. Therefore, arthroscopic management of degenerative joint disease in the MCP and PIP joints represents a logical extension of the arthroscopic technique.

Degenerative joint disease should be divided into posttraumatic indications vs osteoarthritis and inflammatory arthropathy, such as rheumatoid arthritis (RA). In both of these joints, the posttraumatic variant is commonly seen because these are frequently injured joints. However, the treatment of RA may represent the most common indication for this technique, particularly in

Savoie FH III, Field LD, Steinmann SP, eds. *The Elbow and Wrist: AANA Advanced Arthroscopic Surgical Techniques* (pp 387-396).

the MCP joint, which is perhaps the hallmark of rheumatoid disease in the hand. Sekiya et al[4] presented a broad evaluation of arthroscopic rheumatoid synovectomy in the MCP and PIP joints in 2002. To their knowledge, a broad treatise of degenerative joint disease in the MCP and PIP joints had not been performed. This chapter outlines the indications and operative technique for arthroscopy of these critical joints. Arthroscopy of these 2 small joints should likely be grouped into the following 2 major indications: acute and chronic pathology.

Metacarpophalangeal Arthroscopy

Advantages

- Less surgical exposure (extensor hood and capsule protected)
- Excellent joint visualization
- Short learning curve
- Nearly immediate postoperative joint mobilization
- Shorter rehabilitation period

Indications

- Joint synovectomy and biopsy
- Removal of foreign or loose bodies
- Locked MCP joint (articular causes)
- Capsular debridement and release/capsulectomy
- Osteochondral lesions
- Traumatic (juxta-articular lesions, intra-articular fractures, collateral ligament repair, and debridement)[5]
- Late trauma (arthrolysis, chondral debridement, chondroplasty)
- Rheumatoid synovectomy
- MCP infection irrigation and debridement

A primary indication for MCP arthroscopy is for chronic pain, which likely suggests degenerative joint disease of these small joints. Acute indications include management of acute fractures or ligamentous lesions. Chronic degenerative indications are ideally suited for arthroscopic management due to few other options. Only patients with advanced disease and low-demand patients can be considered for implant joint arthroplasty. Another indication is limited function, almost always accompanied by pain, that has failed to respond to appropriate nonoperative treatment. Even when radiographic changes are not significant, a staged arthroscopic treatment may benefit the patient.

Contraindications

Relative contraindications include the following:

- Severe radiological signs of MCP joint space narrowing, which would make the procedure technically demanding.
- This includes large marginal osteophytes or joints that distract little under live fluoroscopy with traction applied to the digit.

- The most volar aspect of the metacarpal head is not accessible to arthroscopy and should be approached by open means.[6]

Pertinent Physical Findings

Before indicating an arthroscopic MPC treatment, the entire upper extremity is evaluated.

- The wrist is assessed for static deformity (radial deviation in RA) that would affect the result of a probable future MCP joint surgery.
- Excessive ulnar drift or, in particular, volar subluxation, would not be well suited for arthroscopic debridement, and the deformity would supercede any attempt at articular modification.
- The skin over the predicted portals should be evaluated to rule out any potential source of infection, particularly in patients with psoriatic arthritis.
- Motion of the MCP joint is assessed to determine if there are any extension or flexion lags, ulnar or radial deformities, and if they can be easily corrected.
- PIP joint motion and alignment should be evaluated.
- Evaluate for any boutonniere and swan-neck deformities, radial or ulnar deviations, and degrees of contracture.
- Flexor and extensor tendons should be checked to rule out any limitation.
- Involvement of lower extremities in patients with inflammatory arthritis must also be considered because the upper limbs may play an important role in ambulation assistance.

Pertinent Imaging

- It is essential to obtain anteroposterior, oblique, and lateral x-rays of the hand and wrist to assess alignment, congruence, and joint integrity.
- Computed tomography and magnetic resonance imaging might better outline the pathology but are seldom needed.[7]
- Fluoroscopy is helpful in that live fluoroscopic assessment of passive and active joint motion can be determined.
- Diagnostic ultrasound is playing an increasing role, permitting assessment of the extensor tendon positioning, degree of effusion or joint capsular thickening, and collateral ligament integrity.

Equipment

A 1.9- or 1.5-mm arthroscope is generally essential to explore the MCP joint. Typically, a 30-degree scope, which is commonly used by maxillofacial surgeons for temporomandibular pathology, is used, and careful attention to minimizing scope damage is used. A 2.0-mm mini-shaver system with a 2.0-mm cutter or full-radius shaver is the workhorse operative instrument. Small radiofrequency (RF) probes (2 to 2.5 mm) for ablation and shrinkage are frequently used. A small joint grabber, as well as small basket forceps, are also needed for more aggressive debridement and loose body removal. A small hook probe is useful, as are small K-wires, because they are often used in acute trauma indications.

Figure 38-1. MCP arthroscopy setup. Distraction is applied using a single Chinese finger trap.

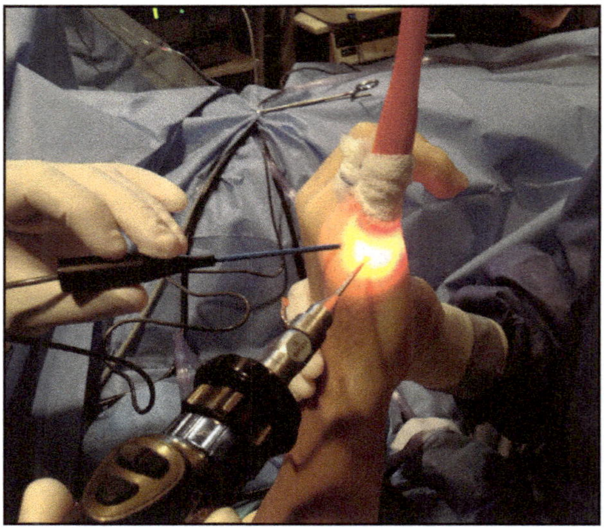

Step-by-Step Description of the Procedure

In the small joints, these procedures can be performed on an outpatient basis under regional block or field block/portal local anesthesia using a fast-acting local anesthetic. In the authors' experience, it is more prudent to use local anesthesia and light sedation to minimize patient discomfort from the tourniquet use. The patient is placed in a supine position with the shoulder abducted and the elbow flexed to 90 degrees, suspending the hand using a single Chinese finger trap on the affected digit and 2.5 to 4.5 kg of traction. A small gauze is usually tied around the finger trap/skin junction to minimize the chance of slippage, which occasionally occurs (some authors prefer manual traction; Figure 38-1). A shoulder holder may be used so that 360-degree access is available for fluoroscopy to come in and visualize pinning, but a standard wrist traction tower can also be used. The monitor should be well positioned in front of the surgeon because minimal motion by the arthroscopist can lead to loss of visibility or inadvertently exiting the joint (Figure 38-2). Adequate sedation is then achieved to allow elevation of the tourniquet for the necessary time period. The surgeon should be comfortably seated facing the joint with the shoulders above joint level to minimize arm fatigue and subsequent unwanted motion. This requires an adjustable stool and a good assistant to frequently support the scope while the instruments are switched to minimize joint exit of the scope. The latter can also be minimized by holding the arthroscope in the surgeon's first webspace, maintaining the index finger on the patient's hand dorsum to provide feedback and control the depth of arthroscope/instrument penetration.

The dorsal joint line is best located by palpation, and the MCP joints are best located by inspection of 2 depressions alongside the central extensor tendon under traction (vacuum sign). A syringe with a 25-gauge needle containing 2 to 3 cc of lidocaine is introduced into the joint and around the capsule depending on whether the regional block is in place. The joint is insufflated with a lidocaine mixture and/or saline to distend it with an 18-gauge needle and also to determine the scope trajectory angle. Two longitudinal dorsal portals, 2 to 3 mm in length, are developed on both sides of the central extensor tendon on the palmar digits and the extensor pollicis longus on the thumb. A #11 blade is used to open the skin and sagittal shroud fibers. Care should be taken not to injure the central extensor tendons or dorsal sensory nerves. Even with distraction, the space between metacarpal head and proximal phalanx base is narrow, and it is recommended to find the appropriate level and insertion angle. It is particularly important to introduce the blunt trocar or a Mosquito clamp into the joint in atraumatic fashion because it is possible to cause considerable iatrogenic injury to the articular cartilage if care is not taken.

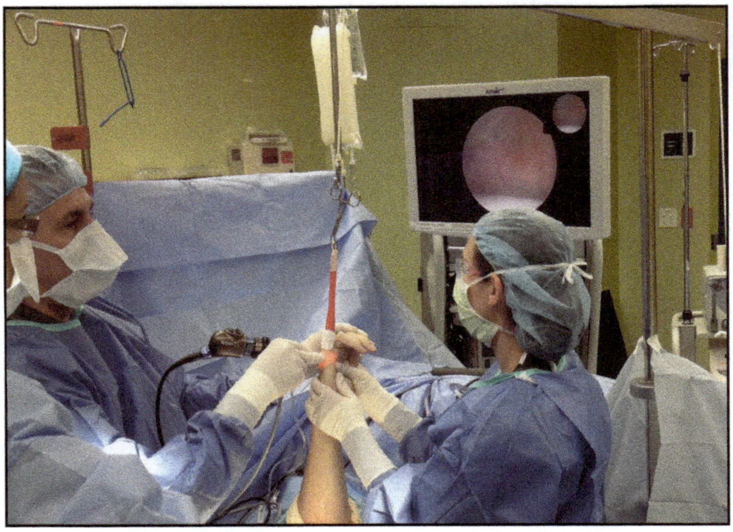

Figure 38-2. The monitor is correctly positioned in front of the surgeon.

Inside the Joint

The arthroscopic cannula is then introduced at this same angle and a thorough joint inspection is performed. The portals are simple; they lie on either side of the often palpable extensor tendon, and one can feel the indentation just underneath the proximal phalanx base. Occasionally, a third portal might be used for outflow and is placed by palpating the capsule, identifying the interval as seen on the monitor, and then passing an 18-gauge needle.

The arthroscope is placed initially into the most comfortable portal for the surgeon, often indicated by hand dominance. Then, irrigation is established, with a continuous saline infusion using 3 L of normal saline bag under gravity, occasionally using a pressure bag. Outflow is not established until the 2.0-mm shaver is placed in the opposite portal. Joint examination is started following an organized method that allows the surgeon to rule out pathological changes.

Synovectomy

Synovectomy must always be initially performed to allow good joint visualization and then identification of pathology. This is done with the 2.0-mm full-radius shaver, allowing the capsule and ligamentous structures to become more apparent. Although effective in providing symptomatic relief, it may not alter the disease progress in cases of inflammatory arthritis.[8]

Use of Radiofrequency

An RF ablator probe expedites the synovectomy but must be done sparingly because the joint capsule is relatively thin and subcutaneous, and thermal injury can occur to the capsule, articular cartilage, and skin.

Anatomic and Pathologic Evaluation

Once synovectomy is performed, the surgeon can identify any abnormal findings in a methodical fashion to avoid missing a lesion. The articular surfaces of the metacarpal head and proximal phalangeal base are examined from radial to ulnar, from the dorsal capsule to the volar plate. The metacarpal head is wider at the volar end. The surgeon should also asses the lateral recesses where the collateral ligaments originate. The surfaces are examined for integrity of the cartilage and for the presence of degenerative changes. The collateral ligaments are easily visible, with their fibers originating in the metacarpal head and running obliquely to the base of the proximal phalanx. Volar to the collateral ligament lies an amorphous fibrous layer leading to the volar plate, which

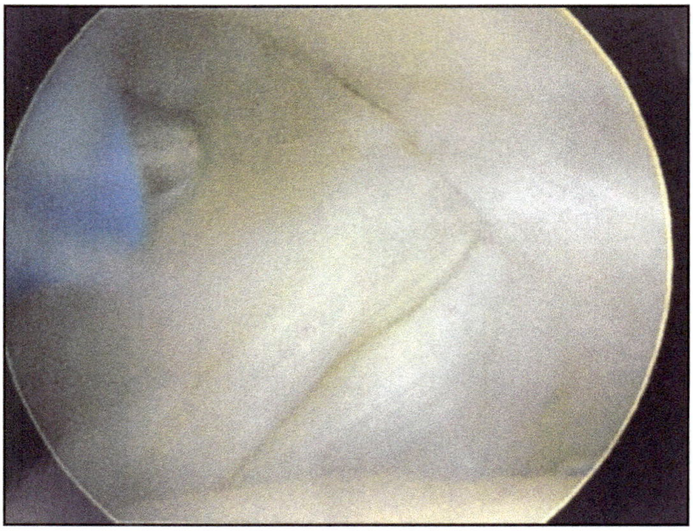

Figure 38-3. The MCP collateral ligament submitted to RF shrinkage.

should be evaluated next, along with the sesamoid bones. The dorsal capsule begins at a well-defined dorsal boundary of the main collateral ligaments, with its fibers running longitudinally; the surgeon should check its integrity along with the extensor mechanism. There is a recess proximal to the dorsal capsule fibers that is filled with areolar and synovial tissue and is easily entered and explored in full digital extension. On each side of the metacarpal head lies a narrow recess also filled with areolar tissue and synovial folds where the collateral ligaments are born.

Some anatomic particularities should be mentioned in MCP arthroscopy of the thumb. The volar plate is covered by a layer of synovium that, once resected, reveals the articular surface of the sesamoid bones. The radial and ulnar recesses are deeper, wider, and easily accessible.[9] Lax, frayed, or redundant collateral ligaments are ideally treated with judicious use of RF shrinkage, ensuring that no pain is caused to the tissue; rather, a striping technique should be used to tighten the tissue and eliminate fraying, which can secondarily promote synovitis (Figure 38-3).

Treatment of Cartilage Injuries

Degenerative changes in the articular cartilage are treated by mechanical resection of any cartilage fibrillation, loose/unstable fragment excision, and RF annealment of the lesion edges to try to limit further flaking (Figure 38-4). Full-thickness cartilage loss can be managed by drilling the subchondral bone and encouraging the formation of fibrocartilage. Loose bodies may be encountered lodged in synovial recesses, including the volar plate recess. Examination of the MCP joint is not complete without visualizing or probing into the recesses.[8]

Closing

Once the pathology is identified and appropriately addressed, the arthroscope is removed and portals are closed with benzoin and Steri-Strips. Any suturing of portals will lead to scars that will be apparent on the dorsum of the hand or thumb.

Postoperative Protocol

The thumb MCP is protected with a short-arm thumb spica splint in extension, and the other digits usually require a dorsal MCP block splint in flexion. This allows the collateral ligaments to heal in their most taut elongated position so that there is no resultant extension contracture. The

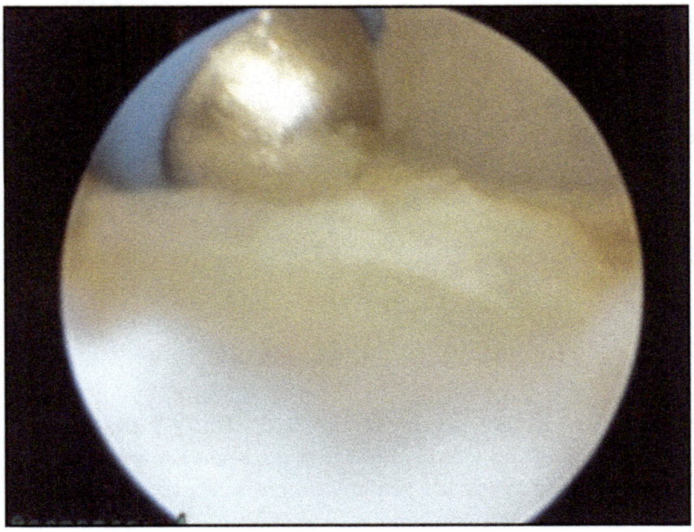

Figure 38-4. Use of RF to achieve annealment of the lesion edges.

period of immobilization is largely determined by the type and extent of pathology found during the arthroscopic procedure. Postoperative therapy is usually minimal, might begin days after the procedure, and focuses on maximizing range of motion, followed by strengthening. Edema control is minimal and contractures are rare.

Potential Complications

Complications are rare in MCP and PIP arthroscopy because no motor nerves or critical soft tissues structures surround the dorsal aspect of these joints. RF thermal injuries can occur if adequate fluid flow is not maintained throughout use of this modality, and the skin can be burned if the depth of probe penetration is not controlled.

The most common potential complication is iatrogenic articular injury, which is usually caused by surgeon inexperience. Ensuring the correct entry trajectory of the blunt cannula/trocar minimizes this. Equipment damage is more common and caution needs to be exercised.

Proximal Interphalangeal Joint Arthroscopy

Little has been written about PIP joint arthroscopy, and some consider it an experimental procedure. However, Chen presented one clinical case in a rheumatoid patient.[1] In 2002, Thomsen et al reported findings, including suggested portal placement, in 8 cadaveric PIP joints and 2 clinical cases.[3] They concluded that the technique was possible, although technically demanding, and that indications needed to be defined.

Sekiya et al[4] presented a thorough analysis in 21 rheumatoid patients. Twenty-seven PIP joints underwent rheumatoid synovectomy. They concluded that it was a worthwhile procedure because biopsies could easily be performed and synovectomies yielded clinical improvement. However, the technique was limited by joint morphology and the equipment used. The rigid nature and size of the arthroscope would not allow visualization of the palmar half of the middle phalanx base, and the condyles could only be seen by flexing the joint. The study focused on rheumatoid disease, but the PIP joint is typically involved more in osteoarthritis.

Indications

Indications remain limited for PIP arthroscopy and include the following:

- Dorsal synovectomy, predominantly in rheumatoid or osteoarthritic patients
- Joint lavage for infection
- Loose or foreign body excision
- Drilling of focal chondral lesions

Pertinent Physical Findings

- Before indicating an arthroscopic PIP treatment, the entire upper extremity is evaluated to ensure there are no concomitant pathologies that would alter the surgical indication. The skin over the predicted portals should be evaluated to rule out any potential source of infection, especially in patients with psoriatic arthritis.
- Motion of the PIP joint is assessed, taking note of any extension or flexion lags, ulnar or radial deformities, and collateral ligaments incompetency. Noting boutonniere and swan-neck deformities will help the surgeon obtain a correct surgical indication. Flexor and extensor tendons will also be checked to rule out any injury.
- Involvement of the lower extremities in patients with inflammatory arthritis must also be considered because upper extremities may play an important role in ambulation.

Pertinent Imaging

- It is essential to obtain anteroposterior, oblique, and lateral x-rays of the involved finger to assess alignment, congruence, and joint integrity.
- Computed tomography and magnetic resonance imaging could better outline the pathology but are seldom needed.

Equipment

The relatively large size and rigidity of the scope is a limiting factor within this bicondylar joint. The palmar aspect of the joint is not visualized adequately, but flexible microarthroscopes might allow passing over the condyles to give more visualization. This would necessitate smaller shavers to enter this confined space and remains a challenge. Current 2.0-mm shavers are limited in tissue resection due to the small level of suction that can be generated due to size constraints.

Positioning and Portals

The anatomic constrictions of the PIP joint require that this arthroscopy be done horizontally, with free motion of the digit during the procedure to allow surgeon visualization of the different joint segments. This would be difficult with traction that would not facilitate joint flexion.

The joint should be insufflated with about 2 cc of lidocaine once adequate digital block anesthesia is achieved. All of this is done dorsally, which allows the dorsal recesses to distend and permits 1.9- or 1.5-mm arthroscopic insertion. The portals are on either side of the central slip, generally just between that critical structure and the lateral bands. Sekiya et al[4] described a more lateral portal that passes through the transverse retinacular ligament and is 1 to 2 mm dorsal to the mid-axial line.

Step-by-Step Description of the Procedure

The joint is distracted by using a finger trap for PIP joint arthroscopy or a skin hook glued to the nail for DIP joint arthroscopy. Usually, 1 to 2 lb of traction is sufficient to distract the joint. Medial and lateral portals are established on either side of the extensor tendon. A 1.9-mm arthroscope is used with inflow on the arthroscope. A small 2-mm shaver or a small laser can be used to perform synovectomy, chondroplasty, or removal of small spurs on the dorsum of the joint. This is best accomplished by switching the viewing and shaver portals as needed to complete the procedure. Technical details regarding more advanced PIP joint arthroscopy are in their infancy. The joint is directly subcutaneous, so RF and/or other cautery type devices should be avoided.

Postoperative Protocol

After a short period of immobilization (5 to 7 days depending on the lesions found), a rehabilitation program should be started to increase range of motion.

Potential Complications

Complications are rare in MCP and PIP arthroscopy because no motor nerves or critical soft tissues structures surround the dorsal aspect of these joints. RF thermal injuries can occur if adequate fluid flow is not maintained throughout use of this modality, and even the skin can be burned if the depth of probe penetration is not controlled.

The most common potential complication is iatrogenic articular injury, which is usually caused by surgeon inexperience. Ensuring the correct entry trajectory of the blunt cannula/trocar minimizes this. Equipment damage is more common, and caution needs to be exercised.

Top Technical Pearls for the Procedure

1. Ensure adequate traction and comfortable surgeon hand positioning at the joint level.
2. Insufflate the joint with saline/lidocaine, with an 18-gauge needle determining the level/trajectory of insertion.
3. Perform ample synovectomy to allow clear identification of joint pathology.
4. Judicious use of RF helps manage tissues and using continuous motion avoids thermal injury.
5. Close portals with Steri-Strips and immobilize the hand in an anatomic position using a plaster splint, allowing early digit motion.

References

1. Chen YC. Arthroscopy of the wrist and finger joints. *Orthop Clin North Am.* 1979;10(3):723-733.
2. Vaupel GL, Andrews JR. Diagnostic and operative arthroscopy of the thumb metacarpophalangeal joint. A case report. *Am J Sports Med.* 1985;13(2):139-141.
3. Thomsen NO, Nielsen NS, Jørgensen U, Bojsen-Møller F. Arthroscopy of the proximal interphalangeal joints of the finger. *J Hand Surg Br.* 2002;27(3):253-255.
4. Sekiya I, Kobayashi M, Taneda Y, Matsui N. Arthroscopy of the proximal interphalangeal and metacarpophalangeal joints in rheumatoid hands. *Arthroscopy.* 2002;18(3):292-297.
5. Badia A. Arthroscopic reduction and internal fixation for bony gamekeeper's thumb. *Orthopedics.* 2006;29(8):675-678.
6. Thaller J. Metacarpophalangeal arthritis. In: Chhabra AB, Isaacs JE. *Arthritis and Arthroplasty: The Hand, Wrist and Elbow.* Philadelphia, PA: Saunders Elsevier; 2010:163-166.
7. Terrono AL, Feldon P, Kimball HL III. Metacarpophalangeal joint synovectomy and extensor tendon centralization in the inflammatory arthritis patient. In: Hunt TR III, Wiesel SW. *Operative Techniques in Hand, Wrist and Forearm Surgery.* Philadelphia, PA: Lippincott Williams & Wilkins, 2011:637-643.
8. Choi AK, Chow EC, Ho PC, Chow YY. Metacarpophalangeal joint arthroscopy: indications revisited. *Hand Clin.* 2011;27(3):369-382.
9. Rozmaryn LM, Wei N. Metacarpophalangeal arthroscopy. *Arthroscopy.* 1999;15(3):333-337.

Please see videos on the accompanying website at

www.routledge.com/9781630910013

39

Arthroscopic Management of Acute Scaphoid Fractures and Nonunions

William B. Geissler, MD and Aaron M. Weber, DO

Introduction

The scaphoid is the most frequently fractured bone in the carpus and accounts for approximately 70% of all carpal fractures.[1] This fracture typically occurs in young men between the ages of 15 and 30 years.[2] In addition, a scaphoid fracture is a common athletic injury occurring in contact sports, particularly football and basketball. It is estimated that 1 in 100 college football players will sustain a scaphoid fracture.[3] It is a common scenario when an injured athlete continues to compete and eventually presents to the treating physician after the season is over with a scaphoid nonunion.

Acute nondisplaced scaphoid fractures have traditionally been managed with cast immobilization.[4,5] Nondisplaced scaphoid fractures have been reported to heal in approximately 8 to 12 weeks when immobilized in long- and short-arm spica casts.[4-6] Although cast immobilization has been successful in up to 85% to 90% of cases, it must be asked as to what cost to the patients, particularly in athletes, who may not be able to tolerate a lengthy course of immobilization during the season or while actively training.[4-6] Prolonged immobilization may lead to muscle atrophy, disuse osteopenia, joint contracture, and financial hardship. The athlete may be inactive for 6 months or longer until the fracture unites. The duration of cast immobilization also varies dramatically according to the fracture site. A fracture of the scaphoid tubercle may be healed within a period of 6 weeks, or a fracture of the waist of the scaphoid may take 3 months or more in immobilization. A fracture of the proximal third of the scaphoid may take 6 months or longer to heal with a cast due to vascularity of the scaphoid.[7] This may result in potential loss of an athletic scholarship or, in a worker, loss of employment.

Displaced scaphoids have a reported nonunion rate of up to 50%.[2] Factors that decrease the prognosis for healing include the amount of displacement, the presence of associated carpal ligament instability, and delayed presentation greater than 4 to 6 weeks.[1] Traditionally, acute displaced fractures of the scaphoid and scaphoid nonunions have been managed by open reduction and internal fixation.[1,2,8] Complications that have been reported in association with open reduction and fixation include avascular necrosis, carpal instability, donor site pain, infection, screw protrusion, and reflex sympathetic dystrophy due to the required significant soft tissue dissection.[4,9]

Savoie FH III, Field LD, Steinmann SP, eds. *The Elbow and Wrist: AANA Advanced Arthroscopic Surgical Techniques* (pp 397-413).

Table 39-1. Scaphoid Nonunion Classification

Slade and Geissler	
Type I	Delayed presentation 4 to 12 weeks
Type II	Fibrous union, minimal fracture line
Type III	Minimal sclerosis less than 1 mm
Type IV	Cystic formation, between 1 and 5 mm
Type V	Humpback deformity, greater than 5 mm cystic change
Type VI	Wrist arthrosis

Arthroscopic stabilization of selected scaphoid nonunions is indicated in fracture types I through IV. Once a humpback deformity is present, arthroscopic stabilization is not recommended, and open reduction is recommended to correct the humpback deformity and dorsal intercalated segment instability rotation of the lunate.

The most commonly reported complication in one series was hypertrophic scarring.[2] Although jigs have been designed to assist an open reduction, they are frequently difficult to apply and may require further extensive surgical dissection.[10] Arthroscopically assisted fixation has also been shown to be beneficial in cases of type I to IV scaphoid nonunions by the classification scheme of Slade and Geissler (Table 39-1).[11] In patients with a stable fibrous nonunion, stabilization with a screw alone has been shown to be effective. In cystic changes, Geissler[12] has shown good success with arthroscopic stabilization and percutaneous injection of demineralized bone matrix into the nonunion site. Percutaneous bone grafting may be another option.

Wrist arthroscopy has revolutionized the practice of orthopedics by allowing surgeons to examine and treat intra-articular wrist joint abnormalities under bright light and magnified conditions.[13] The scaphoid is well visualized from the radiocarpal and midcarpal spaces. Scaphoid fractures are best visualized with the arthroscope in the midcarpal space. Fractures of the proximal pole of the scaphoid are best seen with the arthroscope in the ulnar midcarpal portal, whereas fractures of the wrist are best visualized with the arthroscope in the radial midcarpal portal. Arthroscopic reduction of scaphoid fractures allows for direct visualization and reduction of the scaphoid as the guide wires and percutaneous screws are being inserted. In addition, any associated soft tissue injuries that may occur with a fracture of the scaphoid may be arthroscopically detected and managed at the same setting.

The purpose of this chapter is to review the indications and techniques by arthroscopic management of acute scaphoid fractures and selected nonunions. Arthroscopic stabilization provides direct visualization of the fracture reduction, screw insertion, and limited surgical dissection, which may allow for a greater range of motion (ROM) and earlier return to competition or employment.

Indications

- Displaced scaphoid fractures that are reducible
- Fractures of the proximal pole of the scaphoid
- Nondisplaced fibrous and cystic nonunions
- Concomitant injuries to the wrist, such as transscaphoid perilunate dislocations or distal radius fractures

Controversial Indications

- Nondisplaced scaphoid fractures in individuals who wish for an early return to sports or work

Contraindications

- Humpback deformity in scaphoid nonunion

Pertinent Physical Findings

- Tenderness with palpation of the anatomic snuff box
- Swelling along the radial aspect of the wrist
- Volar tenderness at the level of the scaphoid tubercle
- Pain with scaphoid compression testing: axial load is applied through the scaphoid in line with the first ray

Pertinent Imaging

- Standard posteroanterior (PA) and lateral wrist x-rays
- Semisupinate and pronated wrist x-rays
- PA x-ray in ulnar deviation
- Computed tomography (CT) studies parallel to the longitudinal axis of the scaphoid

Equipment

- Wrist arthroscopy traction tower set
- 2.3-mm, 30-degree arthroscopy set with shaver
- Cannulated drill set
- 14- and 18-gauge hypodermic needles
- Headless cannulated screw set with guide wires
- C-arm or mini C-arm fluoroscopy

Positioning and Portals

The patient is positioned supine with the arm outstretched on a stable, radiolucent arm table.

Step-by-Step Description of the Procedure

Various arthroscopically assisted and percutaneous techniques for scaphoid fractures have been reported in the literature. Haddad and Goddard[14] popularized the volar approach, whereas the dorsal approach has more recently been popularized by Slade et al.[15] Geissler and Slade[16] recently described a new technique in which the starting point of the guide wire and the eventual screw insertion is determined arthroscopically to limit any guesswork of the insertion point.

Volar Percutaneous Approach

Using this technique as popularized by Haddad and Goddard,[14] the patient is placed supine with the thumb suspended in a Chinese finger trap. The thumb under suspension allows ulnar deviation of the wrist, which improves access to the distal pole of the scaphoid. Under fluoroscopic control, a longitudinal 0.5-cm skin incision is made on the most distal radial aspect of the scaphoid. Blunt dissection is used to expose the distal pole of the scaphoid. It is important to protect the cutaneous nerves with this technique. A percutaneous guide wire is introduced into the scaphoid trapezial joint and is advanced proximally and dorsally across the fracture site. The position of the guide wire is easily checked under fluoroscopy on anteroposterior, oblique, and lateral planes by rotating the forearm under fluoroscopy. This provides nearly a 360-degree view of the position of the guide wire within the scaphoid. The length of the guide wire within the scaphoid is determined by placing a second guide wire next to the initial guide wire, and the difference is measured between the two. A drill is inserted through the soft tissue protector to protect the surrounding soft tissues, and the scaphoid is reamed. A headless cannulated screw is then placed over the guide wire after drilling. A second guide wire may be useful to protect against rotation of the fracture fragments while the screw is being inserted.

Haddad and Goddard[14] reported their initial results in a pilot study of 15 patients with acute scaphoid fractures. Union was achieved in all patients within an average of 57 days (range, 38 to 71 days). The ROM was equal to that of the contralateral limb after union had been achieved, and grip strength averaged 90% at 3 months using this percutaneous technique. The patients were able to return to sedentary work within 4 days and manual work within 5 weeks.

The advantage of this technique is that it is fairly simple and straightforward and requires minimal specialized equipment. The disadvantage is that the screw is placed potentially slightly oblique to the mid-waist fracture line in the scaphoid.

Dorsal Percutaneous Approach

Slade et al[15] and Slade and Jaskwhich[17] have popularized the dorsal percutaneous approach. This technique has become popular because of its similar limited surgical dissection, and it allows for arthroscopic evaluation and reduction of the scaphoid fracture. The patient is placed in the supine position on the table with the arm extended. Several towels are placed under the elbow to support the forearm so it is parallel to the floor. The wrist is then flexed and pronated under fluoroscopy until the distal and proximal poles of the scaphoid are aligned to form a perfect cylinder. Continuous fluoroscopy is recommended as the wrist is flexed to obtain a true ring sign as the proximal and distal poles are aligned. Under fluoroscopy, a 14-gauge needle is placed percutaneously in the center of the ring sign and parallel to the fluoroscopy beam. A guide wire is then inserted through the 14-gauge needle and is driven across the central axis of the scaphoid from dorsal to volar until the end of the guide wire comes in contact with the distal scaphoid cortex. The position of the guide wire is then evaluated under fluoroscopy in the PA, oblique, and lateral planes while maintaining the wrist in flexion. It is important not to extend the wrist at this time, which would potentially bend the guide wire. A second guide wire is then placed parallel to the first so it touches the proximal pole of the scaphoid, and the difference of the length of the 2 guide wires is measured to determine the length of the screw. It is recommended that a screw 4 mm shorter than what is measured be used.

The primary guide wire is then advanced volarly through a portion of the trapezium along the radial side of the thumb metacarpal until it exits the skin on the volar aspect of the hand. The wire continues to be advanced out volarly until it is flush with the proximal pole of the scaphoid dorsally, and the wrist is extended.

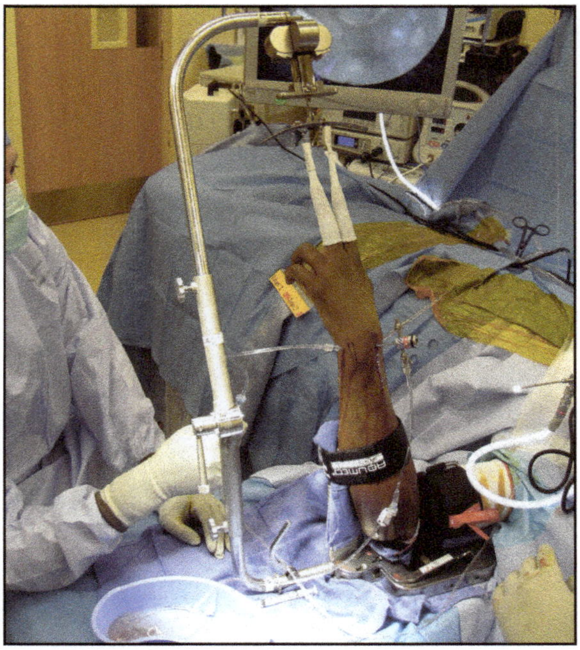

Figure 39-1. The wrist is suspended in 30 degrees of flexion in the Acumed wrist traction tower.

The wrist is then suspended in a traction tower and the radiocarpal and midcarpal spaces are arthroscopically evaluated. The radiocarpal space is evaluated for any additional associated soft tissue injuries. The reduction of the scaphoid is best seen with the arthroscope in the midcarpal space. The primary guide wire is advanced back dorsally and proximally with the wrist flexed once the reduction of the scaphoid fracture is felt to be satisfactory as viewed with the arthroscope in the midcarpal space. It is important to leave a portion of the guide wire out the volar and dorsal aspects of the wrist so that if the guide wire breaks, it is easy to remove it. Blunt dissection is then continued around the guide wire dorsally to minimize the risk of soft tissue injuries, particularly the extensor tendons, as the scaphoid is reamed and the screw is inserted over the guide wire. Through a soft tissue protector, the scaphoid is drilled over the guide wire and a headless cannulated screw is inserted.

The dorsal approach has the advantage that the screw is able to be inserted down the central axis of the scaphoid. This allows for compression directly across the fracture site compared to the more oblique orientation of the screw using the volar technique. The concern with the dorsal percutaneous approach is that the wrist is hyperflexed, which may displace the scaphoid fracture to a humpback deformity if it is unstable. It is important to evaluate the reduction of the scaphoid with the arthroscope in the midcarpal space when this technique is used to ensure the fracture is not hyperflexed.

Arthroscopic Reduction (Geissler Technique)

Most recently, Geissler[18] described his arthroscopic technique for reduction of acute scaphoid fractures and select scaphoid nonunions. The advantage of this technique is that the starting point for the guide wire is viewed directly arthroscopically, and there is no guesswork about where the insertion point of the headless cannulated screw will be. In the authors' opinion, this is a simple approach compared to the dorsal percutaneous approach with the ring sign. In addition, the wrist is not hyperflexed, which could potentially distract the scaphoid fracture and cause a humpback deformity.

In this technique, the wrist is initially suspended in a wrist traction tower (Acumed; Figure 39-1). The arthroscope is initially placed in the 3-4 portal to evaluate any associated soft

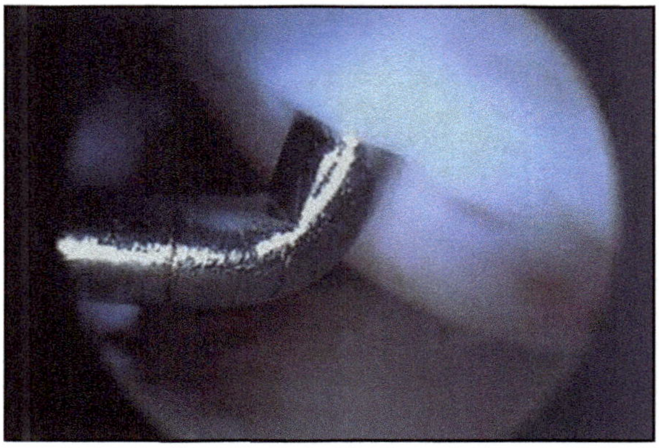

Figure 39-2. Following arthroscopic evaluation of the wrist with the arthroscope in the diagnostic 3-4 portal, the arthroscope is switched to the 6-R portal, and the junction of the SL interosseous ligament to the proximal pole of the scaphoid is palpated with a probe.

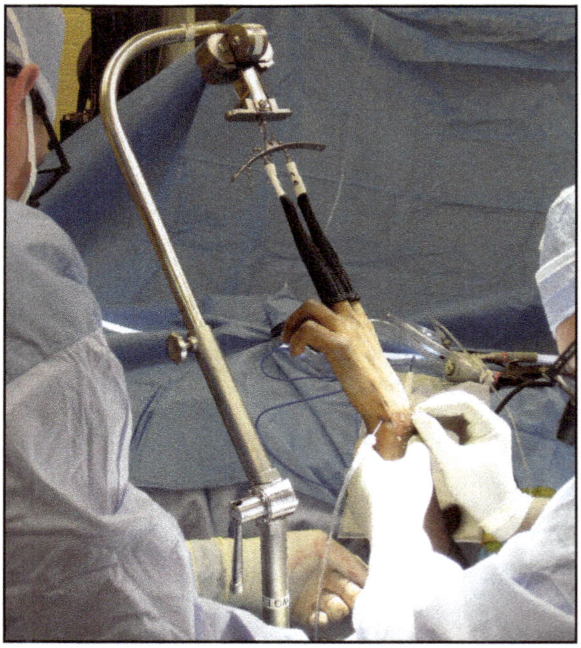

Figure 39-3. A 14-gauge needle is inserted through the 3-4 portal at the junction of the SL interosseous ligament to the proximal pole of the scaphoid.

tissue injuries, which may occur with a scaphoid fracture. Upon evaluation and treatment of any associated soft tissue injuries, the arthroscope is then transferred into the 6-R portal. The wrist is flexed approximately 30 degrees in the traction tower. A 14-gauge needle is then inserted through the 3-4 portal, and the junction of the scapholunate (SL) interosseous ligament is palpated as it inserts onto the proximal pole of the scaphoid. The junction of the SL interosseous ligament onto the scaphoid along the middle third is the most ideal starting point for the screw (Figure 39-2). A 14-gauge needle is advanced and impaled into the proximal pole of the scaphoid right at the insertion of the SL interosseous ligament (Figures 39-3 and 39-4). Occasionally, some dorsal synovitis may block visualization of the starting point and may need to be debrided.

The traction tower is then flexed and the starting point of the needle is evaluated under fluoroscopy (Figures 39-5 and 39-6). Using this technique, the starting point is consistently determined to be at the most proximal pole of the scaphoid. The needle is simply aimed toward the thumb under fluoroscopy and a guide wire is advanced through the needle down the central axis of the scaphoid to abut the distal pole. The position of the guide wire is checked under the PA, oblique, and lateral planes under fluoroscopy by rotating the forearm in the traction tower (Figures 39-7 and 39-8).

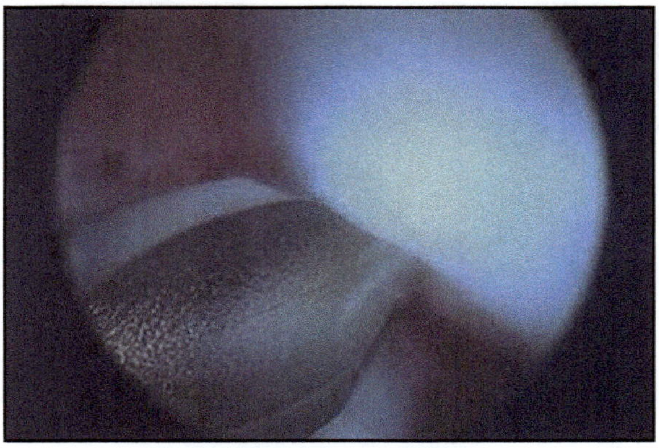

Figure 39-4. Arthroscopic confirmation of the 14-gauge needle as it impales the proximal pole of the scaphoid at the junction of the SL interosseous ligament.

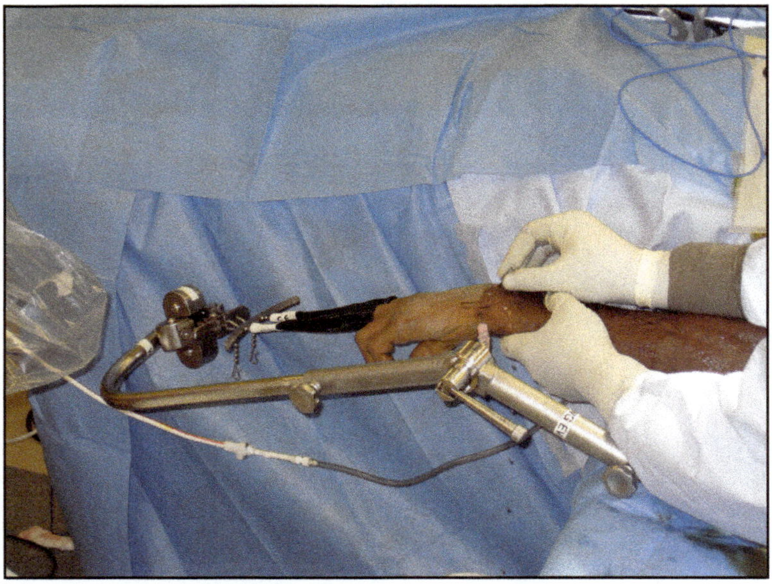

Figure 39-5. The Acumed wrist traction tower is then flexed and fluoroscopic confirmation of the ideal starting point is confirmed.

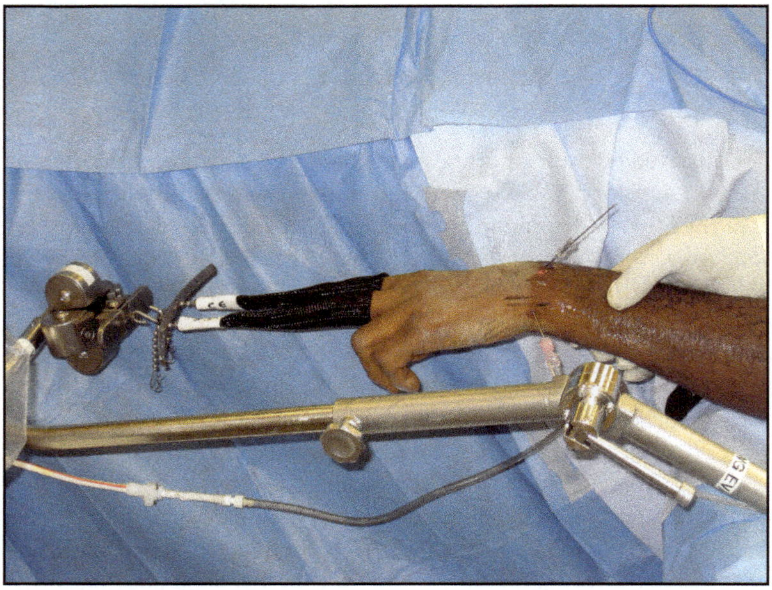

Figure 39-6. Once this has been performed, the needle is aimed toward the thumb and a guide wire is advanced down the central axis of the scaphoid.

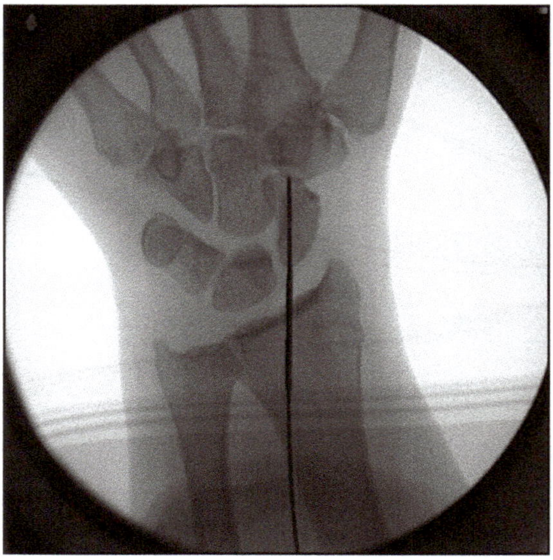

Figure 39-7. Fluoroscopic PA view confirming the ideal starting point of the guide wire and placement of the wire down the central axis of the scaphoid.

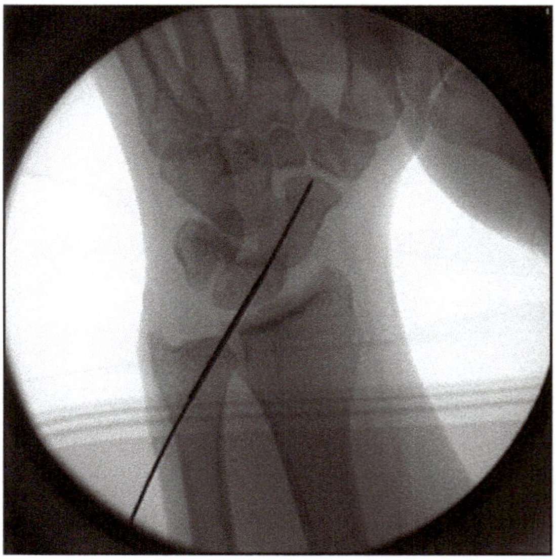

Figure 39-8. Fluoroscopic oblique view confirming ideal placement of the guide wire down the central axis of the scaphoid.

The fluoroscopic image is not hindered by the support beam of the tower, which is off to the side rather than down the central axis. A second guide wire is advanced against the proximal pole of the scaphoid, and the length of the screw is determined by the difference of the 2 guide wires. It is important to remember that a screw at least 4 mm shorter is recommended. The reduction of the scaphoid is evaluated with the arthroscope in the radial and ulnar midcarpal portals. If reduction is not satisfactory, the guide wire is advanced volarly across the wrist but still within the distal pole of the scaphoid. An additional K-wire may be placed in the proximal pole of the scaphoid. These may be used as joysticks to further reduce the fracture anatomically as viewed directly with the arthroscope in the midcarpal portal. It is also helpful to manipulate the wrist in the traction tower, usually with the wrist in extension, which further reduces the fracture. Once the fracture is judged to be satisfactory, the guide wire is then advanced back proximally into the proximal pole of the scaphoid. The scaphoid is then reamed with the cannulated drill (Figure 39-9).

In acute fractures or in stable fibrous nonunions, demineralized bone matrix is not used, and a headless cannulated screw is inserted over the guide wire (Figure 39-10). The position of the

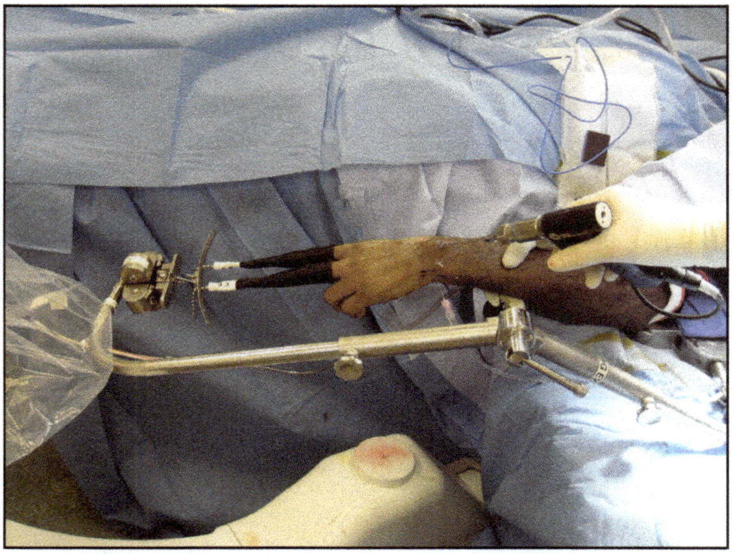

Figure 39-9. Once the length of the screw has been determined, the guide wire is advanced out of the volar aspect of the wrist and the scaphoid is reamed with a cannulated drill.

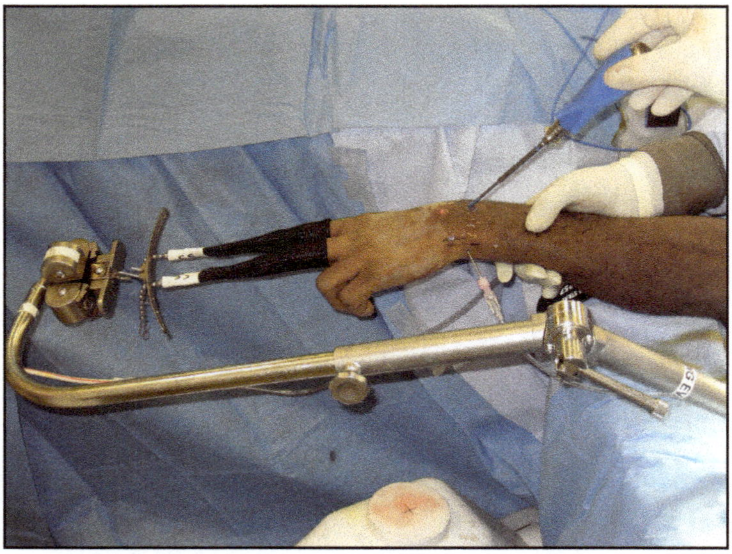

Figure 39-10. The headless cannulated screw is then inserted over the guide wire down the central axis of the scaphoid.

screw is checked in the PA, oblique, and lateral planes under fluoroscopy in the traction tower (Figures 39-11 and 39-12). The wrist is re-evaluated from the radiocarpal and midcarpal spaces. It is important to check from the radiocarpal space that the headless screw is inserted up into the scaphoid and is not protruding to potentially injure the articular cartilage of the scaphoid facet and the distal radius. The final reduction of the scaphoid fracture may be viewed with the arthroscope in the midcarpal space (Figures 39-13 and 39-14).

Arthroscopic fixation limits the guesswork and location of the exact starting point of the screw compared to percutaneous fluoroscopic techniques. The guide wire starting point is at the most proximal pole of the scaphoid of the junction of the SL interosseous ligament. It is reproducible as confirmed under fluoroscopy. In addition, the wrist is not hyperflexed, which may potentially flex the fracture fragment into a humpback deformity. The dorsal insertion of the screw allows for central placement down the axis of the scaphoid. Early arthroscopic evaluation allows for detection and management of any associated soft tissue injuries (Figures 39-15 to 39-18).

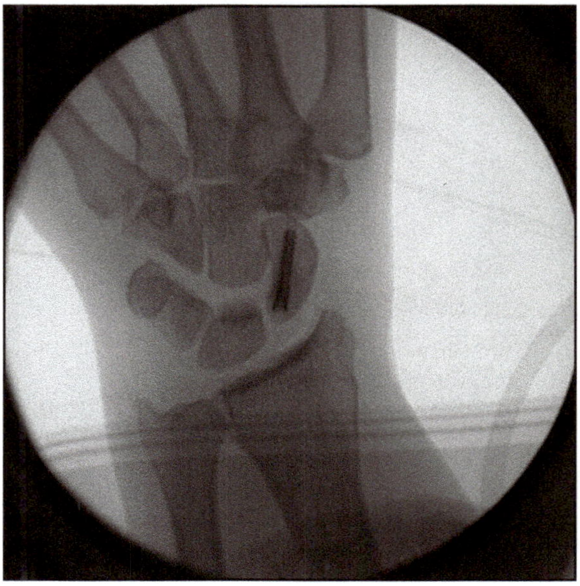

Figure 39-11. Fluoroscopic confirmation on the PA view showing ideal placement of the screw and reduction of the scaphoid.

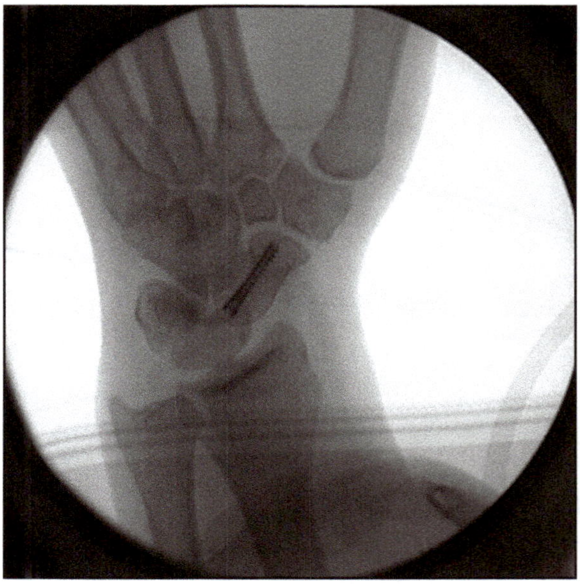

Figure 39-12. Fluoroscopic oblique view showing ideal placement of the headless cannulated screw.

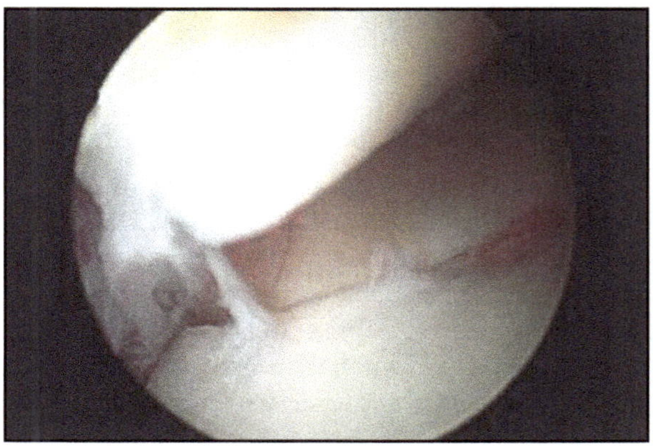

Figure 39-13. Arthroscopic confirmation in the radial midcarpal space showing good compression of the scaphoid fracture and anatomic reduction with no rotation.

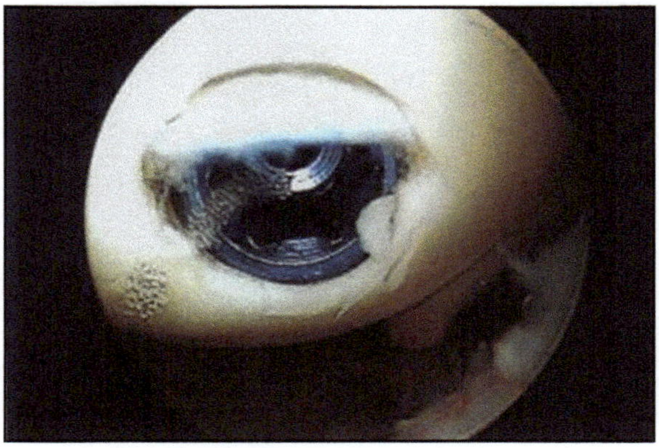

Figure 39-14. Arthroscopic view with the arthroscope in the 3-4 portal confirming the screw placement in the scaphoid.

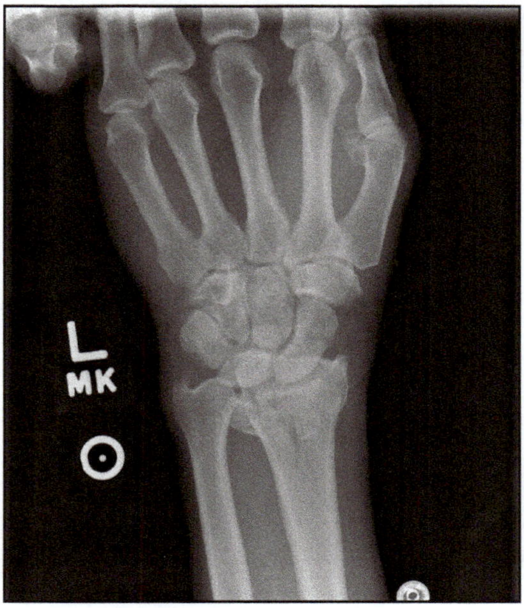

Figure 39-15. PA x-ray of a 42-year-old male with distal radius and scaphoid fractures.

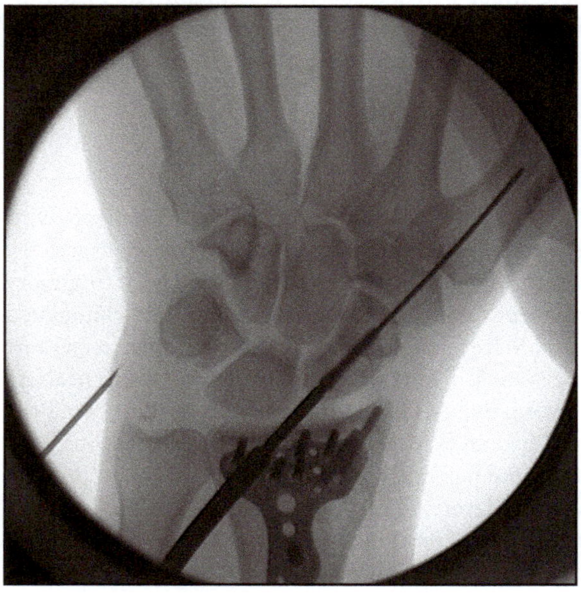

Figure 39-16. The distal radius fracture has been stabilized with an Acumed distal radius plate through the volar approach. Once the distal radius fracture is stabilized, the scaphoid is arthroscopically reduced using the technique previously described.

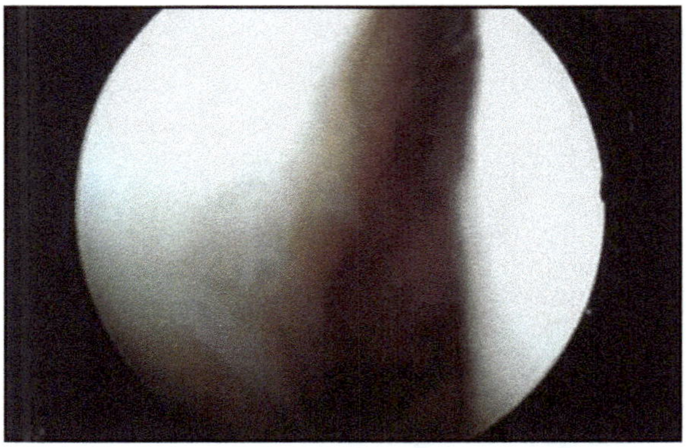

Figure 39-17. Arthroscopic evaluation of the wrist confirming a Geissler grade III tear to the SL interosseous ligament. This was not apparent on plain x-rays.

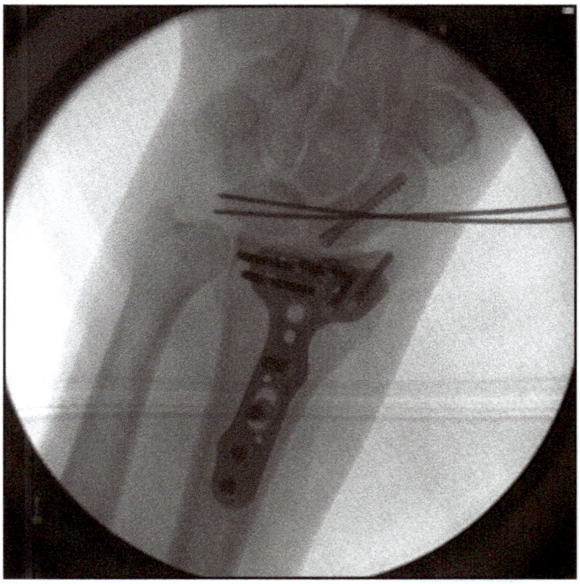

Figure 39-18. The SL interosseous ligament tear is arthroscopically reduced and percutaneously stabilized with K-wires following reduction of the distal radius and scaphoid fractures.

When the scaphoid is reduced arthroscopically or percutaneously, it is important to realize these techniques are not indicated for patients who have a severe humpback deformity, which is not correctable, or in patients with advanced arthrosis of the radiocarpal joint (scaphoid nonunion advanced collapse).[16]

Scaphoid Nonunions

Geissler[18] described using Slade's dorsal percutaneous fixation technique in 15 patients with stable fibrous nonunion of the scaphoid. In the series, there were 12 horizontal oblique fractures, 1 transverse fracture, and 2 proximal pole fractures. The average presentation time prior to surgery was 8 months. All patients underwent percutaneous dorsal fixation with a headless cannulated screw with no accessory bone grafting procedure. All 15 patients healed their fractures in an average of 3 months. Eight of the 15 patients underwent CT evaluation to further document healing. The patients had excellent ROM at final follow-up due to minimal surgical dissection. Using the modified Mayo wrist scale, 12 of the 15 patients had an excellent result. Dorsal percutaneous fixation without bone grafting is recommended for those patients with a stable fibrous nonunion with no signs of humpback deformity without extensive sclerosis of the fracture site. Using the scaphoid nonunion classification scheme proposed by Slade and Geissler, patients with type I through III scaphoid nonunions were included in the study, with a 100% success rate.

In patients with cystic scaphoid nonunions with no humpback deformity, percutaneous cancellous bone grafting or injection of demineralized bone matrix may be used. In Geissler's technique, the scaphoid is reamed through a soft tissue protector. A bone biopsy needle is filled with demineralized bone matrix putty. The bone biopsy needle is then placed over the guide wire from dorsal to proximal and is inserted through the drill hole directly into the nonunion site. The guide wire is then retracted distally out of the proximal pole of the scaphoid while remaining in the distal pole of the scaphoid. Demineralized bone matrix is then injected by the bone biopsy needle directly into the central hole of the scaphoid at the nonunion site. The guide wire is advanced back through the bone biopsy needle from volar to dorsal. In this manner, the guide wire passes back through the original reamed hole of the proximal pole of the scaphoid and out dorsally, protruding from the skin. The bone biopsy needle is then removed. A headless cannulated screw is then inserted over the guide wire across the scaphoid nonunion. The radiocarpal and midcarpal spaces are then re-evaluated arthroscopically to confirm reduction and placement of the screw.

Geissler[18] described arthroscopic reduction of cystic scaphoid nonunions without humpback deformity using demineralized bone matrix putty. In this technique, 1 cc of demineralized bone matrix (Accell) is injected percutaneously into the nonunion site of the scaphoid. Using the classification scale of Slade and Geissler, the series is composed of type IV cystic scaphoid nonunions. Fourteen of the 15 patients healed their scaphoid nonunions using this technique. Arthroscopic evaluation of the wrist from the radiocarpal and midcarpal spaces showed no extravasation of the demineralized bone matrix into the joint.

Arthroscopic Management Perilunate Dislocations

Although an infrequent injury, perilunate dislocations and fracture dislocations can occur in the setting of high-energy trauma to the wrist. Several case series have shown that a scaphoid fracture is associated with this injury in 61% to 65% of these injuries.[19] For closed injuries in the acute setting, arthroscopic treatment should be considered as a part of the treatment spectrum in the hands of the skilled arthroscopist. If the surgeon wishes to address ligamentous injuries percutaneously, an arthroscopic approach for scaphoid fracture fixation allows for better visualization and assessment of ligaments, fractures, and articular injury, as well as potentially reducing further soft tissue damage associated with open treatment of the injury.

In the case of an associated perilunate dislocation, the lunotriquetral (LT) joint is addressed prior to wrist arthroscopy (Figure 39-19). K-wire fixation may be used to stabilize the joint, but it is associated with potential pin tract infection and limits early rehabilitation. To avoid this and allow early therapy, an articulated cannulated cylinder in cylinder screw (SLIC; Acumed) is used (Figure 39-20). In this technique, a 1-cm skin incision was made centered along the ulnar aspect of the triquetrum. Blunt dissection is carried down to the level of the periosteum to protect the dorsal sensory branch of the ulnar nerve. In oscillation mode, a wire driver is used to pass a guide wire down the center of the triquetrum and the lunate (Figure 39-21). Proper placement is confirmed in the anteroposterior and lateral planes under fluoroscopy. A stepped drill is then used to drill over the guide wire. Three screw lengths are available. The length of the screw is determined radiographically based on the markings on the drill itself (Figure 39-22). The drill is removed and the LT interval is stabilized by the articulated screw that is inserted over the guide wire. The guide wire is removed and the scaphoid fracture is addressed via the Geissler technique previously described (Figure 39-23).

Geissler reviewed his management of 14 patients with perilunate dislocations, which were stabilized without K-wires. Seven patients with transscaphoid perilunate dislocations were managed arthroscopically. For the remaining 7 patients, 6 dislocations were managed by open repair of the radius and stabilization without K-wires. Transscaphoid perilunate patients were managed as described previously with arthroscopic reduction of the scaphoid fracture and percutaneous stabilization of the LT interval with a SLIC screw. The open patients underwent open repair of the SL ligament with stabilization of a SLIC screw, and the LT interval was stabilized with a biodegradable screw.

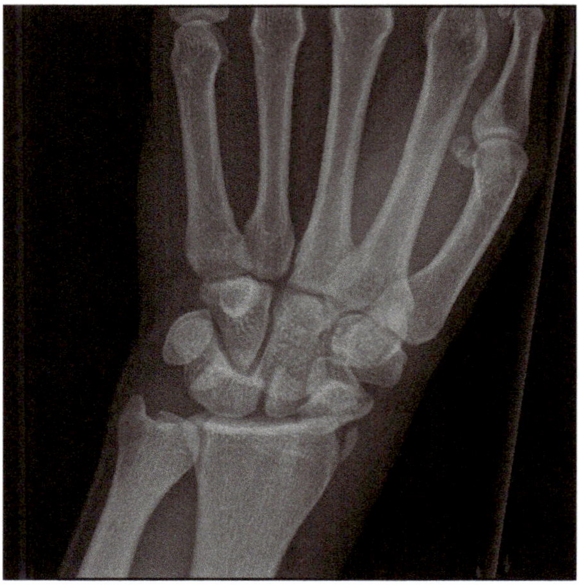

Figure 39-19. PA x-ray demonstrating a transscaphoid perilunate dislocation.

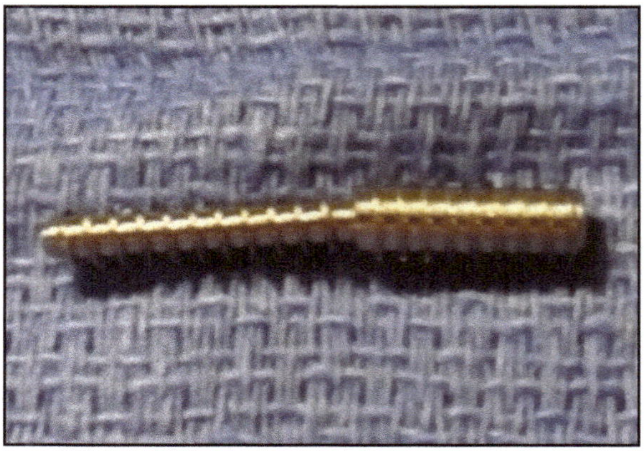

Figure 39-20. The SLIC screw is a cylinder screw that allows full rotation and approximately 20 degrees of toggle. In this manner, after the screw is inserted, it allows prolonged stability of the involved carpal interval while the repaired interosseous ligament heals. The screw allows normal motion between the carpal bones, with full rotation and toggle built into the screw.

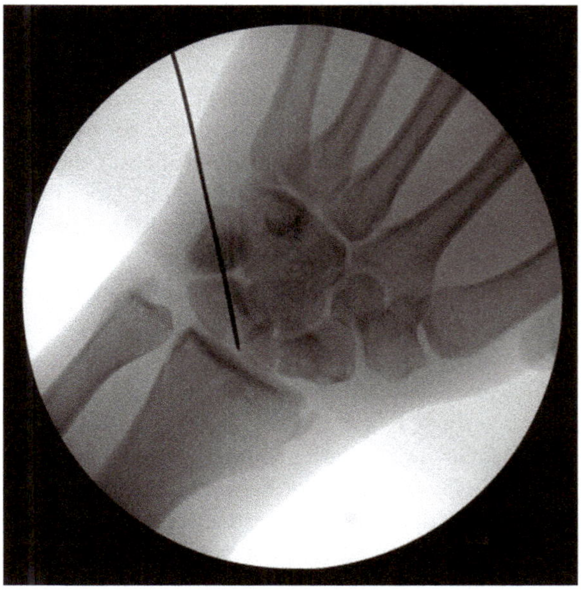

Figure 39-21. PA fluoroscopic image showing percutaneous placement of the guide wire across the LT interval in preparation for the SLIC screw.

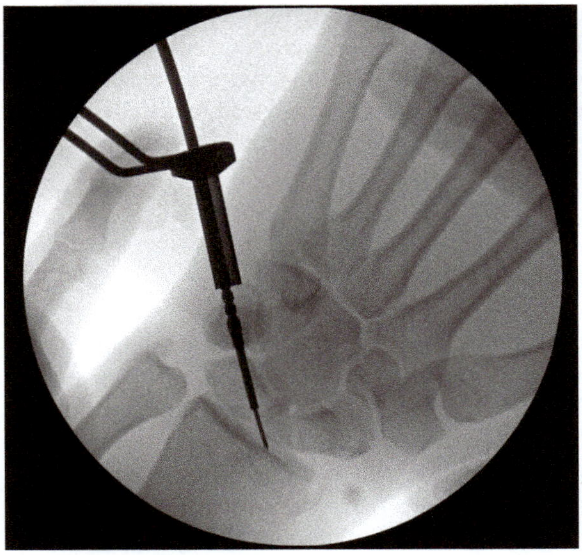

Figure 39-22. Under fluoroscopic observation, the length of the SLIC screw to be placed is measured directly off the step drill indentation. The 3 available sizes are 22, 25, and 28 mm. In this instance, a 28-mm SLIC screw would be inserted.

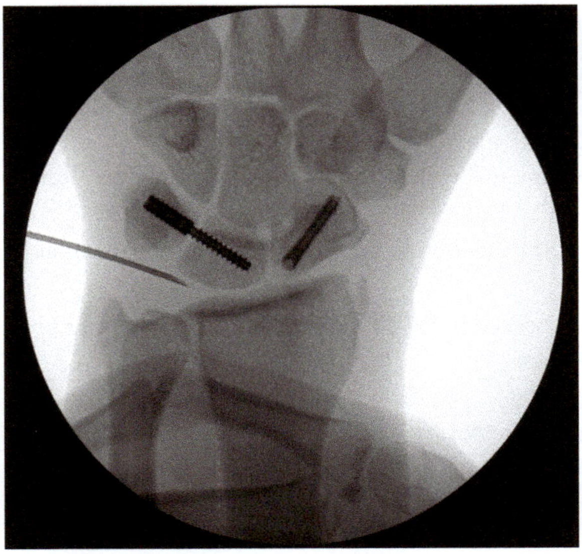

Figure 39-23. PA fluoroscopic image following percutaneous SLIC screw insertion for the LT instability and arthroscopic fixation of the scaphoid via the Geissler technique. With no protruding K-wires, the patient can start early rehabilitation.

ROM exercises were initiated 1 month postoperatively. In the transscaphoid perilunate group, the arc of motion at 3 months was between 70 and 120 degrees. Five patients had no pain. In the open repair group, the arc of motion averaged 60 to 130 degrees. Stabilization of perilunate dislocations without K-wires allowed patients to participate in physical therapy at an earlier stage, which resulted in a functional ROM at 3 months postoperatively. In addition, it resulted in fewer initial postoperative visits for pin tract checks as K-wires were not used.

Postoperative Protocol

Postoperatively, the wrist is placed in a well-padded thumb spica splint to allow for soft tissue rest and immobilization of the fracture. The patient is encouraged to keep the extremity elevated and perform finger exercises to reduce swelling and prevent stiffness. At 2 weeks postoperatively, the splint is removed, plain films are obtained, and any sutures are removed. The patient is placed in a removable thumb spica splint that is worn at all times except to perform gentle ROM exercises. After 4 to 6 weeks postoperatively, the splint is discontinued and exercises focusing on strength and grip are added if fluoroscopic evidence of healing is present in the form of trabeculated bone across the fracture site. At 12 weeks postoperatively, the patient is progressed to activity as tolerated and often may return to contact sports. If there is any question about fracture union, a CT scan may be ordered to further assess the fracture at this time.

Potential Complications

Wrist arthroscopy has a fairly low complication rate, with a recent study demonstrating a 5% complication rate.[20] Complications associated with the arthroscopic portion of the procedure include dorsal sensory neuropraxia, portal infections, formation of a ganglion cyst, and wrist stiffness. Often, these complication can be avoided with good technique and proper portal placement. Complications associated with placement of screw fixation can include pain from a prominent screw, guide wire breakage during drilling or screw placement, avascular necrosis of the fracture fragments, or nonunion of the fracture. Once again, careful technique and taking the proper precautions outlined in this chapter can help to avoid many of these issues.

Top Technical Pearls for the Procedure

1. Clear arthroscopic visualization of the proximal pole of the scaphoid is mandatory. It is important to shave any dorsal synovitis that may obscure visualization.
2. The starting point for the guide wire is the junction of the SL interosseous ligament at the proximal pole of the scaphoid.
3. The position of the guide wire must be checked in PA oblique and lateral planes prior to reaming and insertion of the headless screw.
4. A second guide wire may be helpful to protect against rotation of the fracture fragments as the headless cannulated screw is being inserted.
5. Radiocarpal evaluation following screw insertion should be performed to ensure the headless screw is within the scaphoid and not prominent.

References

1. Gelberman RH, Wolock BS, Siegel DB. Current concepts review: fractures and non-unions of the carpal scaphoid. *J Bone Joint Surg Am.* 1989;71(10):1560-1565.
2. Cooney WP, Dobyns JH, Linscheid RL. Fractures of the scaphoid: a rational approach to management. *Clin Orthop Relat Res.* 1980;(149):90-97.
3. Rettig AC, Ryan RO, Stone JA. Epidemiology of hand injuries in sports. In: Strickland JW, Rettig AC. *Hand Injuries in Athletes.* Philadelphia, PA: WB Saunders; 1992:37-48.
4. Gellman H, Caputo RJ, Carter V, Aboulafia A, McKay M. Comparison of short and long thumb-spica casts for non-displaced fractures of the carpal scaphoid. *J Bone Joint Surg Am.* 1989;71(3):354-357.
5. Kaneshiro SA, Failla JM, Tashman S. Scaphoid fracture displacement with forearm rotation in a short arm thumb spica cast. *J Hand Surg Am.* 1989;71:354-357.
6. Skirven T, Trope J. Complications of immobilization. *Hand Clin.* 1994;10(1):53-61.
7. Gelberman RH, Menon J. The vascularity of the scaphoid bone. *J Hand Surg Am.* 1980;5(5):508-513.

8. Filan SL, Herbert TJ. Herbert screw fixation of scaphoid fractures. *J Bone Joint Surg Br.* 1996;78(4):519-529.
9. Garcia-Elias M, Vall A, Salo JM, Lluch AL. Carpal alignment after different surgical approaches to the scaphoid: a comparative study. *J Hand Surg Am.* 1988;13(4):604-612.
10. Adams BD, Blair WF, Regan DS, Grundberg AB. Technical factors related to Herbert screw fixation. *J Hand Surg Am.* 1988;13(6):893-899.
11. Geissler WB. *Wrist Arthroscopy.* New York, NY: Springer; 2005.
12. Geissler WB. Arthroscopic fixation of cystic scaphoid nonunions with DBM. Presented at: American Association Hand Surgery; January 2006; Tucson, AZ.
13. Whipple TL. The role of arthroscopy in the treatment of intra-articular wrist fractures. *Hand Clin.* 1995;11(1):13-18.
14. Haddad FS, Goddard NJ. Acute percutaneous scaphoid fixation. A pilot study. *J Bone Joint Surg Br.* 1998;80(1):95-99.
15. Slade JF III, Grauer JN, Mahoney JD. Arthroscopic reduction and percutaneous fixation of scaphoid fractures with a novel dorsal technique. *Orthop Clin North Am.* 2000;32(2):247-261.
16. Geissler WB, Slade JF. Arthroscopic fixation of scaphoid nonunions without bone grafting. Presented at: American Society Surgery of the Hand; September 2002; Phoenix, AZ.
17. Slade JF III, Jaskwhich D. Percutaneous fixation of scaphoid fractures. *Hand Clin.* 2001;17(4):553-574.
18. Geissler WB. Arthroscopic assisted fixation of fractures of the scaphoid. *Atlas Hand Clin.* 2003;8:37-56.
19. Budhoff JE. Treatment of lunate and perilunate dislocations. *J Hand Surg Am.* 2008;33(8):1424-1432.
20. Beredjiklian PK, Bozentka DJ, Leung YL, Monaghan BA. Complications of wrist arthroscopy. *J Hand Surg Am.* 2004;29(3):406-411.

Please see videos on the accompanying website at

www.routledge.com/9781630910013

40

The Future
Endoscopic Surgery of the Wrist and Forearm

Gregory Bain, MBBS, FRACS, FA (Ortho)A, PhD
and Bhavin Jadav, MBBS, MS (Ortho)

Introduction

Arthroscopic surgery of the wrist is widely practiced around the world by most upper limb surgeons, but endoscopic surgery for the soft tissues around the wrist is a relatively new form of intervention that has potential for further expansion in the future.

Endoscopic carpal tunnel release was described as early as 1989[1] and has been advanced to become a commonly used technique in clinical practice. Exploration of the Guyon's canal for decompressing the ulnar nerve at the wrist with endoscopic technique has been explored, but concerns remain about the risk to the motor branch of ulnar nerve.[2]

These teething problems are not likely to deter the progress of endoscopic surgical techniques but are to be used as stepping stones in further learning progress. Endoscopic techniques are being applied in release of various nerve entrapment syndromes around the wrist and forearm.[3]

Soft tissue endoscopy has been used more commonly around the elbow, especially with endoscopic ulnar nerve release.[4,5] Around the elbow, endoscopy has also been successfully used in the olecranon bursa[6] and distal biceps tendon.[7,8] In the forearm, endoscopic techniques have been used for decompression of the anterior interosseous nerve[9,10] from pronator syndrome[11] and fasciotomy in cases of chronic exertional compartment syndromes.[12,13]

Hoffman,[14] with manufacturer Karl Storz, developed the fenestrated optical dissector that is an arthroscopic cannula with a hood to lift the soft tissue like a tent post. This creates a working space and makes visualization possible with a standard 30-degree scope. A similar fenestrated endoscope has been used for facelift surgeries as well.

Endoscopic surgeries have the advantage of being minimally invasive while allowing extensile access to the target tissue. For example, an ulnar nerve release can be performed through an endoscopic approach, extended up to 30 cm, and then a transposition can be performed if required.[8] These patients experience less pain, a quicker functional recovery, and return to work.[15]

Endoscopic procedures are developed by modifying accepted open techniques and then performing them with endoscopic methods. Thorough knowledge of regional surgical anatomy, respect for the neurovascular structures, and adhering to the anatomical and biomechanical principles of the original open procedure are paramount for a safe and successful endoscopic procedure.

Savoie FH III, Field LD, Steinmann SP, eds. *The Elbow and Wrist: AANA Advanced Arthroscopic Surgical Techniques* (pp 415-422).

Table 40-1. Therapeutic Endoscopic Procedures About the Wrist

Releases	De Quervain's tenosynovitis, intersection syndrome
	Forearm fasciotomy
	Guyon's canal release
Excision	Tenosynovectomy
	Bursectomy
	Excision of lesions (eg, ganglion)
	Excision of pisiform
Harvesting	Vessel graft (eg, cephalic vein, radial artery for CABG[16])
	Nerve graft (eg, distal PIN, MCNFA)
	Tendon graft (eg, FCR, palmaris longus)
	Bone graft (eg, distal radius)
Stabilization	Fixation of ulnar fractures/ulnar osteotomies
Reconstruction	Tendon transfer (eg, extensor indicis to EPL)

CABG, coronary artery bypass graft; EPL, extensor pollicis longus; FCR, flexor carpi radialis; MCNFA, medial cutaneous nerve of forearm; PIN, posterior interosseous nerve

Indications

There are many potential indications for endoscopic procedures about the wrist (Table 40-1). They can be considered diagnostic or therapeutic procedures. The therapeutic procedures can be considered releases, such as ectomy (excision) procedures, grafting harvesting, stabilization, and reconstructive procedures.

Contraindications

To be able to perform endoscopic procedures, the surgeon needs to be able to create a working space in which to perform the procedure. Therefore, if there is extensive soft tissue scarring, endoscopy is unlikely to be successful. Relative contraindications include infection and previous surgery.

Equipment

The equipment required includes a standard 30-degree scope. The authors prefer the wrist scope because it is easier to maneuverer in the relatively small space. A fenestrated hooded scope cannula is useful but not mandatory. Standard retractors can be used as an alternative. Fiber optic illuminated endoscopic speculums with suction tips can be useful but are also not critical.

Scissors, retractors, and artery clips are used in the same way as in open surgery. Nylon tapes can be placed around tendons to manipulate them. Endoscopic bipolar cautery or sheathed monopolar cautery are also useful.

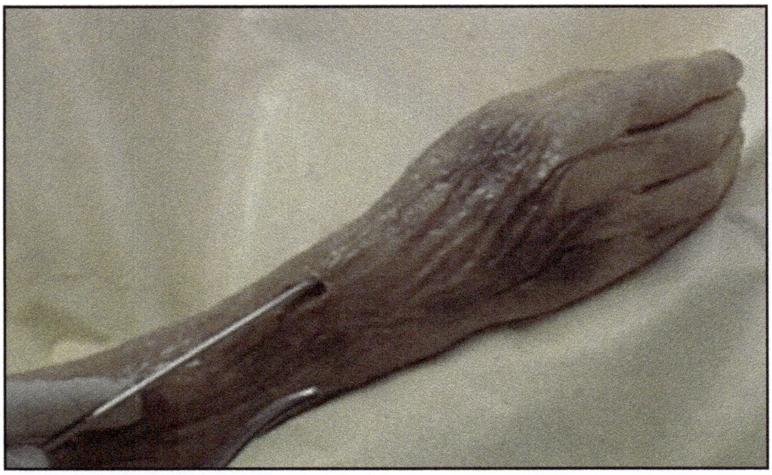

Figure 40-1. Cadaveric specimen used for training. A portal was created proximal to the extensor retinaculum to allow elevation of the subcutaneous tissues and examination of the extensor tendons, and to enable a tenosynovectomy to be performed.

The authors prefer to perform the endoscopy as a dry procedure but, on occasion, use the saline to moisten the tissues or clean the lens. Dry endoscopy provides a better definition of the anatomy and perfusion and prevents soft tissue swelling.

With dry endoscopy, the lens can become fogged or splattered with blood. It can be wiped off on the adjacent tissues, such as the subcutaneous fat. If it remains a problem, wipe the lens with an alcohol or glycerine wipe. The authors added more details on dry endoscopy in Chapter 23 on the future of elbow arthroscopy and endoscopy in this book.

Positioning and Portals

The ideal patient positioning would be with an arm table, with the limb draping (Figure 40-1). Use of an Esmarch bandage and tourniquet will help in obtaining a better clarity in the field. The primary working portal is created at a safe level in line with the target anatomical structures. The skin is incised, the cutaneous nerves are protected, and the deep fascia is visualized. The scope is introduced in the region of the target organ.

Step-by-Step Description of the Procedure

Soft Tissue Releases

De Quervain's tenosynovitis is a painful condition caused by entrapment of the extensor pollicis brevis and abductor pollicis longus tendons within the first extensor compartment. Open surgical release of the first extensor compartment is an accepted surgical treatment.

An endoscopic release of the first extensor compartment is likely to be a successful procedure as long as all of the subcompartments are completely released and the dorsal cutaneous branch of the superficial cutaneous branch of radial nerve is protected (Figure 40-2).

Intersection syndrome presents with pain over the dorsoradial aspect of the distal forearm. It is due to friction between the tendons of the first extensor compartment (extensor pollicis brevis and abductor pollicis longus) and the second extensor compartment (extensor carpi radialis longus and extensor carpi radialis brevis). This condition is less common than De Quervain's tenosynovitis and often does not need surgery. In cases that require surgery, endoscopic release of the intersecting tendons can be performed with a minimally invasive technique.

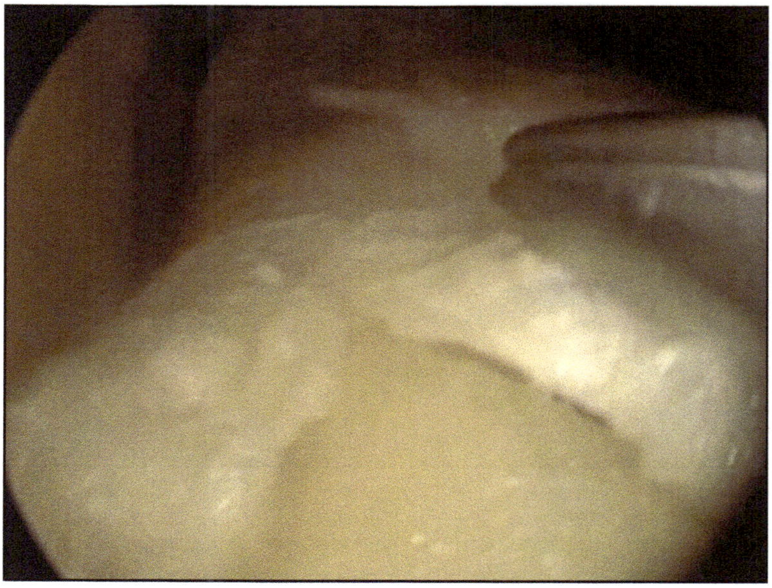

Figure 40-2. De Quervain's release. The cutaneous nerves are safely elevated. An endoscopic release of this cadaveric first extensor compartment was performed, with care to ensure that all separate septae were released.

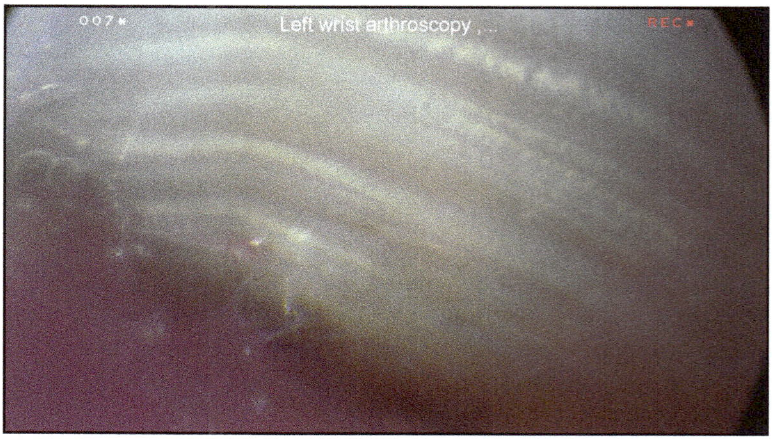

Figure 40-3. Investing layer of the deep fascia of the forearm. This endoscopic view demonstrates the normal deep surface of the investing layer of the deep fascia of the forearm. In the case of compartment syndrome, the subcutaneous tissues would be elevated to expose the outer surface of the investing layer of deep fascia of the forearm, which is then released.

Endoscopic surgical release of an intersection syndrome involves creating a dorsal portal to the wrist, dissection of the subcutaneous tissues, and introduction of the endoscope. The intersection of the offending tendons can be visualized and the fascial tissues that entrap the tendons can be released. This is best performed with the patient awake and with only local anesthetic infiltration so the offending tendons and their intersection can be clearly visualized. The fascia sheath is released using Metzenbaum scissors under endoscopic vision. Release is performed until smooth and undeterred excursion of oblique tendons is visualized.

Chronic (exertional) forearm compartment syndromes are often found in musicians, heavy manual workers, and athletes. Diagnosis of the condition is based on a detailed clinical history and identification of the affected group of muscles and the anatomical compartment that they occupy. Chronic compartment syndromes are often limited to a single compartment, and the elevation of the compartment pressure is relatively lower when compared to acute traumatic compartment syndromes. An endoscopic assessment of the compartment can be performed under local anesthesia (Figure 40-3). The scope can be placed in the subcutaneous tissues and a cannula can be placed into the compartment under endoscopic vision to enable compartment pressure monitoring to be performed. The offending compartment can then be released.

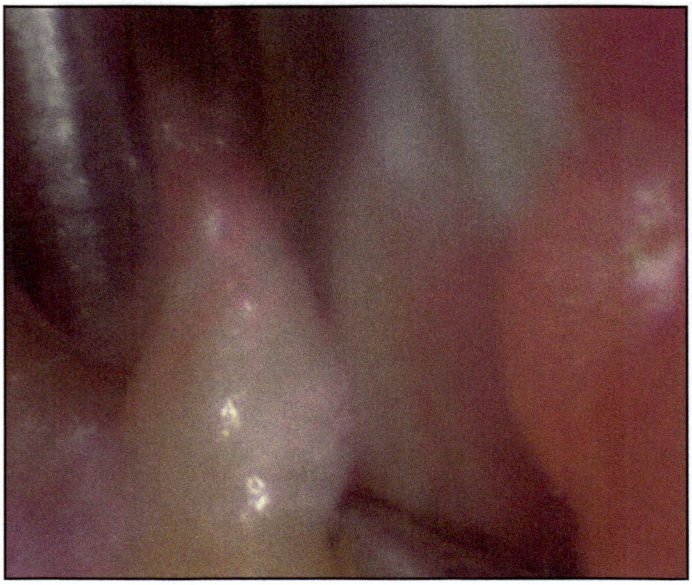

Figure 40-4. Posterior interosseous neurectomy. In this clinical case, the extensor tendons were retracted to expose the posterior interosseous nerve, which is then excised with a rongeur.

Acute compartment syndrome of the forearm or hand demands wide and complete release of all compartments. Endoscopically assisted release of acute compartment syndrome could be performed, but the surgeon needs to be confident that he or she has performed a complete release. This would not be the ideal first case.

Excision Procedures

Many excision procedures are used in hand surgery. Tenosynovectomy of the extensor tendons is a common example. Other examples include excision of ganglions and other soft tissue lesions. The authors have performed neurectomies of the posterior interosseous nerve at the level of the wrist. However, other neurectomies could also be performed (Figure 40-4).

Tissue Harvest

The palmaris longus tendon is a common donor in hand surgery. A preoperative clinical assessment is necessary to establish that the patient has a palmaris longus tendon on the side being operated. After standard surgical preparation for the limb, a primary portal is placed directly over the distal portion of palmaris longus tendon, just proximal to the palmar crease of the wrist. The palmar cutaneous branch of the median nerve is protected. The endoscope is introduced into the forearm, the palmaris longus tendon is identified, and it is then dissected into the forearm. A secondary proximal portal is created and a tenotomy is performed. The tendon is delivered into the distal wound and divided. An endoscopic release of the first extensor compartment is likely to be a successful procedure as long as all of the subcompartments are completely released and the dorsal cutaneous branch of the superficial cutaneous branch of radial nerve is protected (Figure 40-5). The free graft is then used as required.

Fixation Procedures

Fixation of fractures or osteotomies requires that the fracture be reduced (open or closed) and that it then be secured with fixation, such as plates and screws. The ulnar is subcutaneous, so it is ideal for endoscopically assisted fixation of fractures and osteotomies.

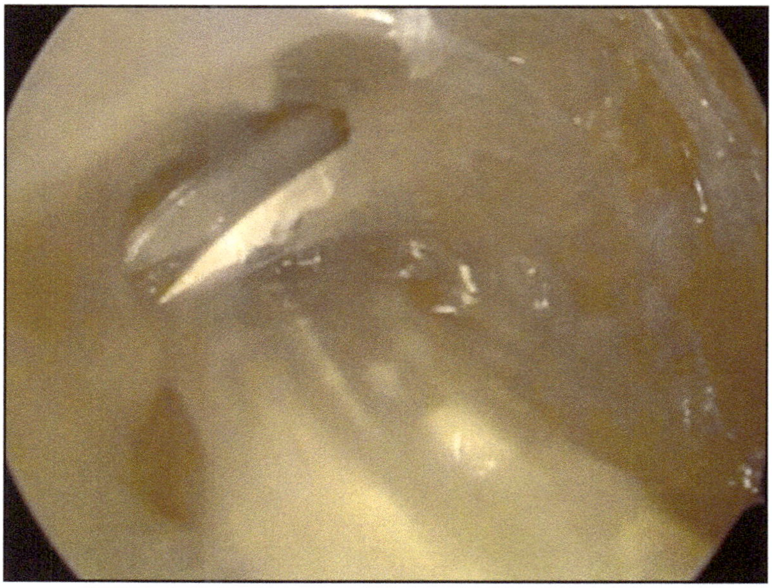

Figure 40-5. Harvesting of the palmaris longus tendon. This cadaveric palmaris longus tendon has been endoscopically dissected into the mid-forearm. It will be cut and retrieved to be used as a tendon graft.

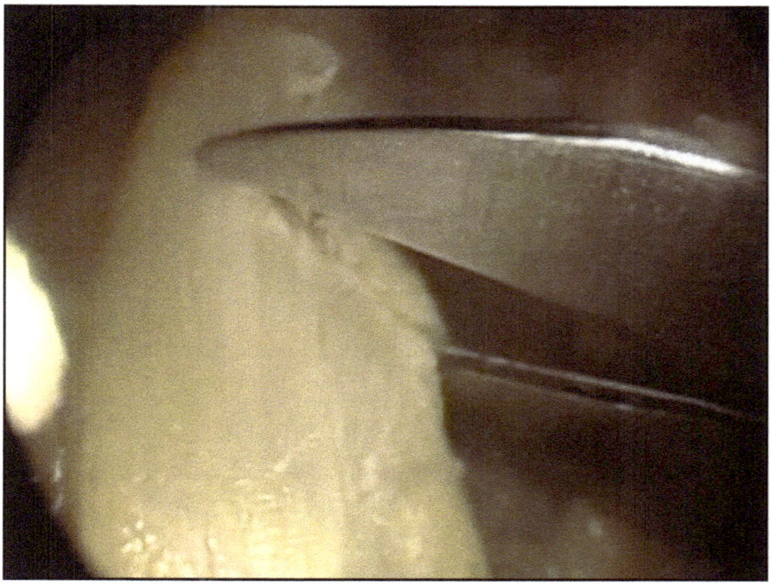

Figure 40-6. EI to EPL transfer. From a central portal, the cadaveric EI tendon has been dissected free of its adjacent structures. It will be divided and retrieved to the central portal, where it will be sutured to the distal stump of EPL tendon.

Reconstructive Surgery

Extensor indicis to extensor pollicis longus (EPL) tendon transfer is a valuable reconstructive technique in hand surgery. A central portal is created over the site of planned extensor indicis (EI) to EPL repair. The subcutaneous tissues are elevated so the 3 components of the procedure can be performed, as they would for an open tendon transfer. From this central portal, the EPL tendon distal to the extensor retinaculum is identified. The third extensor compartment is released and is explored to identify the cause of the tendon rupture. The EI is identified and divided at the level of the index metacarpophalangeal joint (Figure 40-6). A small secondary portal may be required to perform the tenotomy. An endoscopic release of the first extensor compartment is likely to be a successful procedure, as long as all of the subcompartments are completely released and the dorsal cutaneous branch of the superficial cutaneous branch of radial nerve is protected.

The EPL and EI tendons are delivered out of the central portal, and a Pulvertaft weave is performed. The authors ensure that the Pulvertaft repair is a bit tight because it will loosen marginally. If the patient is awake, thumb motion can be assessed actively. If the patient has an arm block or general anaesthetic, the tenodesis effect can be tested. The thumb is protected with a dynamic extension splint for 4 weeks, and then hand therapy is instituted.

Training and Development of New Techniques

This entire surgical field is new and evolving. As a consequence, surgeons need to ensure that the methods are safe and effective. The development and training of these techniques can be demanding. Tips include the following:

1. Become competent with the open procedure (anatomy, principles of the procedure).
2. Develop familiarity with the instrumentation on mock models (eg, sawbones).
3. Perform trials on cadaveric models.
4. Attend cadaveric courses.
5. Visit colleagues who are experienced in the surgical methods.
6. Mind map the procedure (ie, play out all of the steps in your mind before you do it).
7. Commence with diagnostic endoscopic procedures before therapeutic ones.
8. Advance to an endoscopic therapeutic procedure. Have a low tolerance to bail out to an open procedure if the following occur:
   - There are difficulties or concerns with safety.
   - The procedure is taking an undue amount of time. Consider having a time limit, at which point you will convert to an open procedure (eg, 30 minutes).
9. Do not trial a clinical endoscopic case if the following occur:
   - You do not feel safe and confident with the anatomy, instruments, or procedure.
   - There are other significant time, staffing, or logistical issues on that day.
   - It is a revision or complex case.

Potential Complications

The potential complications for endoscopic procedures include infection, cutaneous nerve injury, hematoma, and compartment syndrome. Other potential complications would be directly related to the specific procedure performed (eg, tendon transfer complications include rupture of repair, transfer too tight).

Conclusion

Endoscopically assisted surgeries of the wrist and forearm are in the early experimental phase. The indications are evolving and techniques are developing. With the advent of better-quality optical equipment and endoscopic surgical tools, this promising area has the potential to be more widely used. Being a less invasive modality, the authors expect that it will be progressively adopted.

Top Technical Pearls for the Procedure

1. Be familiar with the anatomy, equipment, and basics of the procedure.
2. Utilise the anatomical principles developed for open surgery.
3. Create a clear working space.
4. Maintain hemostasis throughout the procedure.
5. Bale out to open procedure if having difficulties.

References

1. Okutsu I, Ninomiya S, Takatori Y, Ugawa Y. Endoscopic management of carpal tunnel syndrome. *Arthroscopy.* 1989;5(1):11-18.
2. Noszczyk BH, Zdybek P. Feasibility and limitations of endoscopy in Guyon's canal. *Wideochirurgia Inne Tech Malo Inwazyjne.* 2014;9(3):387-392.
3. Lecĺere FM, Bignion D, Franz T, Mathys L, Vögelin E. Endoscopically assisted nerve decompression of rare nerve compression syndromes at the upper extremity. *Arch Orthop Trauma Surg.* 2013;133(4):575-582.
4. Zajonc H, Momeni A. Endoscopic release of the cubital tunnel. *Hand Clin.* 2014;30(1):55-62.
5. Morse LP, McGuire DT, Bain GI. Endoscopic ulnar nerve release and transposition. *Tech Hand Up Extrem Surg.* 2014;18(1):10-14.
6. Tu CG, McGuire DT, Morse LP, Bain GI. Olecranon extrabursal endoscopic bursectomy. *Tech Hand Up Extrem Surg.* 2013;17(3):173-175.
7. Earnes MH, Bain GI. Distal biceps tendon endoscopy and anterior elbow arthroscopy portal. *Tech Shoulder Elbow Surg.* 2006;7:139-142.
8. Sharma S, MacKay G. Endoscopic repair of distal biceps tendon using an EndoButton. *Arthroscopy.* 2005;21(7):897.
9. Keiner D, Tschabitscher M, Welschehold S, Oertel J. Anterior interosseous nerve compression syndrome: is there a role for endoscopy? *Acta Neurochir (Wien).* 2011;153(11):2225-2229.
10. Damert HG, Hoffmann R, Kraus A, Stowell RL, Lubahn J. Minimally invasive endoscopic decompression for anterior interosseous nerve syndrome: technical notes. *J Hand Surg Am.* 2013;38(10):2016-2024.
11. Lee AK, Khorsandi M, Nurbhai N, Dang J, Fitzmaurice M, Herron KA. Endoscopically assisted decompression for pronator syndrome. *J Hand Surg Am.* 2012;37(6):1173-1179.
12. Hijjawi J, Nagle DJ. Endoscopic-assisted Fascial Decompression for forearm exertional compartment syndrome: a case report and review of the literature. *Hand (N Y).* 2010;5(4):427-429.
13. Pozzi A, Pivato G, Kask K, Susini F, Pegoli L. Single portal endoscopic treatment for chronic exertional compartment syndrome of the forearm. *Tech Hand Up Extrem Surg.* 2014;18(3):153-156.
14. Hoffman R. About Dr. Reimer Hoffmann. *Endoscopic Cubital Tunnel Syndrome.* http://www.endoscopic-cubitaltunnel.com/3-1-about-dr--hoffmann.html. Accessed August 7, 2015.
15. Cobb TK, Walden AL, Merrell PT, Lemke JH. Setting expectations following endoscopic cubital tunnel release. *Hand (N Y).* 2014;9(3):356-363.
16. Dimitrova KR, Dincheva GR, Hoffman DM, DeCastro H, Geller CM, Tranbaugh RF. Results of endoscopic radial artery harvesting in 1577 patients. *Innovations (Phila).* 2013;8(6):398-402.

Please see videos on the accompanying website at

www.routledge.com/9781630910013

Section VII

THE WRIST
Carpal Tunnel Release

41

Endoscopic Carpal Tunnel Release

The Chow Technique

James C. Y. Chow, MD

Introduction

Paget first described median nerve compression after a distal radius fracture in 1854.[1,2] In 1880, Putnam, a neurologist from Boston, reported similar symptoms in a group of his patients.[3] The first formal description of surgical decompression for treatment of this condition was reported in 1933; this was followed by Phalen et al's classic article in 1950.[4] Since then, open carpal tunnel release has been established as the gold standard for surgical treatment of carpal tunnel syndrome.

Chow began working on an endoscopic release of the transverse carpal ligament in 1985. The primary motivation of Chow's concept was to create a method for surgical treatment of carpal tunnel syndrome that could preserve the unaffected surrounding normal anatomic structures of the wrist and hand. Through these pursuits, Chow developed the slotted cannula late in 1986. After a thorough cadaveric trial period, the procedure was completed in May 1987, and it was first performed in a patient in September of that year.

The first 2 reports in the literature on the topic of endoscopic carpal tunnel release (ECTR), written separately by Chow[5] and by Okutsu et al,[6] were published in March 1989. The following year, Chow presented his clinical results after ECTR in 149 cases at the Arthroscopy Association of North America Annual Meeting. In fall 1990 at the American Society for Surgery of the Hand Annual Meeting, Agee et al[7] reported to the clinical results of a multicenter study of the use of Agee's technique for endoscopic release of the carpal ligament.

Anatomy

The carpal tunnel is bounded deeply by the volar surface of the distal radius, ulnarly by the hook of the hamate, radially by the scaphoid, and superficially by the confluence of the stout transverse carpal ligament, palmar aponeurosis, and antebrachial fascia. The carpal tunnel contains the median nerve and 9 tendons (ie, the flexor digitorum sublimus and profundus tendons to all 4 fingers and the flexor pollicis longus).

Savoie FH III, Field LD, Steinmann SP, eds. *The Elbow and Wrist: AANA Advanced Arthroscopic Surgical Techniques* (pp 425-439).

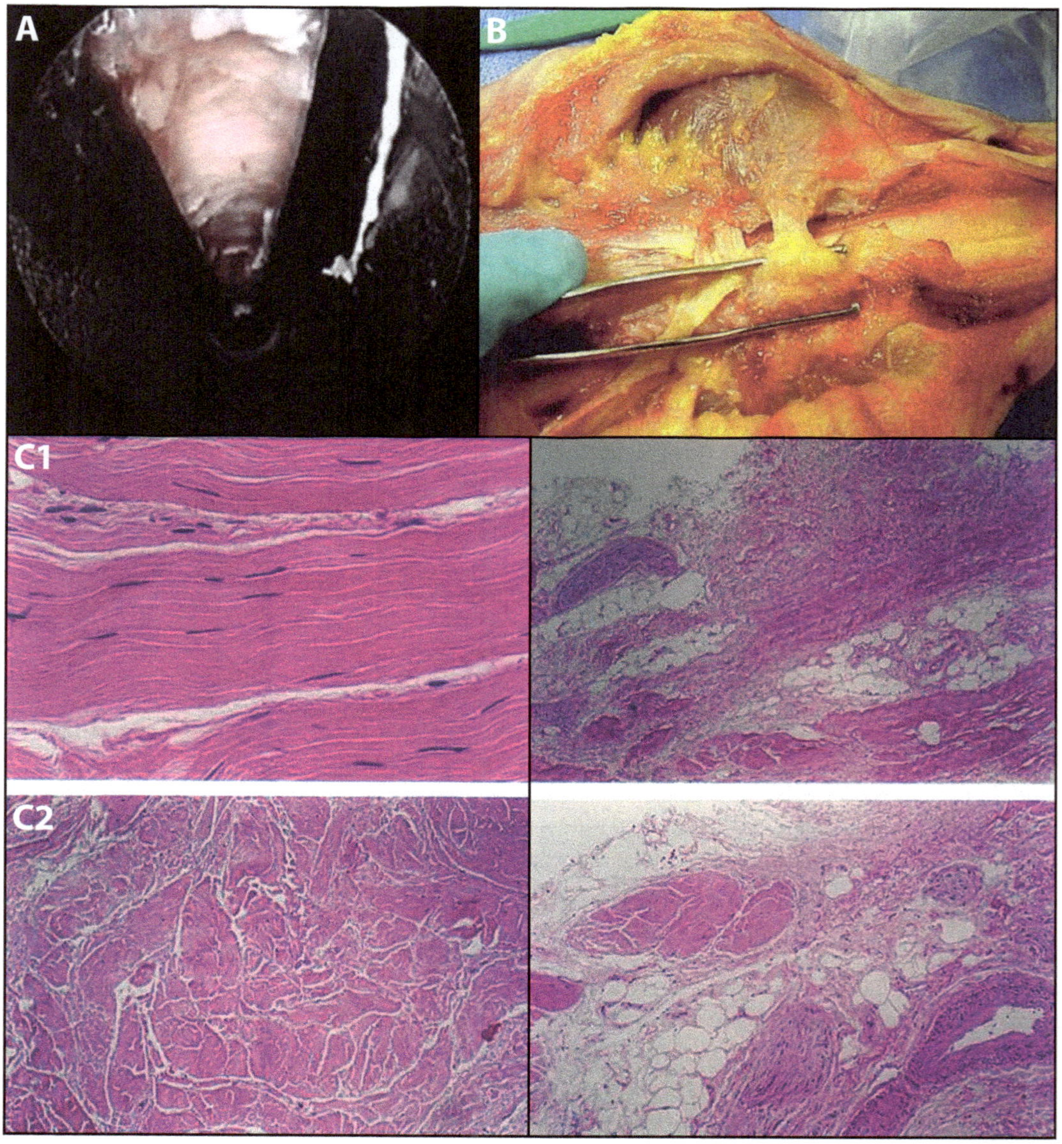

Figure 41-1. (A) Endoscopic view of the interthenar soft tissue band (ISTB). (B) Gross view of the ISTB. (C) Histologic examination of the transverse carpal ligament and the ISTB in (1) longitudinal and (2) cross-sectional views.

Superficial to the transverse carpal ligament lies a sling of vascular and nervous connective tissue, subcutaneous fat, and densely innervated palmar dermis and epidermis. This sling of soft tissue is an interthenar soft tissue band (ISTB; Figures 41-1A and B) that bridges the thenar and hypothenar musculature. It is a histologically distinct structure (Figure 41-1C) that lies volar to the transverse carpal ligament. The ISTB prevents bowstringing of the flexor tendons after surgery, thereby maintaining their strength during contraction.[8-10] It is the goal of ECTR to preserve this natural anatomy while selectively releasing only the transverse carpal ligament.

Pathology

Carpal tunnel syndrome is a compressive neuropathy of the median nerve at the wrist. It can result from any condition that increases intracarpal tunnel pressure, such as irritation and swelling of any of the 9 flexor tendons and their tenosynovium, edema of the median nerve, anatomic abnormality, or scarring of any of the bordering structures of the carpal tunnel, anomalous lumbrical anatomy, an intracarpal tunnel mass (eg, a deep ganglion cyst), or stiffening and contracture of the transverse carpal ligament.

Indications

The primary indication is carpal tunnel syndrome refractory to nonoperative management, including night bracing, therapy, and medication.

Controversial Indications

Acute carpal tunnel syndrome related to edema is a controversial indication.

Contraindications

Evidence of abnormal anatomy is a contraindication.

Pertinent Physical Findings

Patients usually present with a history of characteristic symptoms, including nocturnal pain; paresthesias; numbness in the thumb, index, and middle finger; and thenar muscular weakness. The physician should be aware of the patient's general health condition and family history. Congenital disease or anomalies, connective tissue diseases, systemic and metabolic disorders, and previous injury to the distal forearm or wrist should be taken into consideration.

The physical examination is critical for accurate diagnosis. In an acute case, there is tenderness along the carpal canal area. Light percussion over the median nerve at the wrist produces a sensation of an electric current that radiates to the median nerve distribution; this is known as *Tinel's sign*. The best test is most likely the Phalen's sign; in this test, a positive sign is evoked by holding the wrists at maximum flexion with the dorsal aspects of the hands in full contact (ie, reverse praying position). This position narrows the carpal canal; if it reproduces the paresthesias in the fingers within 60 seconds, the sign is considered positive. As the pathologic condition advances, less time is necessary to evoke a response. Other indicators include the monofilament test, 2-point discrimination, the reverse Phalen's test, and the tourniquet test. In the late stages, with thenar muscle atrophy, the examiner can observe the muscle wasting in the thenar area.[11] Muscle weakness is tested subjectively by resisted palmar adduction of the thumb against the examiner's index finger and comparison of one hand with the other (Strickland's test).

Pertinent Imaging

Electromyography and nerve conduction velocity tests aid in the detection of carpal tunnel syndrome. Indications for surgery should not be decided or altered according to the results of nerve conduction velocity tests, especially when the results are normal but the patient has the clinical signs and symptoms of the syndrome.[12-14] A delay in the distal latency of the median nerve of 7.0 msec or longer represents significant compression of the median nerve; if such a delay is present, surgery should be considered immediately. The most important aspects in diagnosing carpal tunnel syndrome are the history and physical examination results. Electrodiagnostic studies of the median nerve are used adjunctively to confirm the diagnosis and perhaps to suggest how the patient will respond to surgery.

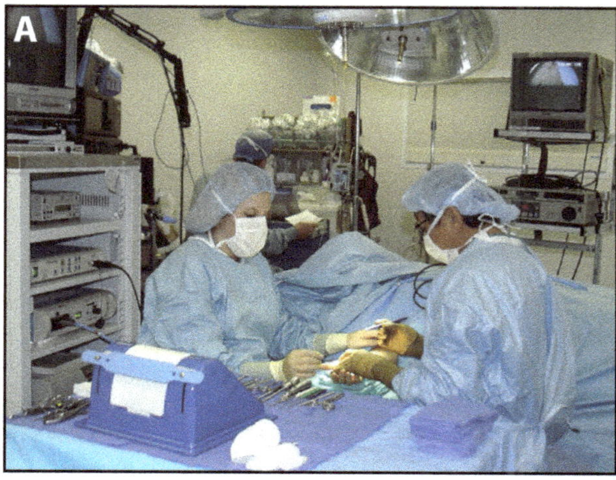

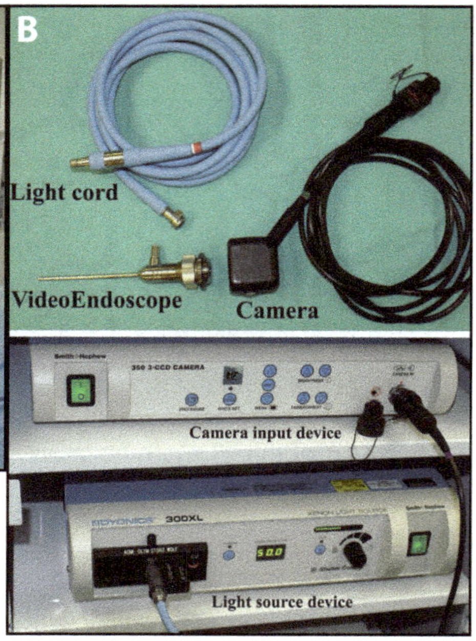

Figure 41-2. (A) Operating room setup for the endoscopic carpal tunnel release using the Chow dual-portal technique. (B) Arthroscopic equipment that is appropriate for the performance of this technique.

Wrist x-rays can rule out the possibility of congenital or acquired bone or joint deformity, abnormality, or pathology. Previously sustained fractures of the distal forearm and wrist should be taken into account. A malunited fracture of the distal radius, previously performed surgery in the wrist area, or a hypoplastic or aplastic hook of the hamate[15] can produce difficulties for the surgeon during placement of and operation through the slotted cannula. Standard anteroposterior and lateral views of the distal forearm and wrist and a tunnel view of the wrist are required. If a more extensive study is indicated, magnetic resonance imaging, computed tomography, ultrasound, bone scanning, or arthrography of the wrist may be necessary.[16,17]

Conservative Management

Conservative management includes daily or nightly wrist splinting, alteration of daily activities, physical therapy, and nonsteroidal anti-inflammatory drugs. Intracarpal tunnel steroid injections have been used with various degrees of success.

Equipment

The equipment needed to perform the procedure includes the standard arthroscopy setup and equipment and the Chow endoscopic carpal tunnel system (Smith & Nephew).

Positioning and Portals

Operating Room Setup

The patient is placed in a supine position and a hand table is used. Two video monitors are preferred, although some surgeons can manage the procedure with one. One of the 2 monitors should face the surgeon, and the other should face the assistant. The surgeon sits on the ulnar side of the patient while the assistant faces the surgeon (Figure 41-2A). The arthroscopic equipment

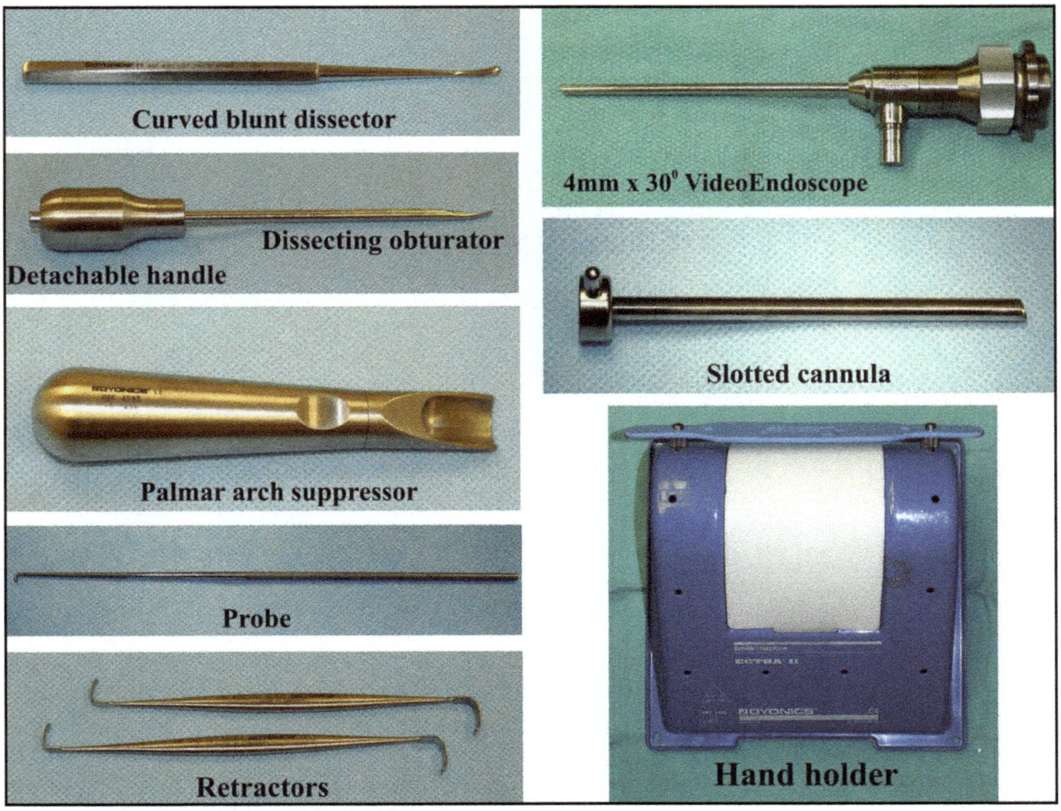

Figure 41-3. Instrumentation included in the ECTRA System Kit.

consists of a short, 4.0-mm, 30-degree video endoscope. The light post is on the same side as the direction of the view, the camera apparatus, the light cord, the camera input device, and the light source (Figure 41-2B). Optional equipment includes a digital video recorder and a video printer for the printing of any captured images. Water pump and shaver equipment are not used.

A standard handset should be available. Specific instrumentation for the procedure, designed by Chow, includes an ECTRA System Kit and an ECTRA Disposable Kit (Smith & Nephew Endoscopy). The ECTRA System Kit includes a video endoscope, slotted cannula, dissecting obturator, curved blunt dissector, palmar arch suppressor, probe, retractors, and hand holder (Figure 41-3). The dissecting obturator is attached with a detachable handle that can also take some other types of obturators included in the kit (eg, conical, boat-nose obturator), but the latter are not used routinely. The ECTRA Disposable Kit includes a probe knife, triangle knife, retrograde knife, hand pad, and swabs (Figure 41-4). These knives allow the surgeon to determine the direction and depth of the cut.

Standard preparations and draping are performed as usual, without the application of a tourniquet. Before local anesthesia is introduced, a skin marker is used to map landmarks for the entry and exit portals.

Anesthesia

Local anesthesia combined with intravenous medication is recommended for the procedure because it allows the patient and the surgeon to communicate. An alert patient can inform the surgeon during the procedure about any abnormal sensation in the hand, which can indicate a potential problem caused by a variance of nerve structure in the wrist and palm region.[18-24] Usually,

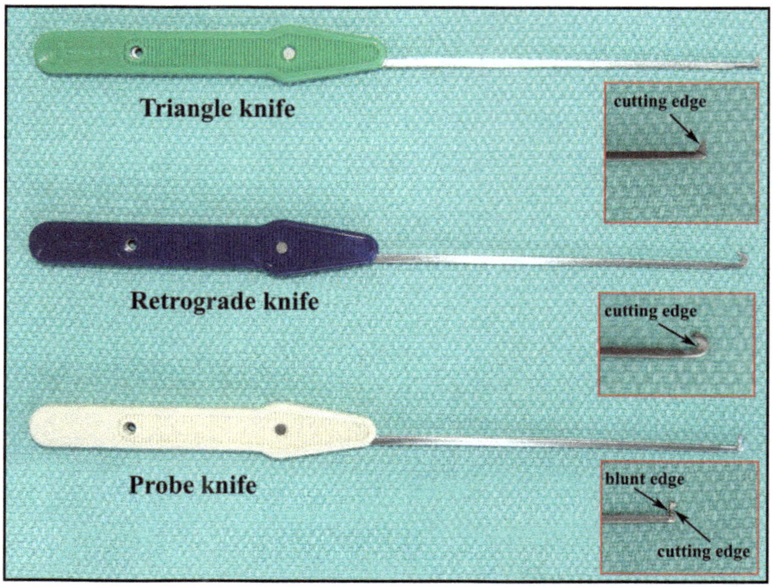

Figure 41-4. Specially designed knives for release of the transverse carpal ligament. The tip of each knife is shown in detail (red squares). This instrumentation is included in the ECTRA Disposable Kit.

when the patient first comes into the operating room, 100 μg of Sublimaze (fentanyl citrate) is given intravenously. This is a narcotic analgesic medication with an onset of 7 to 8 minutes and a peak action of approximately 30 minutes. Usually, the surgical time does not exceed 10 minutes. A 1% solution of Xylocaine (lidocaine) without epinephrine is injected, approximately 2 to 3 mL at the entry portal and 6 to 7 mL at the exit portal (because of the higher degree of sensitivity of the skin on the palmar region). Special care is taken to limit the injection to the skin and subcutaneous tissue and to avoid affecting the nerve by penetrating deeply.

Positioning the Entry Portal

The proximal end of the pisiform bone is palpated on the volar surface of the wrist within the flexor carpi ulnaris tendon at the distal wrist flexor crease and is marked with a small circle. A line from the proximal pole of the pisiform is drawn radially and is approximately 1 to 1.5 cm long. From that point, a second, 0.5-cm line is drawn proximally. A third dotted line, approximately 1 cm long, is drawn radially from the proximal end of the second line to create the entry portal (Figure 41-5). If the palmaris longus muscle is present, the center of the entry portal should be located at the ulnar border of its tendon, almost at the level of the proximal wrist flexor crease. Average dimensions of these lines vary slightly depending on the overall size of the hand.

Positioning the Exit Portal

The patient's thumb is placed in full abduction. A line is drawn across the palm from the distal border of the thumb to the approximate center of the palm, perpendicular to the long axis of the forearm. A second line is drawn from the third web space, parallel to the long axis of the forearm, to meet the first line. These 2 lines should form a right angle. A third line is drawn, bisecting this angle and extending approximately 1 cm proximally from its vertex, which established the site of incision for the exit portal (Figure 41-6). The surgeon should be able to palpate the hook of the hamate. The exit portal should fall into the soft spot at the center of the palm and should line up with the ring finger, just slightly radial to the hook of the hamate.

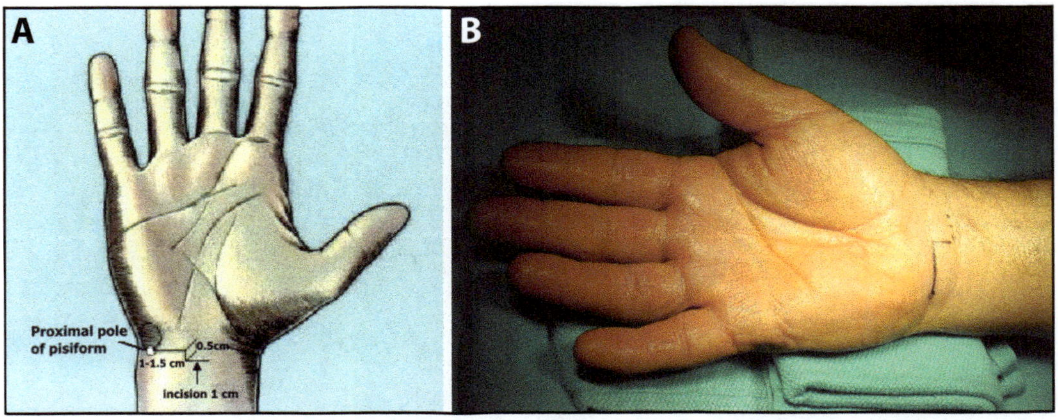

Figure 41-5. (A) Illustration and (B) photograph showing that the entry portal is located by drawing a line 1 to 1.5 cm radially from the proximal pole of the pisiform bone and then drawing a second line of approximately 0.5 cm proximally from the end of the first one. A third line of approximately 1 cm is then drawn radially from the proximal end of the second line to create the entry portal.

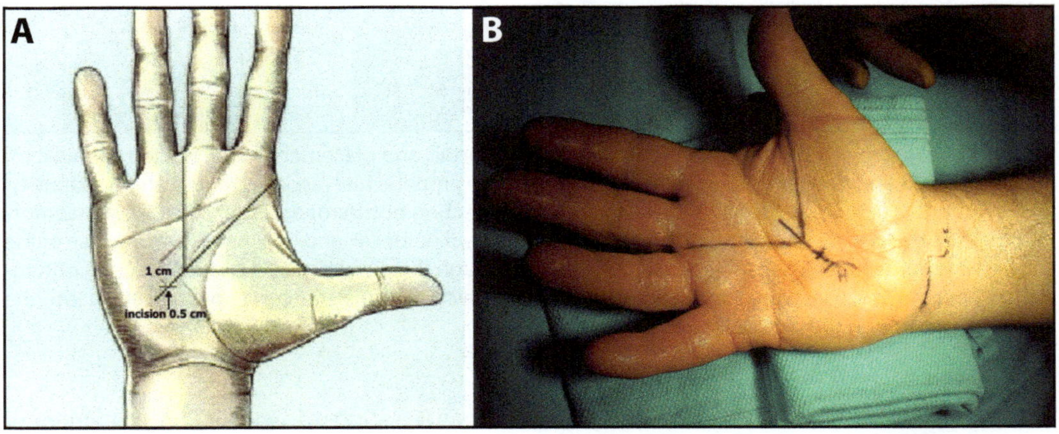

Figure 41-6. (A) Illustration and (B) photograph showing that the exit portal is located by drawing a line from the distal border of the fully abducted thumb perpendicular to the long axis of the forearm. A second line is drawn from the third web space parallel to the long axis of the forearm. These 2 lines form a right angle. A third line is drawn, bisecting this angle and extending approximately 1.0 cm from its vertex to determine the exit portal.

Creation of Portals and Placement of the Cannula

The procedure begins with the creation of the entry portal. A transverse incision of approximately 1 cm (Figure 41-7A) is made at the marked entry portal site, extending just through the skin. Subcutaneous tissue is bluntly dissected off the volar forearm fascia with the use of a hemostat and is retracted with the retractors. Care must be taken to avoid damage to the small subcutaneous blood vessels.

A knife is used to make a small, longitudinal opening of the antebrachial fascia that is extended distally with the use of a Stephen's tenotomy scissors (Figures 41-7B and C). If the palmaris longus muscle is present, the longitudinal cut should be along the ulnar border of palmaris longus tendon. Care should be taken because there are sometimes 2 layers of fascia that must be cut. Retractors are passed just beneath the fascia, with one of them lifting the skin distally to create a vacuum that separates the transverse carpal ligament from the ulnar bursa. A blunt, curved dissector is

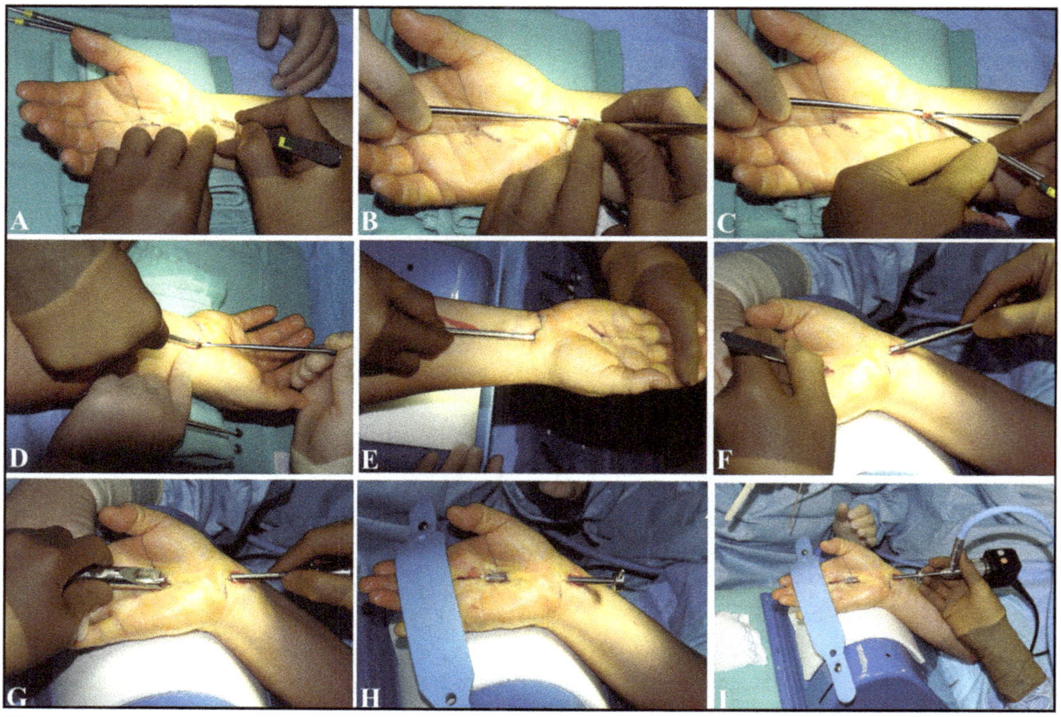

Figure 41-7. Step-by-step procedure for the creation of portals and placement of the slotted cannula. (A) Skin incision. (B and C) A small longitudinal opening of the antebrachial fascia is created and is extended distally using a tenotomy scissors. (D) Insertion of the dissecting obturator and slotted cannula assembly into the carpal canal. (E) Placement of the hand onto the hand holder. (F and G) Skin incision and use of the arch suppressor to allow the cannula assembly to exit through the distal portal. (H) The dissecting obturator has been removed, leaving the slotted cannula into the carpal canal. (I) The scope is inserted into the carpal canal through the proximal portal.

gently slipped into the carpal tunnel, just under the transverse carpal ligament. A gentle pop of resistance should be felt as the blunt dissector punches through the bursal sheath at about midway past the transverse carpal ligament. Maneuvering the dissector back and forth should produce a type of washboard feeling because of the rough undersurface of the carpal ligament. The curved dissector is then removed.

A dissecting obturator and slotted cannula assembly unit can be guided into the space vacated by the curved dissector. The slotted cannula assembly is advanced into the carpal tunnel on the underside of the transverse carpal ligament to the level of the hook of the hamate, staying to the ulnar side of the carpal tunnel (Figure 41-7D). With the tip of this unit touching the hook of the hamate, the surgeon gently picks up and hyperextends the hand. The hand and cannula assembly are now moved as a unit (Figure 41-7E) and placed on the hand holder with the wrist and fingers in full hyperextension. The cannula assembly is advanced along the undersurface of the carpal ligament, while the assistant keeps the hand on the hand holder, until the tip of the cannula assembly can be easily palpated in the palm area where the mark for the exit portal was made.

A small transverse or oblique incision is made just over the palpable cannula assembly tip, cutting only the skin (Figure 41-7F). The palmar skin and soft tissue are depressed with the palmar arch suppressor, and the cannula assembly is pushed into the receptacle of the palmar arch suppressor to exit through the distal portal (Figure 41-7G). The obturator is then removed from the cannula, which should lie just below the transverse carpal ligament, and the hyperextended hand is strapped onto the hand holder (Figures 41-7H and I). Hyperextension of the wrist brings the superficial palmar arch to a level lower than the exiting point of the slotted cannula assembly, thereby protecting if from injury. The creation of 2 portals is essential because they stabilize the slotted cannula while it passes through the portals, ensuring the reproducibility of the technique. The slotted portion of the cannula allows a safe cutting zone, whereas delicate structures, such as the median nerve and flexor tendons, are protected by the walls of the cannula.

Step-by-Step Description of the Procedure

1. Establish adequate general or regional anesthesia.
2. Make a small vertical incision in the proximal volar wrist crease.
3. Make a small incision in the volar wrist fascia and identify the carpal tunnel.
4. Use a blunt freer dissector to evaluate the carpal tunnel for aberrant anatomical structures.
5. Place the wrist on the supplied wrist holding immobilization device.
6. Insert the sheath and blunt trocar into the proximal incision under the transverse carpal ligament and out the skin of the palm at the distal end of the ligament.
7. Using the supplied knives, release the ligament according to the instruction in the surgical technique.
8. Deflate the tourniquet to check for unusual bleeding, then suture each wound with a simple stitch.

Endoscopic Examination

The video endoscope is inserted into the slotted cannula at the proximal portal. The camera and scope should rest comfortably in the first webspace of the surgeon's hand. A cotton swab can be inserted into the tube from the distal portion to clean the lens while focus is adjusted to the best visualization. A blunt probe is then inserted to palpate the undersurface of the transverse carpal ligament proximally to distally; if a thin bursal membrane is seen above the cannula's slotted opening, it is carefully dissected with the probe to gain access to the ligament, which has an ivory white appearance and fibers that run transversely (Figures 41-8A and B). If the median nerve is present in the field (Figure 41-8C), the patient will feel sharp pain radiating to the fingers when the nerve is probed; this response should alert the surgeon to the presence of the nerve. If abundant soft tissue is identified in the opening of the cannula, the procedure should not be performed. The slotted cannula may need to be reinserted to ensure better visualization; however, to avoid irreversible damage, surgery should not be performed if tendons or other important structures are entrapped between the slotted cannula and the undersurface of the carpal ligament (Figure 41-8D).

If there is a minimal amount of synovium obstructing the view, the obturator is replaced into the slotted cannula. The slotted cannula assembly unit can then be rotated radially about 355 to 360 degrees to provide the visualization and protection required. Surgeons should not hesitate to convert an endoscopic procedure to an open one if they cannot obtain adequate visualization.

Technique for Release of the Transverse Carpal Ligament

With the scope in the proximal portal and the probe in the distal portal, the distal border of the transverse carpal ligament is identified. The probe knife, which permits forward cutting only, is inserted into the distal portal. The blunt edge of the knife can be used to probe proximally to distally along the ligament. The cutting edge is then used to release the distal border of the ligament by drawing the knife distally to proximally (Figure 41-9A). Anything beyond the distal border of the carpal ligament should not be excised. The scope is withdrawn proximally about 1 cm, and the triangle knife is used to make a small upward cut in the midsection of the ligament (Figure 41-9B).

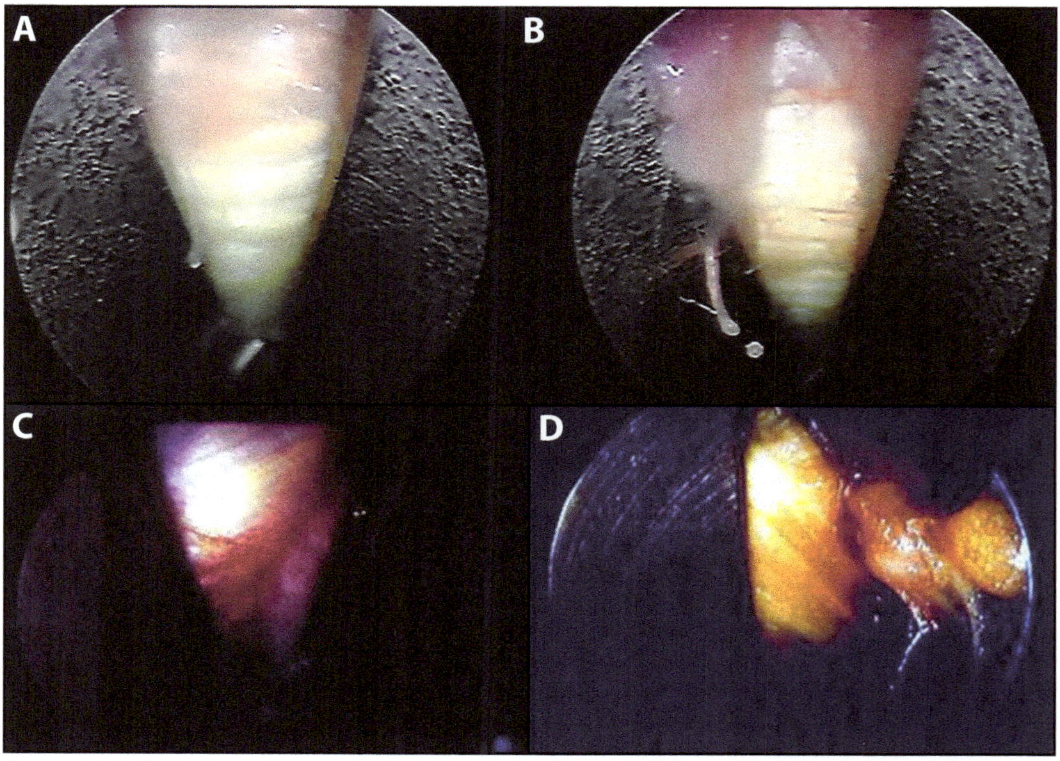

Figure 41-8. (A) Endoscopic normal appearance of the transverse carpal ligament with its fibers running transversely. (B) The thicker bursal membrane that sheaths the undersurface of the proximal portion of carpal ligament has been probed proximally, depicting the fibers of the ligament. (C) The median nerve is present in the field. (D) The tendon is present in the field.

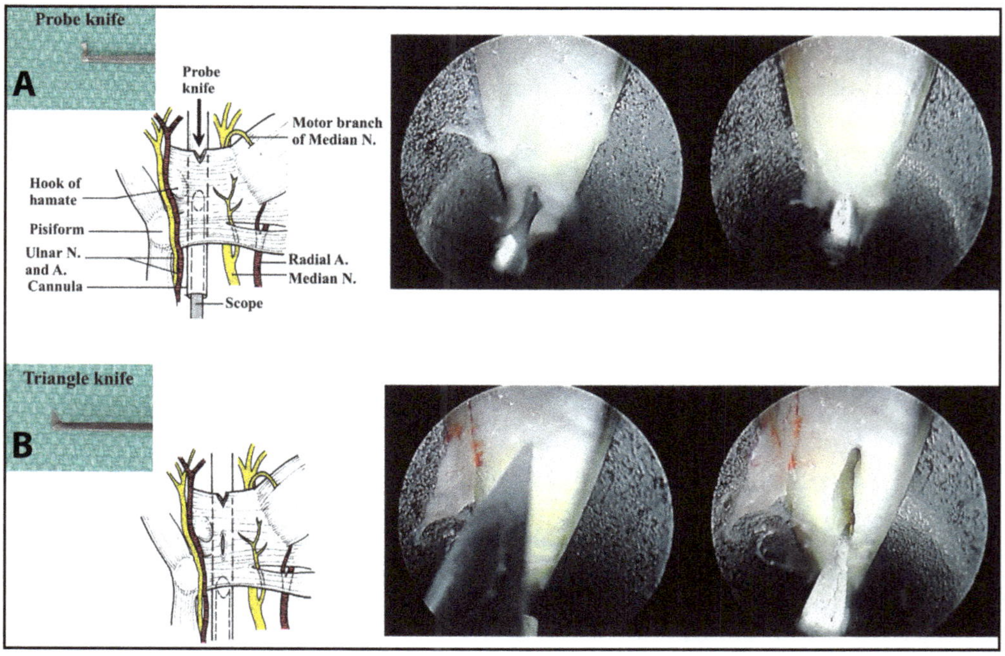

Figure 41-9. (A) After the distal border of the transverse carpal ligament is identified, the probe knife is used to make the first cut distally to proximally. (B) The scope is withdrawn proximally about 1 cm, and the triangle knife is used to make a small cut in the midsection of transverse carpal ligament.

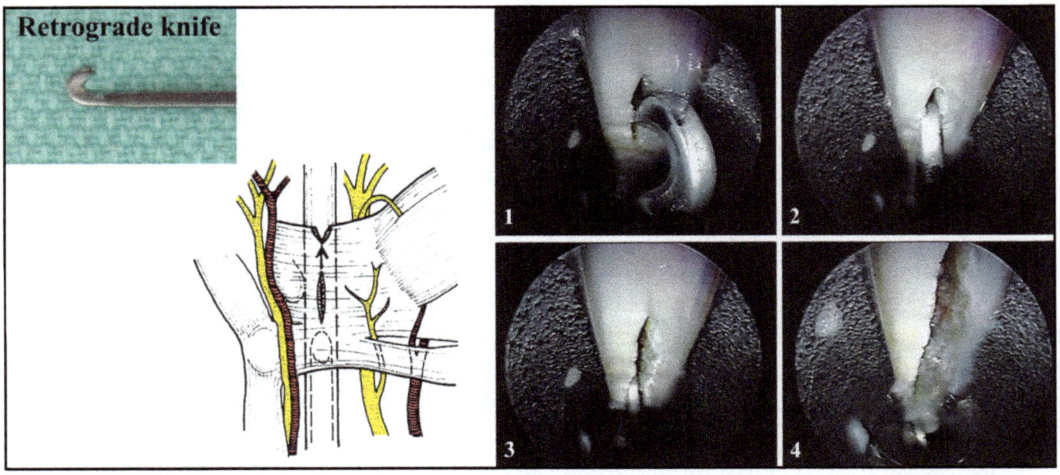

Figure 41-10. The retrograde knife is placed in the incision made by the triangle knife (1 and 2). It is drawn distally to make an incision that joins the previous 2 cuts (3 and 4).

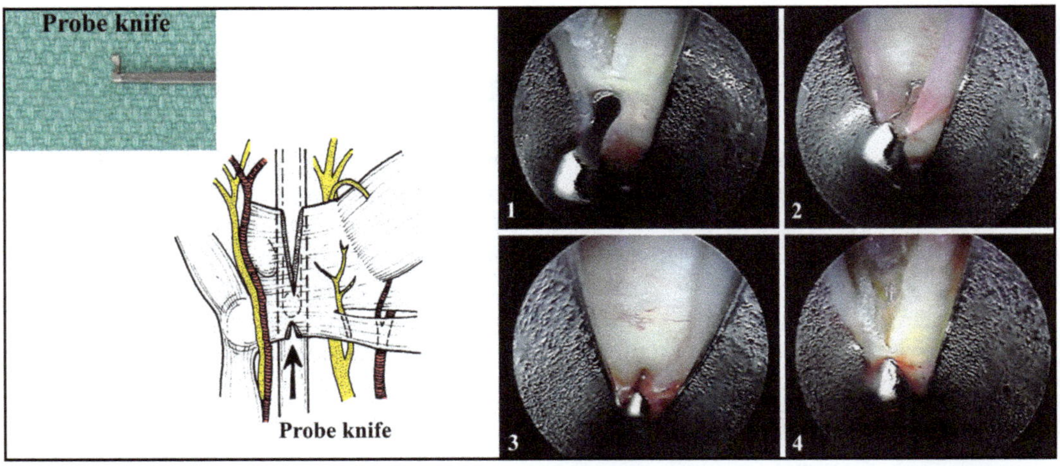

Figure 41-11. After the scope has been switched from the proximal to the distal opening of slotted cannula, the tip of the probe knife is placed just before the beginning of the distal cut (1). From that point, the knife's blunt edge is used to retract the thick bursal membrane distally to proximally (2). After the knife has engaged to the proximal border of transverse carpal ligament, it is advanced distally to complete the release of the ligament (3 and 4).

The retrograde knife is then inserted through the distal portal and its blunt tip is gently positioned at the incision made by the triangle knife (Figure 41-10). The proximal cutting edge of the retrograde knife is drawn distally, making an incision that joins the previous 2 cuts, thereby completing the release of the distal portion of transverse carpal ligament (see Figure 41-10).

The scope is removed from the proximal opening and inserted into the distal opening of the slotted cannula. The camera view on the screen then forms a mirror effect, with the previous ulnar side now being the radial side. By moving the scope proximally and distally, the previous distal cut is identified. The probe knife is inserted into the proximal portal and is drawn toward the level of the previous distal cut with its blunt tip touching the underside of the transverse carpal ligament, just before the beginning of the distal cut (Figure 41-11). From that point, the blunt edge of the knife is used to retract the thick bursal membrane, which sheaths the proximal portion of the carpal ligament, distally to proximally along the ligament's undersurface (see Figure 41-11).

After the cutting edge of the knife has engaged the proximal border of the ligament, the knife is advanced distally to make an incision that joins the previous cut, accomplishing the release of the transverse carpal ligament (see Figure 41-11). This is a slight modification of the technique in which the retrograde knife is used to complete the release of the ligament.[25,26] The thick bursal membrane contains small vessels and should be preserved to avoid bleeding into the carpal canal. The slotted cannula is gently rotated about a few degrees, clockwise and counterclockwise sequentially, enabling the surgeon to view the edges of the transected carpal ligament. If additional fibers remain, the triangle knife, or any other knife that feels appropriate, can be used to release these fibers until the surgeon is satisfied.

Because of the position of the patient's hand, the cut edges of the transverse carpal ligament should spring apart and disappear from the slotted opening of the cannula. If the edges can still be seen through the opening, the release is incomplete. While the assistant fully abducts the patient's thumb, the uncut portion of the ligament can be identified, and the surgeon can complete the transection.

Only one suture is required for closure of each portal. Immediately after the procedure, the surgeon should clinically examine the patient while still in a sterilized environment. If there is any dysfunction indicating intraoperative damage to the median nerve tendons, exposure and exploration of the carpal tunnel can be performed at that time.

Postoperative Protocol

Active range of motion is encouraged immediately after the effects of local anesthesia have subsided. The patient is advised to avoid heavy lifting or pressure on the palm region until the discomfort disappears, usually in 2 to 3 weeks. Active movement of the fingers decreases the formation of scar tissue in the wrist region, preventing adhesions on the tendons and nerves at the surgical site. Sutures are removed after 1 week. If the patient engages in hard occupational activities such as heavy lifting too soon after surgery, there may be swelling and prolonged pain in the palm region. If these occur, fluidized therapy (Fluidotherapy) for 20 minutes daily helps to decrease these symptoms within 1 week.

Potential Complications

Several complications after ECTR by the Chow technique have been reported in the literature. Nagle et al[27] performed a multicenter, prospective review study on a total of 640 cases. The initial transbursal technique was used in 110 cases and the modified extrabursal technique was used in 530 cases. An overall (perioperative and late) complication rate of 11% was found with the transbursal technique, compared with 2.2% with the extrabursal technique. In 21 (3.3%) of the 640 cases, perioperative complications occurred. Fourteen of these 21 cases involved neurapraxia, all of which resolved without sequelae, and no nerves were lacerated or transected. One laceration of the superficial flexor tendon of the ring and small fingers, 4 incomplete releases, 1 case with hematoma, and 1 laceration of the superior palmar arch were reported. Late complications included 3 (0.5%) cases of reflex sympathetic dystrophy. This complication resolved in all cases without the use of sympathetic nerve blocks. The study authors concluded that ECTR performed by the extrabursal, dual-portal technique reliably decompresses the carpal tunnel and can be effectively performed with low perioperative and late complication rates.

In a national study of the complications of 10,246 procedures in 9562 patients treated with the dual-portal Chow technique, Malek and Chow[28] found a complication rate of 2.3% (240 cases with complications were reported). Of these, there were 154 nerve-related complications (ie, median or ulnar nerve neuropraxias, lacerations, or transections), 38 complications related to blood

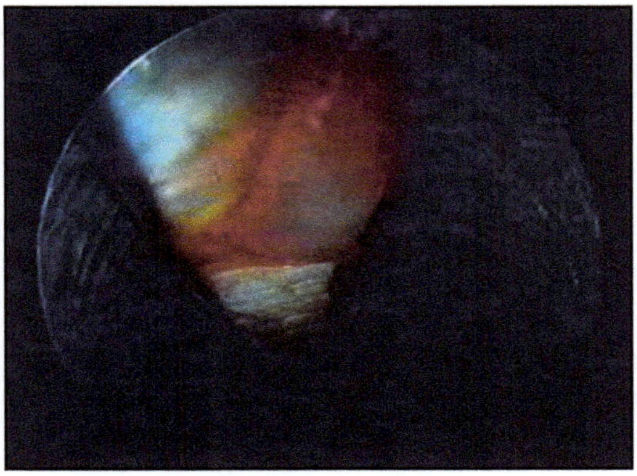

Figure 41-12. Extremely ulnar transligamentous motor branch of the median nerve.

vessels, 15 tendon injuries, 18 incomplete releases of the transverse carpal ligament, and 6 cases of reflex sympathetic dystrophy. The remaining 9 cases were listed as miscellaneous complications and included hematoma and superficial wound infection. Most intraoperative nerve injuries occurred in cases in which general or regional anesthesia was used.

The reported complication rates of ECTR compare favorably with published series of open carpal tunnel release. Complications of the latter include incomplete ligament release, nerve injuries, palmar hematomas, bowstringing of the flexor tendons, adhesions between nerves and tendons, reflex sympathetic dystrophy, deep wound infections, scar tenderness, pillar pain, tendon lacerations, and vascular injuries. The damage to the surrounding anatomic structures that occurs during open or endoscopic carpal tunnel surgery usually requires a second surgical procedure to be repaired.

Results

Chow has successfully performed more than 4350 ECTR procedures since September 1987. During the past 21 years, his experience has included a failure rate of 0.83% (36 cases), a complication rate of 0.11% (5 cases), and a recurrence rate of 0.41% (18 cases). He converted 2 (0.045%) endoscopic procedures to open procedures. There were no instances of laceration or transection of neural, vascular, or tendinous structures during treatment of 4353 hands. Superficial infection in the proximal surgical wound (entry portal) developed in 3 cases and was treated with oral antibiotics and local wound care.

Chow has encountered the anatomic variant of an extreme ulnar transligamentous motor branch of the median nerve in 24 cases (0.55%), or approximately 1 in every 200 patients (Figure 41-12). This variant is easily visualized and accommodated only by ECTR. This anatomic variant is thought to account for the higher rate of nerve injury and nerve-related complications reported for the open procedure.

Conclusion

The advantages of endoscopic over open carpal tunnel release include no hypertrophic scar or scar tenderness, no pillar pain, less compromise to the pinch or grip strength, and an earlier return to work and daily activities. However, the surgeon may face unexpected difficulties (eg, ganglion, neurofibroma, neurilemmoma) that limit visualization in the carpal canal. As with any surgical procedure, safety and success depend on a thorough knowledge of the anatomy of the area, adequate training, and familiarity with the instrumentation. Surgeons who are not familiar with endoscopes and arthroscopic techniques may experience major iatrogenic complications.

Top Technical Pearls for the Procedure

Pearls

1. When administering local anesthetic, preference is given to the subcutaneous regions proximally at the entry portal and distally at the exit portal. These are the areas of greatest pressure from the slotted cannula.
2. To best visualize the fibers of the transverse carpal ligament, the light source often must be dimmed. Chow routinely turns off the auto function on high slight source and dims it according to the available picture. This can markedly improve visualization and thereby increase the safety of the procedure.
3. Because of the symmetric nature of the visual field, it is easy to lose orientation when operating through the slotted cannula. To avoid this, Chow always introduces instrumentation into the cannula with the blade facing ulnarly.
4. It is safest to not use a tourniquet. This allows palpation of the ulnar artery before the skin incision for the entry portal is made so the ulnar neurovascular bundle can be protected.
5. If necessary, the assistant can provide direct pressure to the palm between the 2 portals over the slotted cannula to control bleeding during the operation.

Pitfalls

6. As with any endoscopic procedure, visualization is paramount. Regardless of the circumstance, if the surgeon is unable to obtain a clear view of the undersurface of the carpal ligament, the endoscopic procedure should be abandoned.
7. A common pitfall is ulnar placement of the entry portal. To avoid this situation, the following steps should be taken:
   - ▹ Watch the entire width of the wrist to ensure the central location of the entry portal.
   - ▹ Make sure that the landmarks of the entry and exit portals are aligned along the long axis of the forearm.
   - ▹ Palpate and mark the hook of the hamate. Both portals should be located radially to the hook.
   - ▹ During the entire procedure, surgical instruments that are introduced in the wrist and hand should follow the long axis of the forearm.

References

1. Pfeffer GB, Gelberman RH, Boyes JH, Rydevik B. The history of carpal tunnel syndrome. *J Hand Surg Br*. 1988;13(1):28-34.
2. Paget J. *Lectures on Surgical Pathology: Delivered at the Royal College of Surgeons of England*. 2nd American ed. Philadelphia, PA: Lindsay & Blakiston; 1860.
3. Putnam JJ. A series of paresthesia, mainly of the hand, of periodical recurrence, and possibly of vasomotor origin. *Arch Med (NY)*. 1880;4:147-162.
4. Phalen GS, Gardner WJ, La Londe AA. Neuropathy of the median nerve due to compression beneath the transverse carpal ligament. *J Bone Joint Surg Am*. 1950;32(1):109-112.
5. Chow CY. Endoscopic release of the carpal ligament: a new technique for carpal tunnel syndrome. *Arthroscopy*. 1989;5(1):19-24.

6. Okutsu I, Nonomiya S, Takatori Y, Ugawa Y. Endoscopic management of carpal tunnel syndrome. *Arthroscopy.* 1989;5(1):11-18.
7. Agee JM, Tortsua RD, Palmer CA, Berry C. Endoscopic release of the carpal tunnel: a prospective randomized multicenter study. Paper presented at: 45th Annual Meeting of the American Society for Surgery of the Hand; September 24-27, 1990; Toronto, Canada.
8. Viegas SF, Pollard A, Kaminski K. Carpal arch alteration and related clinical status after endoscopic carpal tunnel release. *J Hand Surg Am.* 1992;17(6):1012-1016.
9. Garcia-Elias M, Sanches-Freijo J, Salo J, Lluch AL. Dynamic changes of the transverse carpal arch during flexion-extension of the wrist: effects of sectioning the transverse carpal ligament. *J Hand Surg Am.* 1992;17(6):1017-1019.
10. Richman JA, Gelberrnan RH, Rydevik BL, et al. Carpal tunnel syndrome: morphologic changes after release of transverse carpal ligament. *J Hand Surg Am.* 1989;14(5):852-857.
11. Phalen GS. The carpal tunnel syndrome. Clinical evaluation of 598 hands. *Clin Orthop Relat Res.* 1972;(83):29-40.
12. Grundberg AB. Carpal tunnel decompression in spite of normal electromyography. *J Hand Surg Am.* 1983;8(3):348-349.
13. Jackson DA, Clifford JC. Electrodiagnosis of mild carpal tunnel syndrome. *Arch Phys Med Rehabil.* 1989;70(3):199-204.
14. Cioni R, Passero S, Paradiso C, Giannini F, Battistini N, Rushworth G. Diagnostic specificity of sensory and motor nerve conduction variables in early detection of carpal tunnel syndrome. *J Neurol.* 1989;236(4):208-213.
15. Chow JC, Weiss MA, Gu Y. Anatomic variations of the hook of hamate and the relationship to carpal tunnel syndrome. *J Hand Surg Am.* 2005;30(6):1242-1247.
16. Murphy RX Jr, Chemofsky MA, Osborne MA, Wolson AH. Magnetic resonance imaging in the evaluation of persistent carpal tunnel syndrome. *J Hand Surg Am.* 1993;18(1):113-120.
17. Richman JG, Gelberman RH, Rydevik BL, Gylys-Morin VM, Hajek PC, Sartoris DJ. Carpal tunnel volume determination by magnetic imaging three-dimensional reconstruction. *Hand Surg Am.* l987;12(5 pt 1):712-717.
18. Mannerfelt L, Hybbinette CH. Important anomaly of the thenar motor branch of the median nerve. *Bull Hosp Joint Dis.* 1972;33(1):15-21.
19. Caffee HH. Anomalous thenar muscle and median nerve: a case report. *J Hand Surg Am.* 1979;4(5):446-447.
20. Ogden J. An unusual branch of the median nerve. *J Bone Joint Surg Am.* l 972;54:1779-1781.
21. Papathanassiou BT. A variant of the motor branch of the median nerve in the hand. *J Bone Joint Surg Br.* 1968;50(1):156-157.
22. Lanz U. Anatomical variations of the median nerve in the carpal tunnel. *J Hand Surg Am.* 1977;2(1):44-53.
23. Johnson RK, Shrewsbury MM. Anatomical course of the thenar branch of the median nerve--usually in a separate tunnel through the transverse carpal ligament. *J Bone Joint Surg Am.* 1970;52(2):269-273.
24. Seradge H, Seradge E. Median innervated hypothenar muscle: anomalous branch of median nerve in the carpal tunnel. *J Hand Surg Am.* 1990;15(2):356-359.
25. Chow CY. Endoscopic carpal tunnel release. In: Chow JCY, ed. *Advanced Arthroscopy.* New York, NY: Springer-Verlag; 2001:271-286.
26. Chow JCY. Carpal tunnel release. In: McGinty JB, ed. *Operative Arthroscopy.* 3rd ed. Philadelphia, PA: Lippincott Williams & Wilkins; 2003:798-818.
27. Nagle D, Fischer TJ, Harris GD, et al. A multicenter prospective review of 640 endoscopic carpal tunnel releases using the transbursal and extrabursal chow techniques. *Arthroscopy.* 1996;12(2):139-143.
28. Malek MM, Chow CY. National study of the complications of over 10,000 cases of endoscopic carpal tunnel release. Paper presented at: 6lst Annual Meeting of the American Academy of Orthopaedic Surgeons; February 24-March 1, 1994; New Orleans, LA.

Please see videos on the accompanying website at
www.routledge.com/9781630910013

SECTION VIII

THE WRIST
Complications

42

Avoiding Complications in Wrist Arthroscopy

Benjamin Graves, MD; D. Nicole Deal, MD;
Cuney Tamam, MD; and Gary Poehling, MD

Preventing Complications

Arthroscopy is a safe and effective method for examining the intra-articular components of the radiocarpal and midcarpal joints and is considered a relatively low-risk procedure in adults and children.[1,2] Complications of wrist arthroscopy can arise, however, and have been reported to occur in 1.1% to 20.5% of wrist arthroscopy cases,[3-6] with a mean compiled complication rate of 4.7% reported in a recent systematic review.[7] As with all surgical procedures, wrist arthroscopy has a learning curve, and surgeons may be particularly vulnerable to error early in their experience.[8,9]

Minor complications that resolve without additional intervention have been reported and include superficial infection, superficial tendon injury from inappropriately placed portals, skin damage from traction devices, transient nerve injury, postoperative stiffness, and complex regional pain syndrome.[3-7,10-12] In addition, complications that cause permanent sequelae or those that require additional surgery to correct have been reported and include deep infection, hematoma, tendon transection, late tendon rupture, vascular injury, and permanent sensory nerve injury.[3-7,13,14] Rare events such as fistula formation,[15] complete transection of the ulnar nerve proper,[16] and radial artery pseudoaneurysm formation[17] have also been reported.

General considerations to keep in mind while performing wrist arthroscopy are patient positioning, traction, and fluid management. Improper or hastily applied drapes, forearm and digit wrapping, and prolonged traction can cause skin injury. Most authors recommend a traction force less than 5 kg/11 lb with continuous monitoring used for as brief a time interval as possible to help prevent traction-related complications. In contrast to the equipment and settings typically used during knee and shoulder arthroscopy, most authors recommend against the use of infusion pumps during wrist arthroscopy.[18,19] Although the authors of this chapter are unaware of a published case report of this potential complication, in theory, high-pressure fluid infusion can lead to extravasation within the compartments of the hand and/or forearm, which could produce a compartment syndrome. Pump infusion is not necessary during wrist arthroscopy, and the authors recommend gravity-fed inflow for these procedures.

Savoie FH III, Field LD, Steinmann SP, eds. *The Elbow and Wrist: AANA Advanced Arthroscopic Surgical Techniques* (pp 443-454).

Figure 42-1. Dorsal arthroscopy portals 3-4, 4-5, and 6-R are relatively safe to use because of their distance from dorsal sensory nerves. MCR, midcarpal radial portal; MCU, midcarpal ulnar portal; STT, scaphotrapeziotrapezoid. (Reprinted with permission of Pau Galano, MD, Barcelona, Spain.)

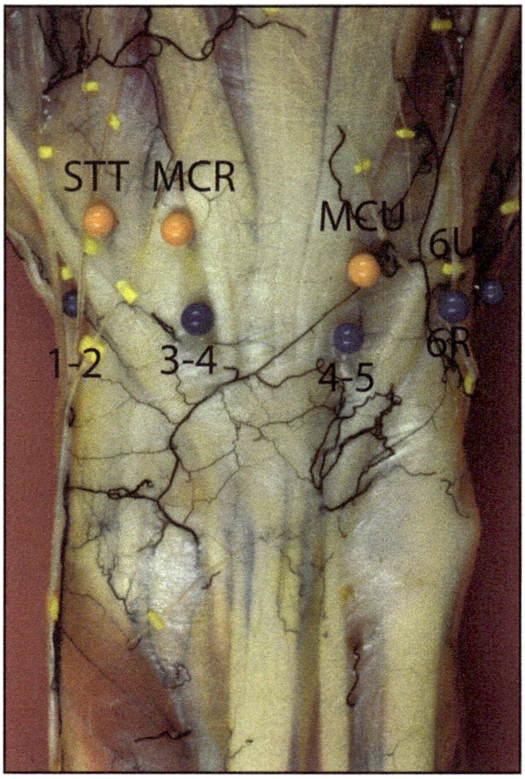

One commonly used technique to facilitate wrist arthroscopy is to place the wrist into traction with slight flexion to distract the joints of the carpus and wrist, making the portal intervals more readily palpable. This facilitates less traumatic trocar and cannula placement in the joint. Typically, the 3-4 portal is established first. Insufflation of the radiocarpal joint with lactated ringer's solution through an 18-gauge needle placed in the 3-4 portal allows distention of the wrist joint capsule. This portal is located just distal to Lister's tubercle and radial to the extensor digitorum communis at the radiocarpal joint line. Additional portals are then established under direct visualization.

To minimize risk while making skin incisions for portals, the authors recommend using a #11 scalpel blade in the vertical/longitudinal orientation. The tip of the blade is inserted through the dermis only. The surgeon then uses digital traction to pull the patient's skin into the cutting edge of the blade. This creates a skin incision without an in-and-out sawing motion, which places deeper structures at risk.

Risks and Complications by Portal Site

Wrist arthroscopy portals are based on the extensor compartments of the wrist.[18-24] Figure 42-1 provides an overview of the dorsal arthroscopy portals with associated structures. Table 42-1 provides a summary of reported complications of wrist arthroscopy in general and by portal site.

1-2 Portal

The structures most at risk during placement and use of the 1-2 portal (ie, extensor pollicis brevis–extensor carpi radialis longus [ECRL] portal) are the radial artery and superficial radial

Table 42-1. Summary of Reported Complications of Wrist Arthroscopy in General and by Portal Site

Portal	Reported Complications
General	Suture abscess, inclusion cyst, skin tearing, postoperative stiffness, tenosynovitis, chondral injury, infection, CRPS[3-7]
3-4	EIP/EDC to index finger tendon laceration,[14] late EPL rupture,[13] tendon sheath fistula formation,[15] posterior interosseous nerve injury[12]
6-R	EDQ/EDC to small finger tendon laceration[14]
6-U	Dorsal sensory branch ulnar nerve laceration,[10,11] ulnar nerve (proper) transection[16]
Palmar	Radial artery pseudoaneurysm formation[17]

Abbreviations: CRPS, complex regional pain syndrome; EDC, extensor digitorum communis; EDQ, extensor digitorum quinti; EIP, extensor indicis proprius; EPL, extensor pollicis longus.

nerve. The radial artery lies deep to the first dorsal compartment and, therefore, should be out of harm's way if the portal is placed correctly. However, if the portal is placed too radially or too distally, this structure is at risk for injury. An easy way to avoid damage to the radial artery as it passes deep to the tendons is to make a small portal incision, bluntly dissect down to the capsule with a hemostat, and insert the trocar through the capsule after ensuring that the artery is not directly under the trocar.

The superficial radial nerve is also at risk because its dorsal branch lies over the 1-2 portal. Injury to the superficial radial nerve as it arborizes ulnarly can be avoided by making longitudinal skin incisions for portals with a #11 blade using the technique described previously. Blunt dissection with a hemostat down to the capsule is recommended to minimize risk of injury to dorsal branches of this nerve as they cross the portal site (Figure 42-2).

3-4 Portal

The structures most at risk during placement of the 3-4 portal (ie, extensor pollicis longus/extensor carpi radialis brevis–index extensor digitorum communis [EPL/ECRB-index EDC] portal) are the tendons of the EPL, ECRB, and EDC. This portal should be placed just distal to Lister's tubercle, around which the EPL tendon passes.

The 3-4 portal is commonly the first portal established and is most easily established by inserting an 18-gauge needle into the wrist joint just distal to Lister's tubercle and insufflating the joint with as much solution as the joint can hold comfortably. Easy backflow of fluid from the wrist into the syringe confirms intra-articular positioning. The needle and syringe are then removed from the joint while maintaining the capsular distention. The information from needle insertion and palpation of the capsular distention guides placement of the 3-4 portal into the radiocarpal joint between the ECRB/EPL and the EDC. As previously described, the skin is pulled over the tip of the blade to establish the portal to lessen the risk of inadvertent tendon laceration. After the skin incision is made, the blunt trocar and cannula are inserted through capsule. The blunt tip is gently moved in a medial and lateral direction for tactile feedback. This helps ensure entry into the joint without iatrogenic articular cartilage injury (Figure 42-3).

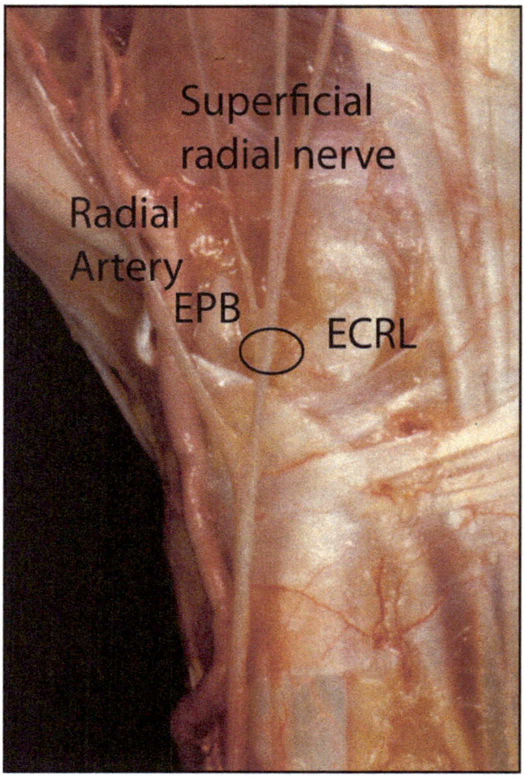

Figure 42-2. The 1-2 portal is near the radial artery and superficial radial nerve. ECRL, extensor carpi radialis longus; EPB, extensor pollicis brevis. (Reprinted with permission of Pau Galano, MD, Barcelona, Spain.)

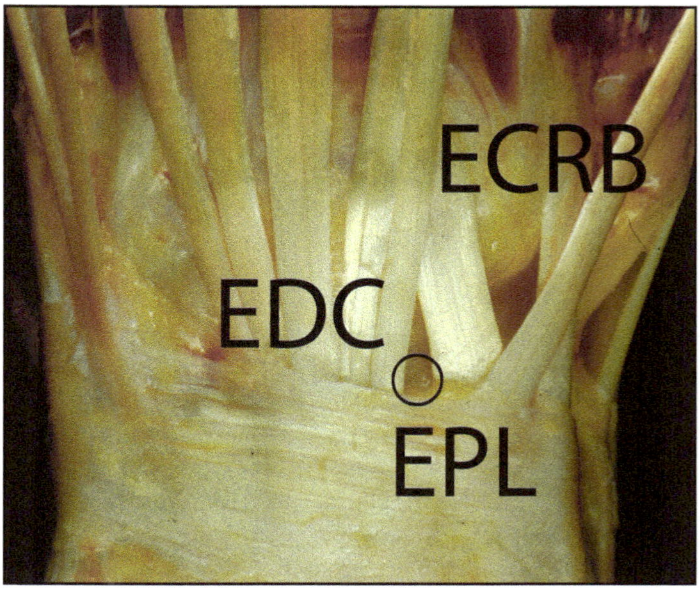

Figure 42-3. The 3-4 portal provides safe access to the radiocarpal joint between the extensor pollicis longus (EPL), extensor carpi radialis brevis (ECRL), and extensor digitorum communis (EDC) tendons. (Reprinted with permission of Pau Galano, MD, Barcelona, Spain.)

4-5 Portal

The structures most at risk during placement of the 4-5 portal (ie, EDC–extensor digiti quinti [EDQ] portal) are the terminal branch of the posterior interosseous nerve (PIN) and the dorsal sensory branch of the ulnar nerve. The PIN is found in the ulnar aspect of the fourth dorsal compartment dorsal to the wrist capsule and provides sensation to the wrist joint. The risk of damage

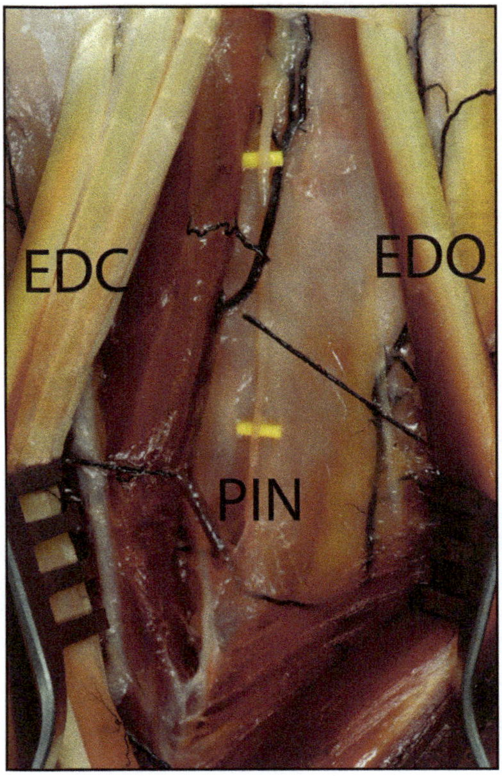

Figure 42-4. The 4-5 interval is close to the terminal branch of the posterior interosseous nerve (PIN). There are no functional consequences of sacrificing this nerve; however, nerve injury should be avoided to minimize the risk of painful neuroma formation. EDC, extensor digitorum communis; EDQ, extensor digiti quinti. (Reprinted with permission of Pau Galano, MD, Barcelona, Spain.)

to this nerve during placement of the 4-5 portal is lessened by placement of the portal in a slightly ulnar position with relation to the EDC tendon, just radial to the EDQ tendon. The loss of the function of this nerve causes no functional deficit, and there is evidence that PIN neurectomy diminishes pain in the wrist joint. However, persistent postoperative mid-dorsal wrist pain attributed to avulsion of the distal PIN has been reported.[12] Care should be taken while establishing this portal to avoid this complication.

The dorsal sensory branch of the ulnar nerve traverses this region and is also at risk during placement of this portal. The transverse branch of this nerve passes distal to the portal and risk of injury may be lessened by placing the portal as proximal as possible in the wrist joint. The authors recommend longitudinal skin incision followed by blunt insertion through capsule to ensure preservation of the nerve (Figure 42-4).

6-R Portal

The structures at most risk during placement of the 6-R portal (ie, EDQ—extensor carpi ulnaris [ECU] portal) are the extensor tendons (EDQ and ECU) and branches of the dorsal sensory branch of the ulnar nerve, which pass ulnar to the portal. The authors stress placement of this portal radial to the ECU tendon with blunt dissection to the joint capsule to help prevent damage to this superficial nerve. The skin incision is made as previously described in a longitudinal fashion with careful blunt dissection down to capsule. The trocar is then safely placed through capsule on the radial side of the ECU tendon (Figure 42-5).

6-U Portal

The structure at most risk during placement of the 6-U portal (ie, ulnar to the ECU tendon) is the main dorsal sensory branch of the ulnar nerve. The authors do not recommend using this

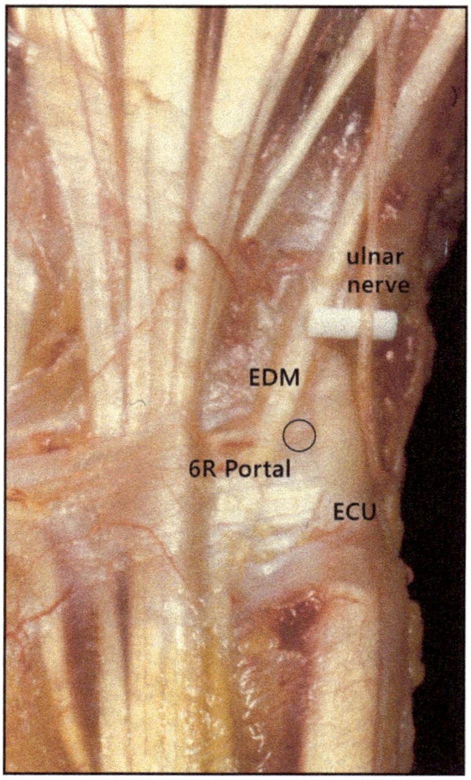

Figure 42-5. The 6-R portal can be safely used to decrease the risk of iatrogenic injury to the dorsal sensory branch of the ulnar nerve. ECU, extensor carpi ulnaris; EDM, extensor digiti minimi. (Reprinted with permission of Pau Galano, MD, Barcelona, Spain.)

portal unless there is no alternative. The dorsal sensory branch of the ulnar nerve predictably traverses the region of this portal. If this portal must be used, one must ensure that the nerve is not lacerated or entrapped during portal placement. The authors stress blunt dissection down to capsule with identification and protection of the nerve to minimize risk of injury, and continued vigilance must be observed throughout the case during instrument exchange and suture placement (Figure 42-6).

Midcarpal Radial Portal

The structures most at risk in the midcarpal radial (MCR) portal (ie, 1 cm distal to the 3-4 portal in line with the radial border of the long metacarpal) are the extensor tendons (Figure 42-7) and the articular cartilage. The space available for portal placement is smaller in the MCR portal compared with the midcarpal ulnar portal (Figure 42-8). For smaller patients, the authors recommend using a 1.8-mm arthroscope in all portals of the midcarpal joint because of this limited space.

Midcarpal Ulnar Portal

The structures most at risk in the midcarpal ulnar portal (ie, 1 cm distal to the 4-5 radiocarpal portal in line with the long axis of the ring metacarpal) are the extensor tendons (Figure 42-9) and the articular cartilage. This portal has more room than the MCR portal, especially in patients with a significant hamate facet of the lunate (Figure 42-10).[20]

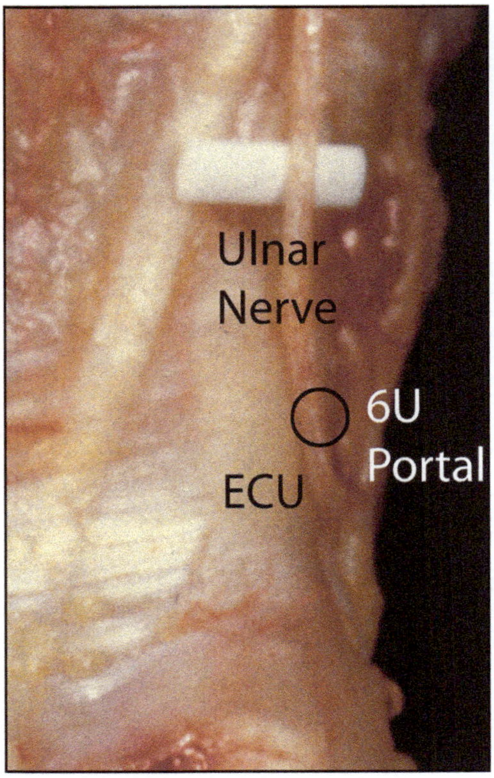

Figure 42-6. The 6-U portal is close to the main dorsal sensory branch of the ulnar nerve. If this portal must be used, dissection and retraction of the nerve must be performed before portal placement. ECU, extensor carpi ulnaris. (Reprinted with permission of Pau Galano, MD, Barcelona, Spain.)

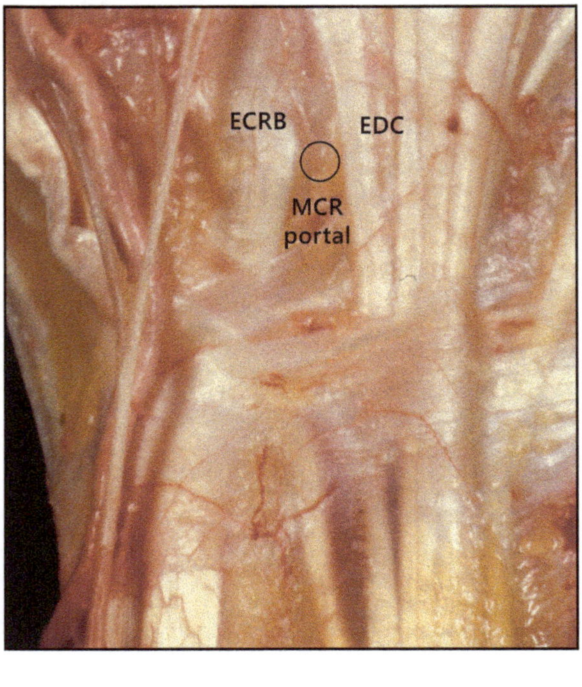

Figure 42-7. The midcarpal radial portal is 1 cm distal to the 3-4 portal and is bordered by the extensor carpi radialis brevis (ECRB) and extensor digitorum communis (EDC) tendons. There are no adjacent nerves or vascular structures. (Reprinted with permission of Pau Galano, MD, Barcelona, Spain.)

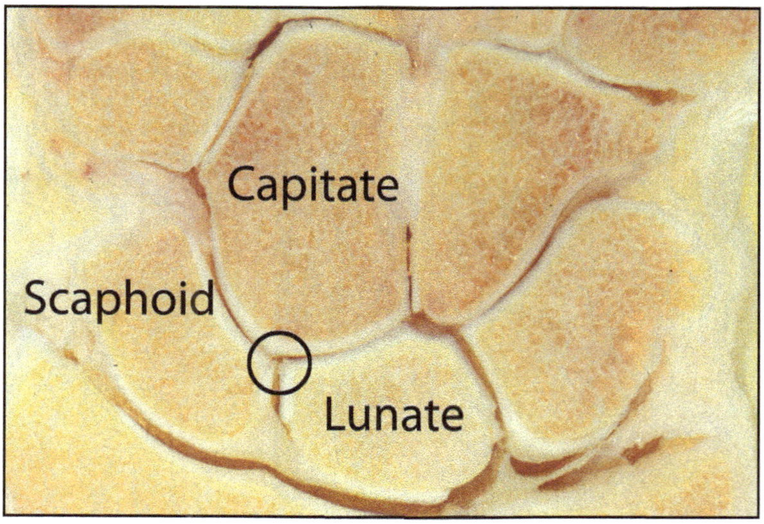

Figure 42-8. Intra-articular section demonstrating the small space available for instrumentation in the midcarpal joints. This increases the risk of iatrogenic articular cartilage damage during placement of the midcarpal radial portal. (Reprinted with permission of Pau Galano, MD, Barcelona, Spain.)

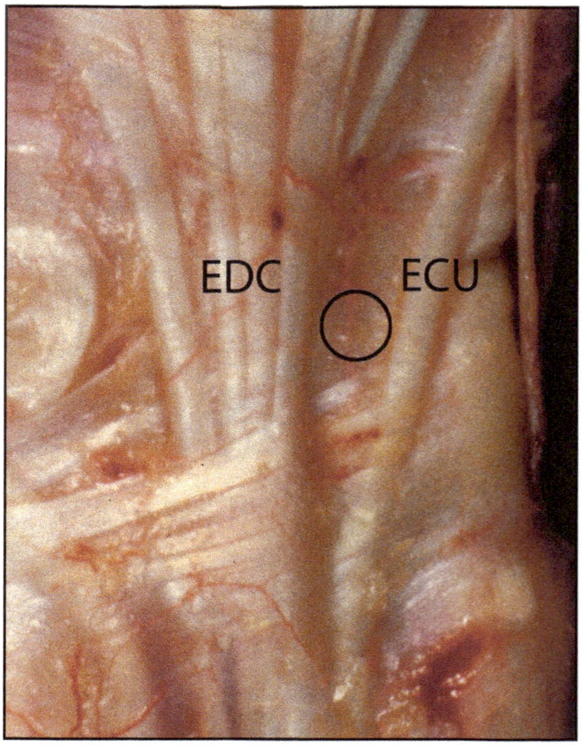

Figure 42-9. The midcarpal ulnar portal is 1 cm distal to the 4-5 radiocarpal portal and is bordered by the extensor digitorum communis (EDC) and extensor carpi ulnaris (ECU) tendons. There are no adjacent nerves or vascular structures. (Reprinted with permission of Pau Galano, MD, Barcelona, Spain.)

Scaphotrapeziotrapezoid Portal

The structures most at risk with placement and use of the scaphotrapeziotrapezoid portal (ie, EDC-EPL distal portal) are the radial artery and superficial radial nerve. The radial artery passes deep to the extensors through the anatomic snuffbox to lie between the 2 heads of the first dorsal interosseous muscle, and it is therefore directly at risk during placement of this portal (Figure 42-11). The easiest way to avoid damage to the radial artery is to approach the space between the ECRL and the ECRB, staying ulnar to the EPL. This approach helps ensure that the artery and the radial nerve are palmar and radial to the portal.

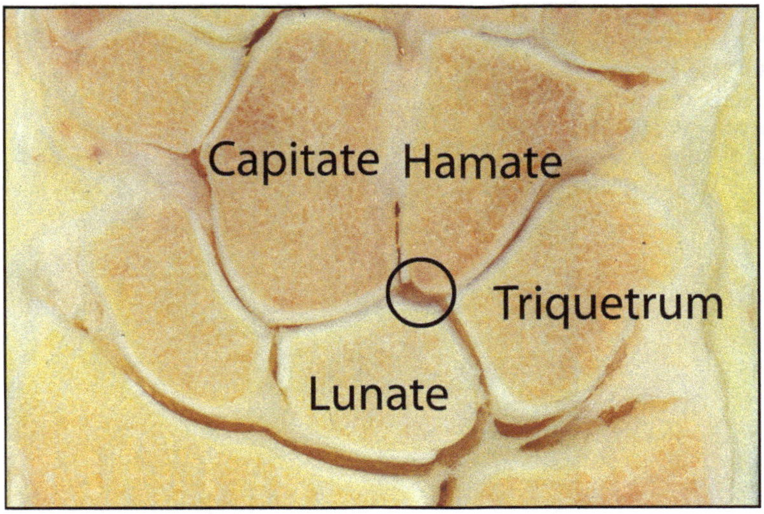

Figure 42-10. This intra-articular section demonstrates the relatively larger space in the midcarpal ulnar portal compared with the midcarpal radial portal. (Reprinted with permission of Pau Galano, MD, Barcelona, Spain.)

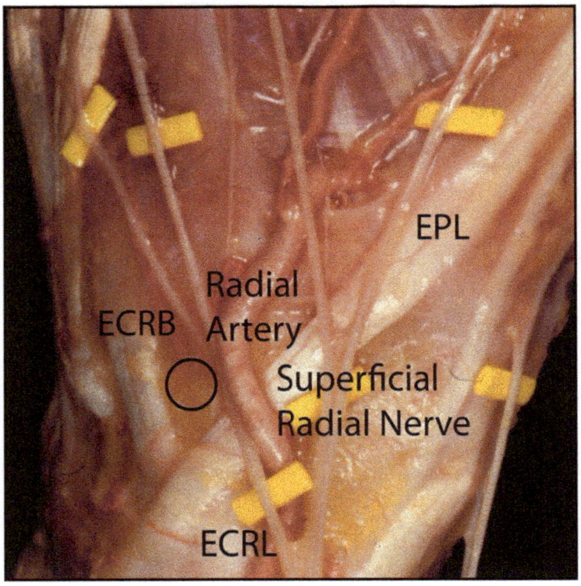

Figure 42-11. The structures most at risk during placement and use of the STT portal are the radial artery and superficial radial nerve. It is safest if the STT portal is made on the radial border of the extensor carpi radialis brevis (ECRB) tendon. ECRL, extensor carpi radialis longus; EPL, extensor pollicis longus. (Reprinted with permission of Pau Galano, MD, Barcelona, Spain.)

Palmar Portal

The palmar portal is the most precarious of the portals discussed because it lies between the radial artery, the median nerve, and the palmar cutaneous branch of the median nerve (Figure 42-12). Whether placed inside-out or outside-in, care must be taken to preserve the radial artery, which lies radial to the flexor carpi radialis (FCR) tendon; the palmar cutaneous branch of the median nerve, which is found superficial between the FCR and palmaris longus tendons; and the median nerve, which lies deep to the palmaris longus and ulnar to the FCR. If placing the portal with an inside-out technique, the switching stick should be placed through the 3-4 portal between the radioscaphocapitate ligament and the long radiolunate ligaments, exiting through an incision radial to the FCR tendon on the volar aspect of the wrist. It is crucial to identify the radial artery and protect it during insertion of the cannula. If the outside-in technique is used with an incision made on the ulnar aspect of the FCR tendon, as described by Slutsky,[23] care must be taken to protect the radial artery and palmar cutaneous branch and median nerve proper.[17]

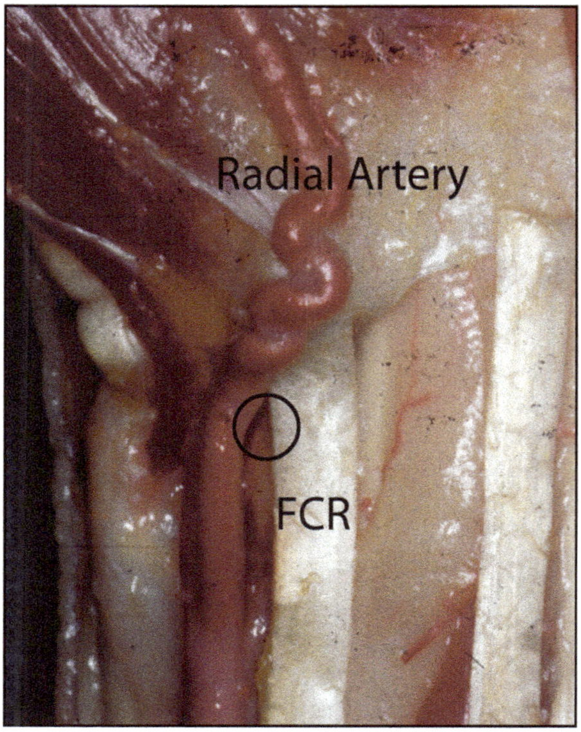

Figure 42-12. The palmar portal is the most precarious of all the portals discussed because it lies directly adjacent to the radial artery. Open dissection is recommended if this portal is used. FCR, flexor carpi radialis. (Reprinted with permission of Pau Galano, MD, Barcelona, Spain.)

Conclusion

Wrist arthroscopy is a safe and effective technique for diagnosing and treating intra-articular wrist pathology. Complications are rare and most can be prevented by using proper technique as described in this chapter.

Top Technical Pearls for the Procedure

Pearls

1. Know the anatomic structures that border specific portals. Small variations in portal placement may lead to injury to adjacent structures.
2. Distend the joint before portal placement.
3. Before establishing a portal, place a needle to ensure unobstructed access and an optimal angle of the approach.
4. Make longitudinal skin incisions using a #11 blade scalpel and apply traction on the skin rather than using a sawing motion with the blade to enlarge the portal.

(continued)

Pitfalls

5. For thin or frail skin, use caution when applying finger traps and watch carefully for skin tearing.
6. Use caution when placing portals to avoid articular cartilage damage, particularly in the midcarpal joints.
7. When evaluating wrist pain, be aware of patients with constant pain, especially if they experience a burning sensation and have difficulty sleeping. These patients should be treated for complex regional pain syndrome (formerly called *reflex sympathetic dystrophy*) before operative procedures to correct mechanical problems.
8. The risk of infection is low with the use of proper sterile technique.
9. Use described techniques to avoid injury to the many superficial nervous structures around the wrist and prevent neuroma formation.
10. Use described techniques to avoid injury to tendons.
11. Bluntly dissect down to the capsule and identify at-risk structures before portal placement.

References

1. Gallego S, Mathoulin C. Arthroscopic resection of dorsal wrist ganglia: 114 cases with minimum follow-up of 2 years. *Arthroscopy.* 2010;26(12):1675-1682.
2. Farr S, Grill F, Girsch W. Wrist arthroscopy in children and adolescents: a single surgeon experience of thirty-four cases. *Int Orthop.* 2012;36(6):1215-1220.
3. Warhold LG, Ruth RM. Complications of wrist arthroscopy and how to prevent them. *Hand Clin.* 1995;11(1):81-89.
4. Culp RW. Complications of wrist arthroscopy. *Hand Clin.* 1999;15(3):529-535.
5. DeSmet L. Pitfalls in wrist arthroscopy. *Acta Orthop Belg.* 2002;68(4):325-329.
6. Beredjiklian PK, Bozentka DJ, Leung YL, Monaghan BA. Complications of wrist arthroscopy. *J Hand Surg Am.* 2004;29(3):406-411.
7. Ahsan ZA, Yao J. Complications of wrist arthroscopy. *Arthroscopy.* 2012;28(6):855-859.
8. Puhaindran ME, Yam AK, Chin AY, Lluch A, Garcia-Elias M. Wrist arthroscopy: beware the novice. *J Hand Surg Eur Vol.* 2009;34(4):540-542.
9. Corella F, Ocampos M, Del Cerro M. Are extensor tendons safe on your first wrist arthroscopy? *J Hand Surg Eur Vol.* 2011;36(9):817-818.
10. McAdams TR, Hentz VR. Injury to the dorsal sensory branch of the ulnar nerve in the arthroscopic repair of ulnar-sided triangular fibrocartilage tears using an inside-out technique: a cadaver study. *J Hand Surg Am.* 2002;27(5):840-844.
11. Tsu-Hsin CE, Wei JD, Huang VW. Injury of the dorsal sensory branch of the ulnar nerve as a complication of arthroscopic repair of the triangular fibrocartilage. *J Hand Surg Br.* 2006;31(5):530-532.
12. Del Piñal F, Herrero F, Cruz-Camara A, San Jose J. Complete avulsion of the distal posterior interosseous nerve during wrist arthroscopy: a possible cause of persistent pain after arthroscopy. *J Hand Surg Am.* 1999;24(2):240-242.
13. Fortems Y, Mawhinney I, Lawrence T, Trial IA, Stanley JK. Late rupture of extensor pollicis longus after wrist arthroscopy. *Arthroscopy.* 1995;11(3):322-323.
14. Cooper AR, Elfar JC. Extensor tendon lacerations from arthroscopic excision of dorsal wrist ganglion: case report. *J Hand Surg Am.* 2013;38(10):1957-1959.
15. Shirley DS, Mullet H, Stanley JK. Extensor tendon sheath fistula formation as a complication of wrist arthroscopy. *Arthroscopy.* 2008;24(11):1311-1312.

16. Nguyen MK, Bourgouin S, Gaillard C, et al. Accidental section of the ulnar nerve in the wrist during arthroscopy. *Arthroscopy.* 2011;27(9):1308-1311.
17. Clerico C, Benatar M, Dumontier C. Radial artery pseudoaneurysm: a rare complication after arthroscopic treatment of a volar wrist ganglion in a hemophilia patient. *Chir Main.* 2014;33(5):361-363.
18. Ekman EF, Poehling GG. Principles of arthroscopy and wrist arthroscopy equipment. *Hand Clin.* 1994;10(4):557-566.
19. Roth JH, Poehling GG, Whipple TL. Hand instrumentation for small joint arthroscopy. *Arthroscopy.* 1988;4(2):126-128.
20. Viegas SF. Midcarpal arthroscopy: anatomy and portals. *Hand Clin.* 1994;10(4):577-587.
21. Bettinger PC, Cooney WP III, Berger RA. Arthroscopic anatomy of the wrist. *Orthop Clin North Am.* 1995;26(4):707-719.
22. Yu HL, Chase RA, Strauch B. *Atlas of Hand Anatomy and Clinical Implications.* St. Louis, MO: Mosby; 2003.
23. Slutsky DJ. Wrist arthroscopy through a volar radial portal. *Arthroscopy.* 2002;18(6):624-630.
24. Buterbaugh GA. Radiocarpal arthroscopy portals and normal anatomy. *Hand Clin.* 1994;10(4):567-576.

Financial Disclosures

Dr. Julie E. Adams is a consultant for Arthrex and Acumed. She also receives royalties from Biomet and an honorarium from Elsevier and Springer.

Dr. David W. Altchek has no financial or proprietary interest in the materials presented herein.

Dr. James R. Andrews is a consultant for Biomet Sports Medicine, Bauerfiend, MiMedx, and Theralase. He holds stock in Connective Orthopaedics and Patient Connection. He is also Medical Director for Physiotherapy Associates and a board member of Fast Health Corporation.

Dr. Alejandro Badia has no financial or proprietary interest in the materials presented herein.

Dr. Gregory Bain has no financial or proprietary interest in the materials presented herein.

Dr. Champ L. Baker III has stock options from Arthrex.

Dr. Champ L. Baker Jr has stock options from Arthrex and Tenex.

Dr. Jonathan D. Brown has no financial or proprietary interest in the materials presented herein.

Dr. James C. Y. Chow receives royalties from Johnson & Johnson.

Dr. Tyler R. Clark has no financial or proprietary interest in the materials presented herein.

Dr. Mark S. Cohen is a consultant for Acumed and Integra, and he receives royalties from Integra.

Dr. Randall W. Culp has no financial or proprietary interest in the materials presented herein.

Dr. D. Nicole Deal has no financial or proprietary interest in the materials presented herein.

Dr. William Desloges has no financial or proprietary interest in the materials presented herein.

Dr. Joshua S. Dines is a consultant for Arthrex, Conmed LInvatec, and Ossur. He receives royalties from Conmed LInvatec. He is also on the Editorial Board for *American Journal of Orthopedics* and *Journal Shoulder Elbow Surgery.*

Dr. Brandon P. Donnelly has no financial or proprietary interest in the materials presented herein.

Dr. Larry D. Field has no financial or proprietary interest in the materials presented herein.

Dr. Michael P. Gaspar has no financial or proprietary interest in the materials presented herein.

Dr. William B. Geissler has not disclosed any relevant financial relationships.

Dr. Benjamin Graves has no financial or proprietary interest in the materials presented herein.

Dr. Bikramjit S. Grewal has no financial or proprietary interest in the materials presented herein.

Dr. Timothy Griffith is a reviewer for *American Journal of Sports Medicine.*

Dr. Jennifer A. Hertz has no financial or proprietary interest in the materials presented herein.

Dr. E. Rhett Hobgood receives consulting income from Depuy/Synthes. He also receives educational support for his fellowship program from Depuy/Mitek, Arthrex, and Smith & Nephew.

Dr. Bhavin Jadav has no financial or proprietary interest in the materials presented herein.

Dr. Graham J. W. King is a consultant for and received royalties from Tornier Inc and Wright Medical Technology for products unrelated to his chapter.

Dr. Brian Klika has no financial or proprietary interest in the materials presented herein.

Dr. Rudy Kovachevich has no financial or proprietary interest in the materials presented herein.

Leonard C. Macrina has no financial or proprietary interest in the materials presented herein.

Dr. Michael L. Mangonon has no financial or proprietary interest in the materials presented herein.

Dr. Murphy P. Martin III has no financial or proprietary interest in the materials presented herein.

Dr. Brent V. McCarty has no financial or proprietary interest in the materials presented herein.

Dr. Robert Nelson Mead has no financial or proprietary interest in the materials presented herein.

Dr. Bernard F. Morrey is Medical Director of Tenex Health.

Dr. Mike Moskal owns stock in Medtronics and Orthofix.

Dr. Daniel J. Nagle has no financial or proprietary interest in the materials presented herein.

Dr. Brian D. Norton has no financial or proprietary interest in the materials presented herein.

Dr. Michael J. O'Brien is on the board/is a committee member of Arthroscopy Association of North America: Board and Association of American Medical Colleges. He is a paid consultant and receives research or other financial or material support from DePuy, a Johnson & Johnson Company, Mitek, and Smith & Nephew.

Dr. Patrick M. O'Brien has no financial or proprietary interest in the materials presented herein.

Dr. Daryl C. Osbahr has no financial or proprietary interest in the materials presented herein.

Dr. A. Lee Osterman is a consultant for Auxillium, Medartis, DJO, Athrex, and Skeletal Dynamics. He is also on the speaker's bureau for Auxillium.

Dr. Stephanie C. Petterson has no financial or proprietary interest in the materials presented herein.

Dr. Joideep Phadnis has no financial or proprietary interest in the materials presented herein.

Dr. Kevin D. Plancher has no financial or proprietary interest in the materials presented herein.

Dr. Gary Poehling is a consultant for Mako, now owned by Stryker.

Dr. Marc Prud'homme-Foster is a consultant and has no financial or proprietary interest in the materials presented herein.

Dr. Matthew L. Ramsey receives consulting fees and royalties as well as research support from Zimmer and Integra. He has stock options in Trice Medical and is on the Board of Directors for Rothman Orthopaedic Specialty Hospital.

Dr. Ashkon Razavi has no financial or proprietary interest in the materials presented herein.

Dr. Juan Manuel Ríos Ruh has no financial or proprietary interest in the materials presented herein.

Dr. Akash Sabharwal has no financial or proprietary interest in the materials presented herein.

Dr. Felix H. Savoie III is on the board/is a committee member of American Shoulder and Elbow Surgeons and Arthroscopy Association of North America. He is on the editorial or governing board for *Arthroscopy* and *Journal of Wrist Surgery*. He is an unpaid consultant for Biomet, Exactech Inc, Mitek, Rotation Medical, and Smith & Nephew. He received IP royalties from Exactech Inc; is a paid presenter or speaker for Smith & Nephew; and is a paid presenter or speaker for and receives research support from Mitek.

Dr. David J. Slutsky has no financial or proprietary interest in the materials presented herein.

Dr. Alex Soneru has no financial or proprietary interest in the materials presented herein.

Dr. Scott P. Steinmann receives royalties from Biomet and Arthrex.

Dr. Sarah Stelma has no financial or proprietary interest in the materials presented herein.

Dr. William B. Stetson has no financial or proprietary interest in the materials presented herein.

Dr. Philipp N. Streubel is a consultant for Acumed.

Dr. Cuney Tamam has no financial or proprietary interest in the materials presented herein.

Dr. Lucas H. B. Walschot has no financial or proprietary interest in the materials presented herein.

Dr. Chris S. Warrell has no financial or proprietary interest in the materials presented herein.

Dr. Aaron M. Weber has no financial or proprietary interest in the materials presented herein.

Dr. Matthew Wert has no financial or proprietary interest in the materials presented herein.

Kevin E. Wilk has no financial or proprietary interest in the materials presented herein.

Dr. Jeffrey B. Witty has no financial or proprietary interest in the materials presented herein.

Dr. Eric S. Wroten has not disclosed any relevant financial relationships.

Index

For Product Safety Concerns and Information please contact our EU
representative GPSR@taylorandfrancis.com
Taylor & Francis Verlag GmbH, Kaufingerstraße 24, 80331 München, Germany

www.ingramcontent.com/pod-product-compliance
Ingram Content Group UK Ltd.
Pitfield, Milton Keynes, MK11 3LW, UK
UKHW052050230926
475702UK00025B/1031
* 9 7 8 1 6 3 0 9 1 0 0 1 3 *